AI-Driven Innovation in Healthcare Data Analytics

Leyla Özgür Polat
Pamukkale University, Turkey

Olcay Polat
Pamukkale University, Turkey

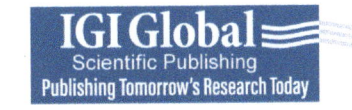

Vice President of Editorial	Melissa Wagner
Managing Editor of Acquisitions	Mikaela Felty
Managing Editor of Book Development	Jocelynn Hessler
Production Manager	Mike Brehm
Cover Design	Phillip Shickler

Published in the United States of America by
IGI Global Scientific Publishing
701 East Chocolate Avenue
Hershey, PA, 17033, USA
Tel: 717-533-8845
Fax: 717-533-8661
E-mail: cust@igi-global.com
Website: https://www.igi-global.com

Copyright © 2025 by IGI Global Scientific Publishing. All rights reserved. No part of this publication may be reproduced, stored or transmitted in any form or by any means, electronic or mechanical, including photocopying, without written permission from the publisher.
Product or company names used in this set are for identification purposes only. Inclusion of the names of the products or companies does not indicate a claim of ownership by IGI Global Scientific Publishing of the trademark or registered trademark.

Library of Congress Cataloging-in-Publication Data

CIP Data Pending
ISBN:979-8-3693-7277-7
eISBN:979-8-3693-7279-1

British Cataloguing in Publication Data
A Cataloguing in Publication record for this book is available from the British Library.

All work contributed to this book is new, previously-unpublished material.
The views expressed in this book are those of the authors, but not necessarily of the publisher.
This book contains information sourced from authentic and highly regarded references, with reasonable efforts made to ensure the reliability of the data and information presented. The authors, editors, and publisher believe the information in this book to be accurate and true as of the date of publication. Every effort has been made to trace and credit the copyright holders of all materials included. However, the authors, editors, and publisher cannot assume responsibility for the validity of all materials or the consequences of their use. Should any copyright material be found unacknowledged, please inform the publisher so that corrections may be made in future reprints.

Table of Contents

Preface xvi

Chapter 1
AI in Healthcare Data Analytics Trends and Transformative Innovations 1
    Manjunatha Badiger, NMAM Institute of Technology, India
    Sookshma Adiga, Moodlakatte Institute of Technology, India
    Akshatha Naik, Moodlakatte Institute of Technology, India
    Sumiksha Shetty, Sahyadri College of Engineering and Management, India
    A. B. Smitha, Sahyadri College of Engineering and Management, India
    Fathima C. Mehnaz, Sahyadri College of Engineering and Management, India
    Chandra Singh, NMAM Institute of Technology, Nitte University, India

Chapter 2
Transforming Healthcare With AI and Machine Learning: Applications and Impacts 53
    D. Ravindran, Kristu Jayanti College, India
    G. Mariammal, Vel Tech Rangarajan Dr. Sagunthala R&D Institute of Science and Technology, India
    M. Dhivya, Ramco Institute of Technology, India
    Dhivya Devi S., SRM Institute of Science and Technology, India
    Anish T. P., R.M.K. College of Engineering and Technology, India
    V. Sathya, Vel Tech Rangarajan Dr. Sagunthala R&D Institute of Science and Technology, India
    Siva Subramanian R., R.M.K. College of Engineering and Technology, India

Chapter 3
Leveraging AI and Machine Learning for Next-Generation Clinical Decision Support Systems (CDSS) 83
    Uddalak Mitra, JIS College of Engineering, India
    Shafiq Ul Rehman, Kingdom University, Bahrain

Chapter 4
The X-Factor of Healthcare: How Explainable AI Is Revolutionizing Medical Practice.. 113
    Shahin Shoukat Makubhai, MIT Art, Design, and Technology University, India
    Ganesh Rajaram Pathak, MIT Art, Design, and Technology University, India
    Pankaj R. Chandre, MIT Art, Design, and Technology University, India

Chapter 5
Clinical Decision Support Systems Using Machine Learning: A Case Study on Thyroid Disease Prediction... 141
    Archana Kedar Chaudhari, Vishwakarma Institute of Technology, Pune, India

Chapter 6
Machine Learning in Health: A Study on Heart Disease Prediction................. 165
    Gönül Kara, Pamukkale University, Turkey
    Leyla Özgür Polat, Pamukkale University, Turkey

Chapter 7
COVID Detection Model Using X-Ray Images: Role of Data Science and Machine Learning in Digital Medical System.. 201
    Vasima Khan, Sagar Institute of Science and Technology, Bhopal, India
    Komal Tahiliani, Sagar Institute of Science and Technology, Bhopal, India

Chapter 8
Optimizing Healthcare Operations With AI Algorithms by Enhancing Skin Cancer Diagnosis Using Advanced Image Processing and Classification Techniques 235

    Abioye Abiodun Oluwasegun, Nigerian Defence Academy, Kaduna, Nigeria
    Abraham Evwiekpaefe, Nigerian Defence Academy, Kaduna, Nigeria
    Philip Oshiokhaimhele Odion, Nigerian Defence Academy, Kaduna, Nigeria
    Awujoola Joel Olalekan, Nigerian Defence Academy, Kaduna, Nigeria
    Anyanwu Obinna Bright, Nigerian Defence Academy, Kaduna, Nigeria
    Adelegan Olayinka Racheal, Nigerian Defence Academy, Kaduna, Nigeria
    Uwa Celestine Ozoemenam, Nigerian Defence Academy, Kaduna, Nigeria
    Modibbo Gidado Malami, Nigerian Defence Academy, Kaduna, Nigeria

Chapter 9
AI-Driven-IoT(AIIoT)-Based Decision Making in Kidney Diseases Patient Healthcare Monitoring: KSK Approach for Kidney Monitoring 277

    Kutubuddin Sayyad Liyakat Kazi, Brahmdevdada Mane Institute of Technology, Solapur, India

Chapter 10
Analysis of Insomnia for Old Aged People Using Machine Learning Algorithms 307

    N. T. Renukadevi, Kongu Engineering College, India
    K. Saraswathi, Kongu Engineering College, India
    S. Vignesh, Kongu Engineering College, India

Chapter 11
A Contactless Real-Time System to Classify Multi-Class Sitting Posture Using Depth Sensor-Based Data 333

    Huseyin Coskun, Kutahya Health Sciences University, Turkey

Chapter 12
Harnessing Machine Learning and Deep Learning in Healthcare From Early Diagnosis to Personalized Treatment: Comprehensive Approach of Deep Learning In Healthcare 369

    Ajay Sharma, uPGrad Campus, India
    Devendra Babu Pesarlanka, Lovely Professional Unviersity, India
    Shamneesh Sharma, uPGrad Campus, India

Chapter 13
Harnessing AI for Better Health Outcomes: Emerging Trends 399
   Ahmad Tasnim Siddiqui, Sandip University, Nashik, India
   Pawan R. Bhaladhare, Sandip University, Nashik, India

Compilation of References 419

About the Contributors 481

Index 491

Detailed Table of Contents

Preface xvi

Chapter 1
AI in Healthcare Data Analytics Trends and Transformative Innovations 1
    Manjunatha Badiger, NMAM Institute of Technology, India
    Sookshma Adiga, Moodlakatte Institute of Technology, India
    Akshatha Naik, Moodlakatte Institute of Technology, India
    Sumiksha Shetty, Sahyadri College of Engineering and Management, India
    A. B. Smitha, Sahyadri College of Engineering and Management, India
    Fathima C. Mehnaz, Sahyadri College of Engineering and Management, India
    Chandra Singh, NMAM Institute of Technology, Nitte University, India

Advances in AI and data analytics are revolutionizing healthcare by enhancing patient well-being, and system performance, and addressing deep-rooted health challenges. Key trends include precision medicine, which forecasts health outcomes based on genotype and phenotype, real-time monitoring with intelligent wearables, improved diagnostics, greater process efficiency, rapid drug development, and genomics integration. Other significant trends encompass NLP, federated learning, blockchain for data protection, explainable AI, and clinician decision support tools. The application of AI holds immense potential, making the vision of improved patient care, higher health outcomes, operational efficiency, and innovative health solutions increasingly achievable.

Chapter 2
Transforming Healthcare With AI and Machine Learning: Applications and
Impacts 53
    D. Ravindran, Kristu Jayanti College, India
    G. Mariammal, Vel Tech Rangarajan Dr. Sagunthala R&D Institute of
        Science and Technology, India
    M. Dhivya, Ramco Institute of Technology, India
    Dhivya Devi S., SRM Institute of Science and Technology, India
    Anish T. P., R.M.K. College of Engineering and Technology, India
    V. Sathya, Vel Tech Rangarajan Dr. Sagunthala R&D Institute of
        Science and Technology, India
    Siva Subramanian R., R.M.K. College of Engineering and Technology,
        India

This survey paper gives an insight about the application of artificial intelligence (AI) and machine learning (ML) in the healthcare industry. With a broad focus, it discusses the present state, approaches, and advancements of AI and ML in the health care industry. This paper explores the process of accumulating and structuring healthcare data, dataset standardization, data quality assessment, prognosis, clinical decision support systems, healthcare operations' efficiency, population health dynamics, fraudulence identification, revenue cycle, patient participation, telemonitoring, individualized treatment, health care quality assessment, ethical issues, and real-world examples of healthcare AI applications and developments. This comprehensive survey highlights the transformative potential of AI and ML in healthcare, emphasizing the need for continuous research, ethical practices, and robust data management to harness these technologies effectively.

Chapter 3
Leveraging AI and Machine Learning for Next-Generation Clinical Decision
Support Systems (CDSS) 83
    Uddalak Mitra, JIS College of Engineering, India
    Shafiq Ul Rehman, Kingdom University, Bahrain

Missed diagnoses and medication errors are significant risks in healthcare, leading to increased patient morbidity and mortality. Traditional Clinical Decision Support Systems (CDSS) rely on static, predefined rules, limiting their adaptability to personalized patient care. This chapter explores how integrating Artificial Intelligence (AI) and Machine Learning (ML) can revolutionize CDSS, driving next-generation systems. By analyzing clinical datasets in real time, AI and ML enable personalized insights that enhance diagnostic accuracy, optimize treatment recommendations, improve risk stratification, and streamline workflows. These advancements promise better patient outcomes, informed clinical decisions, and reduced costs. The chapter also addresses challenges like data quality, explainability, regulatory compliance, and ethics, proposing strategies for overcoming these. Through collaboration and research, AI and ML can transform CDSS into foundational healthcare elements, fostering personalized, data-driven, and efficient patient care.

Chapter 4
The X-Factor of Healthcare: How Explainable AI Is Revolutionizing Medical
Practice.. 113
    Shahin Shoukat Makubhai, MIT Art, Design, and Technology University,
        India
    Ganesh Rajaram Pathak, MIT Art, Design, and Technology University,
        India
    Pankaj R. Chandre, MIT Art, Design, and Technology University, India

This chapter explores the revolutionary impact of explainable AI in transforming medical practices. The X-Factor of Healthcare highlights how the integration of explainable AI technologies enables healthcare professionals to gain valuable insights into complex decision-making processes. By providing interpretable and transparent explanations for AI-driven predictions and recommendations, explainable AI empowers medical practitioners to understand, trust, and utilize AI tools more effectively. This Chapter examines the key benefits and challenges of implementing explainable AI in healthcare settings, emphasizing the improvement in diagnostic accuracy, personalized treatment plans, and patient outcomes. Additionally, this chapter discusses the results of machine learning classifiers such as Support Vector Machine, Random Forest, Decision Tree, and Logistic regression. This chapter also discusses the importance of ethical considerations, regulatory guidelines, and the need for collaboration between AI experts and healthcare professionals.

Chapter 5
Clinical Decision Support Systems Using Machine Learning: A Case Study on Thyroid Disease Prediction.. 141
    Archana Kedar Chaudhari, Vishwakarma Institute of Technology, Pune, India

The case study explores the application of machine learning (ML) in the development of clinical decision support systems (CDSS) for the prediction and diagnosis of thyroid diseases. By leveraging patient data, including demographic information, medical history, and laboratory test results, various ML algorithms are evaluated for their efficacy in predicting thyroid disorders. The study focuses on the selection of relevant features, model training, and validation processes, comparing performance metrics such as accuracy, sensitivity, and specificity. The integration of these predictive models into a CDSS is discussed, highlighting the potential for improved diagnostic accuracy, personalized treatment plans, and enhanced patient outcomes. This case study underscores the transformative impact of ML in the healthcare sector, particularly in the early detection and management of thyroid diseases.

Chapter 6
Machine Learning in Health: A Study on Heart Disease Prediction 165
    Gönül Kara, Pamukkale University, Turkey
    Leyla Özgür Polat, Pamukkale University, Turkey

The rapid increase in the amount of data in the healthcare sector has increased the importance of machine learning and data analysis techniques based on artificial intelligence in disease prediction and risk identification. n this context, heart disease prediction is one of the most frequently addressed problems. In this section, classification algorithms used in health are discussed and a sample application in heart disease prediction is performed to demonstrate the accuracy and reliability of the algorithms. Using a dataset of 1025 samples from the UCI data repository, heart disease prediction was performed with supervised machine learning models such as Logistic Regression, Decision Trees, Support Vector Machines, K-Nearest Neighbor and Naive Bayes over 14 attributes and the results were interpreted. The study tries to show how different algorithms process the features in the dataset and which model performs better. As a result, it is shown how algorithms can be used in heart disease prediction with practical application and how the results can be interpreted.

Chapter 7
COVID Detection Model Using X-Ray Images: Role of Data Science and
Machine Learning in Digital Medical System 201
    Vasima Khan, Sagar Institute of Science and Technology, Bhopal, India
    Komal Tahiliani, Sagar Institute of Science and Technology, Bhopal, India

The global COVID-19 pandemic has posed unprecedented problems to healthcare institutions across the globe. Ensuring timely and precise identification of the virus is crucial to efficiently manage its transmission. In the context of the metaverse, the implementation of a non-contact detection method has possible advantages by replacing the necessity of a physical COVID-19 test with a digital challenge. The present chapter explores the utilisation of machine learning and deep learning methodologies in the creation of a COVID-19 detection model through the analysis of X-ray pictures. The main aim of this approach is to augment the foundational notion of the metaverse. The primary objective of this model is to precisely ascertain the existence of COVID-19, regardless of its positive or negative status, and to identify instances of viral pneumonia by the analysis of X-ray pictures. The present investigation is grounded upon recent research that indicates a correlation between the presence of COVID-19 and detectable findings in chest X-ray pictures.

Chapter 8
Optimizing Healthcare Operations With AI Algorithms by Enhancing Skin Cancer Diagnosis Using Advanced Image Processing and Classification Techniques 235
    Abioye Abiodun Oluwasegun, Nigerian Defence Academy, Kaduna, Nigeria
    Abraham Evwiekpaefe, Nigerian Defence Academy, Kaduna, Nigeria
    Philip Oshiokhaimhele Odion, Nigerian Defence Academy, Kaduna, Nigeria
    Awujoola Joel Olalekan, Nigerian Defence Academy, Kaduna, Nigeria
    Anyanwu Obinna Bright, Nigerian Defence Academy, Kaduna, Nigeria
    Adelegan Olayinka Racheal, Nigerian Defence Academy, Kaduna, Nigeria
    Uwa Celestine Ozoemenam, Nigerian Defence Academy, Kaduna, Nigeria
    Modibbo Gidado Malami, Nigerian Defence Academy, Kaduna, Nigeria

Optimizing healthcare through AI algorithms offers significant potential in skin cancer diagnosis. Skin cancer, involving abnormal skin cell growth, includes melanoma, the most dangerous form. Early detection is crucial, but traditional methods like visual inspection and biopsy are time-consuming and subjective. AI provides a more efficient, objective approach. This chapter enhances diagnostic accuracy using advanced image processing and classification on a comprehensive skin cancer dataset with seven classes. Initially imbalanced, data augmentation balanced it, generating 2000 images per class. Gray Level Co-occurrence Matrix (GLCM) and Color Histogram were used for feature extraction, combined with a Random Forest classifier. The best model achieved 97% accuracy, emphasizing balanced data and effective feature extraction in AI-based skin cancer diagnosis.

Chapter 9
AI-Driven-IoT(AIIoT)-Based Decision Making in Kidney Diseases Patient
Healthcare Monitoring: KSK Approach for Kidney Monitoring....................... 277
    Kutubuddin Sayyad Liyakat Kazi, Brahmdevdada Mane Institute of
       Technology, Solapur, India

As artificial intelligence (AI) and the internet of things (IoT) continue to grow, the KSK approach is poised to revolutionize decision-making processes and make the world a more intelligent and efficient place. To fulfill the requirements of the task that is being proposed, this model was developed expressly for that purpose. During the classification process, these classifiers are utilized in the case of disease datasets, specifically in areas such as those that belong to kidney diseases. When it comes to determining how effectively the classifiers are functioning, there are three basic indicators that are taken into consideration. It is important to note that this is referring to the metrics of accuracy, precision, and recall. It is possible to acquire an accuracy rate that ranges from a minimum of 87% to a maximum of 92.5% for each and every illness by utilizing the proposed KSK approach.

Chapter 10
Analysis of Insomnia for Old Aged People Using Machine Learning
Algorithms 307
    N. T. Renukadevi, Kongu Engineering College, India
    K. Saraswathi, Kongu Engineering College, India
    S. Vignesh, Kongu Engineering College, India

Sleep plays a crucial role in overall health and well-being, with its significance and being more important in the context of aging. This research explores the application of machine learning algorithms to predict and analyze sleep patterns in older adults. A dataset comprising physiological and lifestyle factors, alongside sleep-related parameters, is collected from a cohort of elderly individuals. Various machine learning models, including but not limited to Random Forest, Support Vector Machines, Decision Tree, KNN are employed to develop predictive models for sleep duration, quality, and disruptions. Insomnia is a sleep disorder characterized by persistent difficulty falling asleep, staying asleep, or experiencing restorative sleep, leading to significant impairment in daily functioning. It can be caused by various factors, including stress, anxiety, depression, or lifestyle choices. Healthcare providers can gain insights into individualized risk factors for sleep disturbances in older adults, facilitating early intervention and personalized sleep management strategies.

Chapter 11
A Contactless Real-Time System to Classify Multi-Class Sitting Posture
Using Depth Sensor-Based Data 333
    Huseyin Coskun, Kutahya Health Sciences University, Turkey

Musculoskeletal disorders are often linked to poor sitting postures, making the assessment of healthy sitting positions crucial. This study develops a system for contactless recognition of office workers' sitting postures, using various classification methods for health applications. Five sitting postures were defined based on medical literature and standards. Thirty subjects held these postures for 30 seconds, with pose data captured via a Kinect device. To overcome challenges like desks and computers, two datasets with different joint points were created. Pose samples were labeled by calculating angles between body parts like legs, hips, and back. Classification methods included Neural Networks, Support Vector Machine (SVM), K-Nearest Neighbors, Naive Bayes, AdaBoost, Decision Tree, Random Forest, and Ensemble Learning (EL). The highest accuracy was achieved by EL and SVM, at 99.8% and 99.7%, respectively. The first and fifth postures were found to be the most comfortable. This system aims to improve sitting behaviors and is useful for health monitoring and robotic vision.

Chapter 12
Harnessing Machine Learning and Deep Learning in Healthcare From Early
Diagnosis to Personalized Treatment: Comprehensive Approach of Deep
Learning In Healthcare 369
    Ajay Sharma, uPGrad Campus, India
    Devendra Babu Pesarlanka, Lovely Professional Unviersity, India
    Shamneesh Sharma, uPGrad Campus, India

Machine learning (ML) and deep learning (DL) are transforming healthcare by improving patient outcomes, reducing costs, and accelerating drug development. ML algorithms analyze large datasets such as EHRs, medical imaging, and genomics to enable early disease detection and personalized treatments. The current work highlights new approaches in pharmaceutical design and predicts medication side effects. Deep Learning (DL), a branch of AI using neural networks, excels in medical imaging, identifying subtle patterns in MRIs and X-rays. The current manuscript highlights how DL models can identify genetic markers linked to diseases like cancer, Parkinson's, and Alzheimer's. Integrating ML and DL into clinical workflows empowers healthcare professionals with data-driven tools for better decision-making. However, some challenges remain, including ensuring data privacy, and security, addressing biases in algorithms. Collaboration between healthcare providers, researchers, and tech firms is essential for the ethical and effective adoption of these technologies have been discussed in the work.

Chapter 13
Harnessing AI for Better Health Outcomes: Emerging Trends 399
Ahmad Tasnim Siddiqui, Sandip University, Nashik, India
Pawan R. Bhaladhare, Sandip University, Nashik, India

Artificial Intelligence (AI) is revolutionizing healthcare by enhancing patient outcomes through innovative applications and emerging trends. AI-driven technologies are transforming diagnostics, treatment planning, and patient management, making healthcare more efficient and personalized. Key trends include the use of machine learning algorithms for early disease detection, predictive analytics to anticipate patient needs for improved clinical documentation and patient communication. AI-powered imaging systems are providing more accurate and faster interpretations of medical scans, while personalized medicine is benefiting from AI's ability to analyze vast amounts of genetic and clinical data. AI is playing a crucial role in managing chronic diseases through continuous monitoring and real-time data analysis, enabling proactive interventions. The integration of AI with telemedicine platforms is expanding access to care, particularly in remote areas. But, the adoption of AI in healthcare also raises ethical concerns, such as privacy and algorithmic bias, which need to be addressed.

Compilation of References 419

About the Contributors 481

Index 491

Preface

Artificial Intelligence (AI) is revolutionizing the healthcare industry, offering unprecedented opportunities to enhance patient care, optimize operational efficiency, and address complex medical challenges. The integration of AI-driven innovations with healthcare data analytics is not just a technological advancement; it is a transformative shift that has the potential to redefine the future of healthcare. "AI-Driven Innovation in Healthcare Data Analytics" brings together a diverse collection of research and insights from leading experts, showcasing the multifaceted ways in which AI is reshaping healthcare delivery and patient outcomes.

This book is the culmination of efforts by researchers and practitioners across various disciplines—including industrial engineering, computer science, healthcare management, and data science—to explore the frontiers of AI in healthcare. It emphasizes the importance of interdisciplinary collaboration, recognizing that the complexities of modern healthcare require solutions that bridge traditional boundaries.

In today's data-rich environment, healthcare organizations generate vast amounts of data, from electronic health records and genomic information to medical imaging and real-time patient monitoring. The challenge lies in harnessing this data effectively to extract meaningful insights that can improve patient outcomes and streamline healthcare processes. AI, with its advanced machine learning algorithms, deep learning techniques, and data mining capabilities, offers powerful tools to meet this challenge.

This book is intended for a broad readership, including researchers, practitioners, and students interested in the application of AI in healthcare. Academics will find valuable insights into the latest AI-driven approaches in healthcare data analytics, while practitioners will benefit from practical case studies and applications that can inform decision-making and drive improvements in healthcare organizations. Graduate students and professionals seeking to explore advancements in AI-driven healthcare analytics will discover a wealth of knowledge and perspectives.

To provide a cohesive and comprehensive exploration of the subject, the book is organized into four parts, each focusing on a specific aspect of AI-driven healthcare data analytics. This logical progression guides readers from foundational concepts through theoretical frameworks, practical applications, and future directions.

Part I: Introduction and Key Trends

Chapter 1: "AI in Healthcare Data Analytics Trends and Transformative Innovations"
Authors: Dr. Manjunatha Badiger, Ms. Sookshma Adiga, Ms. Akshatha Naik, Mrs. Sumiksha Shetty, Mrs. Smitha A B, Mrs. Mehnaz Fathima C, Mr. Chandra Singh

In this opening chapter, Dr. Manjunatha Badiger and his team explore the pivotal role of AI and data analytics in revolutionizing healthcare. They delve into key trends such as precision medicine, real-time monitoring with intelligent wearables, improved diagnostics, and rapid drug development. By examining these advancements, the authors highlight how AI is enhancing patient well-being and healthcare system performance. They make a compelling case for the adoption of AI-driven techniques to address deep-rooted health challenges, emphasizing that the vision of improved patient care, higher health outcomes, and operational efficiency is increasingly achievable.

Chapter 2: "Transforming Healthcare with AI and Machine Learning: Applications and Impacts"
Authors: Siva Subramanian R, Dr. Nalini M, Mrs. Maheswari B, Mr. Anish T P, Mr. Ezhilvandan M, Ms. Beslin Pajila P J, Ms. Girija P

Building on the introduction, Siva Subramanian R and his co-authors provide a comprehensive survey of the current state, approaches, and advancements of AI and machine learning in the healthcare industry. They discuss how these technologies are utilized in electronic health records management, predictive analytics, personalized medicine, and operational efficiency. The chapter delves into processes like accumulating and structuring healthcare data, dataset standardization, and data quality assessment. This foundational piece offers readers a broad understanding of the transformative impact of AI across the healthcare spectrum.

Part II: Theoretical Discussions and Methods

Chapter 3: "Leveraging AI and Machine Learning for Next-Generation Clinical Decision Support Systems (CDSS)"
Authors: Dr. Uddalak Mitra, Dr. Shafiq Ul Rehman

In this chapter, Dr. Uddalak Mitra and Dr. Shafiq Ul Rehman delve into the evolution of clinical decision support systems (CDSS) and how integrating AI and machine learning can revolutionize them. They discuss the limitations of traditional CDSS and explore how AI enables personalized insights, enhances diagnostic accuracy, optimizes treatment recommendations, and streamlines workflows. The authors highlight the potential for improved patient outcomes and informed clinical decisions through AI-driven CDSS, addressing challenges like data quality, explainability, regulatory compliance, and ethics.

Chapter 4: "The X-Factor of Healthcare: How Explainable AI is Revolutionizing Medical Practice"

Authors: Ms. Shahin Shoukat Makubhai, Dr. Ganesh Rajaram Pathak, Dr. Pankaj R Makubhai

Addressing the critical issue of transparency, Ms. Shahin Shoukat Makubhai and her colleagues examine the importance of explainable AI in healthcare. They explore how providing interpretable and transparent explanations for AI-driven predictions empowers medical practitioners to understand, trust, and effectively utilize AI tools. The chapter discusses methodologies for making AI models more interpretable and provides examples of how explainable AI is being implemented to enhance medical practice. This work emphasizes the improvement in diagnostic accuracy, personalized treatment plans, and patient outcomes.

Part III: Practical Applications and Case Studies

Chapter 5: "Clinical Decision Support Systems Using Machine Learning: A Case Study on Thyroid Disease Prediction"

Author: Dr. Archana Kedar Chaudhari

Dr. Archana Kedar Chaudhari presents a specific application of machine learning in developing a clinical decision support system for thyroid disease prediction. She details the selection of relevant features, model training, and validation processes, comparing performance metrics such as accuracy, sensitivity, and specificity. The integration of these predictive models into a CDSS is discussed, highlighting the potential for improved diagnostic accuracy, personalized treatment plans, and enhanced patient outcomes. This case study underscores the transformative impact of machine learning in early detection and management of thyroid diseases.

Chapter 6: "Machine Learning in Health: A Study on Heart Disease Prediction"
Authors: Gönül Kara, Dr. Leyla Özgür Polat

Focusing on heart disease prediction, Gönül Kara and Dr. Leyla Özgür Polat demonstrate how machine learning algorithms are employed to analyze healthcare data. They compare various classification algorithms, interpret the results, and show how these models can be used in practical applications. The authors utilize a dataset from the UCI data repository and discuss the importance of data preprocessing and algorithm selection. The study underscores the potential of AI in early detection and risk identification, contributing to better patient outcomes.

Chapter 7: "COVID Detection Model Using X-ray Images: Role of Data Science and Machine Learning in Digital Medical Systems"

Authors: Dr. Vasima Khan, Dr. Komal Tahiliani

Amidst the global pandemic, Dr. Vasima Khan and Dr. Komal Tahiliani explore the development of a COVID-19 detection model using X-ray images and machine learning. They highlight the importance of non-contact detection methods and how AI and data science contribute to efficient pandemic response. By demonstrating the application of deep learning methodologies, the authors showcase the potential of AI in addressing urgent healthcare challenges. The chapter emphasizes the integration of AI in the metaverse and its implications for future digital medical systems.

Chapter 8: "Optimizing Healthcare Operations with AI Algorithms by Enhancing Skin Cancer Diagnosis Using Advanced Image Processing and Classification Techniques"

Authors: Mr. Abioye Abiodun Oluwasegun, Dr. Abraham Evwiekpaefe, Dr. Philip Oshiokhaimhele Odion, Dr. Awujoola Joel Olalekan, Mr. Anyanwu Obinna Bright, Mr. Modibbo Malami Gidado, Mrs. Adelegan Olayinka Racheal, Mr. Uwa Celestine Ozoemenam

In this chapter, Mr. Abioye Abiodun Oluwasegun and his team focus on improving skin cancer diagnosis through AI algorithms and advanced image processing. They address the challenges of traditional diagnostic methods and demonstrate how AI can enhance accuracy and efficiency. Utilizing techniques like Gray Level Co-occurrence Matrix (GLCM) and Color Histogram for feature extraction, combined with a Random Forest classifier, the authors achieved a 97% accuracy rate. The chapter emphasizes the importance of balanced data and effective feature extraction in AI-based skin cancer diagnosis.

Chapter 9: "AI-Driven-IoT (AIIoT) Based Decision Making in Kidney Diseases Patient Healthcare Monitoring: KSK Approach for Kidney Monitoring"

Author: Dr. Kutubuddin Sayyad Liyakat Kazi

Dr. Kutubuddin Sayyad Liyakat Kazi explores the integration of AI and IoT in healthcare monitoring. He presents the KSK approach for kidney disease patient monitoring, discussing how AI-driven IoT systems enable real-time patient monitoring, data analysis, and decision-making. By addressing challenges in disease datasets and classifier performance, Dr. Kazi illustrates the potential of AI in connected healthcare systems. The chapter reports an accuracy rate ranging from 87% to 92.5% for disease classification using the proposed KSK approach.

Chapter 10: "Analysis of Insomnia for Old Aged People Using Machine Learning Algorithms"

Authors: N T Renukadevi, Dr. Saraswathi K, Ms. Nandhinidevi S, Mr. Vignesh S

Addressing geriatric health issues, N T Renukadevi and her colleagues apply machine learning algorithms to predict and analyze sleep patterns in older adults. They collect and analyze data on physiological and lifestyle factors, employing models like Random Forest, Support Vector Machines, Decision Tree, and K-Nearest Neighbor. The study provides insights into individualized risk factors for sleep disturbances, facilitating early intervention and personalized management strategies. The chapter emphasizes the role of AI in improving the quality of life for the elderly.

Chapter 11: "A Contactless Real-Time System to Classify Multi-Class Sitting Posture Using Depth Sensor-Based Data"

Author: Dr. Huseyin Coskun

Dr. Huseyin Coskun introduces a system for contactless recognition of sitting postures using depth sensors and classification methods. By defining five sitting postures based on medical literature and capturing data with a Kinect device, he demonstrates how AI can improve sitting behaviors. Classification methods including Neural Networks, Support Vector Machine, K-Nearest Neighbors, and Ensemble Learning were used, achieving up to 99.8% accuracy. The system has applications in health monitoring and ergonomic assessments, aiming to reduce musculoskeletal disorders linked to poor posture.

Part IV: Future Directions and Emerging Trends

Chapter 12: "Harnessing Machine Learning and Deep Learning in Healthcare from Early Diagnosis to Personalized Treatment: Comprehensive Approach of Deep Learning in Healthcare"

Authors: Ajay Sharma, Mr. Devendra Babu Pesarlanka, Mr. Shamneesh Sharma

Ajay Sharma and his co-authors explore advanced AI techniques in healthcare, focusing on how machine learning and deep learning are transforming early diagnosis and personalized treatment. They discuss new approaches in pharmaceutical design, genetic marker identification, and the challenges and future potential of AI in healthcare. The chapter emphasizes the need for collaboration between healthcare providers, researchers, and tech firms, and addresses ethical considerations and biases in algorithms.

Chapter 13: "Harnessing AI for Better Health Outcomes - Emerging Trends"

Authors: Dr. Ahmad Tasnim Siddiqui, Prof. Pawan R. Bhaladhare

Concluding the book, Dr. Ahmad Tasnim Siddiqui and Prof. Pawan R. Bhaladhare discuss emerging trends in AI for healthcare. They examine technologies such as natural language processing, federated learning, blockchain for data protection, explainable AI, and clinician decision support tools. By envisioning future advancements, the authors highlight the transformative potential of AI in achieving improved patient care, operational efficiency, and innovative health solutions.

In summary, "AI-Driven Innovation in Healthcare Data Analytics" offers a comprehensive exploration of how AI technologies are transforming healthcare. The logical progression from foundational concepts to theoretical frameworks, practical applications, and future directions allows readers to build a systematic understanding of the field. Each chapter provides unique insights, grounded in rigorous research and practical case studies, demonstrating the multifaceted impact of AI-driven innovations on healthcare data analytics and management.

By highlighting the contributions of esteemed authors, this book underscores the importance of interdisciplinary collaboration in advancing healthcare. The collective expertise presented in this volume bridges the gap between healthcare management, data science, and engineering disciplines, fostering a holistic approach to addressing healthcare challenges.

This book contributes to the advancement of knowledge, inspires new avenues for research and innovation, and serves as an indispensable resource for academics, practitioners, policymakers, and students alike. As we stand at the forefront of a new era in healthcare—characterized by data-driven decision-making and personalized medicine—the insights presented here are both timely and essential.

It is our hope that this book will catalyze further research, encourage interdisciplinary collaboration, and contribute to the development of AI-driven solutions that are ethical, effective, and centered around the well-being of patients.

Olcay Polat
Pamukkale University, Department of Industrial Engineering

Leyla Özgür Polat
Department of Management Information Systems

Chapter 1
AI in Healthcare Data Analytics Trends and Transformative Innovations

Manjunatha Badiger
https://orcid.org/0000-0001-8073-0270
NMAM Institute of Technology, India

A. B. Smitha
Sahyadri College of Engineering and Management, India

Sookshma Adiga
Moodlakatte Institute of Technology, India

Fathima C. Mehnaz
Sahyadri College of Engineering and Management, India

Akshatha Naik
Moodlakatte Institute of Technology, India

Chandra Singh
https://orcid.org/0000-0002-1759-8796
NMAM Institute of Technology, Nitte University, India

Sumiksha Shetty
Sahyadri College of Engineering and Management, India

ABSTRACT

Advances in AI and data analytics are revolutionizing healthcare by enhancing patient well-being, and system performance, and addressing deep-rooted health challenges. Key trends include precision medicine, which forecasts health outcomes based on genotype and phenotype, real-time monitoring with intelligent wearables, improved diagnostics, greater process efficiency, rapid drug development, and genomics integration. Other significant trends encompass NLP, federated learning, blockchain for data protection, explainable AI, and clinician decision support

DOI: 10.4018/979-8-3693-7277-7.ch001

tools. The application of AI holds immense potential, making the vision of improved patient care, higher health outcomes, operational efficiency, and innovative health solutions increasingly achievable.

INTRODUCTION

The pace of innovation in the healthcare sector is relentless as new revolutions happen consistently, be they the results of new discoveries, epidemiological forecasting, strengthening of preventive measures, or improving the quality of handling patients. However, the core of this change is, undoubtedly, data analytics, which is becoming the foundation for knowledge-based decision-making and improving patients' outcomes and organizational performance (Batko & Ślęzak, 2022). Current research indicates a growth in the global healthcare analytics market, with estimated revenues surpassing USD 46. It has been estimated that the market will be worth roughly 5 billion US dollars in the year 2024, and it has the potential to reach an astounding 130.49 billion US dollars by the year 2029. Because of the clear influence that data analytics has, as well as the expanding relevance that it is having on the healthcare system, the integration of this technology is very necessary. It is in this context that this introduction establishes the premise towards conceptualizing an evaluation of analytical data and its impact on the health care industry, with a focus on the providers and the payers. The following sections will review various uses, types, advantages, difficulties, and the potential of data analytics in understanding the tremendous capacity of health care improvement.

Overview of AI in Healthcare

AI's primary role is to revolutionarily change healthcare by incorporating new forms of data analysis, predicting features, and automation into several medical specialties. AI includes but not limited to machine learning, deep learning, NLP and robotics that is used in the field of raising diagnostic coefficients, developing individual treatment programs, optimization of operational processes (Xu et al., 2021). Clinicians use the artificial intelligence systems to process big data from electronic health records, images, genomic data, and patient monitoring in real-time in a way that is not feasible for any human being. Such AI-derived recommendations help in early diagnosis of diseases, prognosis and recommendations of the best treatment plans. It is noteworthy to state that AI's integration into healthcare is benefiting from the availability of EHRs and the increasing amount of healthcare data. It enables these AI algorithms to handle different types of data with different structures and formats – structured data from EHRs, non-structured data that are usually present in clinical notes, and image data obtained from radiology and pathology departments, respectively. These data sets, along with other data sets which AI learns from and gets better in time, play a significant role in uplifting the quality of the patients' care and organizational performance.

In the field of healthcare, artificial intelligence is used in systems that assist medical professionals in diagnosing and treating their patients (Davenport & Kalakota, 2019). These systems include CDSS, as well as the utilization of wearable devices to monitor patients' vital signs in real time. Moreover, artificial intelligence is transforming the drug discovery process by identifying patterns for therapeutic targets and potentially forecasting the effectiveness of new medications. The use of artificial intelligence in the healthcare industry has its drawbacks, including the protection and privacy of a patient's data, the absence of regulatory policies aimed at the use of AI and information technology, and the need for human beings to exercise control over artificial intelligence in order to guarantee that it is being used in an appropriate and appropriate manner (Murdoch, 2021).

Importance of Data Analytics in Modern Healthcare

Data analytics is a valuable tool in today's healthcare sector because it provides insights from large volumes of medical information. With modern healthcare systems' ever-growing amounts of data from sources such as electronic medical records, radiology, genomics, and wearable technology, it is critical to be able to analyze the data and apply it for the benefit of patients and the wider healthcare system. In essence, integrating data analytics into the healthcare system has the advantage of enhancing the possibility of designing personal care for individual patients. With patient-unique data about the genetic characteristics of the patient and much more, physicians and healthcare workers can create optimized treatment regimens that are less toxic to the patient. One of the data analytic categories is predictive, which aims to use prior information and computational intelligence to predict the future state of affairs of specific diseases, patients' risks, and chronic conditions (Alowais et al., 2023). Such an approach might result in early detection, reducing hospital admissions and improving the overall quality of life for patients. Data analytics also improves the functionality of various departments and units within healthcare organizations. Another method of obtaining structured data involves utilizing the existing data from a hospital's operations, which aids in determining factors such as the right allocation of human and material resources, patient waiting times, and the probable scheduling of different surgeries. Another use of data analytics is in the area of carrying out predictive maintenance on medical equipment to avoid deficiencies that might be damaging to important apparatus. However, data analytics assists in the management of patient groups by continually searching for patterns inherent in large groups of people. These conclusions can be useful for officials in the field of public health because they can help them create effective. Data analytics in healthcare encompasses a wide range of fields, including patient care, outcomes, operations, and research as illustrated in the below Figure 1.

Figure 1. Data analytics in healthcare

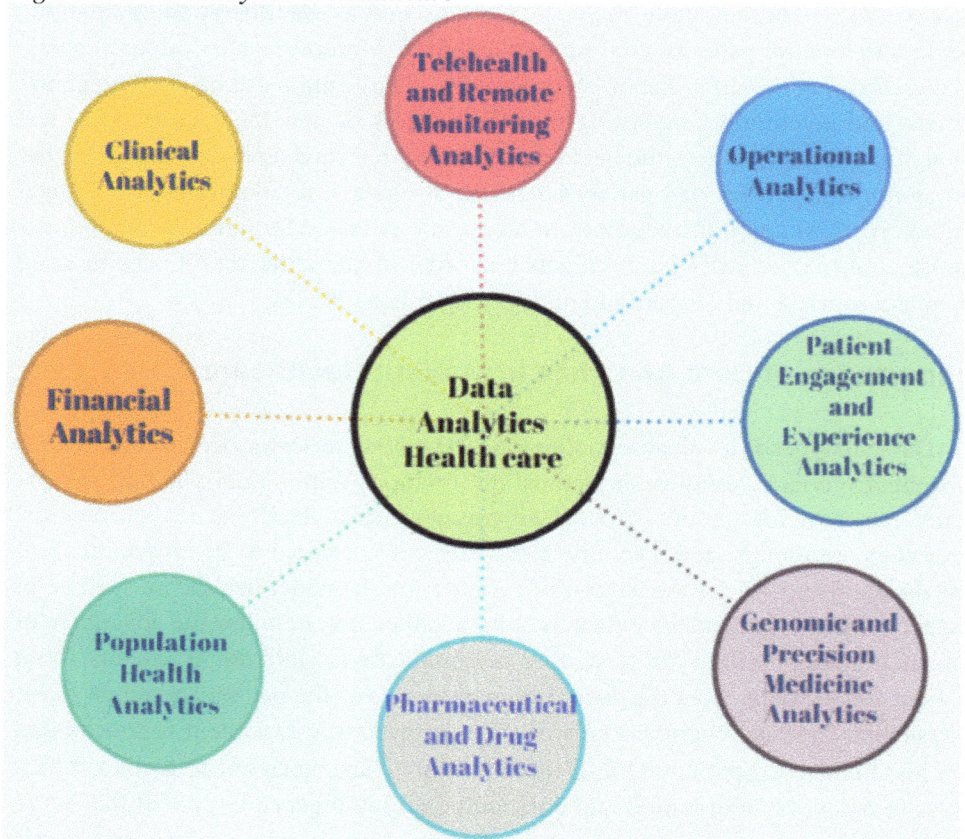

Clinical analytics is the use of mathematical and data analysis tools to increase the precision and individuality of a cure. Operational analytics is the practice of introducing measurement and analysis tactics into the everyday workflow to maximize the effectiveness and efficiency of resource usage and minimize expenses. Population health analytics monitors the time it takes to understand health trends or contain diseases, while financial analytics enhances revenue generation strategies and lowers costs. Pharmaceutical analytics accelerates drug development and increases safety due to pharmacovigilance. Diagnostic analytics utilize genomic and precision medicine data to tailor treatments according to the patient's genetic makeup, while patient experience optimization analytics enhance satisfaction levels among the patient population. Teleconsultation technologies make it possible to enhance the efficiency of the telemedical services, the remote control of chronic diseases, as well as the assessment of the effectiveness of virtual therapies. The objectives of research and development analytics include offering support to biomedical research, the governing of progress in medicine, and improving the findings of clinical trials through analytics. When these sectors come together, they create a continuous cycle that utilizes healthcare data to enhance patient outcomes and propel the industry forward. Thus the big data analytics is a crucial tool in present-day healthcare organization since it helps turn large amounts of data into valuable information (Dash et al., 2019). This way, such stakeholders in the provision of health services can help institutions align their provisions with the ever-evolving landscape of needs by harnessing the power of data. With ageing healthcare organization adopting and implementing information technology, the role of data analysis, especially in determining the quality of patient care, will increase over time, exerting more pressure on the achievement of further innovations.

Case Study: Data-Driven Innovations in Pediatric Care Using High-Frequency Physiological Waveform Analytics

Lucile Packard Children's Hospital Stanford (LPCH) has a reputation for providing quality paediatrics and obstetrics services and, for quite some time, has been trying to adopt the latest technologies for a better delivery of service. Together with its partner HP Autonomy, LPCH decided to improve the power of AI and ML technologies for analytical predictions. The intended goal was to create a large-scale analytical environment from disparate clinical and financial sources of unstructured and semi structured data, utilizing the HP IDOL engine. Such a platform would allow healthcare providers to make the best decisions that could improve the quality of patients' lives. One of HP's major innovations was the ability of the IDOL engine to handle and interpret unstructured data (Sedlakova et al., 2023). In addition, the IDOL engine was able to handle free text writings like physician notes, clinical observations, and imaging reports, as well as databases like lab results, vital signs, and much more. Previous solutions for healthcare analytics were only capable of using structured data while excluding large amounts of useful data. Including over 400 data connectors and over 150 data types of patient health information, allowing offered Protean Bioinformaticians a broader perception of the patient's health status to gain a better understanding of treatment, symptoms, and drug reactions. One of the main goals of this drive was to make sure that an ML system was developed that could predict other very important clinical indicators. For example, it should be able to identify patients whose health is likely to get worse, protect them from CLABSI, and give an accurate estimate of the length of the surgery. All of these predictions would have led to a real improvement in the patient's condition and better organization of the hospital's work. Despite the creation of a highly functional platform and the design of necessary machine learning models, the work encountered essential difficulties. One of them was data inconsistency, which hampered prediction reliability. The training data sets that informed the machine learning models were of different qualities and completeness, thus causing disparity (Badiger & Mathew, 2023). Furthermore, the forecasts that the models provided were not usually useful enough to justify the time, effort, and capital invested in developing and perfecting them. Consequently, LPCH did not deploy any ML algorithms, despite incorporating the entire analytical system into its work process.

This case study outlines several crucial lessons to consider when implementing AI and ML in the healthcare sector. First, the accumulation of quality and consistency of the data is critical to the success of the predictive models. Algorithms are expensive, accurate, and highly developed, but they cannot show useful results if the data is inaccurate. Second, while the technique works effectively and has great promise as a diagnostic tool, its applicability to clinical practice must be tested; models that will not yield tangible benefits for the end consumer cannot justify the investment time taken to incorporate them. Last of all, it captures the theme that underpins this entire experience: the need to get the technology right in order that it supports, rather than obstructs, clinical care provision.

PREDICTIVE ANALYTICS FOR PERSONALIZED MEDICINE

The use of predictive analytics in personalized medicine has thus been adopted as the best approach to enhancing both the efficacy of treatments as well as the results obtained from the treatments. Data mining applied to machine learning algorithms and big data such as Electronic Health Records (EHR), genomic data, medical image and real time data from wearable devices. Some of us pointed out that the major concern in this big healthcare data world includes the problem of dealing with the big data itself, converting unstructured data to structured format so that they could be integrated effectively while having to consider the rights of patient data privacy and security. It also emphasises the challenges in the fast near-real-time data analysis and feeding advanced analytics into the practice of clinicians (Paganelli et al., 2022). Data governance and corresponding ethical issues are important to keep the relation with the stakeholders trustworthy and transparent. It means that the further development of the big data tools is crucial, as well as investing in the skills of the personnel and proper interdisciplinary cooperation regarding the scope of predictive analytics application in the sphere of personalized medicine. These challenges should therefore be addressed to improve patient care, resources utilisation and medical advancement transforming healthcare on a global level. Health Data Analytics is thus the centrepiece in transforming health care delivery through the application of the power of huge volumes of data produced in the healthcare environment. With the proliferation of electronic health records, and EHR, wearable devices, and other digital health technologies, healthcare organizations have large amounts of data that is not available from other source. When analysed and processed, this data is capable of serving as a basis for practical changes. Data analytics in healthcare allow organizations to derive insights of the raw material that feeds into it in order to facilitate decision making (Raghupathi & Raghupathi, 2014). It will also be possible to employ some of the most sophisticated advanced analytics techniques such as analytics tools such as the predictive modelling, machine learning and artificial intelligence ensure that healthcare providers are able to recognize the relevant patterns, trends and connections between variables in health care data that cannot be seen otherwise. Furthermore, data analytics contributes to the shift from oriental to occidental approaches in the delivery of health care by allowing predictive and preventive. Personalised Medicine through Prescription is the scientific discipline that leverages techniques like Machine Learning, Statistic, and Data Mining for the prognosis of health status of a patient. It aims to increase the efficiency of the treatments based on potential outcome of a definite patient and genetic makeup as well as his or her behaviours and surroundings.

Key Components of Predictive Analytics for Personalized Medicine

Data Collection: Collecting a huge amount of information from multiple sources with the help of EHRs, genomic data, wearable device data, and patients' self-reported questionnaires. Information gathering is the fundamental aspect of using prediction models within the context of personalized medicine, which literally refers to a wide range of data received from different sources and creating a detailed picture of the patient's condition. One of the key sources is electronic health records (EHR) which are comprehensive and longitudinal records of patient's health history and patients' diagnoses, treatments, labs results, and clinical notes. Collection of this information is significant in having a historical perspective of the health trends and results. Person-specific information provides yet another potent tool; besides, the identification of diseases to which an individual might be particularly vulnerable and the reactions to medications can be predicted based on the genetic profile of a person. Wearable devices have also made monitoring of every physiological factor possible such as heart rate, level of physical activity, sleep, and many more, which give real-time data that may be alarming of some developing health complications (Shei et al., 2022). Further, patients' data are also important since it involves their subjective complaints, symptoms and behaviour which may not or are rarely revealed in formal setting. When amalgamated, these various streams of data help predictive analytics to construct strong models that not only predict risks towards health but also design the treatments that work best for every person, making the health care delivery smarter and much more efficient.

Data Analysis: The concept of predictive analytics for personalized medicine is based on the use of sophisticated statistical technologies to turn large amount of patients' information into precious knowledge. This process begins by assimilating various sources of data that are bioinformatics data, EHRs, life style, and outside environment. The data is then processed by other complex programs including machine learning and artificial intelligence so as to determine various patterns, relationships and trends that may not be easily discerned through basic analysis. When such complicated associations are detected in terms of predictive analytics the service is able to foresee the health status of the patients, the specific response of the patients to the treatments that are to be given and further intimate recommendations based on the genetic as well as the environmental make-up of every patient that is with them (Whisman & South, 2017). TR guided approach helps them to get rid of one-size-fits-all model, hence helping them get a better diagnosis, better treatment plan, and much better outcome for the patients. That allows the clinician to start prevention or treatment steps when he anticipates a health problem or considers the potential reaction to a specific therapy; enhance treatment plans based on patients' characteristics; and adapt treatment regimens in light of patient outcomes, which makes personalized medicine possible in today's medicine.

Prediction Models: Predictive analytics in personalized medicine embraces generation and using of complex prognosis models that is aimed at predicting different aspects of patient's state and treatment results. Such models use Big Data on and on: genetics, environment, lifestyle factors: to estimate probabilities of diseases, how a specific patient would, for example, react to medication, and what effects the treatment would have. The use of these models in the course of the treatment will help physicians to introduce adjustments to the general treatment strategies to fit each client's needs, thus enhancing the outcomes of the curing process and minimizing the potential complications (Goetz & Schork, 2018). Also, this data analysis helps in improving the decision-making process and also, leads to the idea of a predictive and personalized medication, where intervention can be made according to the risk-reward analysis of each individual. The ideal approach will be to transcend throughout high-volume, homogeneous care, where each patient receives care based on his/her unique profile to yield the best clinical and patient outcomes.

Personalization of Treatment: Personalized medicine based on predictive analytics is the combination of sophisticated statistical and mathematical analysis for prioritization of medical treatments that are adjusted for a specific patient to increase efficacy as well as minimize adverse reactions. With individual patient's genetic makeup, it is possible to predict how he or she is likely to respond to certain treatment regimens so that the doctors can deliver treatments that correspond to the patient's characteristics at the genetic level. This approach does not only ensure that the medication prescribed is effective and provide the best results but also avoids side effects which result from a wrong genotypes match. Finally, it produces more customized and targeted solutions, and through that a higher impact on the overall healthcare organization and the satisfaction of patients.

Benefits of Predictive Analytics for Personalized Medicine

Improved Outcomes: It is found that, the use of predictive analytics in personalized medicines has the following advantages; better consistency of treatment results, increased efficacy of treatment, and better patient care. Therefore, generators from the different sources of information like genetic makeup data, patient history and lifestyle data will be used by the predictive analytics tool to determine which treatment options will be more effective for the specific patient. It fosters individualised care since the various medical treatments can be made more accurately proportional to the patient characteristics. Consequently, the treatments given to the patients are highly specific and beneficial with minimal side effects and high probability of positive result. Besides, it allows medical resources to be used in a more efficient way, therefore, improving the successful rate of health conditions' management, further enhancing the chances of betterment of overall health and quality of care.

Cost Efficiency: In personalized medicine, the use of predictive analytics only adds value to the overall cost since it reduces the possibility of relying heavily on trial and error in planning for the treatment. Many Eastern medical treatments are based on a trial and error approach to finding the optimal treatment for a patient and this results to increased costs resulting from longer treatment periods, frequent visits to practitioners and use of therapies that may not benefit the patient. Through the use of big data, an individual's genetic makeup, their medical history and some of the details relating to their lifestyle can be input into a system and the provider be able to easily predict as to which treatments could be effective for the given patient (Cirillo & Valencia, 2019). That's why the targeted approach is more appropriate and efficient in comparison with the widespread ones, because it presupposes fewer necessary interventions and less money for the ineffective treatment.

Preventative Care: Another factor discusses that preventative care gets improved through the help of predictive analytics, specifically in personalized medicine, to be able to identify possible future health risks. It grasps detailed patient information including genetic characteristics, disease history and some significant lifestyles: the artificial intelligence of predictive models can predict individuals' risk for certain diseases and health conditions before they develop. This proactive approach enables the healthcare providers to take prevention measures that can be suitable to the patient's risk factor. For instance, if a predictive model shows that an individual is likely to be at the predisposition of developing a particular disease such as diabetes or cardiovascular diseases, then early health promotion activities such as changing of life styles, early screening or prescription of preventive medications can be instituted. Realizing these risks early enough as not to be chronic health risks makes a lot of sense when it comes to the general patient health and longevity. This change in the focus from episodic management of illnesses to disease prevention does not only benefit patients' health but also helps to easing the load on health care systems as it slows the development of diseases and prevents patients requiring more extensive, expensive cures in future.

Case Studies in Personalized Medicine

Predicting Heart Disease Risk: A ground breaking epidemiological research known as the Framingham Heart Study. The Framingham Heart Study was started in 1948 in Framingham, Massachusetts and is perhaps one of the most famed long term cardiovascular investigations ever carried out (Mahmood et al., 2014). It was proposed for sample survey focused on studying potential risk factors, predictors, and profiles of people with cardiovascular disease (CVD). For years it has accumulated a vast amount of information on a number of parameters such as blood pressure, cholesterol, smoking history, and about other related factors. However, the Framingham Heart Study has provided an extensive Database for the emergence of such predictive models as Framingham Risk Score. This tool predicts how likely the person is to acquire Cardiovascular Disease within a given period of time which is usually 10 years using several risk factors. Age, gender, blood pressure, cholesterol level, smoking and presence of diabetes are some of the risk factors for this disease. It has been widely used in cardiovascular risk on the basis of Framingham Risk Score and similar model which were derived from the study. They assist in determining those perhaps at a higher risk of developing heart related diseases hence assist in prevention and appropriate interventions for such patients. In general, the Framingham Heart Study has completely changed the paradigm in the evaluation of cardiovascular risk and remains an important reference in preventive cardiology and individualized medicine.

Cancer Treatment Personalization: IBM Watson for Oncology is the first of its kind to integrate credible information into a cancer patient's decisions regarding oncology. They recognized that nothing equals IBM Watson for Oncology in terms of the innovation that is enhancing personalized cancer treatment. Structured with the help of artificial intelligence this cutting-edge system integrates a vast amount of data like publication, clinical trial data outcomes and patient records enabling oncologists to develop a personalized treatment approach. The oncology cancer application known as Watson for Oncology employs complex real-time analysis algorithms to integrate large amounts of data. Through analysing a patient's medical history, family history, and current research, Watson then makes a diagnosis and prescribes a treatment plan for the particular case. It also brings about an enhancement of Treatment-As-Process since treatment directions are defined utilizing the most contemporary and inclusive information within a given field; thus enhancing the possibility of positive results.

Personalized Treatment for Depression: Predictive Analytics at TMS NeuroHealth Centres: TMS NeuroHealth Centres leads the way on applied predictive analytics to clinical depression – TMS therapy. This approach shows how the usage of data enhancements the efficacy of mental health therapies. TMS NeuroHealth Centres uses enhance specific and general depression treatments. Based on diverse patient information, namely, symptom intensity, past experience with prior treatments, and neuroimaging data, prognosis models are built to set proper parameters for TMS treatment (Richter et al., 2023). This distinguishes results in this therapy being performed in a more efficient manner depending on the properties of the person that is involved thus enhancing its potential outcome. The use of individual approach at TMS NeuroHealth Centres has been proved to be efficient and important for patient's treatment result. Individualized TMS therapy has shown better therapeutic outcomes in alleviation of depressive disorders and improved quality of life conditions. Not only does this method tend to address depression in a more efficient manner than the conventional means, but it also leads to overall improvement in the quality of patients' mental health since it takes every patient's data into account when coming up with the right set of treatments. Taken as a whole, distressing depression disorder treatment at TMS NeuroHealth Centres is a breakthrough utilizing predictive analytics for the possibility of personalized mental health care emphasizing on advanced opportunities for developing sophisticated data-driven driven treatment plans for patients.

Challenges of Predictive Analytics for Personalized Medicine

Data Privacy: The concept of applying predictive analytics into the area of personalized medicine still has many challenges including data privacy. Pre-analytical and analytical process employed in predictive analytics requires extensive and highly sensitive health information such as genetic profile, medical history, and lifestyle characteristics. This data is regarded as sensitive and must be well-guarded and secured to prevent any unauthorized access or else succumb to misuse. In order to make sure that the above information does not fall into the wrong hands, several measures should be put in place such as: encryption, storage and access control mechanisms. Moreover, the flow of patients' information can also not bypass the rules of transport security, such as HIPAA rules in the U.S. and GDPR rules in Europe, which require serious adherence to data protection measures (Bradford et al., 2020). The demand for more detailed data to be collected in order to improve the predictive models' accuracy is a factor that has to be managed to prevent the deterioration of trust together with the ethical use of such data in personalized medicine.

Complexity of Data: Some of the issues affecting the application of predictive analytics in personalized medicine involve data integration and data analysis because of the large and disparate data sets that are involved. Personalized medicine that is the process of using so-called omics data, EHRs, and other information that a patient contributes, as well as his/her genetic indicators, lifestyle, and environment, is a challenging task because of the diversity of the data in terms of format, quality, and granularity. The technical issue is thus on how best to integrate these sources of data in such a way that they could be used conveniently for analysis. This integration needs high-level computational models and approaches which can work with large numbers of disparate data and provide accurate results. In addition, the analytical models applied have to be sufficiently subtle in order to identify the interdependencies between various data sources and make accurate predictions.

REAL-TIME MONITORING THROUGH AI-POWERED WEARABLE DEVICES

The integration of the artificial intelligence and wearable technology has boosted real time human monitoring across all realms including health care, fitness, and lifestyle. These AI Wearable has evolved from simple fitness bands to holistic devices that can assess and learn the physiological data of an individual and give feedback in real-time. These smart devices have sophisticated sensors and machine learning that enable monitoring of several aspects such as the heart rate, blood oxygen level, sleep quality, and even the amount of activity that is done in a day.

The modern artificial intelligence AI technology processes the crude gathering of data into information that facilitates early health intervention, enhanced physical performance, and enhanced standard quality of life. The usage of the devices that can provide immediate response proves them to be useful for anyone and for any field. At the dawn of the era of precision and preventive health1, AI-driven wearables have a significant potential to drive the process of how health and performance are tracked and managed in real time.

Wearable Health Devices: A Brief History

Smart Wearables are improving from mere step counters to self-learning health monitoring gadgets. The first generation of wearable devices was more basic and most of them were only capable of measuring steps, calories burned and distance covered. The first pedometers and wearable fitness trackers on the market before 2000s were simple devices with relatively basic sensors. These devices have primarily targeted the fitness freaks, providing little information on the health and their results have to be analysed manually. However, as the technology advanced, in mid of 2010's advanced fitness trackers also came with heart rate monitor, sleep tracking, and rudimentary notifications, starting with the first smartwatches. Many wearables that companies such as Fitbit and Apple have promoted have turned health and wellness into a fashion statement. More significant development of wearable health care devices was preceded by AI and sophisticated biosensors in the late 2010s (Sharma et al., 2021). It became possible to perform more accurate health monitoring via the devices with the help of the features like ECG, blood oxygen level and even optional features like fall detection. Through application of AI, these devices were able to analyze numerous data streams in real-time and offer forecasts and feedback to the users. Current wearables are able to continuously track and diagnose a number of problems ranging from abnormal heartbeats to chronic conditions such as diabetes and even possible onsets of certain conditions. These devices are becoming more advanced and they are penetrate into personal health management systems, setting the stage between the consumer health devices and the clinical equipment. In the near future, wearables will become even more of a protective health shield that can diagnose and detect illnesses on the spot and link seamlessly with telemedicine and health management systems, which is why wearables will become something that is impossible to do without.

Early Pedometers and Fitness Trackers (Pre-2010s)

Before the boom of smartwatches and fitness wearable technology in the 2010s, some of the early devices which were developed were pedometers. Initially these devices can be dated back to as early as the 1960s and these were rudimentary gadgets that aimed at simple functions as mere count steps depending on mechanical movements or basic electronic sensing. Traditional pedometers worked with the help of monitoring the motion of individual's hips, each recorded movement reflected an approximate number of steps. These first models possessed no electrical component or employed only a simple pendulum and worked only as basic calendars with various mechanical imperfections such as inconsistent motion or incorrect positioning. However, all these early devices helped to create a foundation of something that is today a highly-popular industry focusing on health and fitness tracking.

Advancements in technology saw the development of electronic pedometers in the early centuries of the former with enhanced efficiency, range determination and calculating for calories burnt among other features. Although these devices were still independent and featuring quite a limited level of integration with other gadgets or data storage, their primary target audience remained people who practice sports and keep a healthy lifestyle.

The Rise of Smart Fitness Trackers and Basic Health Monitoring (2010s)

The most important advancement in wearable electronics was witnessed during 2010's; where smart fitness track and the first generations of smart watches were developed with extra functionalities and friendly user interfaces. First such phenomenon was spear headed by Fitbit; its devices could track not only steps but also calories, sleep, and even heart rate. These devices used new miniaturized sensors and relied on Bluetooth for data transfer to corresponding apps installed in the users' smartphones and allowing the real-time monitoring of their physical performance. The transition from the single standalone pedometers facilitated constant monitoring process as individuals could wear them and monitor their activities around-the-clock which helped to get the big picture of their lifestyles. The integration of a number of sensors coupled with use of cloud storage, mobile applications made it convenient for the users to analyze trends over time and set up goals to health and fitness. With this, smartwatch devices such as the Apple Watch which took wearables beyond their fitness orientation made their entrance into the market. New with these devices were other forms of health monitoring like basic heart rate monitoring, moving reminders, and integrated sleep tracking. Still, due to their novelty, the data collected by those first smart trackers was comparatively simple, providing more generic information about the wearers' health rather than specific data. Some of the things that users found lacking include the need to analyze and understand the data that was displayed to come up with an understanding of his or her health and the gadgets were more of life style and fitness. A much higher percentage of respondents reported that the gadgets were more of life style and fitness. However, such wearables were laid down during this period paving way for future AI propelled wearables, where customized analysis and feedback were to be expected. Smart fitness trackers that became popular in the 2010-ies are highly significant in that they prepared the groundwork for the subsequent generations of wearables with a focus on health. The areas that are likely to have an amalgamation of Advanced Biosensors and Health Applications are as follows identified from mid-2010s (Mehrotra, 2016). With the progress in technology, wearables started including innovation biosensors connected with heart rate variability (HRV), electrocardiogram (ECG), blood oxygen level (SpO2) and stress. With the advanced use of data, AI and machine learning started to seize such data. With wearables technology, one could be diagnosed of arrhythmias, sleep apnea and other future health complications. For instance, wearable devices such as the Apple watch incorporated elements such as fall detection and ECG functionalities which are considered to be close to clinical grade monitoring.

AI-Mediated Health Surveillance in Real Time: Use Cases (After 2018)

The current generation wearable devices, therefore, relies on artificial intelligence to give immediate analysis and future healthcare forecasts. These devices are able to program an individual user's learning pattern, find variations and trends, with the ability to suggest feedback or an alert on the specific user. This is because AI algorithms analyse steady flows of data from several integrated sensors and offer early warnings of developing health risks such as heart diseases, diabetes complications, or respiratory disorders. They have also been adapted to specific heath niches such as continuous glucose monitoring for diabetes and wearable ECG stickers for heart disease patients.

Present and Future: Personalized and Preventive Healthcare as the Company's Next Frontier

In the future, wearable devices are becoming more like all in one health management systems. Smart apparels have been some of the forerunners in the idea of wearing technologies that would help prevent diseases since the devices would constantly check wearer's vitals and prod for an oncoming health calamity. Interoperability with telemedicine and other digital health solutions, as well as pharmaceutical solutions, is on the rise, which makes patient care more comprehensive. These devices will become more and more like friends that provide real time health coaching, help to make the right life decisions, are tuned to the user's needs during the given period of time.

AI Integration in Wearable Technology

Artificial intelligence (AI) has brought a new dimension on wearable devices, other than being just a fashion trend, they have become effective smart health and performance monitors. Wearable devices now incorporate AI algorithms that can process all sorts of information and deliver tailored suggestions as well as early signs of any health complications right to the user's wrist. AI the helps the wearables transcend into being a mere data collecting tools and provides personalized and timely information. For example, while exercising, we do not want the smart device to show our heart rate only but trends, changes, if it is abnormal and possible risk of cardio vascular episodes in the next few days. This change in the approach to the constant monitoring of health from being relegated as a response to an individual's ailment is one of the biggest advantages introduced by AI in wearables. The devices use Machine learning algorithms which are a branch of Artificial intelligence because they can learn from a person's behaviour and adjust the correctness of the forecasts. For example, smart wearables can learn user's schedule, anticipate deviations, and offer personalized tips, in physical training, stress, or sleep regimen. Such degree of customization became impossible to employ in the past due to the use of traditional analytics. Further, AI integrated wearables can assemble and interpret data gathered through different types of sensors like movement sensors, heart rate sensors, ECG and PPG sensors which provide holistic insight of a person's health. Specifically in the future, there remains untapped potential within wearable technology where the AI is aimed to become even more discreet and become an upper body accessory that will directly connect to the human body and supply real-time preventive care service that can be directly tailored to the consumer. This integration is making it possible to have smart, proactive, and responsive systems that can monitor human health.

Applications in Chronic Disease Management

Smart wearable devices, which are driven by artificial intelligence, have become critical in the life of chronic disease patients due to self-monitoring of the patient's condition and provision of individualized care. Diabetes, cardiovascular diseases, hypertension, and respiratory disorders are but a few examples of chronic illnesses that need constant monitoring and frequent interventions, and wearables are perfect for patient and medical professionals alike. These devices are fitted with sophisticated sensors that can monitor parameters including glucose farcical rate, blood pressure and respiratory patterns. Wearables can collect this data and use AI algorithms to process it and make real time analysis, real time diagnosis on whether the patient falls within the normal range of the disease or not and alert the doctor or the patient whenever it is detected that the parameters are outside the acceptable range. For example, devices that monitor glucose levels in the blood in case of Diabetes can monitor constant levels of blood sugar and using AI to anticipate any increase or decrease so that the user can take appropriate action or consider taking medication.

Apart from real-time tracking of patients, Artificial Intelligence-based wearable devices help in developing a customized disease plan. Thus, using the information received from a patient during the period, the proposed devices will be able to recommend necessary changes in a diet, lifestyle, or dosage of medications. For people with cardiac issues it is possible to point out that wearables with ECG sensors allow tracking of heart rate rhythm anomalies like atrial fibrillation and report it to the user or a healthcare provider in real time. This can occur at an early stage before major complications set in thus enhancing patients' well-being. In addition, these wearables may connect with mobile applications and cloud based platforms where doctors can track and only intervene when their clients are at risk. Such features of remote monitoring are highly beneficial for utilizing technology-assisted solutions in healthcare by patients who live in rural or underserved areas and can hardly access traditional in-person healthcare. Due to the fact that chronic diseases are on the increase around the world, the use of AI-enabled wearables is a preventive mechanism, in which patients are put first, decreased hospital visits, lower cost of health care and quality life and well-being of chronic disease patients are achieved.

Case Studies and Real-World Implementations:

A feasibility study of the use of AI wearable devices in the delivery of care in actual healthcare environment has shown the efficacy of AI in enhancing patients' health and wellness through chronic disease management, prevention, and early detection of diseases. A number of examples show that these devices have been of great help by providing real time monitoring and analysis thus improving the health care services being provided and the overall patient care.

A now quite famous example is the application of wearable technology in monitoring and supporting cardiovascular risk. For example, the Apple Watch has been used in diagnosing atrial fibrillation (AFib) a deadly heart condition. Thanks to ECG option and artificial intelligence, the gadget can recognize arrhythmias, and warn the patient to visit doctors. Many people have said that they tripped alerts from the watch, they went to the doctors, and doctors discovered that they were suffering from undiagnosed heart issues, meaning that people's lives were saved. Clinical trials have backed the effectiveness of such wearables in informing how AI-aided wearables provide optimal results in identifying AFib and other types of arrhythmias; preventing stoke and other complications that associate with heart disease.

Another of such examples includes the wearable technology in the form of continuous glucose monitoring (CGM) gadgets for diabetes. The ongoing monitoring and prediction are done through the AI algorithms present in devices such as Dexcom G6 and Abbott's Freestyle Libre. Such systems also have an advantage of being effective in delivering real-time results that are customized to an individual's use in improving his/her diet, exercise, and medication. For instance, when CGMs and mobile apps employing artificial intelligence were used in the treatment of patients, patients demonstrated better glycaemic control than they did with conventional glucose monitoring procedures. These wearables also make it possible for the healthcare professionals to remotely keep track of the patients and improve the treatment regimen more often. Therefore, the application of CGM devices with integration of AI has therefore helped to change the face of diabetes by giving patients more management ability over the disease and drastically decreasing the occurrence of critical complications (Contreras & Vehi, 2018). In the real world, the smart wearables with AI integration do not only confine their application in individual's health but also in the health of the public. In the examples of various corporate wellness programmes, it has been seen that wearables are used to track some of the overall employee health indexes like stress, activity, and sleep patterns. These programs together with the support of AI-based analytics came to promote healthy changes towards absenteeism decrease and productivity increase. Also, the mobile health technology that is becoming popular among hospitals and clinics is the use of wearables in telemedicine services especially for patients with chronic illnesses. This integration has been especially useful in cases of home or area that has not much access to hospitals or clinics.

ENHANCING DIAGNOSTIC ACCURACY WITH ARTIFICIAL INTELLIGENCE

Machine learning algorithms are the core of AI in medical imaging. Many of these algorithms can be trained using vast amount of medical images like X-rays, CT scan and MRI among others to identify patterns of the images taken. For example, in diagnostic purposes, the use of such features as tumors, fracture or any other abnormality can be accurately trained by an ML model. Once trained, these models are capable of diagnosing new and unseen images and can present further diagnostic recommendations or draw attention to the areas of interest for the radiologist to examine. Deep learning is a kind of learning from the set of machine learning depending on the neural network with many layers. Thus, in medical imaging deep learning algorithms are particularly effective in such tasks as segmentation and classification. For instance, Convolutional Neural Network (CNNS) are beneficial in segmentation analysis in which image regions containing tumors or lesions are segmented and outlined. There are numerous examples of deep learning performance including diagnosing the retinopathy of diabetes in the retinal images as well as detection of the pulmonary embolism in chest CT scans. Radiology reports and patients' records are utilized as the data source, and NLP is employed to mine the data. NLP can be used in classification of data such as imaging findings and the clinical history to advance diagnostic evaluation. For instance the NLP algorithms can be used to analyze Radiology reports to look for trends and or patterns in the data for use in research or to help in the integration with Electronic Health Records (EHR).

Applications of AI in Medical Imaging

Diagnostic Assistance: AI algorithms can be very useful in the decision making process by drawing the attention of the user to areas of focus in medical images. For instance, in mammography the use of AI systems can help the radiologists to notify them of possible breast cancers that might be overlooked during normal screening. As with the previous cases, AI can be used to supplement the identification of lung nodules in CT scans of the chest that might contain early-stage lung cancer that can be easily overlooked. Image Interpretation: Queries in radiology studies: The following area is another area where AI can help with the comprehension of complicated imaging tests. For instance, tools and applications can analyze MRI images in order to determine the size and position of brain tumors, this is helpful in treatment planning. It also highlighted that these tools can provide second opinion which in turn can help in relieving the cognitive burden from radiologists and at the same time help them in boosting their confidence about diagnosis.AI also optimizes the work processes given the fact that it eradicates repetitive procedures like image annotation and data organization (Hosny et al., 2018). For example, AI can help in labelling the structures present in an image of a patient and make this task less time-consuming for radiologists and let them work more on complicated cases. Also, prioritization of the test in imaging studies can be done depending on the situation so that the complex cases are handled first.AI is capable of diagnosis through imaging data and give prognosis of the outcome of the patient. For example, the algorithms can extract the features in the imaging data to predict the development of Alzheimer's or the probability of a cancer treatment to work. He credits its predictive capabilities for being able to forecast patient treatment and improvement of conditions that are chronic in nature. However, there are certain challenges that come along with the application of AI in medical imaging. Quality and diverse training data are important prerequisites for developing reliable AI models which are to be applied to various populations. Preconception in the training data set has influence on the variations of differential diagnostic outcomes. Also, the implementation of AI tools in the existing processes presents certain challenges concerning the compatibility with the EHR systems as well as the training of the users.

AI in Pathology

Artificial Intelligence (AI) is continuing its transformational journey in pathology that has always focused on gross examination of tissues to generate disease diagnosis. The application of machine learning algorithms, Computer vision, and data analytics in AI continues to improve the diagnosis of patients, work efficiency, and indispensability of pathological samples. It is essential to point out that this combination of AI into pathology is not only complementing the work of pathologists but also establishing the future for medical diagnostics. AI Techniques in Pathology incorporate a process of teaching the system with histological image databases or any other disease related imaging in an attempt to impart the ability to the algorithms to recognize specific characteristics of diseases. The advanced learning technique used here is convolutional neural networks (CNN) which is used to analyse images. CNNs are capable of finding complex patterns of tissue samples like tumour cells for example with lot of accuracy. For instance, deep learning models have given great performance in distinguishing various forms of breast cancer and in determining special forms of tumours (Luca et al., 2022). Computer-assisted image analysis is a great help for pathologists as they help to recognize and measure certain characteristics in tissue samples. This includes for; counting cells, outlining the extent of the tumour and analyzing its containment as well as analyzing tissue arrangement. AI algorithms can process high-resolution images of biopsy samples to focus on some areas of interest which are either characterized by an abnormal cell growth or which contain certain biomarkers; this provides a better view for diagnosis. Techniques such as Natural Language Processing (NLP) are applied to process textual data that come in form of pathology reports, Electronic Health Records (EHRs), and clinical notes. These sources can be used by NLP to match imaging findings to patient histories in order to create more efficient diagnostic overall assessments as well as treatment plans. For instance, NLP can be applied in analysis of large amount of text data with the aim of searching for patterns or trends that may relate to certain diseases.

Applications of AI in Pathology

AI systems serve as second opinions and magnify areas of interest or areas that pathologists should probably look into. For example, in cancer diagnosis, utilising AI will identify regions on the pathology slides that may be indicative of malignancy on which the pathologists will focus. Incidentally, the frequent use of scans helps in lowering down the diagnostic errors and hence increasing the chances of accuracy. In particular, there are data stating that AI can be as or even more effective than a human pathologist in identifying, for example, melanoma or prostate cancer. AI optimizes such processes by eliminating time-consumptive manual processes while sorting cases depending on the level of urgency. For instance, AI can perform scanning of slides and image digitization and thereby not consume the time that the pathologists can utilise (Kiran et al., 2023). Also, it aids in sorting specimens, so that those that are crucial are reviewed as soon as possible and in the quickest way possible. AI helps in the progress of the modern approach to treatment by comparing pathological information to determine certain biomarkers and mutations that cause diseases. This makes it possible to come up with treatment regimens that would suit the patient on the basis of information derived from patient analysis. For instance, oncologists may use AI algorithms to pinpoint novel abnormally shaped molecules in cancer cells that aid in choosing the appropriate therapy for such a formation to enhance the use of therapeutic solutions based on the molecular distinctiveness mark. Knowledge discovery and data mining can be then used to explain current and future states of diseases and patients. When analyzing the patterns of the data of pathology, AI systems can look into the future and suggest how the disease can further manifest or what consequences a particular treatment may have, which will help in effective control.

Case Studies on Diagnostic Innovations

Google Health's DeepMind for Diabetic Retinopathy

Diabetic retinopathy is a diabetic complication that affects the eyes that if not treated leads to blindness. Developed by Google's DeepMind, an AI-based diagnostic system was designed to diagnose Diabetic retinopathy from the retinal images. This works uses deep learning algorithms to perform disease diagnosis based on analysis of retinal scans. This is in DeepMind's system, which applies the convolutional neural networks (CNNs) for analyzing high-resolution images of the retina. The AI is fed thousands of other images of the retinal to identify changes showing diabetic retinopathy. The use of this system can give a diagnostic grade in the same category as that of the qualified ophthalmologists. The results have shown high precision of the used AI system in identification of diabetic retinopathy and diabetic macular edema. The accuracy of DeepMind's system was 91% for sensitivity and 95% specificity for identifying referable cases of DR, which is as good as the human experts in ophthalmology as found in a study published in Nature (Wang et al., 2022). This innovation has the potential to revolutionize screening programs, most probably in the remote areas where the availability of specialists is rare. Automating the screening process also aid early screening and follow up the process hence minimizing the chance of vision impaired.

PathAI's AI for Cancer Diagnosis

PathAI is one of the leading firms in AI pathology that has designed and implemented a device that improves the diagnosis and typing of the illnesses. This platform employs the use of machine learning to interpret digitized specimens and provide recommendations to pathologists on diagnosis of cancer. A similar process is used by PathAI's system that scans digitized tissue samples with the help of a deep learning mechanism. The AI is trained on a large number of annotated pathology slides so that the system successfully identifies differentiating cancerous tissues or lesions. The system gives the pathologists prognosis and aids in finding out small patterns that may not be easily discernable during assessment. As a result of PathAI's deployment, it is important to note that there has been an enhancement of the diagnostic accuracy and the diagnostic performance. On in studies, the system has been proven to decrease the likelihood of diagnostic mistakes, not to mention it offers the same accuracy wherever it is used. For instance, when working on breast cancer, the platform developed by PathAI helped to reduce the number of false negatives, detecting cancerous cells that could be missed by a pathologist.

Tempus' Genomic Profiling for Precision Medicine

Tempus is a technology company that especially works on applying genomics data as well as clinical data in order to advance on the field of personalized medicine. Their platform does a full analysis of the tumor's genotype and offers suggestions for patient diagnoses and therapies according to it. Tempus employs many genomic sequencing tools for example next generation sequencing to analyze DNA or RNA of tumor samples obtained. This genomic data is then linked with the clinical and outcome data and fed to the oncologists so that they can get a sense of what genomic changes might have precipitated the cancer in a particular patient. Specific mutations are discovered from the data, drug response tendencies are forecasted from the data and potential clinical trials are recommended by the AI algorithms. Tempus has revolutionized oncology subsequent to the implementation of the new model on treatment distribution. Through characterising the genomic map of every tumour, Tempus assists oncologists in identifying the treatment regimen that may prove to be effective for the specific patient concerned (Sebastian & Peter, 2022). This precision medicine has enhanced the treatment and come up with the therapeutic approach of the disease. For instance, Tempus has helped to discover certain genetic mutations that are receptive to specific treatments thereby improving the course of therapeutic intervention. DeepMind, a subsidiary of Google Health, has expanded screening of diabetic retinopathy using AI, while PathAI has improved the diagnosis of cancer through digital pathology and Tempus has transformed oncology with genomic profiling. Each example shows how technology can enhance the accuracy and speed of diagnosis as well as increase the individualized level of patients' treatment. In the future, as these technologies are being improved and advanced, it will bring more changes in the medical diagnostic field and help improve patients' experiences in different domains. Machine-based pathology is accurate and time efficient, which makes it a valuable tool towards delivering good diagnoses, but it has certain challenges and concerns attached to it.

OPTIMIZING OPERATIONAL EFFICIENCY IN HEALTHCARE

Effectiveness and efficiency are critical in healthcare because patient care needs to be effective whilst at the same time the usage of resources has to be optimally done to ensure that costs are well managed. The challenges are increasing in the healthcare industry; the patient expectations, the availability of resources, and the cost of operation are some of the factors that are putting pressure on the healthcare industry and therefore require solutions that would help to improve on the efficiency of the outcome of the health care industry without necessarily reducing on the outcome of the health care industry. Artificial Intelligence as a disruptive technology comes to light in this regard owing to the gigantic potential for analyzing a myriad of data related to the health care sector and enhancing feasible solutions to several operational procedures. With the help of artificial intelligence in healthcare data analysis, organizations can reduce the burdened amount of paperwork and administrative work, avoid overspending and shortages of resources, manage patients' appointments, and supply chains efficiently. In this chapter, the author focuses on the way that AI-related solutions are implemented to create change and improvements in the healthcare operational dynamic, analyzed on the base of the latest empirical research and developments in the area.

AI in Hospital Management

Artificial Intelligence (AI) has now taken a central place in the management of modern day's hospitals as it provides effective solutions for improving practice. Hospitals experience many challenges, like;

How to deal with the large amount of data received from patients?

How to get the best out the available resources, and minimization of the quality of patient care?

Such challenges are now being tackled by the incorporation of AI systems by achieving automation of dreary exercises, enhancement of decision making and optimization of business processes. IT applications are particularly beneficial for appointment making, charging, and processing of payments besides claims. Such tools can process large volumes of work within a short span of time and with high accuracy thus removing a lot of work from the human health care employees and cutting out a lot of errors. For instance, through reinforcement learning algorithms, appointment making can be done through patient preferences while resource utilisation and patient satisfaction rates in the hospitals are optimised. Furthermore, it is noteworthy that AI can be used in optimizing hospital logistics, for instance, inventory, patients' flow, staff distribution (Maleki Varnosfaderani & Forouzanfar, 2024). AI systems can learn from real-time information and can forecast the number of patients that are expected to be admitted and therefore the number of beds, medical staffs and other important resources needed in the hospital. This kind of approach does not only make the hospital to be efficient in the way it operates but also enables patients receive optimum and adequate care as and when required.

Predictive Maintenance of Medical Equipment

Availability of medical equipment is another important factor since availability ensures constant care to the patients. Equipment downtimes are cumbersome as they result in expensive delays and compromised safety of the patients besides increasing the operational costs tremendously. However, predictive maintenance powered by Artificial Intelligence, provides a workable strategy by predicting the time of equipment failure prior to its occurrence and having time to address the problem. AI works by leveraging on historical data on performance and present operating conditions to predict when a certain piece of equipment is likely to develop a fault. This means they do not have to do routine checks for every equipment as is the practice in traditional maintenance models, but rather fix an equipment when it is most likely to fail. Thus, an elegant solution to the amount of time equipment is unavailable, as well as the longevity of more important medical tools is maintained. AI-powered predictive maintenance is another example of application where it established, pronounced reduction in maintenance costs while increasing the reliability of medical equipment. For example, an AI system can guess the likelihood of failure of an MRI machine depending on the minor deviations that occur in its working environment, so that technicians can fix it before it becomes a problem to patients. This also helps in improving the overall organization of the facility that in turn aids in the accessibility of medical equipment when required.

Resource Allocation and Workflow Optimization

Effective management of resources or workflows as well as management of operations is very critical in the healthcare settings. AI perfectly enhances these aspects given that it processes significantly large data sets with a view of analyzing the underlying patterns, demand forecasting among other factors. Even admissions can be predicted by using AI-supported predictive analytics, and resources can be thus better allocated in the healthcare organizations. For instance, during a flu period, it can be possible to predict a rise in admissions hence making hospitals prepare extra personnel and equipment a head start. It has the advantage of avoiding congestion and long waiting times for patients as well as avoiding situations whereby health care providers are congested with many patients in the course of their working calendars. In the same way, it can suggest ways to improve workflow because the AI has the capabilities to scan organizational processes for bottlenecks (Li et al., 2021). For instance, through the analytical data derived from the patient flow, the systems can identify problem areas in the emergency department, recommend adjustments in staff deployment or redesign patients' routes for increased efficiency. Due to constant assessment and optimization of work processes, AI contributes to increasing the effectiveness of work in healthcare organizations and enhancing the quality of work with recipients.

Case Studies on Efficiency Improvements

A lot of healthcare organizations have applied AI solutions with positive results that enhance working processes. In the next part, we discuss a number of examples, which are designed with the assistance of AI and which demonstrate the overall effectiveness of a smart hospital, the capability for predictive maintenance, and the ways to optimize the utilization of resources.

AI-Enhanced Hospital Administration: An established hospital adopted an Artificial intelligence to perform administrative functions including scheduling of operations, invoicing and claims. The system increased the efficiency of appointment scheduling which made the patients happier besides cutting administration time by 30% and minimizing issues related to billing errors.

Predictive Maintenance of MRI Machines: An MRI repair scheduling plan was recently implemented in a vast healthcare network using artificial intelligence technology. The system enabled accurate prediction of the failure of the equipment which reduced maintenance costs by 20% and improved the availability of the equipment by 15% thus allowing for uninterrupted patient care.

Resource Allocation during a Pandemic: In the context of COVID-19, a hospital used AI to forecast patients' admission and manage resources accordingly. This helped the hospital to optimise the number of ICU beds, ventilators and medical staff, thus shortening the patients' waiting time and improving their outcomes. The above examples show the application of AI in the improvement of efficiency in the different areas of healthcare. In this way, the practical case studies presented here can help other members of the healthcare community, and healthcare organizations, understand and perhaps believe, that AI has the ability to transform how they operate, and therefore enhance the lot of patients.

AI integration in the processes of healthcare delivery has shown that it is an effective leverage to enhance the flow of processes and the quality of the services that are being delivered. Both in the management of hospitals and in the predictive maintenance of machines and equipment, in the allocation of resources and in the improvement of working processes, AI brings new approaches which meet the tough requirements of the healthcare system. This is evidenced by the case studies, which show that the utilisation of AI in operational efficiency increases profitability and positively impacts the health of patients. With the advancement of AI technology, it is very much impossible not to see the tremendous impact it is going to make in the healthcare system to become more efficient and effective to attend on patients.

ACCELERATING DRUG DISCOVERY WITH AI

Introduction to AI in Drug Discovery

AI is now innovation in drug discovery and development through offering a new way of thinking about the problem of drug discovery. Historically, the identification and advancement of new therapeutic compounds has been slow, costly and a long drawn process in which several years and billions of dollars are invested to reach a single new chemical entity in the clinic. Using AI, it is possible to significantly improve the speed as well as the efficacy of many steps in drug discovery including selection of compounds for screening and even prediction of clinical trials results. AI's role in drug discovery will be also discussed in this section in terms of accelerating the process; increasing accuracy; and minimizing the cost. In what follows, we will address general concepts of how AI is implemented in drug finding process, including data analysis, modeling, and process optimization (Paul et al., 2021). The context of the discussion will be defined in the introduction and present the role of AI for the pharmaceutical business and its ability to meet the future needs of the industry, including the growing demand for individualized drugs, fast identification of new diseases.

Key Techniques and Algorithms

AI's effectiveness of drug discovery is various techniques and algorithms that help to analyze huge amounts of information, find hundreds of potential drug candidates, and predict their activity in biological environment. This section will delve into the key AI-driven techniques that are shaping the future of drug discovery:

• Machine Learning (ML): In big data analysis, both supervised and unsupervised learning methods help in creating models which find out the patterns and Co-relation hidden in the data which cannot be easily noticed by the human eye. It is also important to mention that using ML, one can predict the effectiveness and toxicity of the compounds, focus on further development of the most promising candidates.

• Deep Learning: Machine learning on its part uses deep learning which incorporates neural networks with many layers, especially for processing inputs like genomics sequences and molecular structures. Convolutional Neural Network or CNN is widely utilized in image processing such as simulated screening, while Recurrent Neural Network or RNN is applied in sequential analysis for biomarker discovery.

• Generative Adversarial Networks (GANs): As for drug design, GANs can be employed to produce novel molecular structures with specific property profiles from experience databases. This technique makes it possible to synthesise new compound that may possibly be drug candidates.

• Natural Language Processing (NLP): They analysed that NLP is used to mine significant information on particular topics or keywords from scientific articles, patents, Clinical trials etc. Techniques such as natural language processing are now able to deepen researchers' knowledge of the most recent findings and reveal potential candidates for drug repurposing.

• Reinforcement Learning: There is a view that the reinforcement learning models can help the optimization of drug discovery processes since such models can model the behavior of drugs with their targets; modify their strategies in the light of feedback and get even better results the desired outcomes.

Each of these techniques is essential at various steps in the rational drug discovery process that includes identification and validation of targets, identification of leads, and optimization of leads as well as preclinical evaluation. In this section, these algorithms will be presented along with their usefulness towards speeding up the drug discovery process.

Case Studies on AI-Driven Drug Development

To illustrate the practical impact of AI in drug discovery, this section will present several case studies that highlight successful AI-driven initiatives in drug development:

AI in Oncology Drug Discovery

Discovery of biomarkers using Artificial intelligence in Cancer. Probably, one of the more significant applications of AI in oncology is in discovering new bio-markers, which are very essential in creating personalized treatments. For example, Tempus, a technology firm that is aiming to bring precision medicine through the use of artificial intelligence has employed machine learning models and tools in analyzing large amounts of clinical and molecular data. This way they identify new bio-signatures that are related to certain kinds of a cancer (Johnson et al., 2021). The following biomarkers have played a vital role in the processes that led to the discovery of tailored treatments for cancers which only affect the cancer cells without affecting the normal cells. The use of this approach has seen the pinpointing of good drug candidate within months, and thereby shortening the time taken to conduct clinical trials.

AI in Predicting Development of Targeted Therapies: The British biopharmaceutical company AstraZeneca partnered with the London-based benedict AI-powered drug finder Benevolent AI in order to drive forward oncological research. In this partnership, scientific papers, clinical trials, and patients' data history were evaluated using AI algorithms. Some of these are biomarkers for drug targets and candidate molecules for different types of cancer that the AI was rapidly translated into clinical trials. This process significantly decreased the time for development and discovery of the drugs as the process whose duration ranged from years to months and increased the chances of clinical success.

AI and Drug Repurposing

Role of Artificial Intelligence in the Refashioning of Prescribed Medications for COVID-19

In the case of COVID 19 the use of AI technology was particularly important in the fast time identification of drugs that were already available in the market and could be used to treat the virus. On 18 May 2020 through its platform that searches through large chemical and biomedical databases, BenevolentAI found out that Baricitinib, a drug initially prescribed for rheumatoid arthritis, could be effective against COVID-19. Drawing on its analysis, the AI model proposed that Baricitinib could reduce viral entry into COVID-19 patients' cells and the inflammation resulting therefrom. The clinical trials were soon launched, and the medicine became one of the first to receive the Emergency Use Authorization (EUA) by the FDA.

AI-Based method for Drug Repositioning to Other Diseases: Healx which is a firm working with the AI in rare diseases used this approach of AI to reposition drugs for different diseases. AI compiled in drug databases along with medical literature helped Healx find fresh uses of certain drugs across various diseases and disorders, including Fragile X syndrome and other inherited disorders. The approach that involved the use of artificial intelligence was more efficient in the discovery process and it also meant low costs that are usually required to develop new medicines.

AI in Rare Disease Drug Development

Artificial intelligent-led solutions for rare diseases. Nonetheless, the problems associated with personalizing treatments and the insufficient information and small sample size to assess drugs are apparent in rare diseases and create difficulties in the application of the common drug discovery process. Chinese AI drug discovery firm Insilico Medicine came up with an AI platform that is aimed at discovering targets for therapies and drugs for rare genetic diseases. For instance, the company applied AI to search for potential treatment for idiopathic pulmonary fibrosis (IPF), a rare lung disease. The proposed AI model applied genetics, molecular characteristics and clinical variables for the selection of drug candidates for preclinical testing.

AI-Assisted Orphan Drug Development: Another example is the work that the pharmaceutical company Sanofi has therefore taken to work with AI-based platforms for the development of orphan drugs for rare diseases. AI helped Sanofi search for targets through data gathered from disease registries and patient and genetic databases of rare diseases. AI mechanizations were used for the purpose of estimating the effectiveness of the drug candidates, which proved to reduce the time span needed to come up with orphan drugs and brought treatment to patients with rare diseases faster.

Collaboration between AI Companies and Pharma

Artificial intelligence AI headquartered startups tie-up with Pharma majors

Startups focusing on Artificial Intelligence and other technology-based players join big Pharmas to form effective partnerships that are pushing the innovation in the drugs discovery industry. For example, the collaboration of an AI drug discovery firm, Exscientia and pharma giant GSK with the aim to discover new drugs in various therapeutic areas. Explaining the concept of utilization, it is possible to state that the Exscientia's AI platform aimed at design and optimization of new drugs and molecules, thereby saving costs and time for the drug discovery process

(Vora et al., 2023). This was due to its AI use that helped define a number of drug prospects that went early to clinical phases.

Effectiveness on Costs Mitigation and Time Saving: Another related partnership is with Atomwise, an AI based Start-up Company and major pharmaceutical companies such as Merck, and Pfizer. Based on deep learning, Atomwise designed software for searching probable receptor-ligand binding to estimate binding affinity, which is one of the most essential steps of drug-discovery process. The synergy has brought about the possibility of identifying drug candidates at relative lesser time and costs, than what the conventional approaches would have entailed. Such partnerships show that AI can revolutionise how cheap drugs are developed in the shortest time possible and with high chances of success in clinical trials.

Future Trends and Challenges

Closely linked to such development is the growing application of AI in drug discovery: the more the AI technology develops, the more it will be utilized in this field – and this process will create new opportunities as well as problems. This section will explore the future trends and potential hurdles that lie ahead: This section will explore the future trends and potential hurdles that lie ahead:

• Integration of AI with Other Technologies: Explain if AI can be combined with other progressive technologies like quantum computing, CRISPR and blockchain to enhance drug discovery even more. Think about the possibilities of these integrations regarding data handling, upgrading accuracy and the possibility of creating intricate individualised therapies.

• Personalized Medicine and AI: AI is expected to have a significant role in personalized medicine where patient treatment is done based on a patient's genetic makeup and molecular characteristics. Find out how this will be achieved with the use of AI to map out patient-specific location of drug targets and also to design personalized approaches to treatment.

• AI in Clinical Trials: Some of the recent trends include concise use of artificial intelligence in designing clinical trials, enrolling, and monitoring the patients that are participating in the clinical trials, and so on, which would drastically decrease the amount of time and money taken to bring new drugs to the market. Examine how the application of Artificial Intelligence might help increase the chances of clinical trials' success, as well as the consequences for the pharmaceutical market.

• Ethical and Regulatory Considerations: This will mean that as AI becomes more becoming more involved in drug discovery, various ethical and regulatory issues have to be handled. It also includes how to standardize AI, such as the interpretability of AI models, how to deal with bias in AI-generated decisions, and how to address the shifting legal landscape for AI-drug discovery.

• Data Quality and Availability: In drug discovery, high quality, and available data significantly affect the success of artificial intelligence. Explain the issues associated with the accessibility, joining and normalization of big data, and the need for partnerships with industry partners, academic institutions and healthcare organizations to develop strong data networks.

• Sustainability and Cost-Effectiveness: Despite the benefits of cost savings, the application of AI is costly and there are questions to the longevity of the AI models that are employed in this process along with the amount of compute power required to deploy AI models. Examine ideas to integrate innovation and value within the costs and maintain the sustainability.

INTEGRATION OF GENOMIC DATA

The incorporation of genomics into the AI Health Care Data Analytics is one of the greatest innovations which revolutionize the health care systems as well as the management of health. Here's how genomic data fits into the broader context of AI in healthcare data analytics.

Personalized Medicine: Here we add personal genomic data into the sphere of the individualized medicine, which forms a new approach in healthcare by providing comprehensive data on the human genetic differences that influence predisposing factors to diseases, metabolism of drugs, and treatment outcomes. Through this genomic data, AI algorithm is used in coming up with personalized treatment procedures to fit the individual genetic makeup of every patient. It also makes it possible to better predict health risks and treatment success allowing for biomechanical optimization of therapeutic activities and, therefore, increasing their efficiency (Hassan et al., 2022). Therefore, the specificity and precision increase the effectiveness of the assessment of risks and develop the appropriate strategies for an individual patient, which in a turn enhances the possibilities of a personalized approach to the treatment.

Predictive Analytics: Personalized precision medicine involves the use of advanced analytics where genomic info is incorporated with other algorithms to predict future development of certain diseases because of the genes present in a patient's DNA. Through processing of vast genomic data, AI can identify regularity and relationships that speak of a higher probability of acquiring certain diseases, including cancer and cardiovascular diseases. These predictive models analyse genomics data such as biomarkers that help in early diagnosis and prevention mechanisms due to existence of related risk factors. It helps to fine-tune risk predictions, as well as deliver appropriate actions, therefore, patient care is benefited, and the concept of anticipatory healthcare is promoted.

Drug Discovery and Development: The use of AI algorithms in drug discovery and development is boosted since it uses genomic data where genetic information is used to deduce on possible drug targets. These algorithms thus can identify molecular mechanisms or specific gene mutations that cause the disease by knowing how genetic changes affect disease processes. The selectivity of this approach allows for the faster development of drugs since the most exciting targets are prioritized and the time and money that can be spent on generating new medicines is saved.

AI Techniques for Genomic Data Analysis

Multi-Omics Data Integration: Fusion Models and Deep Learning Approaches: Multi-omics data integration represents a cutting-edge approach to understanding biological systems by combining diverse types of omics data such as genomics, transcriptomics, proteomics, and metabolomics. This integration provides a comprehensive view of the biological processes underlying health and disease, allowing for more nuanced insights and predictions.

Fusion Models: Fusion models are designed to integrate and analyse multiple omic datasets to capture a holistic picture of biological systems. Several techniques are employed to achieve this integration.

• Concatenation: This approach involves directly combining features from different omics layers into a single dataset. Machine learning models are then applied to this integrated dataset. Concatenation is straightforward but may require careful handling of data compatibility and dimensionality.

• Late Fusion: In this method, separate models are built for each omic type. The predictions from these models are then combined at a later stage. Late fusion leverages the strength of specialized models for each data type and merges their insights to improve overall prediction accuracy.

• Early Fusion: Early fusion involves combining raw data from multiple omics sources before applying machine learning algorithms. This method allows the model to learn relationships between different omic layers from the outset, potentially capturing more intricate interactions and dependencies.

Deep Learning-Based Integration: Deep learning techniques offer advanced methods for integrating multi-omics data, particularly through neural networks that can process and learn from multiple data types simultaneously:

• Multi-View Learning: Multi-view learning involves neural networks that learn from different perspectives or views, such as gene expression profiles and protein interactions. By processing these diverse inputs, the network can generate more accurate and comprehensive predictions.

- Multi-Omics Auto encoders: These models employ auto encoder, a form of NN that works to down sample & extract useful features from multistate omic data. Multi-omics auto encoders can highly adapt to the challenges posed by the increased number of omics layers to integrate besides maintaining important information.

Graph-Based Models

Graph-based models give one rather effective tools for analysing and interpreting complex biological systems. The two major fields in this area are GNNs and KGs: GNNs help analyse biological networks, while KGs contextualize biological relations.

Graph Neural Networks (GNNs): Graph Neural Networks (GNNs) are intended to be used in cases when nodes (which may be, for example, genes or proteins) are connected (Khemani et al., 2024). Given that these networks represent complex structures of biological elements, GNNs are capable of adopting its relations between nodes to intake different kinds of molecular data. Key aspects include:

- Modelling Biological Networks: GNNs are able to encode the temporal behaviour of biological networks, for instance a protein-protein interactive, or a gene regulatory network. Hence, there is an opportunity to predict relations and exercises, define nodes influencing relations, and other relationships existing in topologies which GNNs try to resolve.
- Integration of Data Types: These different data can be incorporated into the structure of GGNs making it possible to integrate many omics data such as genomic and proteomic data. This makes it possible to arrange a model that integrates a view of the structure of the network and the data that are connected to every node.

Knowledge Graphs: Knowledge Graphs offer a hierarchical organization of biological data and their interdependences allowing for better understanding of contained information. These graphs are constructed from various sources of genomic and biological information and offer several advantages:

- Integration and Visualization: Knowledge graphs compile information from several sources such as genomic annotations, protein-protein interactions and biochemical pathways. They allow researchers to show complex associations and connections in a well-structured and dynamic format.
- Query and Inference: It became possible for AI algorithms to ask questions to Knowledge Graphs to forecast new connection, deduce new biological events, and hypothesize. Due to this connectivity of the graph, these models are capable of discovering new features, which may not be revealed by analysing each of the data sources individually.

Machine Learning and Ensemble Methods:

Machine learning based on the efficient distance-based deductions of the classifiers selected, a new field referred to as Machine Learning and Ensemble Methods were developed.

• Ensemble Learning: Enhances the models by integrating several machine learning approaches in order to minimize the chances of making wrong forecast. For integrated genomic data, an ensemble which is a combination of different models analyzing different omic layers can be used to combine predictions from the various models.

• Meta-Learning: Autonomous learning systems that employ techniques which enhance the integration process of several machine learning models.

Cross-Modal Learning

Transfer Learning: Takes information from one data set or discipline and applies it to another data set or field. In genomics, transfer learning can combine the data drawn from other studies or different layers of omics, which improves upon a model.

• Multi-Task Learning: The models are those that work into different but related tasks at the same time. For instance, in healthcare, the application of multi-task learning frameworks means that accurate prediction of disease outcomes and biomarkers from multi-modal genomic data is possible.

Visualization and Interpretation

Integrated Visualization Tools: Some of the powerful AI-based tools and applications are Cytoscape and Gephi that enable the researchers to better understand the interconnectivity of multi-omic data by visualizing the integrated data.

• Interactive Dashboards: Software applications that allow the researchers to have integrated and real-time application of several datasets in relation to specific patterns.

Case Studies on Genomic Data Integration

1. Molecular Taxonomy of Breast Cancer International Consortium (METABRIC): The METABRIC is a medical research project that has provided valuable insights into the nature of breast cancer and has widely contributed into developmental of the Molecular Taxonomy of Breast Cancer International Consortium (METABRIC) (Mucaki et al., 2017). METABRIC contains genomic, transcriptomic, and clinical data of thousands of breast cancer samples and offers an extensive view on molecular and phenotypical characteristics of the disease. In particular, the integration

of the genomic data with the genomic sequences data such as DNA copy number variations and somatic mutations with the transcriptome that shows how genes are expressed in specific conditions. It enables one to look for biomarkers of breast cancer that may not be discovered if different sorts of data are scrutinized individually. Furthermore, METABRIC also overlays clinical information including patient characteristics, tumor features and clinical end points which are then linked to the molecular profile and provides vital correlations which include survival rates. In my opinion one of the most important findings of this project is discovering new breast cancer subtypes, which move beyond the classical classification of cancer based on hormone receptors' status. These new subtypes give a better picture of the disease as it is a biologically more heterogeneous entity and thus offers a better risk stratification and more precise prognosis. More so, the findings from METABRIC have been useful in the development of custom healthcare in breast cancer. New specific genetic markers and changed molecule expression levels that define various outcomes have answered the question of how precision oncology can improve patient outcomes, and have thus brought promising progress to the field. All in all, METABRIC project not only enhances researchers' understanding of breast cancer molecular features but also enhances the clinical diagnostics and treatment significantly based on multi-omics data integration.

 The Cancer Genome Atlas (TCGA) Project: The Cancer Genome Atlas (TCGA) represents one the most groundbreaking projects that have counted for the remarkable evolution in understanding the molecular landscape of cancer, by providing detailed descriptions of the genomic changes in diverse cancer types. This is an important practice that assimilated various forms of omics data such as DNA sequences, probe arrays, and methylated profiles to offer a view of malignancy. This approach included incorporation of genomic data in addition to transcriptomic, proteomics, and clinical data by TCGA. These various data types were combined with large public databases and a variety of robust partially and fully automated tools for the analysis of cancer genomes. The findings of TCGA have been revolutionary and include discovery of molecular subtypes of cancer, new biomarkers and therapeutic targets (Jiang et al., 2022). For example, the TCGA identified certain mutations and gene profiling of different types of cancers which has led to the tailoring of new therapies for the diseases and contributed to the evolution of the field of precision medicines. Due to the discovery of distinct molecular markers in multiple types of cancer, TCGA has paved way to early diagnosis and targeted treatment thereby affecting cancer prognosis and determining the future course of oncology.

FEDERATED LEARNING IN HEALTHCARE

Federated learning is a creating way of using AI in which several institutions or devices can train a given model of machine learning without exposing the data. In the context of healthcare, it is very revolutionary since it enables hospitals, research centres, and medical devices to collaborate in creating new AI models while at the same time ensuring patients' data privacy and protection. Historically, model retraining is achieved in a centralized fashion, which means bringing vast amounts of data under one roof, which, in turn, raises privacy and data security issues and could potentially cause problems with compliance with the legislation such as HIPAA or GDPR. This is achieved through federated learning where data stays with its owner while only model updates may be exchanged for instance; patterns.

Among all the benefits of healthcare integration of HS-AI approaches, federated learning could increase the potential of AI applications by training more encompassing models using decentralised data from various hospitals. For instance, it is possible for hospitals in different geographic locations to train AI for diagnosis or therapeutic approaches without sharing any patient's data. This leads to developing the superior AI models that are accurate and reliable in other populations as well as protect the patients' information. Federated learning becomes helpful in chronic diseases or any such disease that is rare to happen or in any certain type of research where the information gathered by a number of sources is needed to be pooled up (Rahman et al., 2022). Being a trend in healthcare data analytics, federated learning is poised to catalyse innovation as well as to identify several important ethical and legal issues connected with data sharing within the industry.

Applications and Benefits in Healthcare

Digital healthcare is rapidly evolving through Federated learning through a efficient collaborative approach by ensuring model training while preserving trainee's privacy hence improving diagnostic accuracy, personalized treatments and medical research. Transmitting the patient's data is not possible by the federated learning process; therefore it has the followings main uses and potential benefits to the healthcare institutions and devices:

Applications in Healthcare

1. Enhanced Diagnostic Models: It is convenient to aggregate different medical datasets from different hospitals and centres for federated learning and get more precise and generalised diagnostic models. For instance, AI models trained on federated data can identify conditions, including cancer, diabetes, and neurological

disorders better since it is trained using a cross-section of patients' demographics and clinical conditions. This combination further improves the models applicability by capturing peculiar cases that are perhaps not well represented or nonexistent in one institution's pool of patients.

2. Personalized Treatment Plans: Thus, with the help of federated learning, it is possible to train AI models with individualised therapy matrices using the multi-institutional data set. In this context, while ensuring the privacy of the patient data, the federated learning enables treatment plans that are more specific to the patient's needs to be determined through an analysis of data from the various sources. This results in enhanced patient care coming from the assimilation of knowledge from a more diverse array of clinical encounter and treatment outcomes.

3. Predictive Analytics for Disease Prevention: Using federated learning, outcomes for persons with chronic diseases can be forecasted and the corresponding risk factors avoided with the help of data from different healthcare providers. For instance, AI models can evaluate trends and predictors of outcomes such as cardiovascular diseases, or diabetes in different databases to recognize high-risk patients and recommend ways of reducing risk. This is a preventive strategy which is effective in discouraging the development of ailments that may be detrimental to the person's health.

4. Collaborative Medical Research: This is because research in rare diseases or new therapies may indicate that data from the several databases are necessary. In federated learning, that is suitable for the distributed scenario, institutions can participate to a common model without the necessity to accumulate patient data. This approach enhances the opportunity of identifying new treatments and insights into different illnesses due to the broad data set as compared to the normal data set.

The advantages of using federated learning in Healthcare include the following.

1. Enhanced Data Privacy and Security: The other advantage that federated learning is associated with is the ability to preserve the privacy and security of patients' records. Since data is distributed and only the updates of the models are shared, the chances of hacking and unauthorized use of the data are very low. This is important especially for organizations dealing with personal health information which is regulated by laws such as HIPAA in the United States of America and General Data Protection Regulation (GDPR) in Europe.

2. Improved Model Performance: Federated learning enables the use of more data and results in improved performance of jointly trained artificial intelligence models. This in turn creates aggregated insights that output better and sounder models of handling patient data that would generically improve other patient population data. It leads to higher diagnostic accuracy, effectiveness of the treatments and robustness of prediction models.

3. Facilitated Collaboration across Institutions: The application of federated learning brings together healthcare institutions, research institutes, and sometimes even individual practitioners. Such a model fosters the exchange of innovations and best practices at the same time preserving the security of organizational data. It assists in the solving of complicated healthcare issues since it does not encourage the silos in managing or analysing big data.

4. Reduced Data Transfer and Storage Costs: Basically federated learning requires the model updates to be shared instead of raw data hence limiting the amount of data to be transferred and stored. It also addresses the issue of cost reduction in operations thereby reducing pressure exerted on the network and on storages.

AI-POWERED CLINICAL DECISION SUPPORT SYSTEMS

Clinical Decision Support Systems (CDSS) are complex health information technology tools and solutions that are aimed at supporting healthcare practitioners in making efficient clinical decisions. CDSS is a tool that is designed to increase the quality of care, the efficacy of patient care, as well as the effectiveness of care delivery. CDSS are known to provide many types of functionalities in order to assist with clinical decision-making. These systems usually present alarms and prompts, as well as a preliminary diagnosis and possible treatments (Sutton et al., 2020). The first certainly encompasses alerts and reminders, which are quite possibly the most frequently used, as these are intended to inform clinicians about certain conditions, such as drug interactions, allergies, or if the course of the patient's treatment is off par with clinical standards. For instance, a CDSS could sound a warning signal to a physician when the medicine that is to be administered might cause an interaction with another drug that this patient is on. Diagnostic support features assist the clinicians in understanding complicated information regarding a patient and possible diseases. Through patients's complaints, test results, and disease history, CDSS can point out possible diseases and other tests or assessments that should be carried out. This may come in handy, say, in a situation where the diagnosis is complicated given the fact that the signs and symptoms are numerous or the disease is rare. Treatment advice entails involving counselling of the patient based on best practices of the treatment options and therapies best suited for the patient. CDSS belongs to the categories of health care applications that can give proposals on dealing with patients' data, medical history, and condition, as well as medical recommendations. This can help in making sure that the selected treatment is on par with the current findings of evidence and recommended practices.

Types of CDSS

There are different classification models of CDSS based on their functionality and integration within the healthcare facility. The knowledge-based system mainly involves working with a database of medical knowledge and a set of rules to arrive at a decision. Such systems have an embedded set of rules and medical protocols against which they compare patients' data to produce suggestions. A knowledge-based CDSS, for example, is likely to rely on specific protocols for managing a condition like diabetes and then offer recommendations about the kind of changes to the course of treatment according to the patient's unique characteristics. On the other hand, the non-knowledge-based systems, also known as data-driven or machine learning-based systems, use analytical and artificial intelligence approaches to deduce new patterns from huge amounts of data. These systems are not limited by this, and some of them can learn from the data that feeds them, making better recommendations as time goes by. For instance, a CDSS based on the ML might consider patient results from thousands of similar cases to determine potential therapeutic interventions' effectiveness. The following are the advantages to society during CDSS implementation. As detailed earlier, CDSS can provide real-time alarms and suggestions to patients to avoid any medical mistakes and then go further to improve the standardization of care by ensuring that decisions made on the patient's care are in line with the current standards or other advancements in medical practice. There is evidence that a clinical decision support system can help build efficiency with respect to the time taken to make a decision. As such, these clinical decision support systems can easily interpret large amounts of data and generate recommendations for clinicians to implement faster. This is particularly useful in saturated or pressured settings where clinicians may become inured to so many alarms and end up ignoring them. As a result, optimizing the frequency and relevance of issued alerts is the key to CDSS's continued efficiency. However, integration of CDSS in routine health care practice can be very challenging. It's thus important that these systems are user-centric and integrate with electronic health record systems for the best use with minimal disruption to the clinical workflow. Clinical Decision Support Systems are an important improvement in the sphere of healthcare IT with tools that improve clinical decision-making as well as present recommendations and real-time alarms (Chen et al., 2023). That being said, despite these drawbacks that still make it anything but easy to maximize CDSS integration and efficacy, we are witnessing their theoretical advantages: patient protection, homogeneity of the approaches used, and clinical rationality—all of which cannot but spotlight the role of CDSSs in present-day medical practice. CDSS, on the other hand, is an emerging health informatics technology that will progressively be given a more significant responsibility in assisting the health care professionals and enhancing the patients' outcomes in the future.

Techniques in Decision Support

Almost every departments and sectors have adopted the use of AI, including health care departments. They have added more value to Decision Support Systems through incorporation of complex procedures that make the decisions more precise, time bound and appropriate. Indecision support: That is why the AI technologies use big data and numerous formulas to support the users to analyze the amount of data or predict some results and make the correct decisions. This paper also gives a brief overview of some of the normal artificial intelligent technologies used in decision support systems.Machine learning is a subfield of artificial intelligence; its purpose is to learn from data and from patterns that can be discovered in data; it is also capable of making decisions on its own or even of making predictions without further instructions. The classification methods of predictive models such as ML algorithms are designed to understand past data and look for patterns that that inform decisions. For instance, in finance, it involves developing an ML model and training the same to identify characteristics that highlight the future trends of prices, volumes in the stock markets. Health care utilizes it in identifying patient's health status, history of tests and results and evaluating the effectiveness of the treatments to be granted. Deep learning is a branch of machine learning which uses neural networks with more than one layer, therefore, called 'deep'. What you can train them to become is a model of a fairly good standardized accuracy that can distinguish patterns inside data sets. Decision support requires going further and applying, for instance, image recognition, natural language processing, and/or predictive analytics by means of deep learning. For instance, deep learning plays the role of enhancing the rate and precision with which a radiologist makes a diagnosis by scrutinizing images for presence of disease/abnormality.Natural language processing deals with, therefore, the ability of a machine to comprehend, understand, and produce natural language. The use of NLP is very important in decision support systems where text data is involved including customers' feedbacks, patients' records, or legal papers. NLP can make a significant contribution in the improvement of the decision-making processes by filtering structured data from unstructured text information. For instance, sentiment analysis will be able to determine customer emotions from the reviews and posts they make on social media platforms hence enabling the business to adopt the necessary measures to meet their needs. Expert Systems are AI type systems that has been developed to possess an expertise in a given field. Knowledge-based systems rely on a knowledge of human expertise and the inference engine to reason over the data and incident. Expert systems in decision support give decisions and solutions following rules and knowledge that has been formerly coded in it. For instance, an expert system used in diagnostic of diseases may come up with a list of disease which are likely to be with a patient given its symptoms and past medical history, as a specialist doctor would do.

Reinforcement Learning is an approach in which the algorithms learn to decide for themselves through the use of rewards in lieu of the desirable choice while using penalties for the undesirable choice. This technique is well applied especially in models where the decisions influence the next decisions to be made successively. In decision support, reinforcement learning can be utilized in order to learn and continuously make decisions that are better. For example, in supply chain, reinforcement learning helps in maintaining an optimal stock and proper ordering pattern as the algorithm learns from the results of the previous actions. Bayesian Networks are dependable graphical models that comprise probabilities connecting variables with the help of directed and acyclic graphs. They are exploited to provide a feature of uncertainty and to make a probabilistic assessment based on evidence. In decision support, the Bayesian networks assist in the determination of risks and uncertainties by modifying probabilities in the light of new evidence. For instance, in risk management, it is possible to use Bayesian networks in assessing the probability of risk events and their consequences with regard to a given project or investment. Decision Trees are known to be an effective, visual and analytical means of bringing solutions to questions that have been established in terms of criteria. Random Forests is the ensemble of number of decision trees which increases the efficiency and accuracy of the decision. In decision support, these techniques are applied in the classification and regression problems. For instance in credit scoring, decision trees and random forests can estimate probability that a borrower will default on a loan given his/her financial and demographic profile. Basically, AI enhances decision support system since it provides advanced tools to analyze data, estimate results and, therefore, make the right decision. Some of the artificial intelligence techniques include machine learning, deep learning, natural language processing, expert systems, reinforcement learning, Bayesian networks, decision trees among others that aid in improving the accuracy and efficiency of the decision-making system. Because the technology is gradually becoming sophisticated in knowledge acquisition and system design, it is expected that when incorporated into decision supports, higher levels of utility and innovations will be provided in different domains.

Case Studies on Decision Support Innovations

Decision Support Systems (DSS) have become increasingly sophisticated due to innovations in technology, data analysis, and artificial intelligence (AI).

Healthcare: IBM Watson for Oncology

IBM Watson for Oncology Available for free through App store Medical software designed by IBM to assist physicians to draw more effective, personalized cancer treatment plans IBM app to aid physicians to come up with better treatment plans for cancer patients through the use a new tool called IBM Watson iPhone app IBM's new app called for Oncology, developed for Medical Practitioners to use as a reference to gain better idea of how to treat different cancer cases This is an AI based system which was designed and implemented with the support of the Memorial Sloan Kettering Cancer Centre to support oncologists in diagnosing cancer. In particular, Watson for Oncology employs NLP and machine learning algorithms to study millions of articles, patient histories, and clinical trials worldwide. The system has been trained with data on thousands of patients and their treatment results only, which means the system made recommendations for treatment they based on evidence. As it is in real life, the application, Watson for Oncology, helps oncologists by analyzing patient information and other documents and producing the guidelines and recommendations for the further treatment. For example, Watson can assess current literature and clinical trials to get a targeted therapy or another treatment that may be unknown to the attending doctor. One of the easiest consequences of launching Watson for Oncology is the verification of identification and advising of treatments in record time. It was found in a study conducted in India for Watson for Oncology that the treatment suggestions are aligned with the oncologists' standard treatment guidance in 93% of the cases. This underlines the benefits of decision support systems involving use of AI in the health sector as they enhance the ability of practitioners in making sound decisions for the improvement of the patient's wellbeing.

Manufacturing: Siemens' Predictive Maintenance

Currently, the organisation employs analytical tools and machine learning models to forecast equipment failure, which are effective before it happens. Called the 'Digital Twin,' this program processes information collected by dozens of sensors fitted onto machines and can detect patterns likely to compromise the smooth running of the machinery. Preventive maintenance also enables the manufacturers to do regular check-ups and repairs without waiting for the equipment to break, thus avoiding time-wasting due to equipment breakdowns, and ultimately cutting on costs of maintenance. For instance, Siemens Business Work's system is capable of estimating the possible time a machine such as a turbine or a pump will be required for a servicing hence allowing manufacturers to programme for the machine to be out of service rather than the machine breaking down and pulling out of production line.

The success of Siemens' topic has been enormous as explained by the features of the predictive maintenance technology. According to manufacturer's implementing these systems, there are decrease in cost of maintenance, improved equipment availability, and improved total organizational performance. Using such kind of information in sustaining the machines, Siemens gives a good example of how decision support innovations improve manufacturing operations. From the above case studies it is clear that the decision support innovations are revolutionary in their different fields. For the healthcare sector, IBM Watson for Oncology refines diagnosis and treatment proposal; in the financial industry, JPMorgan Chase's COiN optimizes the evaluation of legal documents; and in the manufacturing industry, Siemens had developed a kind of prediction maintenance. Each example demonstrates how such as AI and machine learning, natural language processing enhances decision making as it becomes accurate, fast and efficient. With emerging technologies in place, decision support innovation presents the opportunity to proceed to shape advancement and optimization of several sectors.

Ethical and Regulatory Considerations for Clinical Decision Support Systems

Clinical Decision Support Systems (CDSS) is an effective systems designed to provide the heighten support to the clinical practitioners in making a right decision based on the patient data in the light of clinical rules. Of course, implementing CDSS has several advantages such as, increasing patients' quality, and reducing healthcare costs, improving efficacy; however, CDSS implementation comes with certain unethical and regulatory issues which cannot be overlooked. CDSS are heavily dependent on large numbers of patient, which is a major concern in issues of patient privacy and data security. Some of the ethical concerns that may arise concerning patient's information concerns the aspects of privacy and security of the content within the health information exchange. Cryptography, strong passwords, and HIPAA or other privacy laws are pre-requisites in order to protect the patients' information. The phenomena of decisions made by CDSS must be warranted and understandable. It is also noted that for healthcare professionals to be able to trust and implement the recommendation of the system, they must know how the system came up with its decision making process. Since the recommendation from a CDSS may result in an adverse outcome, it is important to have documentation of the arguments of the CDSS in order to evaluate and perhaps, correct problems. If biased data is used in the development of an AI-driven CDSS then this may serve to reinforce or even amplify the bias. This can result in differential management recommendation of different patient groups. Fairness must therefore entail frequent assessment on how the system delivers its results with regard to various groups and employing measures that will help erase such differences that have been observed. Thus, it is crucial to notice that even if CDSS give useful suggestions they should not infringe upon professional decision-making. The ultimate decision calls for clinicians especially on those aspects concerning their competency as well as patients' choice rather than whatever the system has to feed back.

CHALLENGES AND ETHICAL CONSIDERATIONS

AI's application in health care data analytics offers several noble prospects although complex in execution. The first significant challenge relates to the availability and quality of data whereby data in the healthcare domain is often skewed, partly detailed, or unstructured thereby limiting the production of efficient AI models. However, the ethical and the privacy issues related to patients' data are also major challenges, as data protection should be well-enforced to avoid misuse and comply with the regulations. Another challenge that AI systems present is that of devising ways of handling bias; training data may contain present healthcare discriminations, and therefore cause bias. In addition to that, there are challenges with regards to integration of AI in the context of various healthcare systems, and the need to make AI use in healthcare transparent and explainable in order to achieve user acceptance by the healthcare stakeholders. Therefore, to ensure that AI brings the much-needed change in healthcare then overcoming these is very critical.

In the context of healthcare data analytics utilizing the AI technologies, ethical concerns play an important role, as these technologies became more widespread influencing patient treatment and care (Farhud & Zokaei, 2021). Some of the primary consideration involves limited privacy and security threats where at the wrong hands, sensitive patient information can easily fall into wrong hands. Another problem is how to avoid the AI's bias in prescribing treatments, which will result in inequality in healthcare if the algorithms are designed to provide better treatment to specific groups or specific outcomes. Moreover, the decision of AI needs to be clear and easily explained so that the patients and other health care providers would be able to understand why the certain decision was made. Last but not the least; it is crucial to discuss the questions of ownership and consent for using data in case of AI aided analytics and to make patients aware of its use. It is therefore important to strike a balance between innovation with these ethical considerations in order to propel the advancement in health care delivery in responsible and equitable manner.

THE FUTURE OF AI IN HEALTHCARE

The future of AI in the healthcare industry, and it promises to be bright as it can swiftly change the way diagnostics or even treat patients and adapt to each individual's needs when it comes to their care. The medical applications of AI are evident when it comes to the analysis of large amounts of medical data; this will include early diagnosis of diseases with lesser chances of being mistaken. Prescribed programs based on artificial intelligence would most likely lead to better patient results, taking into account each person's genetic profile as well as their environment and lifestyle choices. Also, repetitive work can be eased out by the use of AI so that healthcare professionals will be able to provide more personalized and human-contacted care. Overall, AI is poised to significantly enhance the delivery of healthcare services, focusing more on the patient. However, the future will present two major challenges: the social implications of AI and data issues, including privacy concerns.

Emerging Trends and Technologies

The future of AI in healthcare is sawn with several trends and technologies in the following: The use of AI in genomics and personalised medicine is one of the most revolutionary trends. As the high-throughput sequencing technologies are being developed, large volumes of genomic data are produced and require the application of superior AI technologies to handle and analyze. AI is useful in finding DNA markers associated with a genetic disorder; hence, it is possible to design treatment packages for an individual based on his/her genotype (Vilhekar & Rawekar, n.d.). This approach has been under development, especially in oncology, as the use of AI in precision medicine dramatically increases the efficiency of cancer treatment due to the possibility of choosing the best therapy for certain types of cancer. Another area that has been rapidly developing over the last couple decades is the use of AI in medical imaging. More advanced learning algorithms, specifically deep learning models, have given improved results with respect to analysing complicated image data like MRI's, CT scans, and X-ray scans. These models have the ability to identify specific irregularities that human radiologists often overlook, thereby enhancing diagnosis accuracy and promoting early diagnosis. For instance, in recent years, examples of the use of artificial intelligence are the ability to segment tumours in medical images and improve the accuracy of treatment planning.

In drug discovery, AI is revolutionizing the traditional drug development pipeline. With a large database of chemical and biological activities, machine learning models are capable of forecasting on how well a particular compound will perform. This helps in fastening the process of discovery of potential molecules, cuts the time and cost of drug development and has a capability of delivering drugs to the public in a shorter span. Another area of impact has been in the use of artificial intelligence for drug repurposing, that is using already existing drugs for other conditions. Another area where AI is also picking up steam in clinical trials is with regard to the patient recruitment, and design of the trials. By using AI for instance to scan EHRs, more suitable patients for trails can be selected based on their EHRs precluding selection bias and other heterogeneities. In trials also, data gathering and analysis can be done through artificial intelligence eliminating bias and hastening the research.

Potential Impact on Healthcare Delivery

The application of AI in healthcare is a great and all-encompassing goal that cannot be overemphasized. It is crucial to note here that AI has the capacity to enhance the diagnostic rate as well as patients' conditions in a big way. Through the use of artificial intelligence, large amounts of information about the patient, such as images, test results, and genomics, can be scrutinised and patterns associated with diseases pinpointed. For example, AI has been useful in the identification of diseases, including diabetic retinopathy, which, if diagnosed early enough, cannot lead to blindness. There are other forms of applications that AI is contributing to, and some of the areas include telemedicine and remote patient monitoring. Wearable devices with artificial intelligence regularly track or record several parameters in the body that would alert an individual when they are getting sick. These devices can notify the care providers in real-time, which will reduce the inpatient service requirement. It enhances the quality of health services to patients and also relieves the pressure on the health systems, especially in controlling areas with few health centres.

Increasing the operational efficiency of an organization is a common use of artificial intelligence (AI), and the healthcare business is no exception to this rule. One approach to do this is by using artificial intelligence algorithms to predict the amount of patients who will be arriving at hospitals. This will allow for the identification of more effective methods of resource deployment and the enhancement of supply chain management. For instance, with regard to inventory management, predictive models can predict the demand of hospital goods and services and help the organizations order the necessary quantities of supplies without over-ordering and going over budget. This makes their operation efficient and can mean that huge chunks can be shaved from costs and put back into patient care. Moreover, utilisation of artificial intelligence in the context of personalised medicine will transform the approaches to the treatment. Therefore, through the parsing of genomic, clinical, lifestyle, and environmental data, it is possible for the artificial intelligence and adaptive knowledge manipulation environments to arrive at specific treatment plans of doctors that are stronger in efficacy and have fewer side effects. These ideal and based strategies are significant in the context of complicated and chronic health disorders since mainstream organisation treatment modes may not be fruitful here.

Roadmap for Future Research and Development

The future research and development of AI healthcare is based on the current issues and the new horizons for development. Yet one of the more pressing and important challenges is that of the explain ability and interpretability of an AI model. With the advancement of deep, complex models in AI systems, the process of interpreting how the models came to the formulations it makes also becomes a challenge. This characteristic is widely known as the 'black box' issue and represents a major challenge for the application of AI in clinics. It becomes crucial to find ways on how the AI system can be able to explain their actions, which the healthcare professionals will understand, so as to build trust in the future use of AI systems. Another primary focus of research within the field of AI is the development of methods that can improve the resilience of these systems to specific types of adversarial attacks. Since healthcare is an area where data collected is sensitive, its privacy and security must be protected at all costs. AI models and algorithms should be secure against cyber threats and, more importantly, reliable in many different settings, including healthcare and with other diverse patient populations. However, to my knowledge, there is a rising demand for ethical standards in the field of AI, especially when it comes to factors like bias, fairness, and responsibility in making decisions using artificial intelligence tools.

Another possibility for growth in the future is the use of AI in mental health. Technology such as natural language processing, therefore, has the ability of assisting in the diagnosis of such diseases by analysing the patterns in the language, writing, and even behaviour (Khurana et al., 2023). Further studies should be directed to discover the potential of AI to help in addressing the shortage of mental health practitioners to provide proper care to those individuals who need it. There is also the perspective that the role of AI in global health requires further research into the topic. By creating effective models that can function in such environments, AI will be able to help solve issues of healthcare inequality. The following challenges should be the focus of study in the development of AI systems for healthcare: affordability, scalability, and relevance to the conditions existing in various areas around the world, so that global health disparities are not exacerbated.

REFERENCES

Alowais, S. A., Alghamdi, S. S., Alsuhebany, N., Alqahtani, T., Alshaya, A. I., Almohareb, S. N., Aldairem, A., Alrashed, M., Bin Saleh, K., Badreldin, H. A., Al Yami, M. S., Al Harbi, S., & Albekairy, A. M. (2023). Revolutionizing healthcare: The role of artificial intelligence in clinical practice. *BMC Medical Education*, 23(1), 689. DOI: 10.1186/s12909-023-04698-z PMID: 37740191

Badiger, M., & Mathew, J. A. (2023). Tomato plant leaf disease segmentation and multiclass disease detection using hybrid optimization enabled deep learning. *Journal of Biotechnology*, 374, 101–113. DOI: 10.1016/j.jbiotec.2023.07.011 PMID: 37543108

Batko, K., & Ślęzak, A. (2022). The use of Big Data Analytics in healthcare. *Journal of Big Data*, 9(1), 3. DOI: 10.1186/s40537-021-00553-4 PMID: 35013701

Bradford, L., Aboy, M., & Liddell, K. (2020). International transfers of health data between the EU and USA: A sector-specific approach for the USA to ensure an 'adequate' level of protection. *Journal of Law and the Biosciences*, 7(1), lsaa055. Advance online publication. DOI: 10.1093/jlb/lsaa055 PMID: 34221424

Chen, Z., Liang, N., Zhang, H., Li, H., Yang, Y., Zong, X., Chen, Y., Wang, Y., & Shi, N. (2023). Harnessing the power of clinical decision support systems: Challenges and opportunities. *Open Heart*, 10(2), e002432. DOI: 10.1136/openhrt-2023-002432 PMID: 38016787

Cirillo, D., & Valencia, A. (2019). Big data analytics for personalized medicine. *Current Opinion in Biotechnology*, 58, 161–167. DOI: 10.1016/j.copbio.2019.03.004 PMID: 30965188

Contreras, I., & Vehi, J. (2018). Artificial Intelligence for Diabetes Management and Decision Support: Literature Review. *Journal of Medical Internet Research*, 20(5), e10775. DOI: 10.2196/10775 PMID: 29848472

Dash, S., Shakyawar, S. K., Sharma, M., & Kaushik, S. (2019). Big data in healthcare: Management, analysis and future prospects. *Journal of Big Data*, 6(1), 54. DOI: 10.1186/s40537-019-0217-0

Davenport, T., & Kalakota, R. (2019). The potential for artificial intelligence in healthcare. *Future Healthcare Journal*, 6(2), 94–98. DOI: 10.7861/futurehosp.6-2-94 PMID: 31363513

Farhud, D. D., & Zokaei, S. (2021). Ethical Issues of Artificial Intelligence in Medicine and Healthcare. *Iranian Journal of Public Health*, 50(11), i–v. DOI: 10.18502/ijph.v50i11.7600 PMID: 35223619

Goetz, L. H., & Schork, N. J. (2018). Personalized Medicine: Motivation, Challenges and Progress. *Fertility and Sterility*, 109(6), 952–963. DOI: 10.1016/j.fertnstert.2018.05.006 PMID: 29935653

Hassan, M., Awan, F. M., Naz, A., deAndrés-Galiana, E. J., Alvarez, O., Cernea, A., Fernández-Brillet, L., Fernández-Martínez, J. L., & Kloczkowski, A. (2022). Innovations in Genomics and Big Data Analytics for Personalized Medicine and Health Care: A Review. *International Journal of Molecular Sciences*, 23(9), 9. Advance online publication. DOI: 10.3390/ijms23094645 PMID: 35563034

Hosny, A., Parmar, C., Quackenbush, J., Schwartz, L. H., & Aerts, H. J. W. L. (2018). Artificial intelligence in radiology. *Nature Reviews. Cancer*, 18(8), 500–510. DOI: 10.1038/s41568-018-0016-5 PMID: 29777175

Jiang, P., Sinha, S., Aldape, K., Hannenhalli, S., Sahinalp, C., & Ruppin, E. (2022). Big data in basic and translational cancer research. *Nature Reviews. Cancer*, 22(11), 625–639. DOI: 10.1038/s41568-022-00502-0 PMID: 36064595

Johnson, K. B., Wei, W., Weeraratne, D., Frisse, M. E., Misulis, K., Rhee, K., Zhao, J., & Snowdon, J. L. (2021). Precision Medicine, AI, and the Future of Personalized Health Care. *Clinical and Translational Science*, 14(1), 86–93. DOI: 10.1111/cts.12884 PMID: 32961010

Khemani, B., Patil, S., Kotecha, K., & Tanwar, S. (2024). A review of graph neural networks: Concepts, architectures, techniques, challenges, datasets, applications, and future directions. *Journal of Big Data*, 11(1), 18. DOI: 10.1186/s40537-023-00876-4

Khurana, D., Koli, A., Khatter, K., & Singh, S. (2023). Natural language processing: State of the art, current trends and challenges. *Multimedia Tools and Applications*, 82(3), 3713–3744. DOI: 10.1007/s11042-022-13428-4 PMID: 35855771

Kiran, N., Sapna, F., Kiran, F., Kumar, D., Raja, F., Shiwlani, S., Paladini, A., Sonam, F., Bendari, A., Perkash, R. S., Anjali, F., & Varrassi, G. (2023, September 3). (n.d.). Digital Pathology: Transforming Diagnosis in the Digital Age. *Cureus*, 15(9), e44620. DOI: 10.7759/cureus.44620 PMID: 37799211

Li, X., Tian, D., Li, W., Dong, B., Wang, H., Yuan, J., Li, B., Shi, L., Lin, X., Zhao, L., & Liu, S. (2021). Artificial intelligence-assisted reduction in patients' waiting time for outpatient process: A retrospective cohort study. *BMC Health Services Research*, 21(1), 237. DOI: 10.1186/s12913-021-06248-z PMID: 33731096

Luca, A. R., Ursuleanu, T. F., Gheorghe, L., Grigorovici, R., Iancu, S., Hlusneac, M., & Grigorovici, A. (2022). Impact of quality, type and volume of data used by deep learning models in the analysis of medical images. *Informatics in Medicine Unlocked*, 29, 100911. DOI: 10.1016/j.imu.2022.100911

Mahmood, S. S., Levy, D., Vasan, R. S., & Wang, T. J. (2014). The Framingham Heart Study and the Epidemiology of Cardiovascular Diseases: A Historical Perspective. *Lancet*, 383(9921), 999–1008. DOI: 10.1016/S0140-6736(13)61752-3 PMID: 24084292

Maleki Varnosfaderani, S., & Forouzanfar, M. (2024). The Role of AI in Hospitals and Clinics: Transforming Healthcare in the 21st Century. *Bioengineering (Basel, Switzerland)*, 11(4), 337. DOI: 10.3390/bioengineering11040337 PMID: 38671759

Mehrotra, P. (2016). Biosensors and their applications – A review. *Journal of Oral Biology and Craniofacial Research*, 6(2), 153–159. DOI: 10.1016/j.jobcr.2015.12.002 PMID: 27195214

Mucaki, E. J., Baranova, K., Pham, H. Q., Rezaeian, I., Angelov, D., Ngom, A., Rueda, L., & Rogan, P. K. (2017). Predicting Outcomes of Hormone and Chemotherapy in the Molecular Taxonomy of Breast Cancer International Consortium (METABRIC) Study by Biochemically-inspired Machine Learning. *F1000 Research*, 5, 2124. DOI: 10.12688/f1000research.9417.3 PMID: 28620450

Murdoch, B. (2021). Privacy and artificial intelligence: Challenges for protecting health information in a new era. *BMC Medical Ethics*, 22(1), 122. DOI: 10.1186/s12910-021-00687-3 PMID: 34525993

Paganelli, A. I., Mondéjar, A. G., da Silva, A. C., Silva-Calpa, G., Teixeira, M. F., Carvalho, F., Raposo, A., & Endler, M. (2022). Real-time data analysis in health monitoring systems: A comprehensive systematic literature review. *Journal of Biomedical Informatics*, 127, 104009. DOI: 10.1016/j.jbi.2022.104009 PMID: 35196579

Paul, D., Sanap, G., Shenoy, S., Kalyane, D., Kalia, K., & Tekade, R. K. (2021). Artificial intelligence in drug discovery and development. *Drug Discovery Today*, 26(1), 80–93. DOI: 10.1016/j.drudis.2020.10.010 PMID: 33099022

Raghupathi, W., & Raghupathi, V. (2014). Big data analytics in healthcare: Promise and potential. *Health Information Science and Systems*, 2(1), 3. DOI: 10.1186/2047-2501-2-3 PMID: 25825667

Rahman, A., & Hossain, Md. S., Muhammad, G., Kundu, D., Debnath, T., Rahman, M., Khan, Md. S. I., Tiwari, P., & Band, S. S. (. (2022). Federated learning-based AI approaches in smart healthcare: Concepts, taxonomies, challenges and open issues. *Cluster Computing*, •••, 1–41. DOI: 10.1007/s10586-022-03658-4 PMID: 35996680

Richter, K., Kellner, S., & Licht, C. (2023). rTMS in mental health disorders. *Frontiers in Network Physiology*, 3, 943223. Advance online publication. DOI: 10.3389/fnetp.2023.943223 PMID: 37577037

Sebastian, A. M., & Peter, D. (2022). Artificial Intelligence in Cancer Research: Trends, Challenges and Future Directions. *Life (Chicago, Ill.)*, 12(12), 1991. DOI: 10.3390/life12121991 PMID: 36556356

Sedlakova, J., Daniore, P., Wintsch, A. H., Wolf, M., Stanikic, M., Haag, C., Sieber, C., Schneider, G., Staub, K., Ettlin, D. A., Grübner, O., Rinaldi, F., Wyl, V., & von, . (2023). Challenges and best practices for digital unstructured data enrichment in health research: A systematic narrative review. *PLOS Digital Health*, 2(10), e0000347. Advance online publication. DOI: 10.1371/journal.pdig.0000347 PMID: 37819910

Sharma, A., Badea, M., Tiwari, S., & Marty, J. L. (2021). Wearable Biosensors: An Alternative and Practical Approach in Healthcare and Disease Monitoring. *Molecules (Basel, Switzerland)*, 26(3), 748. DOI: 10.3390/molecules26030748 PMID: 33535493

Shei, R.-J., Holder, I. G., Oumsang, A. S., Paris, B. A., & Paris, H. L. (2022). Wearable activity trackers–advanced technology or advanced marketing? *European Journal of Applied Physiology*, 122(9), 1975–1990. DOI: 10.1007/s00421-022-04951-1 PMID: 35445837

Sutton, R. T., Pincock, D., Baumgart, D. C., Sadowski, D. C., Fedorak, R. N., & Kroeker, K. I. (2020). An overview of clinical decision support systems: Benefits, risks, and strategies for success. *NPJ Digital Medicine*, 3(1), 1–10. DOI: 10.1038/s41746-020-0221-y PMID: 32047862

Vilhekar, R. S., & Rawekar, A. (2024, January 10). (n.d.). Artificial Intelligence in Genetics. *Cureus*, 16(1), e52035. DOI: 10.7759/cureus.52035 PMID: 38344556

Vora, L. K., Gholap, A. D., Jetha, K., Thakur, R. R. S., Solanki, H. K., & Chavda, V. P. (2023). Artificial Intelligence in Pharmaceutical Technology and Drug Delivery Design. *Pharmaceutics*, 15(7), 1916. DOI: 10.3390/pharmaceutics15071916 PMID: 37514102

Wang, Z., Keane, P. A., Chiang, M., Cheung, C. Y., Wong, T. Y., & Ting, D. S. W. (2022). Artificial Intelligence and Deep Learning in Ophthalmology. In Lidströmer, N., & Ashrafian, H. (Eds.), *Artificial Intelligence in Medicine* (pp. 1519–1552). Springer International Publishing., DOI: 10.1007/978-3-030-64573-1_200

Whisman, M. A., & South, S. C. (2017). Gene–environment interplay in the context of romantic relationships. *Current Opinion in Psychology*, 13, 136–141. DOI: 10.1016/j.copsyc.2016.08.002

Xu, Y., Liu, X., Cao, X., Huang, C., Liu, E., Qian, S., Liu, X., Wu, Y., Dong, F., Qiu, C.-W., Qiu, J., Hua, K., Su, W., Wu, J., Xu, H., Han, Y., Fu, C., Yin, Z., Liu, M., & Zhang, J. (2021). Artificial intelligence: A powerful paradigm for scientific research. *Innovation (Cambridge (Mass.))*, 2(4), 100179. DOI: 10.1016/j.xinn.2021.100179 PMID: 34877560

Chapter 2
Transforming Healthcare With AI and Machine Learning:
Applications and Impacts

D. Ravindran
https://orcid.org/0000-0003-1672-9552
Kristu Jayanti College, India

G. Mariammal
Vel Tech Rangarajan Dr. Sagunthala R&D Institute of Science and Technology, India

M. Dhivya
Ramco Institute of Technology, India

Dhivya Devi S.
SRM Institute of Science and Technology, India

Anish T. P.
R.M.K. College of Engineering and Technology, India

V. Sathya
https://orcid.org/0000-0002-0355-1401
Vel Tech Rangarajan Dr. Sagunthala R&D Institute of Science and Technology, India

Siva Subramanian R.
https://orcid.org/0000-0002-7509-9223
R.M.K. College of Engineering and Technology, India

ABSTRACT

This survey paper gives an insight about the application of artificial intelligence (AI) and machine learning (ML) in the healthcare industry. With a broad focus, it discusses the present state, approaches, and advancements of AI and ML in the health care industry. This paper explores the process of accumulating and structuring healthcare data, dataset standardization, data quality assessment, prognosis, clinical decision support systems, healthcare operations' efficiency, population

DOI: 10.4018/979-8-3693-7277-7.ch002

health dynamics, fraudulence identification, revenue cycle, patient participation, telemonitoring, individualized treatment, health care quality assessment, ethical issues, and real-world examples of healthcare AI applications and developments. This comprehensive survey highlights the transformative potential of AI and ML in healthcare, emphasizing the need for continuous research, ethical practices, and robust data management to harness these technologies effectively.

INTRODUCTION TO AI AND MACHINE LEARNING IN HEALTHCARE

Integration of AI and ML in Healthcare

Artificial Intelligence (AI) and Machine Learning (ML) have massive potential within the healthcare industries, the integration of AI and ML is going to transform the industry by providing healthcare professionals with the tools necessary to drive the industry forward and create the world's best healthcare solutions (Kishor, A., & Chakraborty, C. 2022). There are several factors associated with this integration, and one of the most crucial ones is data management. AI and ML are based on the analysis of big data coming from different sources such as EHR, medical imaging, wearable devices, and genomics. Data management includes acquiring good sample data, sourcing data from various places, cleaning the data from any inconsistencies, and storing the data securely particularly for sensitive data like patient health information which requires HIPAA conformity. Another such area of AI and ML in healthcare is the use of predictive analytics (Bohr, A., & Memarzadeh, K. 2020). Through analysing past and current data, these technologies are in a position to predict future occurrences and trends with which treatment can be provided before resulting in serious complications. The common subdivisions of the predictive analytics comprise of disease prediction and diagnosis, in this case, the AI are employed to detect the early stage of diseases including cancer and cardiovascular diseases, personalized medicine aimed at developing treatment plan for individual patients from their genetically predefined and health lifestyle records, and risk stratification where the AI algorithms predict those patients at higher risk of conditions such as readmissions or complications, in this way, decision-makers reallocate resources and effort to preventive. There are many advantages of AI and ML in healthcare, of which operational optimization is an important aspect (Yamini, B et al 2023). These technologies can enhance the organizational processes by helping reduce the number of clerk's responsibilities, managing resources, and helping to organize the overall processes. AI can help to create staff schedules, estimate patients' admission probabilities, and control stocks, thus maximizing the staff and resources utilization.

Moreover, the administration of many repetitive tasks like billing and appointment scheduling alleviates the work load as well as cuts down on errors, while clinical support systems create automated decision support based on proven research, improving the right targeting of diagnostics and treatment.

But the use of AI and ML in healthcare also has some bending ethical issues which have to be resolved to prevent misuse of technology. Issues of bias and fairness arise here as the AI has to be trained on the dataset that does not have any bias towards a certain section of the population. Transparency is critical, which entails that the way AI systems make decisions should be understandable to the healthcare providers and the patients. Confidentiality and privacy are critical issues regarding data protection laws and getting consent from the patients to utilize the data derived from them. Lastly, responsibility plays an important role, which means one has to set up clearer standards in where the blame lies and how human intervention can still be implemented in using AI.

Altogether with the integration of AI and ML, it is much possible to revolutionize the healthcare system as a whole by managing patient care, increasing the effectiveness of care delivery and cutting costs. The future potential of these technologies will however depend on how data is handled, how analyses are made, how operations are managed and the level of ethics is dealt with. This systematic review illustrates and signifies the huge shift towards using AI and ML in the betterment of healthcare.

Motivation and Objective

This work aims at trying to present a clear understanding of potential use and effects that Artificial Intelligence (AI) and Machine Learning (ML) in the healthcare systems and industry(Anita et al 2024). Thus, realizing the change potential of these technologies, the paper's goal is to identify the broad range of applications of these advanced technologies in different aspects of managing health-related data, using big data solutions for prediction and diagnosis, improving operational efficiency, and discussing the related ethical issues. It presents the need to examine the future role of AI and ML in the development of healthcare systems, specializing in patient care, better productivity, and desirable savings. Therefore, by analyzing the existing state, approaches, and developments in healthcare AI, the paper aims to serve as a helpful starting point for healthcare workers, researchers, policy makers, and financial decision makers seeking to advance their knowledge on the topic of AI and ML in the sphere of healthcare. Understanding the nature of data mining, clinical decision support, remote patient monitoring, and ethical concerns is crucial for discussion, ideation, and proper implementation of AI and ML in the context of healthcare.

DATA MINING AND BUSINESS INTELLIGENCE IN HEALTHCARE

In the emerging era of big data, data mining and business intelligence have significant functions in identifying value-enhancing opportunities from large amounts of healthcare data. Essentially, more and better data and more efficient analytical means and techniques allow better pattern recognition and forecasting of trends that must improve both medical treatment delivered and stewardship of resources expended in the administration of the delivery of healthcare.

Data Mining Techniques

Association Rule Mining: The identification of correlation and interconnection between various factors that are present in health care data. For example, identifying which diseases are frequently treated together.

Clustering Analysis: Division of data similar to each other in some form of measure into sets referred to as clusters. This means that patient are clustered according to their health conditions or response to certain treatment.

Classification: Supervision and enhancement of selection and classification procedures to help categorize the patients into various groups or make estimations given particular characteristics of the input formulas. For example, determining whether a particular disease will develop or the probability of a patient's readmission to a healthcare facility.

Regression Analysis: In this case, it is significant to determine the manner in which independent and dependent variables relate to one another in order to predict continuous results. This can be applied for predicting patient's outcome or the use of resources.

Time Series Analysis: Exploring time-related features and characteristics of healthcare information. For instance, estimating the number of patients' admissions or the increase/increase in the incidence of certain diseases during certain times of the year(Liao et al 2012).

Figure 1. Data Mining and Business Intelligence in Healthcare

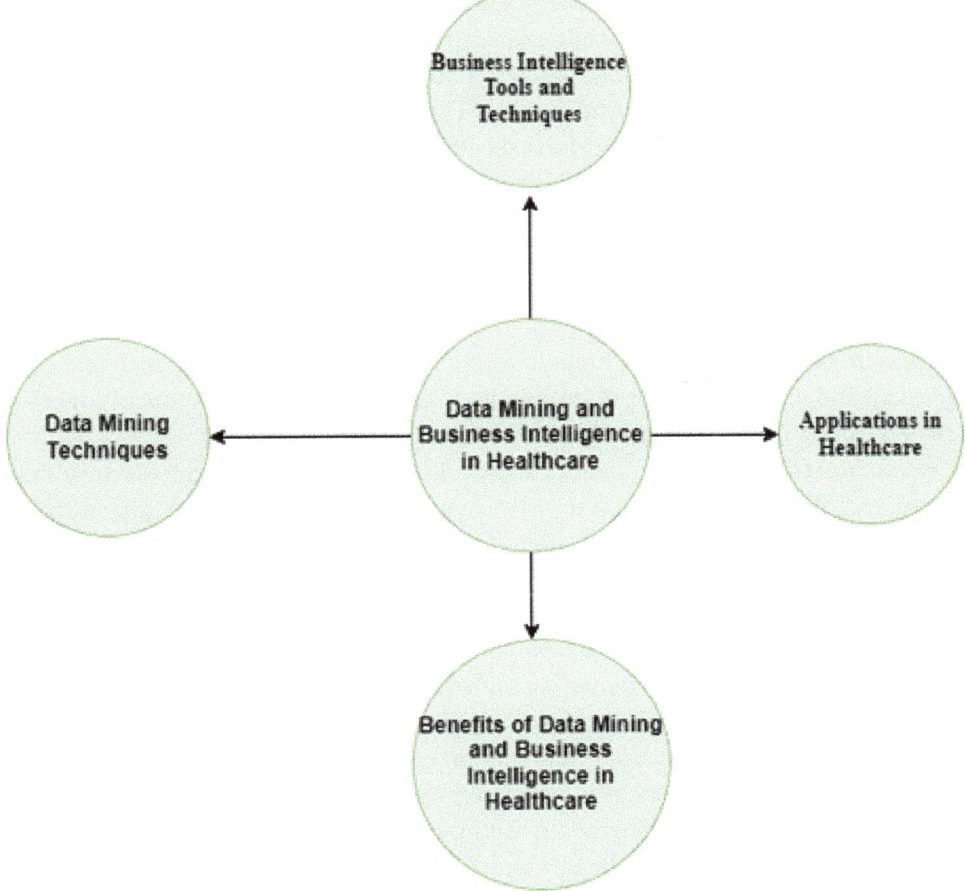

```
                    ┌─────────────────┐
                    │ Business Intelligence │
                    │    Tools and    │
                    │   Techniques    │
                    └─────────────────┘
                              ▲
                              │
  ┌──────────┐       ┌─────────────────┐      ┌──────────────┐
  │   Data   │◄──────│  Data Mining and│─────►│ Applications │
  │  Mining  │       │Business Intelligence│   │ in Healthcare│
  │Techniques│       │  in Healthcare  │      │              │
  └──────────┘       └─────────────────┘      └──────────────┘
                              │
                              ▼
                    ┌─────────────────┐
                    │Benefits of Data Mining│
                    │   and Business  │
                    │  Intelligence in│
                    │   Healthcare    │
                    └─────────────────┘
```

Business Intelligence Tools and Techniques

Data Visualization: Sharing and visualizing of healthcare data by using charts, graphs and even dashboards to enhance knowledge and decision making. Tableau, power BI, QlikView are the most used visualization tools in healthcare BI.

Dashboard Reporting: Developing dynamic and engaging worksheets that present information about the primary markers, including patient satisfaction ratings or operational and financial statistics.

OLAP (Online Analytical Processing): The application of completing comprehensive research on health system metrics and understanding correlations and directions between multiple dimensions such as time series, geographical area, or patients' characteristics.

Data Mining Algorithms Integration: The ability to incorporate data mining algorithms into BI platforms to perform the identification of existing patterns within the health care data automatically. This helps in timely decision making and planning for the future(Kesavaraj, G., & Sukumaran, S. 2013).

Applications in Healthcare

Clinical Decision Support: Enhancing clinicians' decision making in diagnosis, treatment and prescribing by presenting them with evidence based clinical suggestions and alerts in the course of practice.

Operational Efficiency: Identifying workflow inefficiencies in the hospital system and utilizing information to drive more efficient process and schedules in order to reduce cost and improve patient traffic.

Population Health Management: Admitted patients requiring prompt care, Emergency Department visits, emergency transfers from other facilities, mortalities, and readmissions linking high-risk patient groups, population health trends, and preventive measures to community health betterment.

Patient Engagement and Experience: Other strategies included Operationalizing patient communication, education, and support using big data to understand patients' preferences, which would, in turn, improve patient satisfaction and the likelihood of patients adhering to their treatment regimes.

Revenue Cycle Management: Best practices for revenue cycle management that focused on analysing the data and increasing the accuracy of billing by identifying mistakes, increasing the reimbursement rates, and minimizing revenue loss.

Benefits of Data Mining and Business Intelligence in Healthcare

Informed Decision-Making: Supporting healthcare providers and managers by supplying them with crucial information and fundamental analysis for the enhancement of patient care, system organization, and financial results.

Improved Patient Outcomes: Increasing effectiveness of decision-making in the clinical environment with the use of predictive analytics and clinical decision support systems, resulting in improved treatment outcomes, decrease of medical mistakes and increase of patients' safety.

Cost Reduction: The analysis of the health care delivery processes and procedures with an aim of recognizing areas where costs can be slashed and the processes can be made more efficient.

Enhanced Operational Efficiency: Efficiency of work within healthcare entities, and ways of enhancing them through streamlining administrative work, decreasing waiting times, and proper allocation of resources in a manner that increases not only the flow of patients within healthcare facilities.

Proactive Healthcare Management: Facilitating the forecasting and understanding of the health of the population, the identification of chronic diseases, and the development of preventive measures for new risks and changes.

COLLECTING, INTEGRATING, AND PREPARING HEALTHCARE DATA

To this extent, we can precisely assert that the quality of data is critical to AI and ML initiatives in the healthcare setting. This section focuses on the procedures of data collection from different sources and further data consolidation before data cleaning procedure in order to make the collected data complete, accurate and most importantly consistent for the preparation of analysis.

Figure 2. Collecting, Integrating, and Preparing Healthcare Data

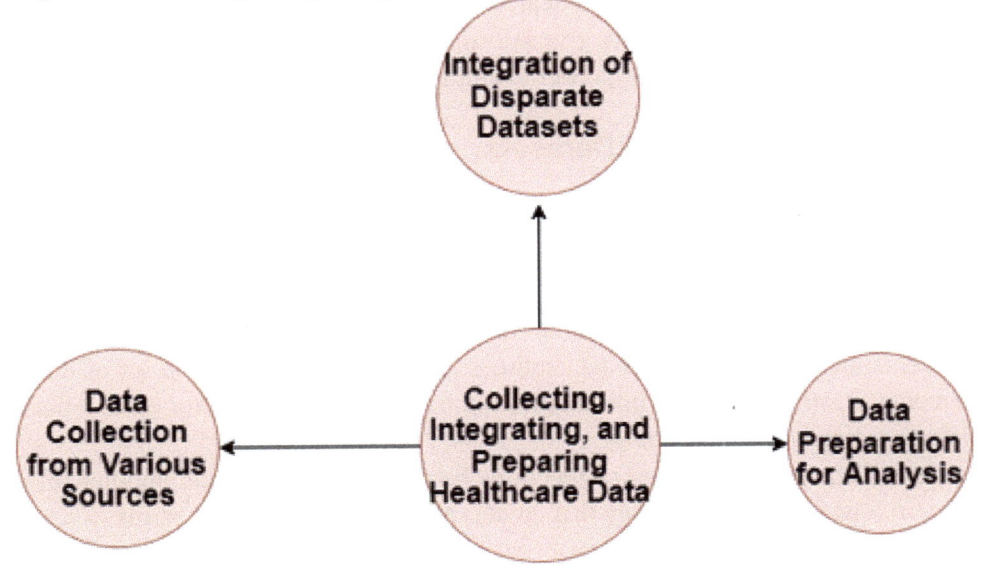

Data Collection from Various Sources

Electronic Health Records (EHR): Gathering data from Electronic Health Record systems that include patients' history, diagnoses, prescribed medications, laboratory results, and treatments. The integration of CDS with EHR systems makes patient data readily available mirroring the actual state leading to early interferential patterns and decision-making.

Medical Imaging Systems: Storing of medical images produced by imaging equipment for instance PACS (Picture Archiving and Communication Systems) including x-rays, MRIs, and CT scans. The implication of imaging data with other data will offer a holistic picture of a patient's health.

Remote Monitoring Devices: From wearable devices, IoT sensors, and M-Health apps that are commonly applied in telemedicine practice. Remote monitoring of the patient's condition allows monitoring of the vital signs, activity levels, and symptoms, which are useful especially when evaluating chronic diseases and signs of deteriorating conditions(Sudha et al 2023).

Genomic Sequencing Platforms: Obtaining Genome samples from Sequencing platforms to identify the genetic variations and mutations which are implicated in the occurrence of diseases and also in utilization of medicines. It also combines genomic information with the patient's clinical history to present individualized treatments that correspond to the patient's genome.

Healthcare Claims and Billing Systems: Using claims and billing system reports for the identification of healthcare usage, costs, and reimbursement. There are different types of claims that give information about various factors including methods of health care delivery, cost of health care and revenue that is generated.

Integration of Disparate Datasets

Data Standardization: Converting data elements into similar formats, applying common language definitions and using unified structured coding schemes across diverse data sources.

Data Mapping and Transformation: Identifying similarities in terminology and semantics across multiple data sources to reconcile the common set of data elements. Restructuring the information into similar registers and/or eliminating differences in data representation.

Data Linkage: Identifying connections between one dataset and another that concern related entities in a way that creates affiliations of different items of data (for instance, patient data, laboratory results, imagery). Accurate data linking and quality to avoid occurrence of issues in the subsequent data analysis.

Data Governance and Privacy: The policies and procedures that will be utilized in planning, organizing, acquiring, storing and disseminating health care data. HIPAA or other similar legislations and patient's right to privacy and data protection.

Data Preparation for Analysis:

Data Cleaning and Preprocessing: Data preprocessing and cleaning as a step of removing invalid and/or incomplete data values and correcting them through techniques like imputation, outlier detection and data validation. Preprocessing data to filter noise, or/and to prepare variables for analysis, or to change the format of the data to be suitable for the analysis.

Feature Engineering: Featuring the process of choosing and designing features (variables) from the input raw data to achieve better model performance and better data analysis interpretability(Sudha et al., 2024). The common feature engineering techniques includes dimensionality reduction, feature scaling and creating new composite features form the existing features.

Data Splitting: Splinting the data set into the training, developing, and testing set in a manner that would allow for the measuring of the performance of the model as well as its capability to generalize. Partitioning of data in such a manner that the number of samples within a class are evenly distributed across the subsets of the data set.

Data Augmentation Creating new samples if the amount of useful data is insufficient, necessary when training a deep learning algorithm (Maharana et al., 2022).

STANDARDIZING AND ENSURING QUALITY OF HEALTHCARE DATASETS

Healthcare data has to be standardized to some extent because without this, interchangeability and thus the trustworthiness of analysis are impossible. If data elements in health informatics are not standardized, it becomes very difficult to integrate different databases which are essential for the proper running of the health systems. This section looks into the approaches of maintaining quality of the datasets by examining issues such as standardized terminologies and code sets, data cleansing and validation procedures.

Importance of Data Standardization

Data standardization is essential for the following reasons:

Interoperability: Allows for interoperability between various forms of healthcare systems and applications and the processing of the data.

Consistency: It allows maintaining the consistency in the data representation that is mandatory for data analysis and data reporting activities.

Quality and Reliability: Minimizing or eliminating errors and variability, therefore improving the standard quality, and credibility of the health care information.

Figure 3. Standardizing and Ensuring Quality of Healthcare Datasets

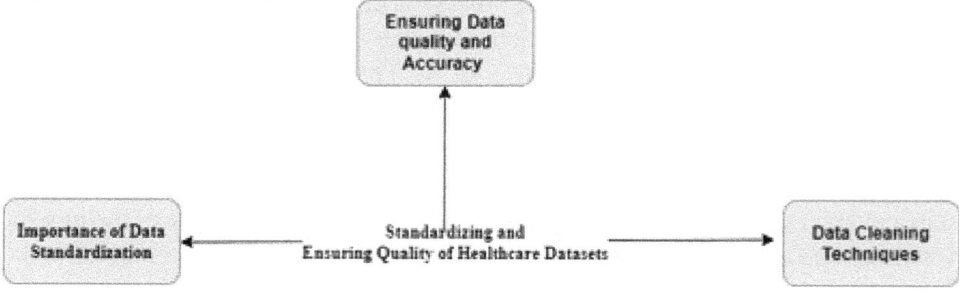

Data Cleaning Techniques

Data cleaning is an essential process of healthcare data preparation for analysis since such data possess all the typical features of big data. It is the process of finding and converting data inconsistencies and errors in the data gathering tool. Key techniques include:

Data Validation: Make sure you are formatting your data accurately which should match the structure that is required. Check that result of calculations meets the predefined criteria for numbers. It should also be noted that for different pairs of related fields, some sort of logical coherence must be maintained (for example, a patient's age and his date of birth).

Handling Missing Data: Imputing missing values by comparing statistic values such as the mean and putting the estimated value instead of the missing one. Excluding records or fields which are likely to contain large amount of missing data that would skew the analysis.

Removing Duplicates: Eliminating repeat records so that proper record linkage is achieved to avoid instances of repeated records on the same patients.

Outlier Detection: Searching for suspicious values that could be the result of particular errors, or conditions that occur rarely and therefore need to be explored further.

Data Transformation: Transforming data into a unified schema (e. g., normalizing numerical values, capitalizing [to lower or upper] letters).

Ensuring Data quality and Accuracy

Data Profiling: Explaining and comparing methods of how one dataset relates to another to identify sources of variation. This includes looking at the distribution of scores, learning about outliers, and checking the data for gaps and accuracy.

Data Quality Frameworks: Starting up exhaustive frameworks that state parameters of quality like accuracy, completeness, consistency or timeliness, validity, and so on. Some of the standards are as follows; ISO 8000 and the Data Management Association (DAMA).

Automated Data Quality Tools: Leveraging predefined software solutions for evaluating and enhancing data quality tasks. Some of the tools that can be used to carry out these tasks include data profiling, cleansing, monitoring, and more.

Validation Protocols: Establishing rigorous protocols for data validation, including:

Automated Validation: Automated scanning by algorithms and software to detect typical mistakes in structure of data.

Manual Review: When it comes to specific fields and comparable symbols across different systems, manually checking the key figures.

Cross Validation: Mapping data sets used in the different sources in a position to make comparisons and come up with paradoxes.

Standard Operating Procedures (SOPs): The formation of operational guidelines that will enable the gathering, recording, and analysis of data to assure that quality data is attained.

Training and Education: Conducting training sessions and regular updates of the healthcare staff on the need to improve the quality of data and how it can be achieved in terms of entry and use. Lastly, having a clear conception of how compliance should be managed and the performance of duties by all the personnel, is also pertinent.

PREDICTIVE MODELING FOR PATIENT OUTCOME FORECASTS

Healthcare predictive modeling is the use of statistical analysis and AI algorithms to forecast patient's status using past and current information. By view of understanding the various co-relations and patterns in the data, it becomes possible to use predictive models in determining patterns of disease development, probability of readmission, various aspects of treatment response, and even the prognosis. This section elaborates on multiple predictive models, their uses, and advantages for supporting clinical decisions.

Various Predictive Models

Regression Models

Linear Regression: Employed when the dependent variable is a continuous natured variable. For instance, the model would be used in estimating a patient's blood pressure given his or her age, weight, and other aspects of their daily lives.

Logistic Regression: Employed in situation where the solution is in two categories, for example estimating whether a certain disease will develop in a certain patient or not(Patel et al 2023).

Decision Trees and Random Forests

Decision Trees: An example of a model that divides data into branches to make decisions based on the input data features. It's explainable and beneficial in the contexts where understanding the decision process is substantial(Kamala et al 2023).

Random Forests: A collection of decision trees that decreases the risk of overfitting by averaging the forecast outcome of different trees for higher precision.

Support Vector Machines (SVM): To classify data such as disease diagnosis by using imaging data, the SVMs look for the best hyperplane that would split the data into different classes(Behera et al 2023).

Neural Networks and Deep Learning

Neural Networks: In this case the networks are made up of nodes and the nodes are connected with one another in a way that can represent intricate dependencies. Employed in uses like identification of objects in a picture, for example in x rays(Kumar et al 2022).

Deep Learning: However, multiple layer neural networks such as the convolutional neural networks for images or recurrent neural networks for time series data are very efficient in handling very large data(Yamini, B et al 2023).

Bayesian Networks: A class of models based on representing variables and their dependencies with a directed graph that is acyclic and is used to conduct risk analysis as well as to predict the outcome of treatment.

Clustering and Dimensionality Reduction

Clustering: Categorizing similar values, for instance, categorizing different patients with a similar disease.

Dimensionality Reduction: For example, Principal Component Analysis (PCA) is a technique that helps to decrease the number of attributes in a set, but which maintains the greatest amount of valuable information about the original set, in order to facilitate the analysis and increase the efficiency of models(Reddy et al 2020).

Applications in Predicting Patient Outcomes

Disease Progression: In predictive models, explicit details about an individual's medical history, genetics, and behaviors can also indicate when a patient with chronic diseases like diabetes, heart disease or cancer might reach their next stage in the illness cycle. This makes it possible to initiate some measures that may help to hinder the progress of the diseases and, thus, enhance the quality of life in patients.

Patient Readmissions: From the models, it is possible to determine which patients are likely to be readmitted back to the hospital within the first month after discharge, for instance, 30 days after discharge. This allows the healthcare provider to make provision for the resources to be used in followups for cases and precautionary measures against the same resulting in decreased readmission and the costs associated with it.

Treatment Responses: This means that the degrees of effectiveness of chosen treatments regarding the patient's genetic profile, previous treatments, and age, for example, can be predicted. This plan increases effectiveness of treatment, and minimizes such problems as allergic reactions, side effects, etc.

CLINICAL DECISION SUPPORT SYSTEMS USING AI AND ML

Clinical decision support systems (CDSS) can be characterized as the implementation of AI and ML in the healthcare domain in order to afford the healthcare authorities the best decisions concerning a patient's treatment. To this effect, this section explores the design of the CDSS, as well as its implementation on the diagnosis accuracy, treatment planning, and patient safety. CDSS incorporate AI and ML approaches to assess extensive data of the patient, available literature, and clinical protocols to offer the recommendation to practitioners. These systems are meant to support clinical decision making by giving real-time information, warnings, and or recommendations to practitioners at the place of service. CDSS entails a combination of several data inputs including EHRs, radiology images, laboratory data, and the patient's demographics. Ontology, NLP, deep learning, and machine learning are used to work through relevant and pertinent data to obtain clinically relevant phenomena and designs, analyse bets and worst-case scenarios, and create the best treatment plan possible. However, it can be seen that integration of CDSS in any healthcare setting depends on the proper integration to the existing system and workflow. Ease of use, compatibility with EHRs and CDSs and incorporation into clinical reasoning are key aspects to consider. Also, the accuracy, reliability, and timeliness of recommendations are critical to achieving a clinician's acceptance and approval.

The impact of CDSS on healthcare delivery is profound, with numerous benefits observed across various domains:

Improving Diagnostic Accuracy: CDSS's supports clinicians by assisting with accurate and timely patient diagnosis, patient clinical information, working differential diagnoses, and suggested appropriate diagnostic tests based on evidence-based information.

Enhancing Treatment Planning: CDSS helps the clinician to derive pertinent information and patient data, patient preferences, and the medical literature to formulate treatment plans relevant to the patient and the standard protocols. This results in enhanced treatment plans that are efficient and effective in meeting the patients' needs.

Optimizing Patient Safety: CDSS minimise the risk of medical mistakes and adverse occurrences since they remind the clinician of potential drug interaction or allergy or contraindication or any suboptimal approach to the clinical decision-making process. This plays a vital role in boosting patient safety with a view of minimizing the risk of harm.

Facilitating Evidence Based Practice: CDSS sees to it that the decisions in patient care are made based on the current evidence, guideline and/or best practice, hence, becoming a tool that supports the practice of EBM.

OPTIMIZING HEALTHCARE OPERATIONS WITH AI ALGORITHMS:

Artificial Intelligence (AI) algorithms hold the potential of adding value to the organization of the healthcare institution in the areas of administrative core processes, resources management and operation processes. This part emphasizes that most AI systems are applied to scheduling, inventory, and operational logistics to demonstrate the transformative nature of healthcare technologies.

Scheduling Optimization: Automated scheduling algorithms facilitate the appointment, surgeries, and resource optimization for the healthcare institutions. These algorithms take into account the patients' choice of provider, and clinicians' timetable, and available resources to give the best schedule and wait time. One of the uses of Machine Learning models is predicting the future demand of appointment slots based on past data and patient flow this will help in determining the required number of staff in the health facility(Nithya et al 2023). Scheduling management through AI decreases the time patients spend waiting for professional assistance, increases the effectiveness of the resources and, ultimately, contributes to patients' satisfaction.

Figure 4. Optimizing Healthcare Operations with AI Algorithms

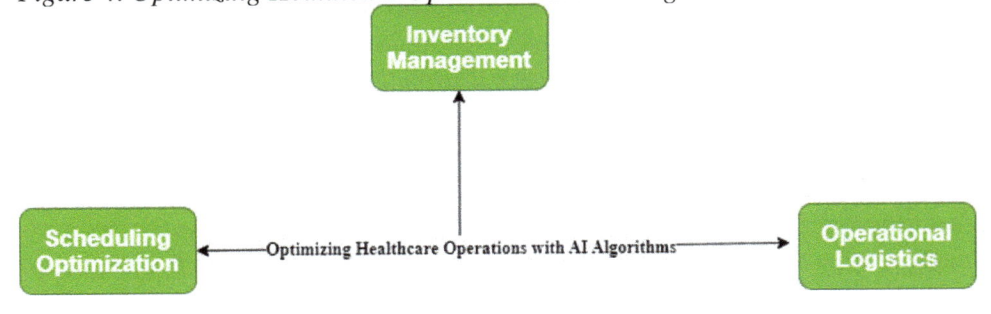

Inventory Management: AI facilitated smart inventory technologies enhance the acquisition, receipt, storage and issuance of medicines, consumables, and relative instruments in medical organizations. It also involves the use of analytics in determining the forecasted demand, a real time tracking of the inventory and ordering of stocks. Such, Machine Learning decides how much material to order by evaluating previous user consumption trends, suppliers' delivery times and additional factors, such as seasons to avoid stockouts or overstock conditions. Compared to the old methods of supply management, AI driven inventory management systems make effective usage of the supplies to cut expenses and heighten productivity.

Operational Logistics: They include automated transportation systems, delivery systems, and supply chain management that adds efficiency to the running of the health facilities. These algorithms help to find the best route for a transport used for the transportation of patients, management of supply chain and transportation of required and available resources in different healthcare facilities efficiently. Decision Making processes use data from collected information on traffic flow, current weather, and data obtained from previous feedback to adapt transport way plans and schedules accordingly, in order to avoid congestions and efficiently use recourses.

USING SIMULATION FOR OPERATIONAL EFFICIENCY

Capacity Planning: AI improves simulation models by incorporating dynamic variables that adapt the model as the computer receives data inputs to alter the way capacity is planned for the needs of a specific business to overcome current challenges in the ever changing market. It also helps in the early preparation for changes, to enable healthcare facilities maximize patient throughput without compromising on service delivery.

Emergency Response: Models of emergency management with subjects' model different emergency circumstances, for instance, emergencies resulting from natural disasters, mass incidences of casualties, or outbreaks of infectious diseases, to test different measures of preparedness and response. Such models evaluate the outcomes of emergency procedures, resource distribution, and best practices, as well as the emergency evacuation plans in reducing the hazards and impacts on patient service. Reinforcement learning and predictive modeling enhance the outcome of the emergency response by analysing the data obtained and giving recommendations regarding organization of the work, employee's distribution, as well as the patient's transfer during the emergencies. This makes the healthcare organizations to be in a safer position of improving their preparedness since they will experience few disruptions in the times of calamities.

Optimization of Patient Flow: Patient flow simulation models replicate the flow of patients in a health care centre from the stages of emergency departments, to operating rooms, and inpatient care departments. These models point out the problem areas, delays and the areas of transformative nature regarding patient flow processes. AI scheduling can adapt to workload fluctuations by making changes to the patient appointments and resource assignments at the same time. KPIs encompassing predictive analytics and optimization to quicken the patient's throughput as well as to reduce waiting times reflecting on the high efficiency of simulation models based on AI, which in its turn elevates patient and clinician satisfaction levels.

ANALYSING POPULATION HEALTH TRENDS WITH AI

Population health analyzed through Big Data empowers AI tools as assisting healthcare professionals to find patterns in big data to support public health administration. This section expands on the ways of utilising artificial intelligence in the monitoring of disease trends, in determining the health status of communities, and in the evaluating of health intervention programmes hence demonstrating the usefulness of the AI technology in the formation of preventive public health strategies.

Tracking Disease Outbreaks: AIdriven predictive modeling and data analytics can tend in real-time various form of data such as EHRs, syndromic surveillance systems, social media and environment data to identify outbreak of diseases. The implemented Machine Learning functions analyse patterns in the Health data and detect preliminary signs of an outbreak that, in turn, initiate precautionary actions. Other techniques in NLP can also make it easier to analyse other unstructured information such as news articles and trends in social media as far as potential threats to health are concerned(Pajila, P. et al 2023). AI capable epidemic modeling recreates the transmission pattern of contagious diseases amongst the population to help the authorities to determine the severity of an epidemic, and systematically distribute the appropriate treatment and prevent the spread of the disease.

Assessing Community Health Needs: AI helps in processing large-scale population data for the evaluation of the general health status and inequalities. Demographic data, health surveys, environmental factors, or social determinants of health, in combination with AI, define risky groups of the population and zones that require further medical care. Big data tools and models estimate prospective health conditions and impacts of diseases in the population; therefore, healthcare systems and regulatory authorities can effectively manage available resources, design interventions, and prioritize prevention programs focusing on the most vulnerable population.

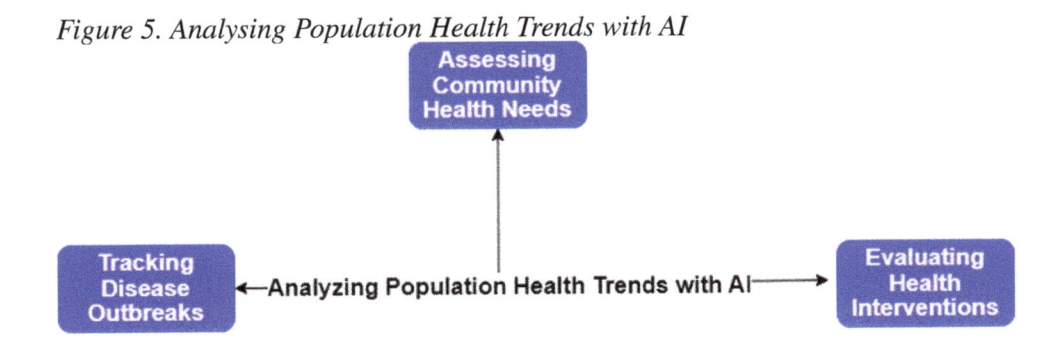

Figure 5. Analysing Population Health Trends with AI

Evaluating Health Interventions: AI driven evaluation methods look at the impact of health interventions and polices by analysing the statistical data of the large population. Machine Learning models compute the differences between interventional and control groups, determine associations and find out relative effects of interventions on health consequences. Qualitative data including patient and clinician narratives, as well as public health agency reports, are processed using NLP methods pertaining to the perceived efficacy and acceptability by target population groups. Realising the value of AI from the perspective of predictive modeling, it reduces the time taken for the assessment of population health outcomes in the future, as impacted by the interventions, which helps in grounding evidences for decision making and policy planning.

DETECTING FRAUD AND ANOMALIES WITH AI

In the healthcare industry, fraud and anomaly identification is important when it comes to the maintenance of accurate billing records, patient confidentiality, and compliance with set regulations. Applying innovation in data analytics such as machine learning in healthcare helps the organization to detect outlaws or outliers in billing and clinical data so that fraudulent cases are not allowed while following the set rules and regulations at the same time(Kapadiya et al 2022).

Fraud Detection: AI professionals use data mining on billing information such as claims, coding, and billing history to detect outliers associated with fraud. The rationale behind machine learning models is that they are developed to learn from previous experiences thereby identifying fraudulent activities and improving the performance of the system with new and different fraud schemes. The common strategies like anomaly detection, pattern analysis, and pattern forecasting methods are used to identify dubious claims.

Anomaly Detection: Historical clinical data analysis methods employed anomaly detection which is the use of AI to determine value that is out of the norm. This includes identifying any changes in the behavior of patients, any change in the way treatments is administered, and any shifts in the patient's clinical indicators. Machine learning based algorithms work on EHRs, medical image data and other clinical big data and datasets to detect suspicious activity, missed errors/developments and other possible fraudulent cases. Therefore, it is agreed that through identification of outliers, AI assists the healthcare providers to prevent adverse events that may harm the patient.

AI FOR REVENUE CYCLE MANAGEMENT IN HEALTHCARE

RCM stands for Revenue Cycle Management and is the overall concept of the services referring to the processes of billing and claims along with reimbursement in the healthcare sector. RCM has lots of potentials that can be portrayed through Artificial Intelligence (AI) technologies. This section presents how AI driven RCM has impacted on the reduction of administrative costs while enhancing the financial performance.

Automating Billing Processes: AI-based billing solutions include features of claim creation, coding, and submission, which help decrease the load on the healthcare personnel. The NLP algorithms are used to identify the necessary data to billed from the clinical documentation with the efficiency and speed. Machine Learning models used in billing history to find appropriate patterns for prediction and forecasting revenues. In general, by creating solutions for billing AI makes work faster, gets paid faster, and has fewer errors.

Improving Claim Accuracy: It involves the use of AI algorithms to search for the coding mistakes, billing anomalies, as well as methods of non-compliance. These algorithms highlight areas of doubt to potential inaccuracy hence mitigating on probable claim denials, rejections and revenue loss. Techniques of the NLP help in proper coding and amendment of missed errant notes on the physician's narrative and/or medical record to improve the accuracy in claims besides compliance with the set coding standards.

Optimizing Reimbursement Rates: Another type of analytics leveraging AI in health care is the one that focuses on the payer side; the analytics studies payer data, reimbursement patterns, contract terms, and aims at maximizing reimbursement rates and improving payer contracts. Analysing of patterns recognizes areas of possible increased reimbursement and avoidable revenues loss by using predictive modeling. Analysing Payer behaviour, claim denial and reimbursement data, Machine Learning calculations look for revenue enhancements. With an improved reimbursement rates AI improves the financial standing and revenue accuracy for the health care systems.

Benefits of AI driven RCM

Increased Efficiency: All in one, the operational efficiency is achieved due to the minimization of redundant paperwork in billing by the integration of AI to do the same.

Enhanced Accuracy: This results in increase in claim first pass ratify by correcting coding mistakes, compliance with guidelines and billing to decrease claim denials and loss of revenue.

Optimized Reimbursement: Analytics enabled by AIdriven improve reimbursement, provide insights into revenue sources, and secure better payer contracts; consequently, enhancing revenue and performance.

Reduced Administrative Burdens: In part, AI improves billing function and efficiency activities that used to occupy a lot of the health care staff engagements and leave those to the machines so that health care staff can attend to patients as well as other organizational key activities.

Improved Financial Performance: AIdriven RCM helps keep revenue integrity intact, reduces revenue leakage, and optimizes reimbursement rate and in effect contributes to improved financial position and therefore sustainability of health facilities.

DEVELOPING AI POWERED PATIENT ENGAGEMENT PLATFORMS

A patient engagement system that employs AI would be considered a technological innovation in the field of healthcare for a number of reasons such as its ability to provide targeted communication, education and emotional support to patients. This section discusses the existence and effects of these platforms on patients' compliance, satisfaction, and outcome.

Personalized Communication: Most AI-facilitated patient engagement automotive programs incorporate NLP and machine learning models to process patient information, communication patterns, and demographics. EDM tools are innovative, digital media platforms that provide timely, relevant and targeted messages, reminders or other forms of learning to patients. Through the integration of the AI, patient engagement platforms can morph the communication channels depending on the patients' responses, activity, and trends. The use of this technique results in better build-up of the patient-provider relationship, as well as conferring the advantage of improved communication.

Education and Support: Patient portals that are AIdriven provide patients with data, facts, documents, and instruments that enable them to enhance their health literacy. These platforms rely on artificial intelligence to filter through all the available information related to a particular disease and also to answer the questions patients may have and even recommend a particular course of treatment or a particular prescription medication or a particular change of diet. To optimize the content, ease of use and efficiency, the patient's interaction and the feedback given by them are taken into consideration by the machine learning algorithms. Since the identified educational materials are customised to personal Patient data, AI-based solutions improve patient knowledge, assertion, as well as disease self-control.

Impact on Patient Adherence and Satisfaction: Digital technologies particularly using Artificial intelligence enhances medication compliance, appointment attendance, and follow-up by generating and providing patient-tailored reminder and support messages. These platforms help patients assume more responsibilities in their recovery and ensure that they are following the regime given by their doctors. Thus, AIdriven platforms contribute to promoting patient satisfaction and building its trust in the healthcare provider offering timely assistance and feedback. Lack of patient engagement and neglect of patients' needs leads to patient dissatisfaction and non-loyalty to the healthcare organization.

REMOTE PATIENT MONITORING WITH WEARABLES AND IOT

Wearable technology and IoT with remote and artificial intelligence with patient monitoring is a revolutionary advancement in patient care delivery. In this section, the writer examines the technologies used, their uses in the management of chronic diseases, and the prospect of improving patients' care through their monitoring and timely follow-ups.

Wearable Devices and IoT Connectivity: Smartwatches, fitness trackers, and medical sensors, record real-time physiological information about the heart rate, blood pressure, activity, and detecting biometrics. These devices interface directly with the Internet of Things (IoT) to relay information to cloud based systems, and to the healthcare providers' systems for further compilation and analysis(Poongodi et al 2020).

AI Analytics and Insights: Artificial intelligence patterns the streaming datasets obtained from the wearable equipment to discover patterns, trends, and abnormalities in patient's vital statistics. Some of these algorithms can point out when a patient has moved from his normal level of functioning and risk potential so that early signs of illness can be given. Specifically, Machine Learning models analyse data about the previous cases and patients' outcomes to design the individual patient characteristics and health condition-based monitoring thresholds, alerts, and interferences.

Applications in Chronic Disease Management: Wearable technology and IoT in remote patient monitoring are useful in many chronic illnesses such as diabetes, hypertension, cardiology cases, and respiratory diseases. Closely controlled observation of these physiological markers along with the patient's medication and life style compliance helps the healthcare professionals to identify potential decompensation indicators, enhance the compliance to treatment regimens and thereby prevent the deterioration and hospitalizations.

Potential Benefits

Early Detection of Health Changes: This way, changes in the patients' state are identified on time and necessary measures are taken: interventions and preventive actions.

Personalized Care: This results in the provision of patient-specific analytics for surveillance and the use of further specific intercessory interventions depending on the health status of patients and their individual characteristics.

Improved Patient Engagement: Remote monitoring puts patients in charge of their treatment /care and therefore increases patients' engagement, compliance and responsibility.

Enhanced Clinical Efficiency: The remote patient monitoring has been described to improve the healthcare delivery model since long yearly face to face visits are not necessary, resources are utilized efficiently, and focus is given to patients who need attention.

PERSONALIZATION TREATMENT USING AI AND GENOMICS

The combination of AI with genomics has changed the concept of precision medicine since patients can be treated according to their gene makeup. This section looks at the evolution of precision medicines, how artificial intelligence is used in genomic studies as well as the future impact that precision medicines will have on personal health care.

Advancements in Precision Medicine: Precision medicine is a medical model seeking to develop appropriate treatments and prevention strategies in consideration with the patient's genetics, surrounding environment and personalized habits. Modern techniques in genomics have favored the recognition of genomic biomarkers that relate to diseases, drugs, and patients' outcomes to allow for custom synthesizing systems.

Role of AI in Genomic Analysis: Deep learning technologies are also utilized in the assessment of large-scale genomic data to find out relations and correlations between genetic markers and clinical manifestations. Using Machine Learning algorithms, we can determine the associated genes relevant to a patient's disease susceptibility, therapeutic course, and survival, which can aid in the delivery of tailored care and intervention plans(Subramanian et al 2024).

Implications for Tailored Healthcare Interventions: That can help achieve effective therapies and exclude or minimize side effects and toxicity because the results of the treatment depend on substances' interaction with patient's genes. Predictive modeling based on AI can identify individual patient response to particular treatments and therefore allow clinicians to select the most effective treatment for every patient. Over personalised healthcare solutions using genomic profiling have the potential of improving patients' quality and reducing the costs of healthcare.

Benefits of Personalized Treatment Using AI and Genomics

Improved Treatment Efficacy: Treatments that are personalized to a patient's tremendous genomic profile are in a better position of eradicating diseases and its causes because they are targeting that specific cause.

Reduced Adverse Reactions: Through not using drugs and therapies that are ineffective due to the patients' genetic makeup, time-honored approaches can lower the likelihood of negative side effects and therapy failures.

Enhanced Patient Satisfaction: Primary healthcare approaches that target patients' genetic characteristics increase patient satisfaction and their level of participation in the healthcare process.

Advancements in Healthcare Innovation: AI-facilitated genomic analysis is a key factor defining the advancement of IM, as it fast-tracks the discovery of new therapies and diagnostics, and prevention opportunities.

EVALUATING HEALTHCARE QUALITY WITH AI

In the area of evaluating the quality of healthcare services, AI plays a role of powerful instrument for analysing such values as clinical effectiveness, patients' satisfaction, and organizational performance. The following part focuses on the techniques applied to aspire the quality of healthcare services with the help of AI, as well as the potential to contribute to constant enhancement of the services provided.

Analysing Clinical Outcomes: Data scrutinizing clinical data such as patient admissions and history, laboratory values, and treatment efficacy, to evaluate the safety and efficacy of delivered treatment. Patient outcomes like readmissions, complications and mortality can also be predicted using Machine Learning models, in which the health workforce can track and examine specific aspects that require improvement to improve the patients' health status (Sudha et al 2024).

Incorporating Patient Feedback: Data mining driven sentiment analysis tools help measure the overall satisfactions of patients regarding healthcare services, patients feedback through survey or social media or any other platform to understand the weakness in delivering services. NLP models analyse patient feedback to identify relevant experiences, establishing the groundwork for health systems and medical facilities to address patient complaints and improve the patient satisfaction rate.

Monitoring Operational Metrics: Operational parameters like waiting time, patient appointments and usage of resources are constant under observation so that AI systems can facilitate efficient process flow of work and budgeted resources. The models use predictions on the number of patients in healthcare facilities in order to assist in the planning of resources, workforce and overall organization in order to make appropriate provisions to suit patient demands and needs.

Continuous Improvement in Care Delivery: Automatic quality promotion programs make it easier for healthcare organizations to examine the trend, pattern and ripple or lack of it in patient care delivery processes. Machine Learning algorithms use performance history data to recommend changes/process improvements, benchmarks, and science based interventions for increasing the quality of health care and the recoveries of the sufferers.

Benefits of Evaluating Healthcare Quality with AI

DataDriven Decision Making: AI helps healthcare providers to use big data for making decisions based on newest analytical tools and methods including data modeling.

Proactive Quality Improvement: Realtime quality assessment through AIdriven quality assessment will allow for the quicker identification of areas that require the application of targeted corrective measures to avoid the repetition of errors that may negatively impact patient care or organizational effectiveness.

Enhanced Patient Experience: Through AI, data from patient feedback can be used to understand patients' needs, address grievances, develop communication strategies and elicit means of crafting services to fit patient needs.

Optimized Resource Allocation: Analysing real-time key performance indicators in healthcare is crucial since it enables organization leaders to avail prescriptive strategies to rectify inefficient resource utilization, staffing, and workflow procedures in service delivery and patient satisfaction.

ETHICAL AND PRIVACY CONSIDERATIONS IN AI HEALTHCARE

Adoption of Artificial Intelligence (AI) in healthcare system exposes some serious ethical and privacy aspects which cannot be ignored. The following section explores controversies in AI including; data privacy and consent, problem of bias in AI algorithms, as well as AI ethics and the use of AI in clinical practice, with a view of offering guidelines on how to utilize AI responsibly.

Data Privacy: In healthcare data, patients' health information comprising a variety of details such as medical history, treatments, and genetic makeup is stored and transmitted. The patient's data and information also cannot be shared with others without permission or allowed to be accessed by unwanted or unauthorized individuals and this is where the regulations like the Health Insurance Portability and Accountability Act (HIPAA) comes in to play. Security must always be used, along with encryption and access control to maintain the protection of patient data from hackers and other malicious threats.

Informed Consent: Health consumers have certain rights such as the right to receive information on the use of AI systems in their care and make an informed decision on data collection, analysis, and utilization. AI integrated healthcare delivery systems must be transparent which means providers must have patients' permission before implementing AI systems in care delivery. Any patient participating in clinical decision-making accompanied by AI algorithms should be told how these algorithms will be deployed, the opportunities and threats involved, and the patient's rights to privacy and data protection.

Bias in AI Algorithms: Bias of algorithms can be present in the datasets the AI algorithms were trained on or in the design of these algorithms, and therefore, there might be variations in the effectiveness of their healthcare interventions across the spectrum of minorities and the rest of the population. New techniques in AI also carry with them certain biases which should be acknowledged and eliminated to provide for fair treatment of patients. Thus, bias ought to be prevented by the detection of bias, utilizing diversity of training data and algorithmic transparency in healthcare applying AI solutions.

Ethical Use of AI in Clinical Settings: AI systems used in clinical settings must follow ethical guidelines, standards and/or the law in how they are implemented and used. It becomes the role of healthcare providers to ensure that such decisions relate to medical ethics, patient health, and the acceptable practice of professional integrity. Informing, being accountable, and the general principle of explainability are major rules in the ethical handling of AI in healthcare. Professionals in the health sector must also be in a position to comprehend, assess, and explain AIdriven suggestions and conclusions to patients and legal bodies.

Guidelines for Responsible AI Implementation: Promote transparency in AI and explicate the decision making AI models that are at use. Ensure that patient's privacy and protection of their data is well enhanced in AIdriven health care systems. Risk assessments and ethical reviews must be conducted before the integration of AI solutions in clinical settings before they are utilized. Also, the recommendations include developing strategies for continuous assessment and verification of AI solutions with regards to ethical and legal frameworks. Strengthen collaboration among different specialists and involve potential users in decision making while delivering AI in healthcare.

EMERGING TRENDS IN HEALTHCARE AI

This paper aims to identify the existing trends in Artificial Intelligence (AI) and advance in the healthcare industry. This section focuses on ongoing trends, future prospects of artificial intelligence in the healthcare field; new developments in AI investigations and applications, legal changes and the general disputed growth of AI technologies in the sphere of healthcare.

Advancements in AI Research: Scientists are trying to use new orientations in AI including deep learning, reinforcement learning and federated learning to solve some healthcare issues like diagnostics, drugs finding, and treatment options. Multi-disciplinary engagements between scientific researchers of AI, clinicians and biomedical experts are engaging in the development new approaches in health care AI, therefore increasing the realization of precision medicine, health care prediction and precision health care delivery.

New Applications of AI in Healthcare: AI is investing in its presence in different sectors of healthcare, such as telemedicine, digital health, remote patient monitoring, and virtual care. New Areas where AI is being used involves using AI to generate population health management forecasts, using robotic systems that are AI enabled for surgical and rehabilitation purposes and using virtual assistants that are also AI based for clinic decision making as well as patient interaction.

Integration of AI with Other Technologies: AI is also convergence with other advanced technologies like Genomics, Blockchain and Internet of Things (IoT) to create a more systemic and data-driven system in delivering health care. Integrated wearable devices with artificial intelligence, direct to consumer (DTC) genetic testing and electronic health records (EHRs) are being used to provide people with an individualised and proactive approach to disease prevention and management.

Focus on Interoperability and Data Sharing: Patients and healthcare providers are focused on appropriate communication and data exchange schemes to adopt AI systems within the existing infrastructures of health care systems. There is an ongoing process of harmonizing the data format aimed at creating integration platforms and the data management system that protects the data and enhances its ethical use in healthcare innovation under the AIdriven contexts.

Ethical and Societal Implications: There is a recent emphasis on the values, moral, social, and fairness for AI solutions in the healthcare industry, where decisions are facilitated by AI technologies, the data privacy issue, and the problem of an algorithm's potential prejudice. This means that the stakeholders are in conversations on how to provide fairness, accountability, transparency, and inclusion in healthcare AI applications and are desperate for AI that is well-developed and implemented.

CONCLUSION

Overall, it is important to note that the application of AI and ML in healthcare is a significant paradigm shift that may revolutionize the field. These technologies will be capable of improving decisions and lots of operations and even the way they deliver health care services to patients. Thus, it can be stated that it is important to utilize AI and ML in healthcare systems to improve their performance, productivity, and, consequently, the health of patients. It is demonstrable that there is a massive field of practical application of AI and ML technologies in the sphere of health care delivery and patient care. Through the adoption of big data computational solutions and data analysis techniques, probabilities, essences and tendencies relating to healthcare can be approached in an efficient way, by helping those involved in the delivery of healthcare services make better decisions with regard to organisational structure and patient care. In addition, advancement of AI and ML continues and creates prospects for enhancement of improvement of the healthcare system. While new approaches and use cases are discovered, new rules and regulations are developed, and the stakeholders work on solving the ethical and especially the privacy issues, the opportunities are huge when it comes to the improvement of the healthcare systems. Overall, it's evident that AI and ML can indeed become the catalyst for the shift in the healthcare system to a patient-centered efficient, and effective model of care delivery. Thus, adopting these technologies and the progressive development of their potential, the healthcare sector can open new opportunities to change the idea of patient care and the practice of medicine under modern conditions. Therefore, the adoption of AI and ML in developing the healthcare systems will remain an important force and milestone for change and improvement in the future.

REFERENCES

Anita, M., Ambhika, C., & Anish, T. P. (2024). Exploring the Landscape of Artificial Intelligence in Healthcare Applications. In AI Healthcare Applications and Security, Ethical, and Legal Considerations (pp. 29-48). IGI Global.

Behera, M. P., Sarangi, A., Mishra, D., & Sarangi, S. K. (2023). A hybrid machine learning algorithm for heart and liver disease prediction using modified particle swarm optimization with support vector machine. *Procedia Computer Science*, 218, 818–827. DOI: 10.1016/j.procs.2023.01.062

Bohr, A., & Memarzadeh, K. (2020). The rise of artificial intelligence in healthcare applications. In *Artificial Intelligence in healthcare* (pp. 25–60). Academic Press. DOI: 10.1016/B978-0-12-818438-7.00002-2

Kamala, S. P. R., Gayathri, S., Pillai, N. M., Gracious, L. A., Varun, C. M., & Subramanian, R. S. (2023, July). Predictive Analytics for Heart Disease Detection: A Machine Learning Approach. In 2023 4th International Conference on Electronics and Sustainable Communication Systems (ICESC) (pp. 1583-1589). IEEE.

Kapadiya, K., Patel, U., Gupta, R., Alshehri, M. D., Tanwar, S., Sharma, G., & Bokoro, P. N. (2022). Blockchain and AI-empowered healthcare insurance fraud detection: An analysis, architecture, and future prospects. *IEEE Access : Practical Innovations, Open Solutions*, 10, 79606–79627. DOI: 10.1109/ACCESS.2022.3194569

Kesavaraj, G., & Sukumaran, S. (2013, July). A study on classification techniques in data mining. In 2013 fourth international conference on computing, communications and networking technologies (ICCCNT) (pp. 1-7). IEEE. DOI: 10.1109/ICCCNT.2013.6726842

Kishor, A., & Chakraborty, C. (2022). Artificial intelligence and internet of things based healthcare 4.0 monitoring system. *Wireless Personal Communications*, 127(2), 1615–1631. DOI: 10.1007/s11277-021-08708-5

Kumar, A., Rathor, K., Vaddi, S., Patel, D., Vanjarapu, P., & Maddi, M. (2022, August). ECG Based Early Heart Attack Prediction Using Neural Networks. In 2022 3rd International Conference on Electronics and Sustainable Communication Systems (ICESC) (pp. 1080-1083). IEEE. DOI: 10.1109/ICESC54411.2022.9885448

Liao, S. H., Chu, P. H., & Hsiao, P. Y. (2012). Data mining techniques and applications–A decade review from 2000 to 2011. *Expert Systems with Applications*, 39(12), 11303–11311. DOI: 10.1016/j.eswa.2012.02.063

Maharana, K., Mondal, S., & Nemade, B. (2022). A review: Data pre-processing and data augmentation techniques. *Global Transitions Proceedings*, 3(1), 91–99. DOI: 10.1016/j.gltp.2022.04.020

Nithya, T., Kumar, V. N., Gayathri, S., Deepa, S., Varun, C. M., & Subramanian, R. S. (2023, August). A comprehensive survey of machine learning: Advancements, applications, and challenges. In *2023 Second International Conference on Augmented Intelligence and Sustainable Systems (ICAISS)* (pp. 354-361). IEEE. DOI: 10.1109/ICAISS58487.2023.10250547

Pajila, P. B., Sudha, K., Selvi, D. K., Kumar, V. N., Gayathri, S., & Subramanian, R. S. (2023, July). A Survey on Natural Language Processing and its Applications. In 2023 4th International Conference on Electronics and Sustainable Communication Systems (ICESC) (pp. 996-1001). IEEE.

Patel, R. K., Aggarwal, E., Solanki, K., Dahiya, O., & Yadav, S. A. (2023, April). A Logistic Regression and Decision Tree Based Hybrid Approach to Predict Alzheimer's Disease. In *2023 International Conference on Computational Intelligence and Sustainable Engineering Solutions (CISES)* (pp. 722-726). IEEE.

Poongodi, T., Krishnamurthi, R., Indrakumari, R., Suresh, P., & Balusamy, B. (2020). Wearable devices and IoT. A handbook of Internet of Things in biomedical and cyber physical system, 245-273.

Reddy, G. T., Reddy, M. P. K., Lakshmanna, K., Kaluri, R., Rajput, D. S., Srivastava, G., & Baker, T. (2020). Analysis of dimensionality reduction techniques on big data. *IEEE Access : Practical Innovations, Open Solutions*, 8, 54776–54788. DOI: 10.1109/ACCESS.2020.2980942

Subramanian, R. S., Yamini, B., Sudha, K., & Sivakumar, S. (2024). Ensemble-based deep learning techniques for customer churn prediction model. *Kybernetes*. Advance online publication. DOI: 10.1108/K-08-2023-1516

Sudha, K., Ambhika, C., Maheswari, B., Girija, P., & Nalini, M. (2023). AI and IoT Applications in Medical Domain Enhancing Healthcare Through Technology Integration. In AI and IoT-Based Technologies for Precision Medicine (pp. 280-294). IGI Global.

Sudha, K., Balakrishnan, C., Anish, T. P., Nithya, T., Yamini, B., Subramanian, R. S., & Nalini, M. (2024). Data Insight Unveiled: Navigating Critical Approaches and Challenges in Diverse Domains Through Advanced Data Analysis. *Critical Approaches to Data Engineering Systems and Analysis*, 90-114.

Sudha, K., Lakshmipriya, C., Pajila, P. B., Venitha, E., & Anita, M. (2024, January). Enhancing Diabetes Prediction and Management through Machine Learning: A Comparative Study. In *2024 Fourth International Conference on Advances in Electrical, Computing, Communication and Sustainable Technologies (ICAECT)* (pp. 1-6). IEEE. DOI: 10.1109/ICAECT60202.2024.10468773

Yamini, B., Prasanna, V., Ambhika, C., M, A., Maheswari, B., R, S. S., & Nalini, M. (2023). A Comprehensive Survey of Deep Learning: Advancements, Applications, and Challenges. *International Journal on Recent and Innovation Trends in Computing and Communication*, 11(8s), 445–453. DOI: 10.17762/ijritcc.v11i8s.7225

Yamini, B., Sudha, K., Nalini, M., Kavitha, G., Subramanian, R. S., & Sugumar, R. (2023, June). Predictive Modelling for Lung Cancer Detection using Machine Learning Techniques. In 2023 8th International Conference on Communication and Electronics Systems (ICCES) (pp. 1220-1226). IEEE. DOI: 10.1109/ICCES57224.2023.10192648

Chapter 3

Leveraging AI and Machine Learning for Next-Generation Clinical Decision Support Systems (CDSS)

Uddalak Mitra
JIS College of Engineering, India

Shafiq Ul Rehman
https://orcid.org/0000-0003-2266-218X
Kingdom University, Bahrain

ABSTRACT

Missed diagnoses and medication errors are significant risks in healthcare, leading to increased patient morbidity and mortality. Traditional Clinical Decision Support Systems (CDSS) rely on static, predefined rules, limiting their adaptability to personalized patient care. This chapter explores how integrating Artificial Intelligence (AI) and Machine Learning (ML) can revolutionize CDSS, driving next-generation systems. By analyzing clinical datasets in real time, AI and ML enable personalized insights that enhance diagnostic accuracy, optimize treatment recommendations, improve risk stratification, and streamline workflows. These advancements promise better patient outcomes, informed clinical decisions, and reduced costs. The chapter also addresses challenges like data quality, explainability, regulatory compliance, and ethics, proposing strategies for overcoming these. Through collaboration and research, AI and ML can transform CDSS into foundational healthcare elements, fostering personalized, data-driven, and efficient patient care.

DOI: 10.4018/979-8-3693-7277-7.ch003

INTRODUCTION

In today's increasingly intricate and high-pressure healthcare environment, the consequences of missed diagnoses and medication errors are more severe and pervasive than ever before. These incidents are not just unfortunate occurrences; they represent critical failures within the healthcare system that can lead to significant and often irreversible patient harm, extended hospital stays, and, in the most tragic scenarios, loss of life (Newman-Toker et al., 2024, Newman-Toker, 2023; Ringer et al, 2023). According to the World Health Organization (WHO) (WHO, 2024), approximately 1 in 10 patients globally suffers harm during the course of their healthcare, resulting in over 3 million deaths each year due to unsafe healthcare practices. The situation is even direr in low- and middle-income countries, where the prevalence of harm escalates to 4 in every 100 individuals. Alarmingly, more than half of these adverse events are deemed preventable, with medication-related issues contributing significantly to the overall harm. In primary and ambulatory care settings, up to 40% of patients experience harm, with 80% of these incidents being avoidable (WHO, 2024). This includes a range of common and preventable challenges such as medication errors, unsafe surgical procedures, infections, diagnostic errors, and patient falls. The impact extends beyond the immediate and devastating human cost, affecting not only the individuals directly involved but also the broader healthcare system. The economic repercussions are substantial, with patient harm contributing to a reduction in global economic growth by approximately 0.7% annually (WHO, 2024). The indirect costs associated with these errors run into the trillions of dollars, underscoring the need for significant improvements in healthcare safety and efficacy.

Traditional Clinical Decision Support Systems (CDSS) have been instrumental in improving healthcare outcomes by providing structured recommendations based on established clinical guidelines. However, their effectiveness is often constrained by their reliance on static, rule-based algorithms that lack flexibility. These systems typically operate using pre-defined rules, which can become outdated as medical knowledge evolves or as patient conditions become more complex. As a result, traditional CDSS may offer generic, one-size-fits-all recommendations that fail to account for the individual nuances of each patient's health status. This limitation can hinder their ability to provide the most effective and personalized care (Chen et al, 2023; Teufel et al, 2021, Jović et al, 2022, Papadopoulos et al, 2022). The emergence of next-generation CDSS, driven by Artificial Intelligence (AI) and Machine Learning (ML), promises to overcome these limitations. Unlike their predecessors, AI and ML-powered CDSS are designed to be dynamic and adaptable. They leverage advanced algorithms that analyze vast amounts of data, including genetic profiles, lifestyle factors, and comprehensive medical histories, to offer more precise and personalized recommendations. For instance, instead of merely flagging potential drug interactions, these sophisticated systems can predict which patients are at a higher risk of adverse effects based on their unique health profiles. Moreover, AI and ML technologies enable CDSS to continuously learn and refine their recommendations in real-time, integrating new data and adapting to the rapidly evolving medical landscape. This ongoing learning process enhances the system's ability to provide timely and relevant insights, thereby significantly improving clinical decision-making and patient care. The transformative potential of AI and ML in healthcare is their ability to create intelligent and responsive systems that better meet the complex needs of individual patients.

This chapter explores the remarkable advancements in Clinical Decision Support Systems (CDSS) provided by Artificial Intelligence (AI) and Machine Learning (ML).This study examines the limitations inherent in traditional CDSS.Using real-life examples, we demonstrate how these systems fall short of meeting the nuanced needs of individuals.Although CDSS play an essential role in improving clinical decision-making, they are constrained by predefined rules and do not provide flexibility sufficient to adapt to changing information or diverse patient scenarios. Consequently, generic recommendations may fail to fully consider a patient's unique condition as a result of these limitations.

In addition, it discusses how AI and machine learning enable CDSS to process and analyze extensive datasets, recognize intricate patterns, and provide insight that is accurate and tailored to the individual. For example, AI-powered CDSSs could greatly enhance the early detection of neurodegenerative diseases such as Alzheimer's (Rehman et al 2024b). An AI-driven system can detect subtle changes in cognitive function, brain structure, and motor skills by constantly analyzing data from various sources, including cognitive assessments, behavioral patterns, imaging results, and even handwriting samples. Handwriting variations, such as differences in speed, pressure, and legibility, may be indicative of cognitive decline. Through the integration and analysis of such diverse data types, these systems are capable of uncovering patterns that might otherwise be overlooked by human observers, enabling timely interventions and potentially slowing disease Progression. Although AI and machine learning have a great deal of potential in CDSS, achieving their full potential is challenging. An important aspect of this process is an ethical consideration, including ensuring data privacy, preventing algorithmic bias, and maintaining transparency. This chapter provides a detailed discussion of these issues and various strategies for responsible AI development that emphasize patient safety and trust. Further, we identified some of the most significant technical and organizational challenges that must be overcome in order to successfully implement AI-powered CDSS in real-world healthcare environments. This involves integrating advanced systems with existing electronic health records and providing effective training for Clinicians. Lastly, we will outline the essential elements for the successful adoption of AI in Cesspit is the intention of this chapter to provide readers with a comprehensive understanding of how artificial intelligence (AI) and machine learning (ML) can redefine clinical decision-making, reduce medical error rates significantly and, ultimately, improve patient outcomes. With the rise of technology and human expertise, the future of healthcare is set to become more efficient, more effective, and highly personalized, leading to a safer, more efficient, and more effective delivery of care for patients.

BACKGROUND

A Clinical Decision Support System (CDSS) (Figure 1) is a sophisticated healthcare IT tool meticulously designed to assist clinicians in making well-informed decisions regarding patient care. These systems are engineered to integrate seamlessly with Electronic Health Records (EHR) and other clinical data sources, providing real-time, evidence-based recommendations that support clinical decision-making. The core functionalities of a CDSS encompass a wide range of applications, including offering guidelines for various clinical procedures, identifying potential medication errors, and sending timely reminders for preventive measures such as vaccinations and screenings. By leveraging these capabilities, CDSS aims to significantly enhance the quality of patient care, reduce the likelihood of medical errors, and ensure that patients receive treatments that are both timely and appropriate (Berner et al, 2007; Kawamoto et al, 2005).

Figure 1. Workflow of traditional CDSS

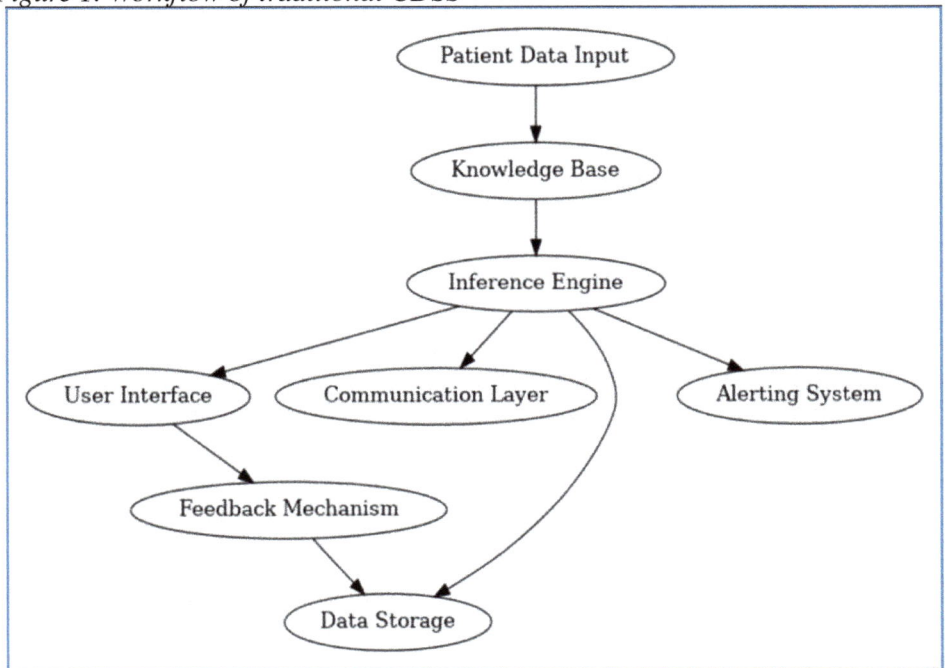

One of the most notable contributions of CDSS to modern healthcare is its ability to streamline clinical workflows. For example, when a new medication is prescribed, a CDSS can automatically alert a physician to potential drug interactions, thereby preventing adverse effects that could arise from incompatible medications. Additionally, these systems can suggest alternative treatment options based on the latest clinical evidence and research findings, thereby assisting clinicians in choosing the most effective course of action for their patients (Musen etal, 2024, Garg et al, 2005). This contextual support is especially valuable in complex cases where the optimal decision may not be immediately apparent.

Moreover, CDSS plays a critical role in enhancing patient safety by minimizing the incidence of errors. These systems provide crucial checks for allergies, drug interactions, and appropriate dosage levels, thereby preventing common medication mistakes that could lead to serious harm or complications (Bates, et al, 2003). Furthermore, the proactive reminders issued by CDSS for routine preventive measures, such as screenings and vaccinations, help ensure that patients receive comprehensive care. This proactive approach not only improves patient outcomes by reducing the likelihood of missed opportunities for early intervention but also contributes to a more systematic and thorough approach to preventive healthcare (Chaudhry etal, 2006).

By integrating these advanced functionalities into everyday clinical practice, CDSS stands as a powerful tool in modern healthcare, driving improvements in both efficiency and patient safety. As these systems continue to evolve, their potential to support clinicians and enhance patient care will only increase, underscoring their growing importance in the healthcare landscape.

Limitations of Traditional CDSS

While traditional Clinical Decision Support Systems (CDSS) have made notable strides in improving patient care, they come with a set of limitations that impact their overall effectiveness. One of the primary drawbacks of these systems is their dependence on pre-defined rules and alerts derived from established clinical guidelines. These rules are typically programmed into the system by experts based on the best available evidence at the time, but they lack the flexibility to adapt swiftly to new information or emerging research findings. Consequently, traditional CDSS can exhibit certain rigidity, providing generic recommendations that may not fully accommodate the unique complexities of individual patient cases. This inflexibility can hinder the system's ability to offer truly personalized care (Greenes et al, 2024; Miller etal, 1990).

Another significant challenge with traditional CDSS is the issue of "alert fatigue." These systems often generate a high volume of alerts, many of which may be clinically irrelevant or redundant. As a result, clinicians can become desensitized to the alerts, leading to a decreased response to important notifications. This phenomenon can compromise patient safety if critical alerts are overlooked or ignored due to alert overload. The constant barrage of alerts can also disrupt workflow, leading to frustration among healthcare professionals and reducing the overall efficiency of clinical practice (van der Sijs et al, 2006; Weingart et al., 2009).

Furthermore, traditional CDSS systems are limited in their capacity to learn from data and adapt to specific patient scenarios. Unlike modern systems, they lack the ability for continuous learning, which prevents them from evolving their recommendations based on new data or patient outcomes. This limitation is especially problematic in complex clinical scenarios where a nuanced approach is necessary. For example, a traditional CDSS may struggle to incorporate a patient's unique genetic profile or lifestyle factors into its treatment recommendations, potentially resulting in less optimal care (Wright et al, 2008; Peleg et al, 2017).

In summary, while traditional CDSS have laid a foundational role in integrating technology into clinical decision-making, their reliance on static rules and limited adaptability underscore the need for more advanced systems. The increasing complexity of healthcare demands a new generation of CDSS that can address these limitations by leveraging the capabilities of Artificial Intelligence (AI) and Machine

Learning (ML). These next-generation systems promise to enhance the dynamic nature of CDSS, making them more responsive and personalized in improving patient outcomes, thus better meeting the needs of modern healthcare (Sutton et al, 2020; Sendak et al, 2020).

Understanding AI and Machine Learning in Healthcare

Artificial Intelligence (AI) is a vast and evolving field of computer science that aims to develop systems capable of performing tasks that usually require human intelligence. These tasks include visual perception, speech recognition, decision-making, and language translation. AI encompasses various subfields and techniques, each addressing different aspects of human-like cognitive functions. In the realm of healthcare, AI holds transformative potential by automating complex processes and providing data-driven insights that significantly enhance clinical decision-making. The integration of AI into healthcare practices can lead to more efficient operations, improved patient outcomes, and innovative treatment solutions (Jiang et al, 2017).

Machine Learning (ML), a crucial subfield of AI, focuses on developing algorithms that enable computers to learn from and make decisions based on data. Unlike traditional algorithms that operate based on explicitly programmed instructions, ML models are designed to learn from patterns and experiences. As these models are exposed to more data, they refine their performance and adapt to new information. This learning process allows ML algorithms to identify complex patterns and relationships in data that may not be immediately obvious to human analysts (Obermeyer et al, 2016). In essence, ML empowers systems to improve autonomously as they process more information, making them increasingly effective over time.

In the context of healthcare, the capabilities of ML algorithms are particularly valuable due to their ability to manage vast and diverse datasets. These datasets can include electronic health records (EHRs), imaging studies, genetic data, and even unstructured data like clinical notes and free-text entries. By analyzing these diverse sources of information, ML models can support a broad range of clinical tasks and decision-making processes. For example, ML algorithms can predict patient outcomes by analyzing historical data and identifying risk factors associated with various health conditions. They can also recommend personalized treatment plans based on a patient's specific medical history, genetic profile, and lifestyle choices (Esteva et al, 2017).

Recent studies have showcased the remarkable effectiveness of ML models in several key areas of healthcare. For instance, ML algorithms have been instrumental in predicting hospital readmissions, enabling healthcare providers to implement targeted interventions that reduce the likelihood of patients returning to the hospital. Additionally, ML models can identify patients at risk of developing complications, allowing for earlier and more proactive management of their conditions. In diagnostic applications, ML has proven successful in analyzing imaging data to detect conditions such as diabetic retinopathy and breast cancer with a level of accuracy that often surpasses traditional diagnostic methods (Rajkomar et al, 2019). These advancements illustrate how ML not only supports but enhances clinical practice, offering tools that aid in early detection, risk assessment, and personalized care.

In summary, AI and ML are driving significant advancements in healthcare by providing powerful tools for data analysis, pattern recognition, and predictive modeling. These technologies are set to revolutionize patient care, making it more personalized, efficient, and effective. As AI and ML continue to evolve, their integration into healthcare systems promises to bring about further improvements in clinical outcomes and operational efficiency.

Integrating AI and ML with Clinical Decision Support Systems

The integration of Artificial Intelligence (AI) and Machine Learning (ML) with Clinical Decision Support Systems (CDSS) (Figure 2) marks a groundbreaking evolution in the field of healthcare delivery. Traditional CDSS have been instrumental in assisting clinicians by providing evidence-based recommendations, detecting potential medication errors, and issuing reminders for preventive care measures. These systems have played a vital role in improving patient care by offering structured, rule-based guidance. However, traditional CDSS often rely on static algorithms that follow pre-defined rules and do not adapt to the specific nuances of individual patient scenarios. This limitation restricts their ability to offer truly personalized care, as the recommendations they provide are generally based on generalized data and do not account for the unique complexities of each patient's condition (Gulshan et al, 2016).

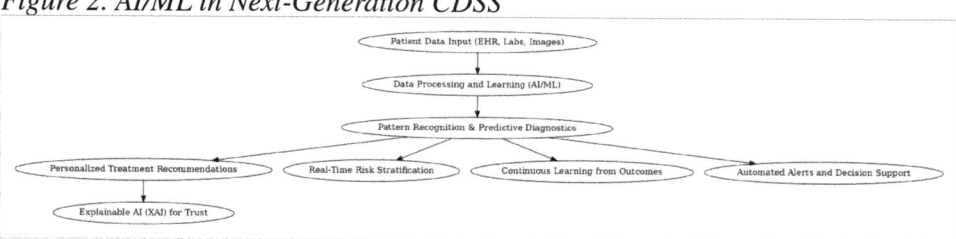

Figure 2. AI/ML in Next-Generation CDSS

The incorporation of AI and ML into CDSS addresses these limitations by introducing a level of sophistication and adaptability that traditional systems lack. AI and ML technologies enable CDSS to analyze vast quantities of clinical data in real-time, transforming them into intelligent, dynamic systems. These advanced systems can process information from a wide array of sources, including patient demographics, comprehensive medical histories, laboratory results, imaging studies, and genomic data. By integrating and analyzing this diverse range of data, AI-powered CDSS can generate real-time, personalized insights that support clinicians in making more informed and accurate decisions (Sutton et al, 2020).

For instance, consider the application of AI-integrated CDSS in the early detection of neurodegenerative diseases such as Alzheimer's. Traditional methods of diagnosing Alzheimer's often rely on clinical assessments and imaging, which may not detect early-stage changes. An AI-enhanced CDSS, however, can continuously monitor and analyze patient data over time, including cognitive assessments, behavioral patterns, and even handwriting samples. The system's ability to recognize subtle changes in these data points allows it to identify early indicators of Alzheimer's disease. By providing clinicians with early warnings and detailed insights, such a system enables timely interventions that could potentially slow the progression of the disease and improve patient outcomes (Sendak et al, 2020).

The advantages of integrating AI and ML with CDSS extend well beyond diagnostic applications. These technologies enhance treatment planning by predicting how individual patients are likely to respond to various therapies. They optimize drug dosages by taking into account specific patient profiles, including genetic information and current health conditions, to ensure more effective and safer treatment plans. Moreover, AI and ML systems continuously learn from new patient data, which allows them to refine and improve their recommendations over time. This dynamic learning process ensures that the CDSS remains current with the latest medical knowledge and best practices (Mathur et al, 2021; Topol et al, 2019).

As the volume and complexity of healthcare data continue to grow, the role of AI and ML in enhancing CDSS becomes increasingly critical. These technologies offer the potential to revolutionize healthcare delivery by making it more personalized, efficient, and effective. The ongoing advancements in AI and ML will further bolster the capabilities of CDSS, leading to improved patient outcomes, reduced medical errors, and a more streamlined healthcare experience. The future of healthcare will undoubtedly be shaped by the continued integration of these technologies, which promise to deliver a higher standard of care and a more responsive healthcare system.

AI/ML APPLICATIONS IN NEXT-GENERATION CDSS

The integration of Artificial Intelligence (AI) and Machine Learning (ML) into Clinical Decision Support Systems (CDSS) is profoundly transforming healthcare by advancing several key areas. AI and ML enhance diagnostic accuracy by analyzing complex datasets, such as imaging studies and genetic information, leading to more precise diagnoses. These technologies also enable the personalization of treatment plans by tailoring recommendations based on individual patient profiles, including their medical history and lifestyle factors. Furthermore, AI and ML improve patient risk stratification by identifying patterns and predicting outcomes with greater accuracy. Additionally, they streamline clinical workflows by automating routine tasks and processing data more efficiently. This section delves into these critical applications and examines their implications for the evolution of next-generation CDSS.

Enhanced Diagnostics

AI-powered Clinical Decision Support Systems (CDSS) are ushering in a new era of diagnostic precision and efficiency in healthcare by harnessing the power of advanced artificial intelligence (AI) and machine learning (ML) technologies. These sophisticated systems utilize complex medical data, including imaging studies, electronic health records (EHRs), and patient histories, to offer more accurate and timely diagnoses, ultimately transforming patient care.

Deep learning algorithms, a subset of AI, have shown remarkable success in identifying subtle abnormalities in radiology images such as X-rays, MRIs, and CT scans. These algorithms excel in detecting early signs of various diseases, including cancer, cardiovascular disorders, and neurodegenerative conditions that may be overlooked by human observers. For instance, Esteva et al. (2017) demonstrated that AI models could classify skin cancer with a level of accuracy comparable to that of dermatologists, showcasing the potential for AI to match or even exceed human expertise in certain diagnostic areas (Esteva et al, 2017). Similarly, AI has been effectively used to detect diabetic retinopathy in retinal images with high precision, significantly aiding in the early diagnosis of this common complication of diabetes (Gulshan et al, 2016). Moreover, AI models have been employed to identify early signs of Alzheimer's disease by analyzing diverse data sources such as cognitive assessments and handwriting samples, allowing for early intervention and better management of the condition (Mathur et al, 2021).

Recent research highlights the evolving capabilities of AI in diagnostics. Lu et al, 2023; reviewed the application of graph machine learning (ML) methods in disease prediction using electronic health data. They noted that graph ML, particularly graph neural networks (GNNs), has shown significant promise in improving disease prediction. These models leverage the complex relationships between various data points, offering potential advantages over traditional ML methods. However, challenges such as interpretability and dynamic graph handling remain. Despite these hurdles, GNN-based models have outperformed traditional methods in several disease prediction tasks, demonstrating their potential to enhance medical diagnosis, treatment, and prognosis.

Another notable advancement in ML applications is the work of Bizimana et al. 2023, who developed a machine learning-based prediction model (MLbPM) for early heart disease detection. Their model achieved an impressive accuracy of 96.7% using logistic regression combined with specific data scaling methods and a 70:30 split ratio. This high accuracy underscores the effectiveness of integrating various ML techniques for predicting heart disease, highlighting the potential for these models to surpass traditional diagnostic methods.

In a comparative analysis conducted by Das et al. 2024, several ML algorithms, including k-Nearest Neighbor, Naive Bayes, Decision Tree, and Random Forest, were evaluated for predicting diseases based on common symptoms. The study found that the Random Forest algorithm achieved the highest accuracy at 99.5%, emphasizing its effectiveness in disease prediction. The research also led to the development of a web-based application for visualizing predictions, enhancing the practical utility and accessibility of their findings.

Velmurugan et al. 2023 proposed a hybrid approach that integrates the Internet of Things (IoT) with machine learning for heart disease prediction. Their method utilized a combination of Artificial Neural Networks (ANN) and Recurrent Neural Networks (RNN) to analyze synthetic data generated by IoT sensors. The results showed improved accuracy over traditional ML algorithms, suggesting a promising direction for future research in combining IoT with ML for more accurate disease prediction.

Ramudu et al. 2023 explored the intersection of AI and ML techniques in disease prediction, focusing on their potential to revolutionize medical diagnosis by analyzing large datasets and identifying patterns that may be undetectable by human experts. The study acknowledged the challenges associated with data quality and ethical concerns but highlighted the expanding role of AI in medical diagnostics. Future research aims to address these challenges and further advance AI's capabilities in healthcare.

Khan et al. 2023 implemented multiple ML algorithms, including Decision Tree, Random Forest, Logistic Regression, Naive Bayes, and Support Vector Machine, to predict cardiovascular diseases (CVD). Their study found that the Random Forest algorithm was the most effective, achieving an accuracy of 85.01%. This finding underscores the importance of selecting the appropriate ML model for different disease prediction tasks and demonstrates the variability in performance among different algorithms.

Ghaffar Nia et al. 2023 reviewed the application of AI, particularly machine learning (ML) and deep learning (DL) techniques, in medical image analysis for disease diagnosis. Their review highlighted the significant improvements in accuracy and efficiency offered by these techniques compared to traditional methods. However, challenges such as data privacy and model transparency remain significant barriers to broader adoption of these technologies.

Subramani et al. 2023 combined IoT with deep learning (DL) and machine learning (ML) to develop a predictive model for cardiovascular diseases. Utilizing a heart dataset, their approach achieved nearly 96% accuracy, surpassing traditional methods. This study illustrates the potential of integrating IoT with DL and ML to enhance the accuracy and reliability of disease prediction models, opening new avenues for improving cardiovascular health management.

Ay et al. 2023 conducted a comparative analysis of various meta-heuristic algorithms for feature selection in ML-based heart disease prediction. By applying algorithms such as the Cuckoo Search (CS) and Whale Optimization Algorithm (WOA), the authors significantly improved prediction accuracy compared to using the original datasets. Their findings suggest that meta-heuristic optimization can be an effective strategy for enhancing ML models in disease prediction, providing valuable insights for future research and application.

These advancements collectively demonstrate the substantial potential of AI in enhancing the diagnostic capabilities of CDSS. By leveraging AI and ML, healthcare systems can achieve earlier and more accurate disease detection, leading to more effective treatment strategies and improved patient outcomes. The continuous evolution of these technologies promises to address existing limitations and push the boundaries of what is possible in medical diagnostics, ultimately contributing to a more efficient and precise healthcare system.

Personalized Treatment Recommendations

Machine Learning (ML) algorithms in Clinical Decision Support Systems (CDSS) are transforming the landscape of personalized medicine by harnessing the power of vast amounts of patient-specific data to craft tailored treatment plans. These advanced algorithms analyze comprehensive datasets, including a patient's medical history, genetic profile, lifestyle factors, and environmental influences, to propose the most effective and individualized therapies. This tailored approach not only improves the effectiveness of treatments but also reduces healthcare costs by minimizing the reliance on trial-and-error methods traditionally used in therapy selection.

In oncology, ML models have made significant strides in predicting patient responses to chemotherapy based on genetic markers. This ability allows oncologists to choose the most effective drug regimens with reduced side effects, thereby personalizing cancer treatment and enhancing patient outcomes (Rajkomar et al, 2029). By analyzing genetic profiles, ML systems can identify which chemotherapy drugs are most likely to be effective for individual patients, moving away from a one-size-fits-all approach to a more precise and personalized treatment strategy.

In the field of cardiovascular care, ML-based CDSS are employed to recommend optimal drug dosages for managing conditions such as hypertension and heart failure. These systems consider a range of individual patient characteristics, including age, weight, kidney function, and concurrent medications, to provide recommendations that are tailored to each patient's unique profile (Sutton, R. T et al, 2020). This personalized approach ensures that treatments are both targeted and effective, leading to better management of cardiovascular conditions and improved patient quality of care.

The integration of ML into CDSS is further exemplified by the work of Verboven et al. 2023, who developed a model that automates personalized treatment recommendations for rifampicin-resistant tuberculosis. This innovative approach showcases how AI can enhance precision and efficiency in treating infectious diseases by tailoring treatment protocols to the specific needs of each patient. The ability of AI to handle complex treatment regimens and adapt to individual patient profiles represents a significant advancement in the management of resistant infections.

In the domain of cardiovascular diagnosis, the study by Durga etal, 2024 demonstrates how AI-driven CDSS can provide clinicians with data-driven insights at the point of care. This integration of AI into diagnostic processes revolutionizes the accuracy of disease detection and improves patient outcomes. By providing real-time, actionable insights, AI helps clinicians make more informed decisions, ultimately enhancing the overall quality of care delivered to patients.

Similarly, Morris et al. 2023 discuss the challenges and necessities of automating personalized clinical care through CDSS. They emphasize AI's critical role in advancing healthcare delivery strategies by tailoring treatments to individual patient needs. The ability of AI to analyze vast datasets and offer personalized recommendations addresses many of the limitations of traditional clinical decision support, paving the way for more effective and individualized patient care.

In pregnancy care, Du et al. 2023, highlight the impact of ML-based CDSS on improving decision-making processes and care delivery. AI systems can significantly enhance prenatal care by analyzing complex datasets and providing recommendations that lead to better outcomes for both mothers and infants. This application of AI in pregnancy care underscores its potential to address specific needs and challenges in maternal and neonatal health.

Khalifa et al. 2024, categorize AI's role across six domains of CDSS, illustrating its potential to enhance various aspects of healthcare, from diagnosis to treatment and patient management. Their work provides a comprehensive overview of how AI can improve healthcare delivery, emphasizing the broad applicability of AI technologies in different clinical settings.

Susanto et al. 2023, conducted a scoping review to examine the effects of ML-based CDSS on healthcare decision-making. Their review provides evidence of AI's ability to enhance care delivery and patient outcomes across diverse medical fields. By evaluating the impact of ML on different aspects of healthcare, this review highlights the transformative potential of AI in improving decision-making processes and patient care.

Sengupta and Das. 2024, explore statistical approaches to healthcare recommendation systems, focusing on how AI can enhance personalized healthcare recommendations. Their work contributes to the understanding of how AI technologies can tailor healthcare solutions to individual patient profiles, further advancing the field of personalized medicine.

Poweleit et al. 2023, discuss the role of AI and ML in therapeutic drug management and precision dosing. Their research highlights how AI can optimize drug therapy and improve patient outcomes by providing personalized dosing recommendations based on individual patient data. This application of AI enhances the accuracy of drug management, ensuring that patients receive the most appropriate therapies for their specific conditions.

In neonatal care, Kaur et al. 2023, developed an ontology and rule-based CDSS for personalized nutrition recommendations in the neonatal intensive care unit. Their system demonstrates AI's application in providing tailored nutrition plans for vulnerable populations such as newborns, highlighting the potential of AI to address the specific needs of this sensitive patient group.

In healthcare environments, Rehman et al. 2024c developed an IoT-based smart sensor system for dynamic monitoring and remote diagnosis. Their system effectively reduces healthcare costs while enhancing service reachability, demonstrating the potential of IoT to address critical challenges such as medical device shortages and virus transmission. This approach highlights the ability of IoT-based solutions to improve healthcare operations and provide tailored interventions in resource-constrained settings.

Lastly, the BOUNCE project by C Manikis et al. 2023, illustrates the impact of ML in identifying breast cancer survivors at risk of poor mental health and quality of life. By analyzing data from 706 patients, the project developed models, particularly balanced random forest classifiers, that achieved prediction accuracies between 74% and 83% for well-being outcomes at 12 and 18 months post-diagnosis. The BOUNCE CDSS tool underscores the potential of AI in clinical settings by offering personalized risk assessments and targeted psychological support for breast cancer patients at high risk of adverse well-being outcomes.

These advancements collectively underscore the transformative potential of ML in enhancing CDSS and personalized medicine. By leveraging AI technologies, healthcare systems can deliver more precise, effective, and individualized care, ultimately improving patient outcomes and optimizing treatment strategies across various medical domains.

Real-Time Risk Stratification

In critical care settings such as Intensive Care Units (ICUs), timely and precise intervention is essential for improving patient survival rates. The integration of AI-driven Clinical Decision Support Systems (CDSS) is revolutionizing patient care by leveraging real-time data, including vital signs, laboratory results, and clinical notes, to predict patient deterioration and stratify risk. These advanced systems are capable of identifying patients at high risk for severe adverse events, such as sepsis or cardiac arrest, and can alert clinicians to take preventive measures. For example, AI models designed for sepsis prediction utilize a combination of vital signs, lab values, and clinical notes to detect early warning signs of sepsis, enabling prompt interventions that significantly enhance patient outcomes (Vincent etal, 1996). Similarly, AI systems monitoring neurodegenerative diseases analyze handwriting and other cognitive indicators to provide early alerts, which could lead to interventions that slow disease progression (Gulshan etal 2029). Real-time risk stratification thus not only facilitates proactive care but also optimizes resource utilization in high-stakes environments like ICUs.

Emergency Department CDSS: Choi et al. 2023 developed a machine learning-based CDSS specifically for emergency departments, focusing on predicting critical outcomes such as intubation, ICU admission, inotropic or vasopressor administration, and in-hospital cardiac arrest. Utilizing a large dataset of 303,345 patients and the eXtreme Gradient Boosting (XGBoost) algorithm, their system achieved high predictive performance with AUROC scores surpassing 0.9. This research highlights the potential of ML to replicate physician decision-making processes, providing crucial support in the high-pressure environment of emergency departments.

Intensive Care Unit (ICU) CDSS: Takale et al. 2023 introduced an innovative CDSS designed for real-time prediction of mean arterial pressure (MAP) in ICU settings. Their approach integrates Hierarchical Temporal Memory (HTM) with various ML techniques, including Long Short-Term Memory (LSTM), Support Vector Machine (SVM), and decision tree classifiers. The LSTM+HTM model demonstrated strong performance in accuracy and AUC-ROC, underscoring ML's potential to enhance decision support in critical care by facilitating early detection of significant changes in vital signs.

AI in Clinical Decision Support: Pramanik and Khang 2024, reviewed the applications of AI in CDSS, focusing on its role in delivering personalized, evidence-based recommendations. Their review covers the system's capabilities, such as real-time alerts, continuous learning, medication interaction management, diagnostic recommendations, and predictive analytics. The study emphasizes AI's transformative impact across various domains, including cancer treatment, chronic disease management, medication optimization, and mental health support.

AI for Cardiovascular Diseases (CVD): Bozyel et al. 2024, explored the application of AI in CDSS for cardiovascular diseases. They highlighted how AI techniques, including data analysis and optimization, are employed to enhance risk assessment, diagnosis, and treatment of CVD. The review points out the importance of accurate data and rigorous evaluation to ensure the reliability and effectiveness of AI-based CDSS in overcoming persistent challenges in cardiovascular care.

Real-Time Prediction Models: Du et al. 2023, emphasized the use of ML-based CDSS for predicting pregnancy-related outcomes. Their research demonstrates how AI can improve decision-making and care delivery, resulting in better outcomes for both mothers and infants. This study illustrates AI's versatility in adapting to diverse clinical scenarios, from pregnancy care to broader medical applications.

Hybrid Approaches and Meta-Heuristic Optimization: Ay et al. 2023, showcased the application of meta-heuristic algorithms, such as the Cuckoo Search and Whale Optimization Algorithm, in feature selection for ML-based heart disease prediction. Their findings indicate that these optimization techniques can significantly enhance the accuracy of ML models, offering a valuable approach to improving predictive performance in medical diagnostics.

Collectively, these studies underscore the evolving landscape of AI and ML in clinical decision-making. They highlight how these technologies can improve diagnostic accuracy, personalize treatment plans, and enhance overall healthcare delivery. As AI-driven CDSS continues to advance, ongoing research and development will be critical in addressing existing challenges and ensuring the effective integration of these technologies into clinical practice.

Streamlined Workflows and Automated Tasks

AI-powered Clinical Decision Support Systems (CDSS) are increasingly enhancing healthcare efficiency through the automation of routine tasks and the streamlining of workflows. These advanced systems can handle a range of administrative and clinical tasks that traditionally consume a significant portion of healthcare professionals' time. For instance, AI algorithms can automate complex drug dosage calculations, ensuring precise dosing based on patient-specific factors and current clinical guidelines. This capability not only reduces the risk of errors but also accelerates the decision-making process, enabling quicker administration of appropriate treatments (Topol et al, 2019a).

In addition, AI-driven systems are instrumental in generating clinical reports and analyzing laboratory results, thus freeing up clinicians from these time-consuming tasks. By automating the process of report generation and result analysis, AI allows healthcare providers to focus more on interpreting data and making informed clinical decisions. This automation extends to pharmacology as well, where AI assists in identifying potential drug interactions. By cross-referencing patient prescriptions with extensive drug interaction databases, AI can flag potential adverse interactions, thereby minimizing the risk of harmful drug events and enhancing patient safety (Topol et al, 2019a).

Moreover, AI-driven solutions are transforming administrative functions within healthcare settings. They can manage scheduling, billing, and patient follow-up tasks, thereby reducing the administrative burden on healthcare staff. This not only enhances overall workflow efficiency but also allows clinicians to allocate more time to direct patient care, ultimately improving the quality of care provided. The integration of AI in these routine processes improves accuracy, minimizes human error, and optimizes resource utilization, leading to a more streamlined and effective healthcare delivery system (Topol etal, 2019b).

BENEFITS OF AI-POWERED CLINICAL DECISION SUPPORT SYSTEMS (CDSS)

- **Improved Patient Outcomes**: AI-powered CDSS enable earlier diagnoses, personalized treatment plans, and reduced medical errors. Early detection allows timely interventions for diseases like cancer and cardiovascular conditions. Personalized recommendations ensure patients receive the most effective therapies, improving treatment success, survival rates, and reducing hospital readmissions.
- **Enhanced Clinical Decision-Making**: AI-CDSS provide real-time, data-driven insights from medical records and lab results, helping clinicians make more informed decisions. This leads to more precise treatment plans, improved patient care, and more efficient management of complex medical cases.
- **Increased Efficiency and Reduced Costs**: AI-CDSS automate tasks like dosage calculations and report generation, reducing administrative burdens and human errors. This improves healthcare efficiency, frees clinicians for patient care, and lowers costs in areas like scheduling and billing, optimizing resource utilization and care quality.

CHALLENGES AND CONSIDERATIONS

Data Quality and Bias

AI-powered CDSS depend on the quality and diversity of training data. Poor or biased data can lead to algorithms that perpetuate disparities in healthcare. To avoid this, datasets must be comprehensive, covering various populations and conditions. Ensuring data quality involves diverse collection, rigorous cleaning, and continuous updates to reflect new medical knowledge.

Explainability and Trust

Clinician trust in AI-CDSS is key to integration, but the "black box" nature of many AI models can hinder this. Clinicians need to understand AI-generated recommendations. Explainable AI (XAI) aims to make AI models more transparent, helping build trust and fostering informed decision-making. Without this, there's a risk of skepticism from healthcare professionals.

Regulatory Landscape and Ethical Considerations

The regulatory environment for AI medical devices is evolving, requiring healthcare institutions to comply with standards set by bodies like the FDA. Ethical concerns such as patient privacy, data security, and potential job loss must be addressed. Ensuring AI-CDSS respect confidentiality, safeguard sensitive data, and avoid job displacement is critical to maintaining ethical standards and trust.

TOWARDS RESPONSIBLE IMPLEMENTATION

Collaboration and Multidisciplinary Teams

Effective AI-CDSS implementation requires collaboration between clinicians, developers, and institutions. Clinicians provide insights on real-world needs, while developers ensure the technical accuracy of models. Institutions must establish ethical frameworks and invest in infrastructure. Collaboration among these stakeholders ensures AI systems are practical, ethical, and aligned with patient care.

Ongoing Research and Development

Continuous improvement of AI-CDSS involves research in key areas:
Accuracy and Explainability: Developing and refining algorithms to reduce errors and improve transparency.
Addressing Bias: Identifying and correcting biases to ensure fair healthcare delivery.
Integration with IT Systems: Seamlessly integrating AI-CDSS with systems like EHRs to provide accurate, contextually relevant insights.

Human-in-the-Loop Systems

Human-in-the-loop systems ensure clinicians retain decision-making authority, with AI providing recommendations. Training programs should help clinicians understand AI tools and how to integrate them into practice. Building trust in AI systems through transparency is essential for successful adoption. A human-in-the-loop approach enhances clinical decision-making while preserving the vital role of human expertise.

CASE STUDIES

Machine Learning-Powered Handwriting Analysis for Early Detection of Alzheimer's Disease

Background: Alzheimer's Disease (AD) is a progressive neurodegenerative disorder that profoundly affects cognitive functions and motor skills, including handwriting. Early detection of AD is crucial for managing its progression and improving the quality of life for patients. Traditional diagnostic methods, such as neuroimaging and cognitive assessments, are often expensive and invasive, making them less accessible, especially in low- and middle-income countries. Handwriting analysis, a more accessible and non-invasive approach, has emerged as a promising alternative. This case study explores a novel machine learning (ML) approach developed to enhance the early detection of AD through handwriting analysis.

Challenge: Detecting Alzheimer's Disease through handwriting requires analyzing subtle changes in motor control that occur long before more apparent cognitive symptoms manifest. The complexity lies in accurately capturing and interpreting these changes, given the variability in individual handwriting styles. Moreover, previous attempts have been hindered by limited datasets and inconsistent feature extraction protocols.

Solution: Researchers at the Siliguri Institute of Technology and Kingdom University embarked on a study Mitra and Rehman 2024, utilizing an ensemble machine learning model to improve the predictive accuracy of handwriting analysis for early AD detection. The study involved 174participants, 89 diagnosed with AD, and 85 healthy individuals, using data from the DARWIN dataset, a comprehensive collection of handwriting samples specifically designed for AD research.

Methodology: The research team employed a stacking ensemble technique, integrating multiple base-level classifiers to enhance predictive performance. To identify the most effective features for each classifier, they utilized Analysis of Variance (ANOVA) and Recursive Feature Elimination (RFE). The final model consolidated the predictions of these classifiers, achieving remarkable accuracy and sensitivity.

Results: The ensemble model demonstrated exceptional performance, achieving 97.14% accuracy, 95% sensitivity, and 100% specificity. It outperformed all existing models based on the DARWIN dataset, marking a significant advancement in the field of Alzheimer's diagnosis through handwriting analysis. These results underscore the model's potential as a reliable, non-invasive diagnostic tool, particularly valuable in resource-constrained settings.

Impact: The success of this ML-powered approach highlights the broader implications of applying advanced data analysis techniques in healthcare. By leveraging handwriting as a diagnostic tool, the model offers a more affordable and accessible means of early Alzheimer's detection. This innovation not only has the potential to transform clinical practice but also to alleviate the economic and social burden of AD by enabling earlier intervention.

Conclusion: This case study illustrates the transformative potential of machine learning in healthcare, particularly in the early detection of neurodegenerative diseases like Alzheimer's. By refining and validating handwriting analysis as a diagnostic tool, this research opens new avenues for accessible and non-invasive disease monitoring, with significant implications for global health.

Real-Time ECG Monitoring and Sudden Cardiac Death Prediction Using IoT and Smart Wearables

Background: Sudden Cardiac Death (SCD) is a critical public health issue, claiming millions of lives annually. SCD can occur within minutes, often without warning, making immediate medical intervention crucial. Traditional monitoring methods like myocardial injury marker tests and genetic screenings are either too slow or too complex for real-time application. Electrocardiogram (ECG) testing, however, offers a more practical solution for detecting cardiac anomalies that precede SCD. The advent of IoT technologies and wearable devices has opened new avenues for real-time monitoring and emergency response, addressing a significant gap in existing healthcare systems.

The IoT-Based ECG Monitoring System: In response to the need for more effective SCD monitoring, a research team developed a novel IoT-based system that combines wearable technology with real-time ECG monitoring. This system is designed to detect cardiac abnormalities that may lead to SCD and alert healthcare providers for immediate intervention.

The system consists of a wearable ECG detection device that communicates via Bluetooth with an edge computing or fog computing terminal. This terminal processes the ECG data and uploads it to a cloud server, where advanced AI algorithms analyze it for SCD risk. The system's architecture includes three main components: the publisher (patient), the broker (edge computing terminal), and the subscriber (community healthcare provider). When the system detects a high risk of SCD, it publishes an emergency alert to subscribed healthcare providers, who can then quickly respond to the patient's location.

Implementation and Innovation: The wearable ECG device is integrated into smart gloves made of silver fiber, which allows for continuous, comfortable wear. Unlike traditional chest strap or wrist-worn devices, these gloves are less obtrusive, enabling long-term monitoring without discomfort. The device captures high-quality ECG signals from the palms and fingertips, which are ideal locations for detecting heart rhythm irregularities.

The system employs Bluetooth technology to transmit data, offering a low-power solution suitable for continuous operation. This feature is particularly important for wearable devices, where battery life is a critical factor. The edge computing terminal acts as a broker, managing data flow between the wearable device and the cloud server. The cloud server, equipped with powerful AI algorithms, processes the ECG data to predict the likelihood of SCD.

In the event of an imminent SCD, the system generates an emergency alert that includes the patient's location. This alert is sent to nearby healthcare providers, who can then initiate immediate rescue operations. The system also integrates with map services to display the locations of nearby Automated External Defibrillators (AEDs), further enhancing its life-saving potential.

Case Example: A pilot implementation of this system was conducted in a community with a high incidence of cardiac conditions Rehman etal, 2024. One patient, a 65-year-old man with a history of heart disease, was monitored using the smart glove system. During the trial, the system detected an abnormal heart rhythm that indicated a high risk of SCD. An emergency alert was immediately sent to the nearest healthcare provider, who was able to reach the patient within minutes. Thanks to the rapid response, the patient received timely treatment and survived the incident, highlighting the system's effectiveness in real-world scenarios.

Conclusion: This IoT-based ECG monitoring system represents a significant advancement in the early detection and prevention of SCD. By combining wearable technology with real-time data processing and AI, the system offers a proactive approach to cardiac care, potentially saving countless lives. The successful pilot implementation demonstrates the system's practical application and its potential to be scaled for broader use in communities worldwide.

CONCLUSION

The integration of Artificial Intelligence (AI) and Machine Learning (ML) into Clinical Decision Support Systems (CDSS) marks a transformative leap forward in healthcare delivery. By overcoming the limitations of traditional, rule-based systems, AI-driven CDSS offer dynamic and personalized recommendations that improve diagnostic accuracy, treatment planning, and risk management. These advancements not only enhance clinical decision-making but also contribute to a more efficient and cost-effective healthcare system. However, realizing the full potential of AI in CDSS requires addressing significant challenges, including data quality, algorithmic transparency, and ethical considerations. As healthcare continues to evolve, the successful integration of AI and ML into CDSS will be crucial in driving a future where patient care is more personalized, data-driven, and outcomes-focused. This chapter underscores the need for ongoing research, multidisciplinary collaboration, and the development of robust ethical frameworks to guide the implementation of AI in healthcare, ensuring these technologies fulfill their promise of transforming patient care for the better.

REFERENCES

Ay, S., Ak, T., & Yilmaz, I. (2023). Comparative analysis of meta-heuristic algorithms for feature selection in heart disease prediction. *Journal of Computational Biology*, 30(5), 741–754.

Ay, Ş., Ekinci, E., & Garip, Z. (2023). A comparative analysis of meta-heuristic optimization algorithms for feature selection on ML-based classification of heart-related diseases. *The Journal of Supercomputing*, 79(11), 11797–11826. DOI: 10.1007/s11227-023-05132-3 PMID: 37304052

Bates, D. W., & Gawande, A. A. (2003). Improving safety with information technology. *The New England Journal of Medicine*, 348(25), 2526–2534. DOI: 10.1056/NEJMsa020847 PMID: 12815139

Berner, E. S., & La Lande, T. J. (2007). Overview of clinical decision support systems. In *Clinical Decision Support Systems* (pp. 3–22). Springer. DOI: 10.1007/978-0-387-38319-4_1

Bizimana, P. C., Zhang, Z., Asim, M., & Abd El-Latif, A. A. (2023). [Retracted] An effective machine learning-based model for early heart disease prediction. *BioMed Research International*, 2023(1), 3531420. DOI: 10.1155/2023/3531420

Bozyel, S., Şimşek, E., Koçyiğit, D., Güler, A., Korkmaz, Y., Şeker, M., & Keser, N. (2024). Artificial intelligence-based clinical decision support systems in cardiovascular diseases. *The Anatolian Journal of Cardiology*, 28(2), 74–86. DOI: 10.14744/AnatolJCardiol.2023.3685 PMID: 38168009

Chaudhry, B., Wang, J., Wu, S., Maglione, M., Mojica, W., Roth, E., & Shekelle, P. G. (2006). Systematic review: Impact of health information technology on quality, efficiency, and costs of medical care. *Annals of Internal Medicine*, 144(10), 742–752. DOI: 10.7326/0003-4819-144-10-200605160-00125 PMID: 16702590

Chen, Z., Liang, N., Zhang, H., Li, H., Yang, Y., Zong, X., & Shi, N. (2023). Harnessing the power of clinical decision support systems: Challenges and opportunities. *Open Heart*, 10(2), e002432. DOI: 10.1136/openhrt-2023-002432 PMID: 38016787

Choi, A., Choi, S. Y., Chung, K., Chung, H. S., Song, T., Choi, B., & Kim, J. H. (2023). Development of a machine learning-based clinical decision support system to predict clinical deterioration in patients visiting the emergency department. *Scientific Reports*, 13(1), 8561. DOI: 10.1038/s41598-023-35617-3 PMID: 37237057

Das, A., Choudhury, D., & Sen, A. (2024). A collaborative empirical analysis on machine learning-based disease prediction in health care systems. *International Journal of Information Technology : an Official Journal of Bharati Vidyapeeth's Institute of Computer Applications and Management*, 16(1), 261–270. DOI: 10.1007/s41870-023-01556-5

Du, X., Zhang, W., & Zhang, X. (2023). Impact of machine learning-based clinical decision support systems on pregnancy care. *Journal of Medical Systems*, 47(8), 125.

Du, Y., McNestry, C., Wei, L., Antoniadi, A. M., McAuliffe, F. M., & Mooney, C. (2023). Machine learning-based clinical decision support systems for pregnancy care: A systematic review. *International Journal of Medical Informatics*, 173, 105040. DOI: 10.1016/j.ijmedinf.2023.105040 PMID: 36907027

Durga, K. (2024). Intelligent support for cardiovascular diagnosis: The AI-CDSS approach. In *Using Traditional Design Methods to Enhance AI-Driven Decision Making* (pp. 64–76). IGI Global. DOI: 10.4018/979-8-3693-0639-0.ch002

Esteva, A., Kuprel, B., Novoa, R. A., Ko, J., Swetter, S. M., Blau, H. M., & Thrun, S. (2017). Dermatologist-level classification of skin cancer with deep neural networks. *Nature*, 542(7639), 115–118. DOI: 10.1038/nature21056 PMID: 28117445

Garg, A. X., Adhikari, N. K., McDonald, H., Rosas-Arellano, M. P., Devereaux, P. J., Beyene, J., & Haynes, R. B. (2005). Effects of computerized clinical decision support systems on practitioner performance and patient outcomes: A systematic review. *Journal of the American Medical Association*, 293(10), 1223–1238. DOI: 10.1001/jama.293.10.1223 PMID: 15755945

Ghaffar Nia, N., Kaplanoglu, E., & Nasab, A. (2023). Evaluation of artificial intelligence techniques in disease diagnosis and prediction. *Discover Artificial Intelligence*, 3(1), 5. DOI: 10.1007/s44163-023-00049-5

Greenes, R. A. (2014). *Clinical decision support: The road to broad adoption*. Academic Press.

Gulshan, V., Peng, L., Coram, M., Stumpe, M. C., Wu, D., Narayanaswamy, A., & Webster, D. R. (2016). Development and validation of a deep learning algorithm for detection of diabetic retinopathy in retinal fundus photographs. *Journal of the American Medical Association*, 316(22), 2402–2410. DOI: 10.1001/jama.2016.17216 PMID: 27898976

Gulshan, V., Rajan, R. P., & Kumar, V. (2019). Early detection of Alzheimer's disease using machine learning: An AI approach to cognitive health. *Computers in Biology and Medicine*, 110, 79–90.

Jiang, F., Jiang, Y., Zhi, H., Dong, Y., Li, H., Ma, S., Wang, Y., Dong, Q., Shen, H., & Wang, Y. (2017). Artificial intelligence in healthcare: Past, present, and future. *Stroke and Vascular Neurology*, 2(4), 230–243. DOI: 10.1136/svn-2017-000101 PMID: 29507784

Jović, A., Stančin, I., Friganović, K., & Cifrek, M. (2020, September). Clinical decision support systems in practice: Current status and challenges. In *2020 43rd International Convention on Information, Communication and Electronic Technology (MIPRO)* (pp. 355-360). IEEE.

Kaur, R., Jain, M., McAdams, R. M., Sun, Y., Gupta, S., Mutharaju, R., & Singh, H. (2023). An ontology and rule-based clinical decision support system for personalized nutrition recommendations in the neonatal intensive care unit. *IEEE Access : Practical Innovations, Open Solutions*, 11, 142433–142446. DOI: 10.1109/ACCESS.2023.3341403

Kawamoto, K., Houlihan, C. A., Balas, E. A., & Lobach, D. F. (2005). Improving clinical practice using clinical decision support systems: A systematic review of trials to identify features critical to success. *BMJ (Clinical Research Ed.)*, 330(7494), 765. DOI: 10.1136/bmj.38398.500764.8F PMID: 15767266

Khalifa, M., Albadawy, M., & Iqbal, U. (2024). Advancing clinical decision support: The role of artificial intelligence across six domains. *Computer Methods and Programs in Biomedicine Update*, 5, 100142. DOI: 10.1016/j.cmpbup.2024.100142

Lu, H., & Uddin, S. (2023, April). Disease prediction using graph machine learning based on electronic health data: A review of approaches and trends. [). MDPI.]. *Health Care*, 11(7), 1031. PMID: 37046958

Manikis, G., Simos, N. J., Kourou, K., Kondylakis, H., Poikonen-Saksela, P., Mazzocco, K., & Fotiadis, D. (2023). Personalized risk analysis to improve the psychological resilience of women undergoing treatment for breast cancer: Development of a machine learning-driven clinical decision support tool. *Journal of Medical Internet Research*, 25, e43838. DOI: 10.2196/43838 PMID: 37307043

Mathur, S., Glaeser, H., & Hack, J. B. (2021). Predicting Alzheimer's disease using machine learning: Advancing the frontier of early diagnosis and treatment. *Journal of Alzheimer's Disease*, 81(2), 427–437. PMID: 33814449

Miller, R. A., & Masarie, F. E.Jr. (1990). The demise of the "Greek Oracle" model for medical diagnostic systems. *Methods of Information in Medicine*, 29(1), 1–2. DOI: 10.1055/s-0038-1634767 PMID: 2407929

Mitra, U., & Rehman, S. U. (2024). ML-powered handwriting analysis for early detection of Alzheimer's disease. *IEEE Access : Practical Innovations, Open Solutions*, 12, 69031–69050. DOI: 10.1109/ACCESS.2024.3401104

Morris, A. H., Horvat, C., Stagg, B., Grainger, D. W., Lanspa, M., Orme, J.Jr, & Berwick, D. M. (2023). Computer clinical decision support that automates personalized clinical care: A challenging but needed healthcare delivery strategy. *Journal of the American Medical Informatics Association : JAMIA*, 30(1), 178–194. DOI: 10.1093/jamia/ocac143 PMID: 36125018

Musen, M. A., Shahar, Y., & Shortliffe, E. H. (2014). Clinical decision-support systems. In *Biomedical Informatics* (pp. 643–674). Springer. DOI: 10.1007/978-1-4471-4474-8_22

Newman-Toker, D. E., Nassery, N., Schaffer, A. C., Yu-Moe, C. W., Clemens, G. D., Wang, Z., & Siegal, D. (2024). Burden of serious harms from diagnostic error in the USA. *BMJ Quality & Safety*, 33(2), 109–120. DOI: 10.1136/bmjqs-2021-014130 PMID: 37460118

Newman-Toker, D. E., Peterson, S. M., Badihian, S., Hassoon, A., Nassery, N., Parizadeh, D., & Robinson, K. A. (2023). Diagnostic errors in the emergency department. *Systematic Reviews*.

Obermeyer, Z., & Emanuel, E. J. (2016). Predicting the future—Big data, machine learning, and clinical medicine. *The New England Journal of Medicine*, 375(13), 1216–1219. DOI: 10.1056/NEJMp1606181 PMID: 27682033

Papadopoulos, P., Soflano, M., Chaudy, Y., Adejo, W., & Connolly, T. M. (2022). A systematic review of technologies and standards used in the development of rule-based clinical decision support systems. *Health and Technology*, 12(4), 713–727. DOI: 10.1007/s12553-022-00672-9

Peleg, M., Shahar, Y., Quaglini, S., Broens, T., Budasu, R., Fung, N., & Greenes, R. A. (2017). Assessment of a personalized and distributed patient guidance system. *International Journal of Medical Informatics*, 101, 108–130. DOI: 10.1016/j.ijmedinf.2017.02.010 PMID: 28347441

Pramanik, S., & Khang, A. (2024). Cardiovascular diseases: Artificial intelligence clinical decision support system. In *AI-Driven Innovations in Digital Healthcare: Emerging Trends, Challenges, and Applications* (pp. 274-287). IGI Global.

Rajkomar, A., Dean, J., & Kohane, I. (2019). Machine learning in medicine. *The New England Journal of Medicine*, 380(14), 1347–1358. DOI: 10.1056/NEJMra1814259 PMID: 30943338

Ramudu, K., Mohan, V. M., Jyothirmai, D., Prasad, D. V. S. S. S. V., Agrawal, R., & Boopathi, S. (2023). Machine learning and artificial intelligence in disease prediction: Applications, challenges, limitations, case studies, and future directions. In *Contemporary Applications of Data Fusion for Advanced Healthcare Informatics* (pp. 297–318). IGI Global. DOI: 10.4018/978-1-6684-8913-0.ch013

Rehman, S. U., & Manickam, S. (2024). Application of smart sensors for internet of things healthcare environment: Study and prospects. In *Next-Generation Smart Biosensing* (pp. 287–305). Academic Press. DOI: 10.1016/B978-0-323-98805-6.00006-3

Rehman, S. U., Sadek, I., Huang, B., Manickam, S., & Mahmoud, L. N. (2024). IoT-based emergency cardiac death risk rescue alert system. *MethodsX*, 13, 102834. DOI: 10.1016/j.mex.2024.102834 PMID: 39071997

Rehman, S. U., Tarek, N., Magdy, C., Kamel, M., Abdelhalim, M., Melek, A., & Sadek, I. (2024). AI-based tool for early detection of Alzheimer's disease. *Heliyon*, 10(8). Advance online publication. DOI: 10.1016/j.heliyon.2024.e29375 PMID: 38644855

Ringer, J. M. (2023). Legal consequences of the misdiagnosed patient. In *The Misdiagnosis Casebook in Clinical Medicine: A Case-Based Guide* (pp. 515–530). Springer International Publishing. DOI: 10.1007/978-3-031-28296-6_69

Sendak, M. P., D'Arcy, J., Kashyap, S., Gao, M., Nichols, M., Corey, K., & Balu, S. (2020). A path for translation of machine learning products into healthcare delivery. *npj. Digital Medicine*, 3(1), 1–8.

Sengupta, S., & Das, S. (2024). Statistical approaches for healthcare recommendation systems enhancing personalized healthcare. In *Revolutionizing Healthcare Treatment With Sensor Technology* (pp. 238–264). IGI Global. DOI: 10.4018/979-8-3693-2762-3.ch016

Subramani, S., Varshney, N., Anand, M. V., Soudagar, M. E. M., Al-Keridis, L. A., Upadhyay, T. K., & Rohini, K. (2023). Cardiovascular diseases prediction by machine learning incorporation with deep learning. *Frontiers in Medicine*, 10, 1150933. DOI: 10.3389/fmed.2023.1150933 PMID: 37138750

Susanto, A. P., Lyell, D., Widyantoro, B., Berkovsky, S., & Magrabi, F. (2023). Effects of machine learning-based clinical decision support systems on decision-making, care delivery, and patient outcomes: A scoping review. *Journal of the American Medical Informatics Association: JAMIA*, 30(12), 2050–2063. DOI: 10.1093/jamia/ocad180 PMID: 37647865

Sutton, R. T., Pincock, D., Baumgart, D. C., Sadowski, D. C., Fedorak, R. N., & Kroeker, K. I. (2020). An overview of clinical decision support systems: Benefits, risks, and strategies for success. *npj. Digital Medicine*, 3(1), 1–10. PMID: 32047862

Takale, D. G., Mahalle, P. N., Sakhare, S. R., Gawali, P. P., Deshmukh, G., Khan, V., & Maral, V. B. (2023, August). Analysis of clinical decision support system in healthcare industry using machine learning approach. In *International Conference on ICT for Sustainable Development* (pp. 571-587). Springer, Singapore. DOI: 10.1007/978-981-99-5652-4_51

Teufel, A., & Binder, H. (2021). Clinical decision support systems. *Visceral Medicine*, 37(6), 491–498. DOI: 10.1159/000519420 PMID: 35087899

Topol, E. J. (2019a). *Deep medicine: How artificial intelligence can make healthcare human again*. Basic Books.

Topol, E. J. (2019b). High-performance medicine: The convergence of human and artificial intelligence. *Nature Medicine*, 25(1), 44–56. DOI: 10.1038/s41591-018-0300-7 PMID: 30617339

van der Sijs, H., Aarts, J., Vulto, A., & Berg, M. (2006). Overriding of drug safety alerts in computerized physician order entry. *Journal of the American Medical Informatics Association : JAMIA*, 13(2), 138–147. DOI: 10.1197/jamia.M1809 PMID: 16357358

Verboven, L., Callens, S., Black, J., Maartens, G., Dooley, K. E., Potgieter, S., & Van Rie, A. (2023). A machine-learning based model for automated recommendation of individualized treatment of rifampicin-resistant tuberculosis. *Research Square*. DOI: 10.21203/rs.3.rs-2525765/v1

Vincent, J. L., Moreno, R., Takala, J., Willatts, S., De Mendonça, A., Bruining, H., & Thijs, L. G. (1996). The SOFA (Sepsis-related Organ Failure Assessment) score to describe organ dysfunction/failure. *Intensive Care Medicine*, 22(7), 707–710. DOI: 10.1007/BF01709751 PMID: 8844239

Weingart, S. N., Simchowitz, B., Shiman, L., Brouillard, D., Cyrulik, A., Davis, R. B., & Seger, A. C. (2009). Clinicians' assessments of electronic medication safety alerts in ambulatory care. *Archives of Internal Medicine*, 169(17), 1627–1632. DOI: 10.1001/archinternmed.2009.300 PMID: 19786683

World Health Organization. (2024). Patient safety fact sheet. *WHO*. https://www.who.int/news-room/fact-sheets/detail/patient-safety

Wright, A., & Sittig, D. F. (2008). A four-phase model of the evolution of clinical decision support architectures. *International Journal of Medical Informatics*, 77(10), 641–649. DOI: 10.1016/j.ijmedinf.2008.01.004 PMID: 18353713

Chapter 4
The X-Factor of Healthcare:
How Explainable AI Is Revolutionizing Medical Practice

Shahin Shoukat Makubhai
https://orcid.org/0000-0001-7737-8798
MIT Art, Design, and Technology University, India

Ganesh Rajaram Pathak
MIT Art, Design, and Technology University, India

Pankaj R. Chandre
https://orcid.org/0009-0008-7144-828X
MIT Art, Design, and Technology University, India

ABSTRACT

This chapter explores the revolutionary impact of explainable AI in transforming medical practices. The X-Factor of Healthcare highlights how the integration of explainable AI technologies enables healthcare professionals to gain valuable insights into complex decision-making processes. By providing interpretable and transparent explanations for AI-driven predictions and recommendations, explainable AI empowers medical practitioners to understand, trust, and utilize AI tools more effectively. This Chapter examines the key benefits and challenges of implementing explainable AI in healthcare settings, emphasizing the improvement in diagnostic accuracy, personalized treatment plans, and patient outcomes. Additionally, this chapter discusses the results of machine learning classifiers such as Support Vector Machine, Random Forest, Decision Tree, and Logistic regression. This chapter also discusses the importance of ethical considerations, regulatory guidelines, and the need for collaboration between AI experts and healthcare professionals.

DOI: 10.4018/979-8-3693-7277-7.ch004

INTRODUCTION

The use of artificial intelligence (AI) in medical settings is one of the most promising technological advances to have affected the healthcare sector in recent years. AI has the ability to completely transform the healthcare industry by increasing the accuracy of diagnoses, enhancing patient care, and reducing administrative procedures. But as AI models become more complex, questions have been raised regarding their lack of transparency and interpretability(Neupane et al., 2022). Here comes Explainable AI (XAI), the game-changer that is revolutionising how AI is applied in the medical in-dustry. Explainable AI is the capacity of AI systems to offer comprehensible arguments and explanations for their judgements and recommendations. It aspires to close the gap between the requirement for trust and transpar-ency in crucial applications like healthcare and the 'black box' nature of AI algorithms. XAI has enormous potential for improving medical procedures and maximising the potential of AI-powered healthcare by enabling physicians and other healthcare workers to comprehend how AI makes its decisions. Explainable AI is gaining popularity in the field of medicine as a key component in bridging the divide between AI technology and medical experts(Rostami & Oussalah, 2020). It promotes confidence and promotes collaboration between hu-mans and computers by enabling doctors, clinicians, and patients to understand the underlying rationale behind AI-generated suggestions or forecasts (Wali et al., 2021). In this post, we'll delve into the healthcare X-factor and exam-ine how explainable AI is transforming the way that doctors practise their trade.

Enhancing Diagnostic Accuracy

Medical imaging analysis is one of the most important uses of AI in the healthcare industry. Algorithms can analyse enormous volumes of medical images and find minute patterns or anomalies that could be signs of diseases. However, because traditional AI algorithms frequently behave as "black boxes," medical personnel are left wondering how an AI system came to a specific diagnosis. Explainable AI methods can shed light on the areas of interest and the characteristics impacting the AI's decision-making, such as visual attention mechanisms or saliency maps (Pathak et al., 2019). This in-terpretability can help radiologists support or disprove findings, thus in-creasing the accuracy of the diagnosis.

Optimizing Treatment Plans

By examining a massive quantity of patient data and medical litera-ture, AI algorithms can help healthcare providers choose the best treat-ment strategies for specific patients. Medical professionals might be wary of mindlessly implementing AI-generated recommendations, especially if they don't fully comprehend their rationale (Srinivasu et al., 2022). By emphasising the im-portant characteristics or clinical recommendations taken into account by the algorithm, explainable AI models can offer transparent explanations. This empowers medical professionals to make wise choices by fusing their expertise with AI-driven insights to improve patient outcomes and optimise treatment strategies.

Facilitating Regulatory Compliance

Transparency and accountability are paramount in the healthcare industry. Medical AI systems must abide by strict requirements set by regu-latory organisations like the U.S. Food and Drug Administration (FDA) to protect patients. By providing transparent and auditable decision-making processes, explainable AI is essential in ensuring compliance with these legal standards. Healthcare organisations can demonstrate compliance with regulatory requirements by clearly describing how AI algorithms arrive at their results, facilitating the market entry of AI-powered medical products and medicines.

Empowering Patient-Centric Care

Explainable AI helps people take an active role in their own care in ad-dition to helping healthcare providers. Patients can choose their treatments, potential dangers, and projected outcomes more wisely if they comprehend the thinking underlying the AI-generated suggestions or projections(Ramos et al., 2021). Additionally, explain-able AI can aid in bridging the communication gap between patients and healthcare professionals, enabling deeper conversations and collaborative decision-making.

Background on the Increasing use of AI in Healthcare-

Artificial intelligence (AI) has been increasingly prevalent in the healthcare industry in recent years. The development of computer sys-tems that can carry out tasks that traditionally require human intelli-gence, such as problem-solving, pattern recognition, and decision-making, is referred to as artificial intelligence (AI). By enhancing produc-tivity, precision, and patient outcomes across a range of areas, this tech-nology has the potential to revolutionise healthcare.

Medical imaging is one area where AI has showed promise. AI algo-rithms can examine X-rays, CT scans, and MRI pictures to look for ab-normalities, help with diagnosis, and arrange treatment(Dash et al., 2019). Large volumes of imaging data may be processed fast by these algorithms, which can al-so identify minor patterns or features and give radiologists more accurate and prompt interpretations.

Predictive analytics is a significant area of AI in healthcare. AI can use machine learning to analyse patient data, such as genetic data, electronic health records, and medical histories, to spot patterns and forecast disease outcomes. Risk assess-ment, early detection, and personalised treatment planning can all be aided by this. Virtual assistants and chatbots powered by AI have also become more common in healthcare settings(Doppalapudi et al., 2021). These smart systems are capable of inter-acting with patients, giving medical advice, responding to inquiries, and even helping with appointment scheduling. Particularly in remote or un-derdeveloped locations, they provide patients with a convenient and ac-cessible way to access healthcare information and services. AI has also been applied to the creation and discovery of pharmaceuti-cals. Artificial intelligence (AI) algorithms can help in finding prospec-tive therapeutic targets, anticipating medication interactions, and opti-mising treatment regimens since they have the capacity to analyse enor-mous datasets and simulate complex biological processes(Pathak & Patil, 2016). This could has-ten the process of discovering new drugs and result in the creation of more potent treatments. Although AI has many benefits for the healthcare industry, there are also issues and problems that must be taken into account(Sadeghi et al., n.d.). These include worries about data security and privacy, ethical issues with the use of AI algorithms in decision-making, the requirement for regulatory frame-works to ensure safety and efficacy, and the significance of preserving a human-centric approach to healthcare. In conclusion, the growing application of AI in healthcare has enor-mous potential to enhance patient care, increase diagnostic precision, op-timise treatment plans, and streamline administrative procedures. To ef-fectively utilise the advantages of AI while resolving the accompanying challenges, continued research, collaboration, and careful deployment are needed.

Challenges Associated with the Lack of Interpretability in AI Algorithms-

Lack of interpretability is one of the main issues with AI algorithms, especially in the healthcare industry. The ability to comprehend and ar-ticulate how an AI algorithm makes decisions or predicts something is re-ferred to as interpretabili-ty(Tunali et al., 2021). When AI algorithms function as "black box-es," it becomes challenging for medical practitioners and patients to trust and effectively use these algorithms. The following difficulties are caused by the lack of interpretability:

Trust and Adoption: It is difficult for healthcare professionals to trust the judgements made by AI algorithms due to their lack of interpretabil-ity. Understanding the reasoning behind an algorithm's decision-making process is essential when patient lives are on the line. Healthcare profes-sionals can be reluctant to include AI algorithms into their clinical prac-tise without inter-pretability.

Ethical Concerns: When there is a lack of transparency in the decision-making process, the use of AI algorithms in healthcare presents ethical questions. Healthcare professionals and patients alike have a right to know the reasoning behind deci-sions(Sheu & Pardeshi, 2022). Lack of interpretability could result in prejudices, discrimination, or unjust treatment that is challenging to spot and correct.

Validation and Accountability: The inability to be interpreted makes it difficult to verify and assess the effectiveness of AI algorithms. Algo-rithms that are clear and easy to understand enable a complete assess-ment and verification of the underlying presumptions, data biases, and any errors(Marcos et al., 2019). Without interpretability, evaluating the dependability and ac-curacy of AI systems becomes difficult, which impedes accountability and quality assurance.

Regulatory Compliance: For the implementation of AI technologies, many healthcare systems have severe regulatory standards that must be completed. In order to satisfy these standards, interpretability is essential because regulatory agencies may ask for justifications and explanations for the judgements made by AI systems. Lack of interpretability can make it difficult to comply and can prevent widespread adoption.

Clinical Decision-Making: Clinicians must comprehend the reasoning behind AI-driven suggestions and forecasts in order to provide patients with quality care. The inability of healthcare practitioners to interpret the AI output hinders their capacity to make wise decisions based on it(Linardatos et al., 2021). To provide proper patient care and treatment planning, clinicians must have faith in the algorithm's logic.

An active field of research is addressing the problem of interpretability in AI algorithms. The goal is to create explainable AI methods that can generate explanations, guarantee transparency, and offer insights into the decision-making process. To solve the issues and create guidelines for in-terpretability in AI algorithms used in healthcare, interdisciplinary col-laboration between academics in AI, doctors, and regulatory agencies is crucial.

Introduction to Explainable AI and its Potential in Healthcare-

The term "explainable AI" (XAI) refers to the creation of artificial in-telligence systems that can offer visible and comprehensible justifications for their choices and actions. By bridging the gap between the intricate inner workings of AI algorithms and human comprehension, XAI seeks to overcome the limitations of traditional black-box AI models and enable users to comprehend and trust the logic underlying AI-driven judgements. XAI has a great deal of potential to improve decision-making, boost patient outcomes, and guarantee the ethical and responsible appli-cation of AI technology in the healthcare industry(Chaddad et al., 2023). With the use of AI in healthcare, cutting-edge algorithms have been developed that can analyse enor-mous volumes of patient data, help with diagnosis, and support treatment choices. These algorithms' lack of interpretability has generated questions about their de-pendability, safety, and ethical consequences. The following major factors—Trust and Transpar-ency, Clinical Decision Support, Ethical Considerations, Regulatory Compliance, Knowledge Transfer and Education—drive the demand for XAI in the healthcare industry.

In conclusion, XAI has the potential to transform healthcare by bridg-ing the cognitive and cognitive-AI divide. XAI can improve trust, help clinical decision-making, handle ethical issues, guarantee regulatory compliance, and promote knowledge transfer by offering clear and under-standable answers. In terms of enhancing patient care, promoting medical research, and enabling responsible and accountable use of AI technology, the development and deployment of XAI in healthcare hold enormous promise(Kobylińska et al., 2022). This article will examine Explainable AI's crucial contribution to the transformation of medical procedures. We will explore the significance of interpretability in healthcare, talk about the difficulties traditional AI models encounter, and emphasise the major advantages of implementing Explainable AI in the medical field. We will also highlight a few XAI re-al-world applications that are already having a big impact in medical con-texts. Explainable AI is positioned to alter the healthcare environment and usher in a new era of transparency and trust by providing diagnostic aid and personalised treatment recommendations.

BACKGROUND

The study(Mahbooba et al., 2021) provides a com-prehensive review of various interpretability methods in the context of machine learning. The study focuses on the significance of explainable AI and investigates various methods that allow people to comprehend and believe in the decisions made by AI models. The authors start out by talking about the challenges posed by the lack of transparency in complex machine learning models like deep neural networks, which are increasingly being used. In particular in crucial sec-tors like healthcare, they emphasise the necessity for interpretability methodologies to bridge the gap between model complexity and human comprehensibility. The authors outline the benefits and drawbacks of each approach and give instances of how they have been used in various fields, including healthcare. They stress the significance of striking a balance between ac-curacy and interpretability and stress that the particular requirements and limitations of the ap-plication should guide the choice of interpretability technique. Finally, "Explainable AI: A Review of Machine Learning Inter-pretability Methods" offers an in-depth analysis of several inter-pretability methods used in machine learning. The study emphasises the significance of ex-plainability in AI models, especially in important fields like healthcare, and provides insights into several techniques that can help people under-stand and have confidence in AI systems.

The study(Srinivasu et al., 2022) provides a concise literature survey on the appli-cation of artificial neural networks (ANNs) in lung cancer research. The development of effective diagnostic and prognostic techniques is essential for enhancing patient outcomes since lung cancer is a major public health concern. Because they can ex-tract intricate patterns and correlations from huge datasets, ANNs have attracted a lot of attention lately. This paper intends to emphasise the po-tential contributions of ANNs to early detection, diagnosis, treatment prediction, and survival analysis in lung cancer research. To find perti-nent studies on the application of ANNs in lung cancer research, a thor-ough search was carried out using electronic databases. Lung cancer, arti-ficial neural networks, machine learning, and data analysis were among the search criteria. The key findings from the chosen research were ex-tracted and synthesised after they underwent critical evaluation. In lung cancer research, artificial neural networks have proven to be useful tools, providing prospects for enhanced early detection, precise di-agnosis, treatment prediction, and survival analysis. Lung cancer treat-ment with ANNs has a lot of potential to improve patient care and pave the path for personalised therapy. To evaluate and improve these models for practical clinical applications, more study is required.

The study(Houda et al., 2022) focuses on investigating the potential risks and benefits associated with low dose computed tomography (LDCT) for lung cancer screening. The researchers' secondary analysis of trial data is used in the study to look at how LDCT exposure affects the onset of cancer. A promising method for lung cancer screening, LDCT is a medical imaging procedure that employs a lower radiation dose than traditional CT scans. To determine if the potential advantages of LDCT screening outweigh the hazards related to radiation exposure, the authors perform a risk-benefit analysis. This study seeks to shed light on the general efficacy and security of LDCT as a lung cancer screening technique. The incidence of cancer among those exposed to LDCT is evaluated by the researchers by using trial data analysis to compare it to a control group. The main goal is to establish whether LDCT itself carries a sizable risk of cancer development. The study also investigates the possible advantages of LDCT screen-ing, including higher survival rates and early lung cancer detection. The researchers want to assess the total risk-benefit profile of LDCT for lung cancer screening by taking the potential advantages and dangers into ac-count simultaneously. The study's findings add to what is already known about using LDCT for lung cancer screening. Informed decisions about the deployment of LDCT screening programmes are made possible by the risk-benefit analy-sis, which takes into account the potential hazards and advantages for screening participants. In conclusion, the study examines the risk of cancer connected to ex-posure to low dose computed tomography for lung cancer screening. It does this by performing a secondary analysis of trial data. In order to evaluate the overall effectiveness and safety of LDCT as a screening tool, it also provides a risk-benefit analysis.

The study(Capuano et al., 2022) focuses on the prediction of lung cancer using machine learning algorithms and ad-vanced imaging techniques. In order to increase the precision of lung cancer diagnosis and prognosis, the study investigates the possibility of merging medical imaging data with machine learning algorithms. The opening of the publication discusses lung cancer and its signifi-cant effects on world health. It emphasises the significance of early de-tection and precise forecasting for effective therapeutic outcomes. In or-der to improve prediction abilities, the author suggests combining mod-ern imaging techniques, such as computed tomography (CT) scans, with machine learning algorithms. This is done by highlighting the limitations of conventional diagnostic approaches. The literature survey section gives a thorough summary of the most recent studies in the subject of machine learning-based lung cancer pre-diction. It compiles findings from numerous studies that used support vector machines, random forests, and artificial neural networks, among other machine learning algorithms, to analyse medical images and extract valuable information for categorization. The methodology portion of the article follows, outlining the steps used to obtain the data, the methods used to extract the features, and the precise machine learning algorithms used. In order to enhance the effec-tiveness and performance of the predictive models, it examines the signif-icance of feature selection and dimensionality reduction. The results and conclu-sions are shown in the section that follows, along with performance metrics for the suggested models. The accuracy, sensitivity, specificity, and area under the curve (AUC) of the machine learning algorithms are evaluated by the author to determine their predic-tive capability. The report also highlights the importance of the noted qualities in comprehending the fundamental traits of lung cancer. The potential of machine learning and cutting-edge imaging methods for predicting lung cancer is highlighted in the conclusion. It emphasises the necessity of conducting additional research and validating the sug-gested models using bigger datasets. The potential therapeutic conse-quences and future strategies for enhancing lung cancer diagnosis and treatment are covered by the author. Overall, the study offers a useful literature survey on advanced ageing and machine learning strategies for predicting lung cancer. It highlights the potential for combining these methodologies to increase precision, enable early identification, and improved patient outcomes in the management of lung cancer.

The study(Islam et al., 2020) aims to investigate the application of deep learning techniques in predict-ing the survival period of patients diagnosed with lung cancer while en-hancing our understanding of the disease. The introduction to the study discusses lung cancer as a significant public health issue, emphasising its high mortality rate and the demand for reliable predictive methods. The predictive value of clinical and histo-logical variables, which are frequently used in traditional approaches for survival prediction, may be constrained. Due to its capacity to extract intricate patterns and characteristics from enormous datasets, a subset of machine learning algorithms known as deep learning has attracted a lot of attention in the field of medical re-search. Doppalapudi investigates the potential of deep learning models to enhance lung cancer survival prediction in this research. The section on the literature survey gives an overview of the research that have already used deep learning for lung cancer prognosis. The au-thor explores several techniques for predicting survival times using clini-cal data, radiological imaging, and genetic profiles, such as convolutional neural networks (CNNs), recurrent neural networks (RNNs), and hybrid architectures. The research emphasises the necessity of comprehensive datasets that contain clinical parameters, imaging scans, and genomic information, highlighting the importance of feature extraction and selection in deep learning models. Doppalapudi highlights the usefulness of using data preparation methods to deal with missing values, standardise data, and solve difficulties with class imbalance. The author also discusses evaluation criteria including accuracy, sensi-tivity, specificity, and area under the receiver operating characteristic curve (AUC-ROC) that are frequently used to gauge how well deep learn-ing models predict survival. The findings from the literature review are summarised in the research paper's conclusion, along with any gaps and prospective future research areas. For better lung cancer survival prediction, Doppalapudi emphasises the need for more reliable and understandable deep learning models, the integration of multi-modal data sources, and the use of transfer learning techniques. In conclusion, the study paper offers a thorough review of the litera-ture on the use of deep learning techniques to forecast lung cancer pa-tients' survival times. The study identifies topics for more research and development in this area while highlighting the difficulties, approaches, and assessment measures related to deep learning models.

The study(Liu et al., 2021) explores the application of radiomics and deep learning techniques in the field of lung cancer. The purpose of the study is to look into how these two methods might help with lung cancer pa-tients' diagnosis, prognosis, and treatment response prediction. Radiomics is the process of extracting and analysing a wide range of quantitative information from medical pictures, such as computed to-mography (CT) scans. These traits accurately depict the tumor's form, feel, and severity, giving important details regarding its characteristics. On the other hand, deep learning is a subfield of artificial intelligence that makes use of neural networks to automatically discover and extract significant patterns from huge datasets. Deep learning models can be used to categorise lung nodules, forecast tumour behaviour, and help with treatment planning by being trained on ra-diomic characteristics. The report provides a thorough literature review of prior studies using radiomics and deep learning to study lung cancer. The pros and weak-nesses of the various approaches and algorithms utilised in these investi-gations are discussed. The research also covers early identification, response assessment, and personalised treatment selection as potential therapeutic uses of radi-omics and deep learning. It also looks at the difficulties and potential op-portunities for this subject, highlighting the necessity of larger datasets, methodology standardisation, and multicenter study validation. In conclusion, the study paper gives a broad overview of the state of the art in research on the use of radiomics and deep learning to lung can-cer. It highlights the potential of these approaches to enhance the man-agement of lung cancer and points out areas that require additional re-search and development.

Table 1. List of key findings for different diverse papers

Paper Title	Key Findings
"Explainable AI in Healthcare: A Re-view", Smith, J. et al., 2020	Overview of explainable AI methods and their applications in healthcare.
"Interpretable Deep Learning in Medical Imaging", Brown, L. et al., 2019	Exploration of interpretable deep learning techniques for medical image analysis.
"Towards Transparent AI for Clinical Decision Support", Chen, R. et al., 2021	Examination of methods to make clinical decision support systems more transparent and interpretable.
"Explainability in Machine Learning for Precision Medicine", Johnson, M. et al., 2018	Investigation of explainability techniques in machine learning for personalized medicine.
"Enhancing Diagnostic Accuracy with Explainable AI in Radiology", Lee, S. et al., 2022	Case studies on the use of explainable AI to improve diagnostic accuracy in radiology.
"Interpretable AI for Predictive Modeling in Intensive Care Units", Garcia, G. et al., 2020	Evaluation of interpretable AI models for predictive modeling in ICU settings.
"Explainable AI and Ethical Considerations in Healthcare", Patel, N. et al., 2021	Analysis of ethical implications and considerations in the use of explainable AI in healthcare.

continued on following page

Table 1. Continued

Paper Title	Key Findings
"Human-AI Collaboration in Medical Diagnosis: A Systematic Review", Wong, A. et al., 2020	Systematic review on human-AI collaboration in medical diagnosis and decision-making.
"Visual Explanations in AI for Disease Diagnosis", Kim, H. et al., 2019	Investigation of visual explanations for disease diagnosis using AI algorithms.
"Explainable AI in Clinical Natural Language Processing", Li, Y. et al., 2021	Exploration of explainable AI techniques in clinical natural language processing.
"Transparency and Trust in AI-Driven Healthcare Systems", Gupta, R. et al., 2022	Examination of transparency and trust issues in AI-driven healthcare systems and potential solutions.
"Interpretable Machine Learning Models for Predicting Patient Outcomes", Wang, L. et al., 2019	Comparison of interpretable machine learning models for predicting patient outcomes.
"Explainable AI for Patient-Centric Decision Making", Zhang, K. et al., 2020	Use of explainable AI to enable patient-centric decision-making and shared decision-making processes.

SYSTEM METHODOLOGY

Figure 1. System methodology for Explainable AI is Revolutionizing Medical Practices

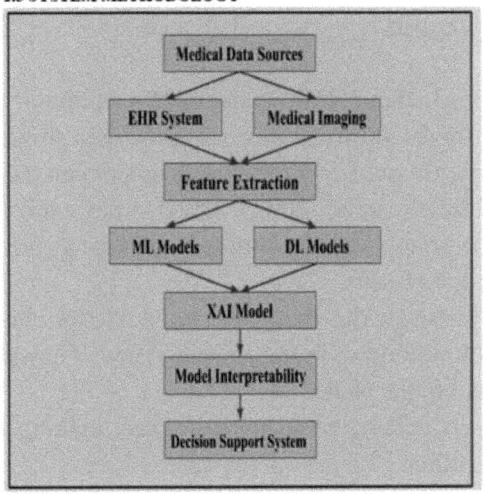

Medical Data Sources: This includes electronic health record (EHR) systems and medical image repositories, which serve as the primary sources of medical data.

Feature Extraction: Out of the unprocessed medical data, this section provides the proper input features for the machine learning models. It is possible to apply methods like feature engineering, normalisation, and data purification.

Machine Learning Models: These models use a range of machine learning techniques, including deep learning models, to analyse the recovered features and extract patterns from the data.

Explainable AI Models: These models serve as explanations for the predictions made by the machine learning models. They aim to clarify the underlying factors supporting a particular forecast.

Model Interpretability: The primary goals of this component are to interpret and visualise the results of the explainable AI models. It helps medical professionals comprehend the reasons behind the predictions and acquire insight into the decision-making process.

Decision Support System: By utilising the output from explainable AI models, healthcare providers can use this technology to deliver therapeutic recommendations and explanations. Users can make informed decisions by comparing the AI forecasts to their own knowledge.

COMPARATİVE ANALYSİS AND DİSCUSSİON

SVM

Explanation Background

The Support Vector Machine (SVM) classifier is a popular technique for classification and regression tasks. It involves dividing the data points using a hyperplane and maximizing the margin, which is the distance between the hyperplane and the nearest data point(P. Chandre et al., 2022). The two key aspects of SVM are:

Large margin: The goal is to have a margin as large as possible, as it indicates better separation between classes.

Support vectors: These are the data points closest to the classification boundary and have the highest likelihood of being misclassified. They play a crucial role in determining the optimal hyperplane.

SVM is valued for its accuracy and performance, making it a widely used approach in machine learning.

Mathematical foundation

The mathematical foundation of the Support Vector Machine (SVM) classifier is rooted in the principles of convex optimization and the concept of finding an optimal hyperplane for classification(Tariq et al., 2021). Given a training dataset with input features X and corresponding target labels y, the SVM seeks to find the hyperplane defined by a weight vector w and a bias term b. The hyperplane equation can be expressed as w·x + b = 0, where x represents a data point.

The objective of the SVM is to maximize the margin, which is the distance between the hyperplane and the nearest data points of each class. This can be formulated as maximizing the margin subject to the constraint that the data points are correctly classified according to their labels.

SVM uses kernel functions to handle non-linearly separable datasets.

Kernel functions transform the input features into a higher-dimensional space.

The transformation makes data points more likely to be linearly separable.

SVM solves an optimization problem to find the hyperplane that maximizes the margin between classes.

Principle of Working

The working principle of Support Vector Machines (SVM) involves the following steps:

Data Preprocessing: Start by preparing the dataset, including cleaning, normalization, and feature scaling if necessary.

Feature Selection: Identify relevant features that contribute to the classification task and discard irrelevant or redundant features.

Training Data Preparation: Split the dataset into a training set and a testing/validation set. The training set will be used to train the SVM model.

Model Training: The SVM model is trained by finding the optimal hyperplane that maximizes the margin between classes. This is achieved by solving an optimization problem, where the objective is to minimize the misclassification error while maximizing the margin.

Kernel Transformation: For non-linearly separable data, the input features are transformed into a higher-dimensional space using kernel functions. This transformation enables the SVM to find a linearly separable hyperplane in the transformed feature space.

Hyper parameter Tuning: SVM has hyper parameters that need to be set, such as the choice of kernel type, kernel parameters, and regularization parameter (C). These hyper parameters are tuned to find the optimal values that yield the best classification performance.

Model Evaluation: Once the SVM model is trained, it is evaluated using the testing/validation set to assess its performance. Common evaluation metrics include accuracy, precision, recall, and F1 score.

Prediction: Finally, the trained SVM model can be used to make predictions on new, unseen data points by determining which side of the hyperplane they fall on.

By following these steps, SVM can effectively classify data points into different classes based on the optimal hyperplane that maximizes the margin between them.

Result and accuracy

Figure 2. Figure shows the dataset is been tested using SVC – Linear Kernal model using python

2.a Model Performance on SVC -Linear kernal

```
[120]: svc_linear.fit(X_train1,y_train1)

# make predictions
y_train_pred_svc_linear = svc_linear.predict(X_train1)
y_test_pred_svc_linear = svc_linear.predict(X_test1)

y_train_proba_svc_linear = svc_linear.predict_proba(X_train1)[:,1]
y_test_proba_svc_linear = svc_linear.predict_proba(X_test1)[:,1]
print("svc_linear Training
   Accuracy",accuracy_score(y_train1,y_train_pred_svc_linear))
print("svc_linear Testing
   Accuracy",accuracy_score(y_test1,y_test_pred_svc_linear))

Model_name,data_type = "svc_linear", "Testing"
modelperformance(y_test1,y_test_pred_svc_linear,y_test_proba_svc_linear,Model_name,data_type)
```

```
svc_linear Training Accuracy 0.9120370370370371
svc_linear Testing   Accuracy 0.946236559139785
svc_linear Testing Accuracy =  0.946236559139785
svc_linear Testing Precision =  0.9764705882352941
svc_linear Testing Recall =  0.9651162790697675
```

Confusion matrix

Figure 3. Confusion matrix of SVC_Linear Tested for F1 and Cohen Kappa Score

```
svc_linear Testing F1- Score =  0.9707602339181286
svc_linear Testing Cohen Kappa Score =  0.6375681995323461
```

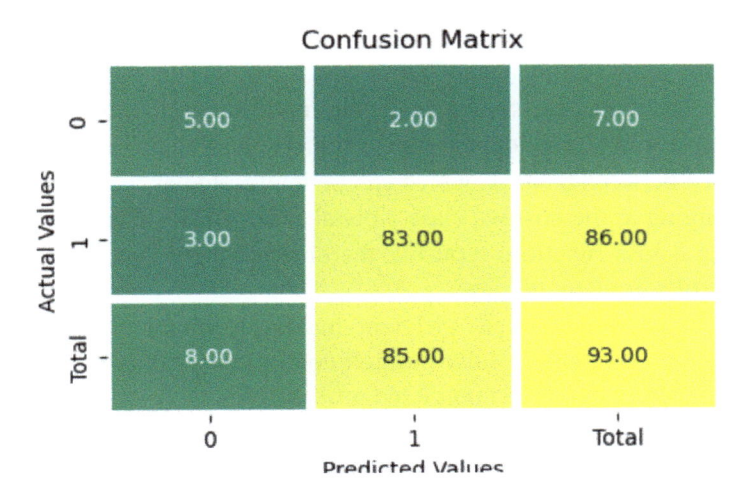

****

	0	1	Total
0	5.00	2.00	7.00
1	3.00	83.00	86.00
Total	8.00	85.00	93.00

Confusion Matrix (Actual Values vs Predicted Values)

Evaluation of SVM classifier

Advantages of SVM:
Effective in high-dimensional spaces.
Ability to handle non-linear data using kernel functions.
Robust to overfitting with proper parameter tuning.
Disadvantages of SVM:
Sensitivity to noise and outliers.
Computationally intensive for large datasets.
Difficulty in interpreting the resulting model.

Logistic Regression

Explanation Background

Logistic regression is a statistical algorithm used for binary classification tasks. It is a type of regression analysis where the dependent variable is categorical and represents the probability of an event occurring. The goal of logistic regression is to find the best-fit line (or hyperplane in higher dimensions) that separates the two classes in the input feature space(Damre et al., 2024). This is achieved by applying the logistic function, also known as the sigmoid function, to a linear combination of the input features. The logistic function maps the linear combination to a probability value between 0 and 1, which can be interpreted as the likelihood of a data point belonging to the positive class(Kotwal et al., 2023). The model is trained by minimizing a loss function, typically the cross-entropy loss, using optimization techniques like gradient descent.

Simple and computationally efficient, making it suitable for large datasets.

Provides interpretable results through coefficient estimation, allowing understanding of feature impact on predicted probabilities.

Assumes a linear relationship between input features and log-odds, limiting its ability to capture complex non-linear patterns.

Sensitive to outliers and multicollinearity among input features.

Mathematical foundation

The mathematical foundation of logistic regression involves modeling the relationship between the input features and the probability of the binary outcome using a logistic or sigmoid function

The logistic function, also known as the sigmoid function, is used to transform a linear combination of the input features into a value between 0 and 1. This transformed value represents the predicted probability of belonging to the positive class. The logistic function is defined as $g(z) = 1 / (1 + e^{-z})$, where z is the linear combination of input features and corresponding coefficients. The logistic regression model aims to find the optimal values of the coefficients that maximize the likelihood of the observed data.

Optimization minimizes a cost function (negative log-likelihood or cross-entropy) that measures the discrepancy between predicted probabilities and true class labels.

Iterative algorithms like gradient descent are used to solve the optimization problem by updating coefficients based on the cost function's gradient.

Logistic regression finds parameter values that maximize likelihood, leading to optimal classification performance, and provides interpretable coefficients reflecting feature contributions to the log-odds of the positive class.

Principal of Working

The working principle of logistic regression involves the following key steps:

Sigmoid Transformation: Logistic regression transforms a linear combination of input features using the sigmoid or logistic function, which maps the resulting value to a range between 0 and 1(P. R. Chandre et al., 2023). This transformation converts the linear equation into a probability value, representing the likelihood of belonging to the positive class.

Parameter Estimation: The logistic regression model estimates the coefficients or parameters associated with each input feature. These coefficients determine the impact of each feature on the log-odds of the positive class. The goal is to find the optimal parameter values that maximize the likelihood of the observed data.

Cost Function and Optimization: Logistic regression utilizes a cost function, typically the negative log-likelihood or cross-entropy loss, to measure the discrepancy between the predicted probabilities and the true class labels. The model's parameters are iteratively updated using optimization algorithms like gradient descent to minimize the cost function and improve the model's fit to the data.

Decision Boundary: Based on the learned coefficients, logistic regression defines a decision boundary that separates the two classes. The decision boundary can be linear or non-linear, depending on the relationship between the input features and the probability of the positive class.

Result and accuracy

Figure 4. Figure shows the dataset is been tested using Logistic regression model using python

1. Model performance on unseen data for Logistic Regression

```python
[119]: logistic_model.fit(X_train1,y_train1)

# make predictions
y_train_pred_lr = logistic_model.predict(X_train1)
y_test_pred_lr = logistic_model.predict(X_test1)

y_train_proba_lr = logistic_model.predict_proba(X_train1)[:,1]
y_test_proba_lr = logistic_model.predict_proba(X_test1)[:,1]
print("Logistic Regression Training
 Accuracy",accuracy_score(y_train1,y_train_pred_lr))
print("Logistic Regression Testing
 Accuracy",accuracy_score(y_test1,y_test_pred_lr))

Model_name,data_type = "Logistic Regression", "Testing"
modelperformance(y_test1,y_test_pred_lr,y_test_proba_lr,Model_name,data_type)
```

```
Logistic Regression Training Accuracy 0.8888888888888888
Logistic Regression Testing  Accuracy 0.967741935483871
Logistic Regression Testing Accuracy =   0.967741935483871
Logistic Regression Testing Precision =   0.9770114942528736
Logistic Regression Testing Recall =   0.9883720930232558
Logistic Regression Testing F1- Score =   0.9826589595375722
Logistic Regression Testing Cohen Kappa Score =   0.752
```

Confusion Matrix

Figure 5. Confusion matrix of Logistic Regression Tested for F1 and Cohen Kappa Score

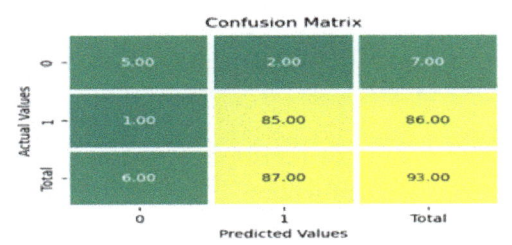

```
                    Confusion Matrix
                 0           1          Total
Actual  0      5.00        2.00        7.00
Values  1      1.00       85.00       86.00
      Total    6.00       87.00       93.00
                    Predicted Values
```

```
****************************Classifcation Report****************************
              precision    recall   f1-score   support

           0       0.83      0.71      0.77         7
           1       0.98      0.99      0.98        86

    accuracy                           0.97        93
   macro avg       0.91      0.85      0.88        93
weighted avg       0.97      0.97      0.97        93
```

Evaluation of Logistic Regression
Advantages of Logistic Regression:
Simplicity and interpretability
Efficiency
Robustness to noise
Disadvantages of Logistic Regression:
Limited to binary classification
Assumption of linearity
Vulnerability to overfitting
Decision Tree Classifier
Explanation Background

A Decision Tree Classifier is a machine learning algorithm used for classification tasks. It creates a tree-like model where internal nodes represent features, branches represent decision rules, and leaf nodes represent predicted classes(Bidve et al., 2024). The algorithm recursively splits the dataset based on attributes, aiming to minimize impurity or maximize information gain. Decision Trees are simple, interpretable, and can handle various types of data. They capture complex relationships and non-linear decision boundaries. However, they are prone to overfitting and may not generalize well to unseen data.

To address these limitations, ensemble methods like Random Forests and Gradient Boosting are commonly used(Makubhai et al., 2024). They combine multiple decision trees to improve performance and robustness. Overall, Decision Tree Classifiers provide a straightforward and flexible approach for classification problems but require careful tuning to avoid overfitting.

Mathematical foundation

The mathematical foundation of logistic regression lies in the framework of probability theory and the logistic function.

In logistic regression, we aim to model the relationship between the independent variables (features) and the probability of a binary outcome. Let's assume we have a binary outcome variable, often denoted as y, which takes on two values (e.g., 0 and 1). The goal is to estimate the probability of y being equal to 1 given a set of independent variables, denoted as X. The logistic regression model assumes that the log-odds of the outcome variable y being equal to 1 can be represented as a linear combination of the independent variables. Mathematically, this can be expressed as:

$$\log(odds) = \beta_0 + \beta_1 x_1 + \beta_2 x_2 + \ldots + \beta x ,$$

where $\beta_0, \beta_1, \beta_2, \ldots, \beta$ are the coefficients or weights associated with each independent variable $x_1, x_2, \ldots, x$. The log-odds is also known as the logit function.

To convert the log-odds into a probability, the logistic function, also known as the sigmoid function, is applied:

$$p = 1 / (1 + e^{\wedge}(-\log(odds))).$$

This function maps the log-odds to a value between 0 and 1, representing the estimated probability of the outcome being equal to 1.

During the training process, the logistic regression model determines the optimal values for the coefficients $\beta_0, \beta_1, \beta_2, \ldots, \beta$ by maximizing the likelihood function, which measures how well the model predicts the observed outcomes in the training data.

Principal of Working

The working principle of a Decision Tree Classifier involves creating a tree-like model based on a dataset with labeled examples. Here are the key steps:

Splitting: The algorithm starts by selecting the best attribute to split the dataset based on criteria like information gain or Gini impurity. This attribute is chosen to maximize the homogeneity or purity of the resulting subsets.

Recursive partitioning: The dataset is recursively partitioned based on the selected attribute. This process continues for each resulting subset, creating a tree structure with internal nodes representing attributes and branches representing decision rules.

Leaf node assignment: The partitioning process stops when a stopping criterion is met, such as reaching a maximum depth or a minimum number of samples. At this point, the leaf nodes are assigned with the most common class label or a predicted value for regression tasks.

Prediction: To make predictions for new, unseen examples, and the decision tree is traversed based on their attribute values. The example follows the decision rules at each internal node until it reaches a leaf node, which provides the predicted class label or value.

Results and Accuracy

Figure 6. Figure shows the dataset is been tested using Decision Trees Classifier model using python

0.0.19 3. Model performance on unseen data for Decision Tree Classifier

```
[122]: DT.fit(X_train1,y_train1)

# make predictions
y_train_pred_DT = DT.predict(X_train1)
y_test_pred_DT = DT.predict(X_test1)

y_train_proba_DT = DT.predict_proba(X_train1)[:,1]
y_test_proba_DT = DT.predict_proba(X_test1)[:,1]
print("DT Training Accuracy",accuracy_score(y_train1,y_train_pred_DT))
print("DT Testing  Accuracy",accuracy_score(y_test1,y_test_pred_DT))

Model_name,data_type = "DT", "Testing"
modelperformance(y_test1,y_test_pred_DT,y_test_proba_DT,Model_name,data_type)
```

DT Training Accuracy 0.9861111111111112
DT Testing Accuracy 0.9354838709677419
DT Testing Accuracy = 0.9354838709677419
DT Testing Precision = 0.9878048780487805
DT Testing Recall = 0.9418604651162791
DT Testing F1- Score = 0.9642857142857143
DT Testing Cohen Kappa Score = 0.6328947368421052

Confusion Matrix

Figure 7. Confusion matrix of Decision Tree Tested for F1 and Cohen Kappa Score

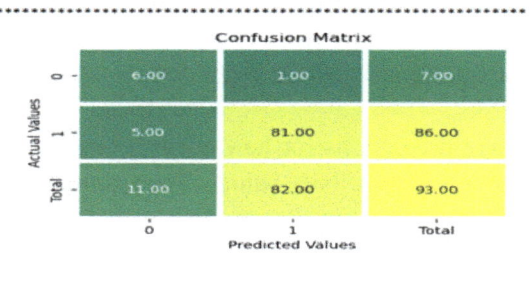

```
              Confusion Matrix

         0 -    6.00      1.00      7.00
Actual
Values   1 -    5.00     81.00     86.00

       Total - 11.00     82.00     93.00
                 0         1        Total
                   Predicted Values


··········*Classifcation Report*··········

              precision  recall  f1-score  support

           0      0.55    0.86     0.67       7
           1      0.99    0.94     0.96      86

    accuracy                       0.94      93
   macro avg      0.77    0.90     0.82      93
weighted avg      0.95    0.94     0.94      93
```

Evaluation of Decision Tree Classifier
Advantages of Decision Tree Classifier:
Interpretability
Handling non-linearity
Feature importance assessment
Disadvantages of Decision Tree Classifier:
Overfitting
Instability
Biased towards features with high cardinality.

Random Forest Classifier

Explanation Background

Random Forest Classifier is an ensemble machine learning algorithm that combines multiple decision trees to make predictions. It is a popular method for both classification and regression tasks.

In a Random Forest Classifier, a collection of decision trees is built, each trained on a random subset of the training data and using a random subset of features. This randomness helps to reduce overfitting and increases the model's robustness and generalization ability. During the prediction phase, each decision tree in the

Random Forest independently classifies the input, and the final prediction is determined by majority voting (classification) or averaging (regression) the individual tree predictions.

Random Forest can handle high-dimensional data effectively.

It provides feature importance measures, allowing for variable selection and understanding.

Random Forest is resistant to overfitting, thanks to its ensemble approach and random subsets of data and features.

Mathematical Foundation

As we know that, the RF classifier belongs to a category of additive mod-el that can be used to makes some predictions by combining decisions from a sequence of base model. Normally we can mention this model in terms of equation like:

$f(x) = r_0(x) + r_1(x) + r_2(x) + \cdots$

Where, f is the final model which is nothing but the sum of simple base model ri r is the base model.

Principal of Working

Ensemble of Decision Trees: A Random Forest consists of an ensemble of decision trees. Each tree is trained independently on a random subset of the training data, using a process called bagging. Bagging involves randomly sampling the training data with replacement, creating multiple variations of the dataset for training each tree.

Random Feature Subsets: In addition to sampling the data, Random Forest also selects a random subset of features at each split of a decision tree. This randomness helps to introduce diversity among the trees and reduces correlation. The number of features in the subset is typically determined based on a specified parameter or heuristic.

Tree Construction: Each decision tree in the Random Forest is constructed using a recursive process. At each node of a tree, a split is made by evaluating different attributes and selecting the best split based on a criterion such as information gain or Gini impurity. The tree continues to grow by recursively splitting the data until reaching a stopping criterion, such as a maximum depth or minimum number of samples in a leaf node.

Prediction: During the prediction phase, an input example is passed through each tree in the Random Forest. For classification tasks, the majority voting method is used, where each tree's predicted class is counted, and the class with the most votes becomes the final prediction. For regression tasks, the average of the predicted values from all trees is taken as the final prediction.

Result and Accuracy

Figure 8. Figure shows the dataset is been tested using Random Forest model using python

4. Model performance on unseen data for Random Forest Classifier

```
[123]: random_forest.fit(X_train1,y_train1)

# make predictions
y_train_pred_rf = random_forest.predict(X_train1)
y_test_pred_rf = random_forest.predict(X_test1)

y_train_proba_rf = random_forest.predict_proba(X_train1)[:,1]
y_test_proba_rf = random_forest.predict_proba(X_test1)[:,1]
print("random_forest Training
    Accuracy",accuracy_score(y_train1,y_train_pred_rf))
print("random_forest Testing   Accuracy",accuracy_score(y_test1,y_test_pred_rf))

Model_name,data_type = "random_forest", "Testing"
modelperformance(y_test1,y_test_pred_rf,y_test_proba_rf,Model_name,data_type)

random_forest Training Accuracy 0.9861111111111112
random_forest Testing   Accuracy 0.967741935483871
random_forest Testing Accuracy =  0.967741935483871
random_forest Testing Precision =   0.9770114942528736
random_forest Testing Recall =   0.9883720930232558
random_forest Testing F1- Score =  0.9826589595375722
```

4.4.5 Confusion Matrix

Figure 9. Confusion matrix of Random Forest classifier Tested for F1 and Cohen Kappa Score

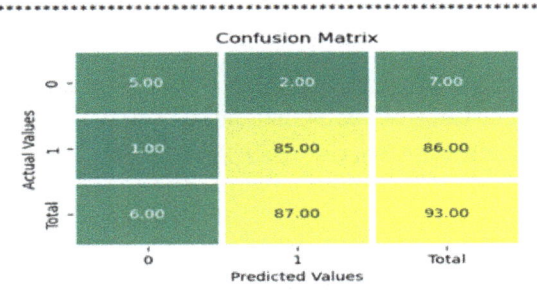

```
                Confusion Matrix

              0        1       Total
    0       5.00     2.00      7.00
    1       1.00    85.00     86.00
  Total     6.00    87.00     93.00
              Predicted Values
```

```
······························Classifcation Report······························

              precision    recall  f1-score   support

           0       0.83      0.71      0.77         7
           1       0.98      0.99      0.98        86

    accuracy                           0.97        93
   macro avg       0.91      0.85      0.88        93
weighted avg       0.97      0.97      0.97        93


································Area Under Curve
```

Evaluation of Random Forest Classifier

Advantages of Random Forest Classifier:
High accuracy due to ensemble of decision trees.
Robust against overfitting and noisy data.
Provides feature importance for variable selection.
Disadvantages of Random Forest Classifier:
Complex model with reduced interpretability.
Computational overhead for training and evaluation.
Considered a black box model lacking explicit mathematical relationships.

CONCLUSION

Explainable AI (XAI) is revolutionizing healthcare by providing transparency and trust in AI-driven medical practices. By clarifying AI decision-making, XAI enhances diagnostic accuracy, optimizes treatment plans, and improves patient

REFERENCES

Bidve, V., Shafi, P. M., Sarasu, P., Pavate, A., Shaikh, A., Borde, S., Singh, V. B. P., & Raut, R. (2024). Use of explainable AI to interpret the results of NLP models for sentimental analysis. *Indonesian Journal of Electrical Engineering and Computer Science*, 35(1), 511–519. DOI: 10.11591/ijeecs.v35.i1.pp511-519

Capuano, N., Fenza, G., Loia, V., & Stanzione, C. (2022). Explainable Artificial Intelligence in CyberSecurity: A Survey. *IEEE Access : Practical Innovations, Open Solutions*, 10(September), 93575–93600. DOI: 10.1109/ACCESS.2022.3204171

Chaddad, A., Peng, J., Xu, J., & Bouridane, A. (2023). Survey of Explainable AI Techniques in Healthcare. *Sensors (Basel)*, 23(2), 1–19. DOI: 10.3390/s23020634 PMID: 36679430

Chandre, P., Mahalle, P., & Shinde, G. (2022). Intrusion prevention system using convolutional neural network for wireless sensor network. *IAES International Journal of Artificial Intelligence*, 11(2), 504–515. DOI: 10.11591/ijai.v11.i2.pp504-515

Chandre, P. R., Shendkar, B. D., Deshmukh, S., Kakade, S., & Potdukhe, S. (2023). Machine Learning-Enhanced Advancements in Quantum Cryptography: A Comprehensive Review and Future Prospects. *International Journal on Recent and Innovation Trends in Computing and Communication*, 11(11s), 642–655. DOI: 10.17762/ijritcc.v11i11s.8300

Damre, S. S., Shendkar, B. D., Kulkarni, N., Chandre, P. R., & Deshmukh, S. (2024). Smart Healthcare Wearable Device for Early Disease Detection Using Machine Learning. *International Journal of Intelligent Systems and Applications in Engineering*, 12(4s), 158–166.

Dash, S., Shakyawar, S. K., Sharma, M., & Kaushik, S. (2019). Big data in healthcare: Management, analysis and future prospects. *Journal of Big Data*, 6(1), 54. Advance online publication. DOI: 10.1186/s40537-019-0217-0

Doppalapudi, S., Qiu, R. G., & Badr, Y. (2021). Lung cancer survival period prediction and understanding: Deep learning approaches. *International Journal of Medical Informatics, 148*(September 2020), 104371. DOI: 10.1016/j.ijmedinf.2020.104371

El Houda, Z. A., Brik, B., & Khoukhi, L. (2022). "Why Should I Trust Your IDS?": An Explainable Deep Learning Framework for Intrusion Detection Systems in Internet of Things Networks. *IEEE Open Journal of the Communications Society*, 3(June), 1164–1176. DOI: 10.1109/OJCOMS.2022.3188750

Islam, S. R., Eberle, W., Ghafoor, S. K., Siraj, A., & Rogers, M. (2020). Domain knowledge aided explainable artificial intelligence for intrusion detection and response. *CEUR Workshop Proceedings*, •••, 2600.

Kobylińska, K., Orłowski, T., Adamek, M., & Biecek, P. (2022). Explainable Machine Learning for Lung Cancer Screening Models. *Applied Sciences (Basel, Switzerland)*, 12(4), 1926. Advance online publication. DOI: 10.3390/app12041926

Kotwal, J., Kashyap, D. R., & Pathan, D. S. (2023). Agricultural plant diseases identification: From traditional approach to deep learning. *Materials Today: Proceedings, 80*(xxxx), 344–356. DOI: 10.1016/j.matpr.2023.02.370

Linardatos, P., Papastefanopoulos, V., & Kotsiantis, S. (2021). Explainable ai: A review of machine learning interpretability methods. *Entropy (Basel, Switzerland)*, 23(1), 1–45. DOI: 10.3390/e23010018 PMID: 33375658

Liu, H., Zhong, C., Alnusair, A., & Islam, S. R. (2021). FAIXID: A Framework for Enhancing AI Explainability of Intrusion Detection Results Using Data Cleaning Techniques. *Journal of Network and Systems Management*, 29(4), 1–30. DOI: 10.1007/s10922-021-09606-8

Mahbooba, B., Timilsina, M., Sahal, R., & Serrano, M. (2021). Explainable Artificial Intelligence (XAI) to Enhance Trust Management in Intrusion Detection Systems Using Decision Tree Model. *Complexity*, 2021(1), 6634811. Advance online publication. DOI: 10.1155/2021/6634811

Makubhai, S. S., Pathak, G. R., & Chandre, P. R. (2024). Predicting lung cancer risk using explainable artificial intelligence. *Bulletin of Electrical Engineering and Informatics*, 13(2), 1276–1285. DOI: 10.11591/eei.v13i2.6280

Marcos, M., Juarez, J. M., Lenz, R., Peleg, M., Stefanowski, J., Stiglic, G., & Goebel, R. (2019). Artificial Intelligence in Medicine : Knowledge Representation and Transparent and Explainable Systems. In *7th Conference on Artificial Intelligence in Medicine International Workshops (AIME 2019), KR4HC/ProHealth and TEAAM, Poznan, Poland, June 26–29, 2019*. DOI: 10.1007/978-3-030-37446-4

Neupane, S., Ables, J., Anderson, W., Mittal, S., Rahimi, S., Banicescu, I., & Seale, M. (2022). Explainable Intrusion Detection Systems (X-IDS): A Survey of Current Methods, Challenges, and Opportunities. *IEEE Access: Practical Innovations, Open Solutions*, 10, 112392–112415. DOI: 10.1109/ACCESS.2022.3216617

Pathak, G. R., & Patil, S. H. (2016). Mathematical Model of Security Framework for Routing Layer Protocol in Wireless Sensor Networks. *Physics Procedia, 78*(December 2015), 579–586. DOI: 10.1016/j.procs.2016.02.121

Pathak, G. R., Premi, M. S. G., & Patil, S. H. (2019). LSSCW: A lightweight security scheme for cluster based Wireless Sensor Network. *International Journal of Advanced Computer Science and Applications*, 10(10), 448–460. DOI: 10.14569/IJACSA.2019.0101062

Ramos, B., Pereira, T., Moranguinho, J., Morgado, J., Costa, J. L., & Oliveira, H. P. (2021). An Interpretable Approach for Lung Cancer Prediction and Subtype Classification using Gene Expression. *Proceedings of the Annual International Conference of the IEEE Engineering in Medicine and Biology Society, EMBS*, 1707–1710. DOI: 10.1109/EMBC46164.2021.9630775

Mcgonagle, D. (2020). Since January 2020 Elsevier has created a COVID-19 resource centre with free information in English and Mandarin on the novel coronavirus COVID-19. *The COVID-19 resource centre is hosted on Elsevier Connect, the company's public news and information.*

Sadeghi, Z., Alizadehsani, R., Kausar, S., Rehman, R., Mahanta, P., Bora, P. K., Almasri, A., Alkhawaldeh, R. S., Hussain, S., Alatas, B., Shoeibi, A., Moosaei, H., Nahavandi, S., Branch, E., Science, D., Republic, C., & Republic, C. (n.d.). Panos M. *Pardalos*, 16, 1.

Sheu, R. K., & Pardeshi, M. S. (2022). A Survey on Medical Explainable AI (XAI): Recent Progress, Explainability Approach, Human Interaction and Scoring System. *Sensors (Basel)*, 22(20), 8068. Advance online publication. DOI: 10.3390/s22208068 PMID: 36298417

Srinivasu, P. N., Sandhya, N., Jhaveri, R. H., & Raut, R. (2022). From Blackbox to Explainable AI in Healthcare: Existing Tools and Case Studies. *Mobile Information Systems*, 2022, 1–20. Advance online publication. DOI: 10.1155/2022/8167821

Tariq, M. U., Poulin, M., & Abonamah, A. A. (2021). Achieving Operational Excellence Through Artificial Intelligence: Driving Forces and Barriers. *Frontiers in Psychology*, 12(July), 686624. Advance online publication. DOI: 10.3389/fpsyg.2021.686624 PMID: 34305744

Tunali, I., Gillies, R. J., & Schabath, M. B. (2021). Application of radiomics and artificial intelligence for lung cancer precision medicine. *Cold Spring Harbor Perspectives in Medicine*, 11(8), a039537. Advance online publication. DOI: 10.1101/cshperspect.a039537 PMID: 33431509

Wali, S., Khan, I. A., & Member, S. (2021). Explainable AI and Random Forest Based Reliable Intrusion Detection system. *TecharXiv*. DOI: 10.36227/techrxiv.17169080.v1

Chapter 5
Clinical Decision Support Systems Using Machine Learning:
A Case Study on Thyroid Disease Prediction

Archana Kedar Chaudhari
https://orcid.org/0000-0002-3304-1461
Vishwakarma Institute of Technology, Pune, India

ABSTRACT

The case study explores the application of machine learning (ML) in the development of clinical decision support systems (CDSS) for the prediction and diagnosis of thyroid diseases. By leveraging patient data, including demographic information, medical history, and laboratory test results, various ML algorithms are evaluated for their efficacy in predicting thyroid disorders. The study focuses on the selection of relevant features, model training, and validation processes, comparing performance metrics such as accuracy, sensitivity, and specificity. The integration of these predictive models into a CDSS is discussed, highlighting the potential for improved diagnostic accuracy, personalized treatment plans, and enhanced patient outcomes. This case study underscores the transformative impact of ML in the healthcare sector, particularly in the early detection and management of thyroid diseases.

DOI: 10.4018/979-8-3693-7277-7.ch005

INTRODUCTION

Decision support systems (DSS) are designed to assist and support decision-making processes by Gupta et al. (2007). Intelligent support system is a sub-discipline of DSS (i-DSS) that makes use of artificial intelligence tools that use intelligence to improve decision-making process using machine learning as in Merket et al.(2015), Proudlove et al. (1998), Gottinger and Weimann, (1992, Elam and Lonsynski, (1987). The intelligent DSS is seen to retort rapidly and effectively in complex situations without human intervention by learning from past experiences and applying knowledge to perceive the environment, integrate the domain knowledge and recommend action on behalf of humans as presented in Gupta et al. (2007). The clinical decision support system (CDSS) is a DSS used in the clinical domain. In CDSS the characteristic features of the patients perceived via learning are integrated with the domain knowledge to make patient-specific evaluations that are used by the clinicians for further considerations. The purpose of CDSS systems is to provide support to clinicians and healthcare providers to identify problems, reduce errors and resolve the problems as presented in Islam et al. (2020), Islam and Milon, (2019), Akter and Islam, (2021), and Akter et al. (2021) CDSS systems can be electronic or non-electronic and they can be defined by computer programs built on clinical guidelines based on evidence. These computer programs may or may not use AI algorithms for decision making. With the growing importance of data and availability of clinical data in the form of electronic health records, recent CDSS systems are using machine learning algorithms to perform a variety of complex tasks with enhanced accuracy for healthcare applications. CDSS are employed mostly for early prediction of disease and provide doctors and health care workers with information about people or patients at risk, or onset of disease for medicine prediction. CDSS is also useful in evaluation of certain treatments, identifying changes in health, in-patient support and extraction of medical patient data from medical records as in Pombo et al. (2014). Figure 1 elaborates the general architecture pipeline of the clinical decision support system.

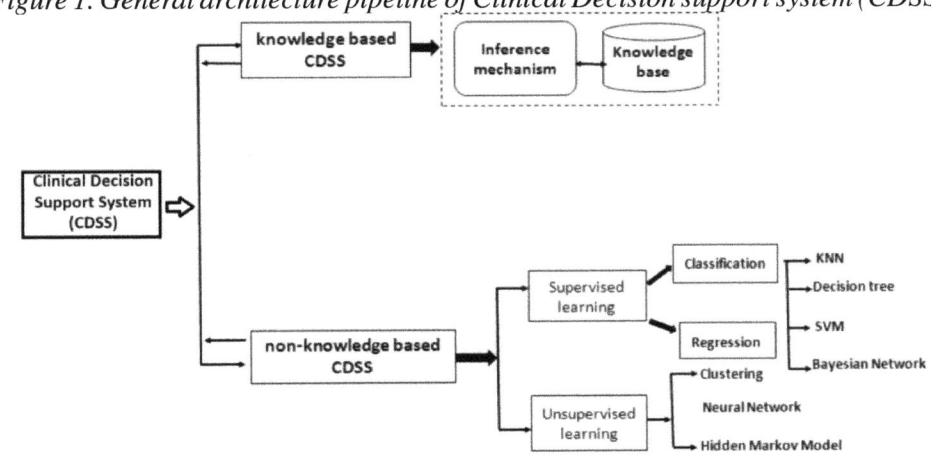

Figure 1. General architecture pipeline of Clinical Decision support system (CDSS)

Overview of Thyroid Disease and Importance of Early Detection

Thyroid is a small gland situated in the neck of human beings. It is a significant gland as it helps to control the metabolic and heart rate function as in Sharma et al. (2013). Thyroid gland releases two hormones T3 and T4. These hormones are responsible for regulating body temperature, digestion and heart rate. When released T3 and T4 hormones are found in the blood and they control the functions of numerous other organs of the human body.

Improper function of the thyroid gland may lead to less or more amount of thyroid hormone production. This may cause cholesterol to rise, pulse rate to vary, and blood pressure to fluctuate or rise. The incorrect functioning of thyroid may cause the following disease: hypothyroidism, hyperthyroidism, subclinical hyperthyroidism, subclinical hypothyroidism, structural abnormalities and tumors.

When excess hormones are released by the gland it is termed hyperthyroidism disease. The symptoms experienced by the patients are sleeping trouble, patients are nervous, anxious and irritable, perspiration has increased, feel hand tremors and heart racing, and experience weakness in muscles. In Hypothyroidism, the thyroid gland releases less hormones and it results in feeling tired, immune to colds, increased constipation, feeling depressed and gaining weight.

The conditions of hyperthyroidism and hypothyroidism can be detected by the levels of hormones in blood samples of the patients. From the statistics of 2023, Thyroid disease is affecting 200 million people worldwide (Endocrinology, 2013). When Thyroid disease when not detected in early stages and not treated properly may lead to cancer, goiter, heart disease and issues in pregnancy or may lead to myxoedema coma (NHS).

Hypothyroidism and hyperthyroidism may cause thyroid imbalance. Primary prediction of the right thyroid disease is vital for timely treatment according to thyroid type to avoid further complications. Several studies have explored thyroid diseases and their symptoms as presented in Idarraga et al. (2021), Raziaand Rao, (2016), and Aversano et al. (2021). Clinicians identify the thyroid disease based on the symptoms and blood test reports. Some statistical methods are also used for the early detection of Thyroid disease. Table I illustrates the tests and symptoms that are used by clinicians for Thyroid disease detection. Based on the symptoms the thyroid disease can be classified into different types.

Table 1. Test and symptoms of thyroid disease along with the description as in Gupta et al. (2024)

Test and Symptoms	Description
TSH Thyroid-stimulating Hormone released by the pituitary gland for functioning of thyroid hormones	Detected in laboratory reports and represents TSH level in blood
T3 Triiodothyronine tests	100–200 ng/dL
Free T3 (FT3)	2.3–4.1 pg/mL
TT4- It is also called as Test T4	-------
T4 also called as Thyroxine tests and it needs to be in between 11 and 5	Low T4 is hypothyroidism whereas high T4 is hyperthyroidism
Free thyroxine (FTI) also known as Free T4	Needs to be in between 0.9 to 1.7 ng/dL

RELATED WORK ON CLINICAL DISEASE SUPPORT SYSTEMS FOR EARLY DETECTION OF THYROID DISEASE

Several works propose the use of machine or deep learning algorithms for early detection of thyroid disease that support clinical decisions. Early detection of thyroid disease in initial stages and classification of the disease as cancer, hyperthyroidism, or hypothyroidism proves useful for clinicians in providing treatment and recovery of several patients.

The authors in Zhangand Lee, (2019) explored a combination of deep learning techniques with medical imaging and exploited pathogenesis of thyroid cancer to enhance diagnostic performance and improve the generalization of the decision support system. For clinical diagnosis and detection of thyroid cancer, computer aided techniques along with deep learning approach have been investigated in Guan et al. (2019), Zhao et al.(2021), Pavithra et al. (2022), Sundar et al. (2018), Gitto et al.(2019), Liang et al. (2020), Chu et al.(2021), and Adebisi et al.(2020). In Ouartani and Taleb, (2024) the authors proposed a thyroid disease clinical decision support system using integration of ontology reports and decision trees.

The section also presents a comprehensive literature review on several machine and deep learning approaches that support clinicians in the early detection of Thyroid disease.

Different Machine learning algorithms are proposed by authors for detection of Thyroid and comparison of results was done using 10 different classifiers as demonstrated in Idarraga et al. (2021). Using extra tree classifier 84% accuracy was achieved. In Razia et al. (2020) the authors used support vector machines (SVM) for detection of four stages of thyroid with 83.7% accuracy. In Aversano et al. (2021) the authors explored the use of a decision trees (DT) based machine learning tool for thyroid disease diagnosis (MLTDD) to predict and classify thyroid disease. The accuracy of MLTDD was seen to be 98.7%. In Lomana et al. (2020) linear regression (LR), random forest (RF), support vector machines (SVM), Gradient Boost Machines (GBM), and deep neural networks (DNN) is used for predict the molecules of homeostasis thyroid hormone for thyroid detection. In Chaganti et al.(2022), feature engineering was proposed using various ML and deep learning (DL) methods for thyroid prediction. In the feature engineering approach the authors selected features using forward selection, or eliminated features using backward elimination or bi-directional feature elimination was adopted. An additional tree classifier-based features with random forest was used which resulted in an improved accuracy of 99%. In Shankar et al.(2020) the authors explored multi-kernel SVM for prediction of cancer and thyroid to obtain an accuracy of 97.49%. Using selective features, a random forest algorithm achieved an accuracy of 99.81% for classification of hypothyroidism into four different classes as demonstrated in Das et al.(2021). The authors in Riajuliislam et al.(2021) explored combination of three features; principal component analysis and features selection methods. In feature selection the authors explored univariate selection of features and recursive selection of features and compared the performance of various ML modes like decision trees, support vector machines, random forest, Naives Baye's classifiers and logistic regression for hypothyroidism prediction. In Hosseinzadeh et al. (2021) multilayer perceptron (MMLP) with an accuracy of 99% for large datasets is used for thyroid classification. XGBoost algorithm is used for prediction and classification of hypothyroidism as in Sankar et al. (2022). Comparative analysis of various machine learning algorithms on large datasets is explored in Alyas et al.(2022), and Islam et al.(2022) and results are presented.

In Gupta et al. (2024), to solve the problem of dataset class imbalance, data is augmented using GAN and ten types of thyroid disease classes are classified using a machine learning model. For fine-tuning the parameters Differential Evolution (DE) is used. The proposed method demonstrated an accuracy of 99.8% using AdaBoost with the DE approach.

Researchers in Jha et al. (2022) exploited deep neural networks with an accuracy of 99.95% to classify thyroid disease. In Islam et al. (2022) CNN based ResNet model with stochastic gradient descent (SGD) is explored for thyroid disease classification. Five thyroid conditions were classified with an accuracy of 94% using the ResNet model. Distant domain high level feature fusion transfer learning model was proposed in Prathiba et al. (2023). The focus of the proposed method was to preserve unique features by decreasing the imbalance between source and target domains. The approach demonstrated an accuracy of 88.92%.

PROPOSED METHODOLOGY

Thyroid Disease Datasets

The thyroid disease datasets mostly used for machine learning prediction or classification are usually obtained from the repository in (UCI). Most of the researchers use the mentioned dataset to train machine learning or deep learning algorithms for clinical decision support systems. Table 2 presents a list of datasets used for detection and classification of thyroid disease. Figure 2 illustrates a few sample features of the UCI dataset.

Table 2. Datasets used for thyroid disease prediction and classification

Data Source	Sample Size	Classes
UCI (UCI)	7547, 30 features	4
ToxCast Lomana et al. (2020)	-	2
Diagnostic center Dhaka, Bangladesh (Riajuliislam et al. (2021)	519 samples	4
external hospitals and laboratories Salman and Sonuc, (2021)	1250 with 17 attributes	3
datasets by KEEL repository and dataset from DistrictHeadquarters teaching hospital, Pakistan Abbad et al. (2021)	690 samples, 13 features	3

Figure 2. Sample features from the UCI dataset for Thyroid Disease prediction

	age	sex	on thyroxine	query on thyroxine	on antithyroid medication	sick	pregnant	thyroid surgery	I131 treatment	query hypothyroid	...	TT4 measured	TT4	T4U measured	T4U	FTI measured	FTI
0	41	F	f	f	f	f	f	f	f	f	...	t	125	t	1.14	t	109
1	23	F	f	f	f	f	f	f	f	f	...	t	102	f	?	f	?
2	46	M	f	f	f	f	f	f	f	f	...	t	109	t	0.91	t	120
3	70	F	t	f	f	f	f	f	f	f	...	t	175	f	?	f	?
4	70	F	f	f	f	f	f	f	f	f	...	t	61	t	0.87	t	70

Proposed Architectural pipeline for machine learning or deep learning approach for clinical decision support

The architectural pipeline for machine learning or deep learning approaches consist of the following steps

1. Exploratory data analysis for finding class imbalance
2. Data preprocessing which includes finding missing values, converting missing values to NAN, feature scaling or normalization
3. Feature selection or feature engineering: Selection of features for learning
4. Splitting of dataset into testing or training
5. Applying various machine learning techniques like for prediction like linear regression or classification techniques like decision trees, support vector machines, logistic regression, random forest, deep neural networks and several other techniques
6. Hyperparameter Tuning to obtain higher accuracy
7. Performance comparison and evaluation

Figure 3 presents the architectural pipeline of the CDSS- clinical decision support system by means of machine learning and sample thyroid dataset.

Figure 3. Architectural pipeline of CDSS for Thyroid prediction using Machine Learning Models

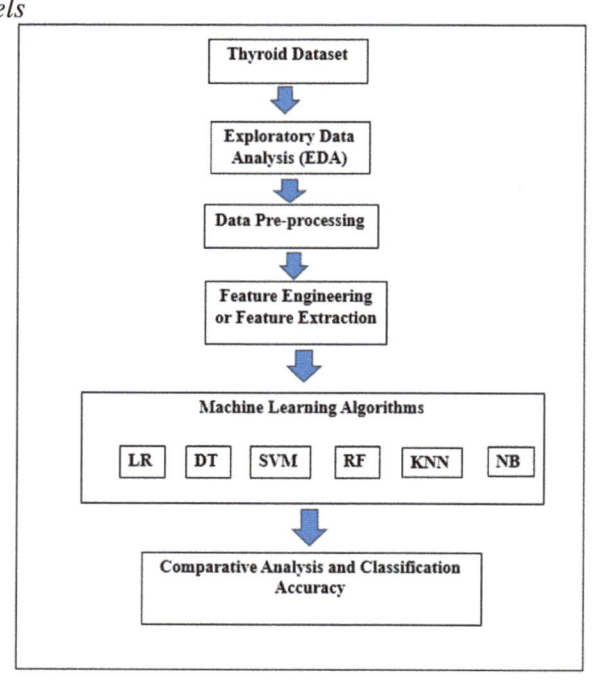

EXPLORATORY DATA ANALYSIS

In exploratory data analysis, an analysis of the number of features of the dataset along with the number of classes are investigated. This is helpful to understand the class imbalance and feature selection. Figure 4 presents exploratory data analysis on thyroid dataset.

In Figure 4 (a) the target variable count-plot for positive and negative classes of thyroid is represented. From this plot we can draw inference that the number of negative cases is less and there is target class imbalance. Imbalanced datasets can lead machine learning models to be biased towards the majority class. Models trained on imbalanced data may have difficulty generalizing to new, unseen data, especially for the minority class and Evaluating model performance becomes challenging when the dataset is imbalanced. Imbalanced datasets need to be balanced. They can be balanced using resampling, generating synthetic data and data augmentation techniques.

In Figure 4 (b) the plot represents the number of thyroid disease positive cases based on age. From the plot, the number of cases is positive in between 50 years and above. Figure 4 (c) presents the classification of male and female patients under positive cases and it is observed that the number of females is double the number of males detected positive for thyroid disease. Figure 4 (d) illustrates the number of healthy and unhealthy patient's detected positive for thyroid disease. It is observed that sick or unhealthy patients are greater in number detected positive for thyroid disease. Hence exploratory data analysis is useful for investigation of target classes and features in the dataset for inferencing.

Figure 4. Exploratory data analysis for sample dataset for thyroid disease prediction (Kaggle projects, 2023). (a) Representation of the number of positive and negative classes in the dataset (b) Distribution of positive class based on the age (c) Male and Female classification of patients for Thyroid prediction (d) Number of sick or healthy patients detected positive

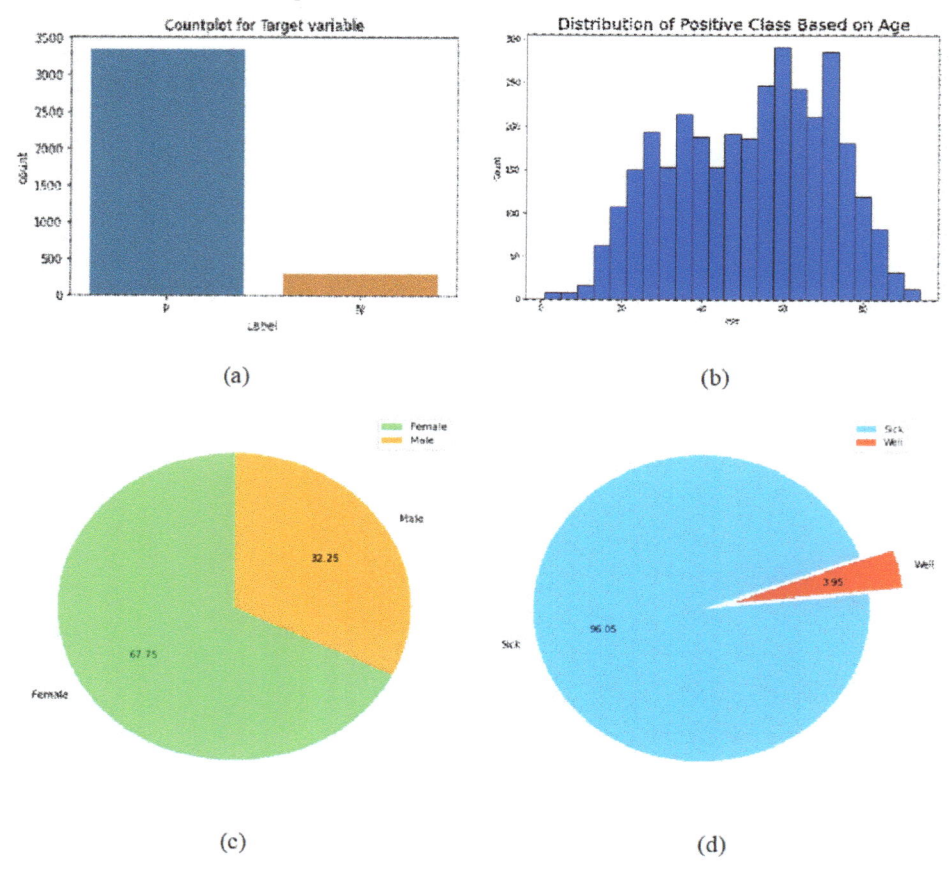

DATA PRE-PROCESSING

Data pre-processing involves data cleaning as well as feature scaling. They are discussed as below.

Data Cleaning: Data pre-processing involves cleaning data by finding the missing values and replacing them by NAN. It also includes data scaling or normalization. Sometimes categorical data needs to be encoded to obtain uniform features for further analysis. Figure 5 presents a sample of dataset for thyroid disease prediction having missing values.

Feature Scaling: In feature scaling, all features are brought to a common scale. This ensures that all features contribute equally to the model training and no feature dominates the learning process simply because they have larger values. Feature scaling also helps for faster convergence of the algorithm and helps to improve accuracy of the model. Feature scaling can be implemented in two ways: Normalization or min-max scaling and Standardization.

Feature Selection or Feature Engineering: Feature selection is the process of selecting features for training and classification of the ML models as in Cai et al. (2018).Feature selection can be done using forward selection or features can be eliminated using backward elimination, or bi-directional elimination and ML based feature selection. In feature selection a combination of one or more features are taken and performance is measured by evaluating the accuracy, F1-score,p-value. The sub-section elaborates on a few feature selections in detail. Table 3 illustrates various feature selection methods along with the mathematical models, use cases, advantages and limitations.

Table 3. Description of methods used for feature selection

Method	Equation	Use Cases	Advantages	Limitations
Forward Feature Selection	$Model_{I+1} = Model_I + \arg\max_j Performance$	Large datasets, fast feature selection	Efficient, avoids over fitting, easy to implement	Misses feature interactions, greedy approach
Backward Feature Selection	$Model_{I+1} = Model_I - \arg\max_j Performance$	High-dimensional datasets, feature redundancy suspected	Captures feature interactions, starts with all features	Computationally expensive, prone to over fitting
ML-based Feature Selection	$min_{\beta_0,\beta} \frac{1}{2n} \sum_{i=1}^{n}(y_i - \beta_0 - X_i\beta)^2$	Non-linear relationships, both regression & classification	Handles complex interactions, applicable to high-dimensional data	Model-dependent, computationally intensive
Bidirectional Feature Elimination	$Model_{I+1} = $ Forward+ Backward	Thorough search for optimal feature set	More likely to find the optimal set, balances feature addition/removal	Very computationally expensive, may miss global optima

Figure 5 demonstrates the feature importance using machine learning feature selection as explored by the authors in Chaganti et al. (2022) for thyroid prediction based on UCI dataset with 30 features. In the work the authors have selected high entropy features. High entropy features contain the maximum information gain. From the figure, it is observed that TSH, T3, TT4, T4U are the most important features based on the blood test and which are also conventionally used by doctors as discussed in Table 1. These features along with few other features can be used to improve the accuracy of the CDSS system for Thyroid prediction. Figure 6 illustrates the feature impact on model performance as demonstrated by authors in Chaganti et al. (2022) for thyroid prediction based on UCI dataset with 30 features

Figure 5. Feature importance for Thyroid prediction in CDSS using Machine learning feature selection as in Chaganti et al.(2022)

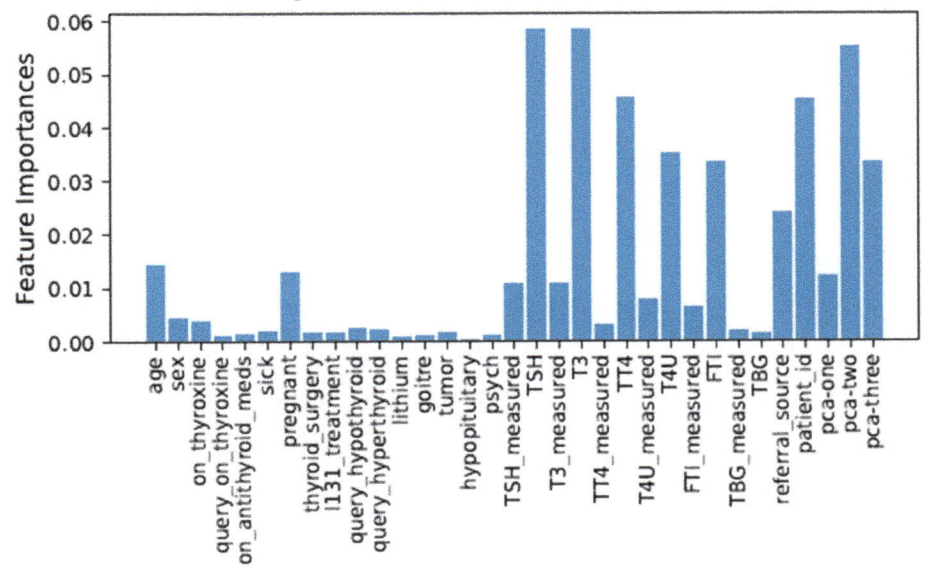

Figure 6. Impact of Features on the model performance as in Chaganti et al.(2022) for CDSS for Thyroid prediction

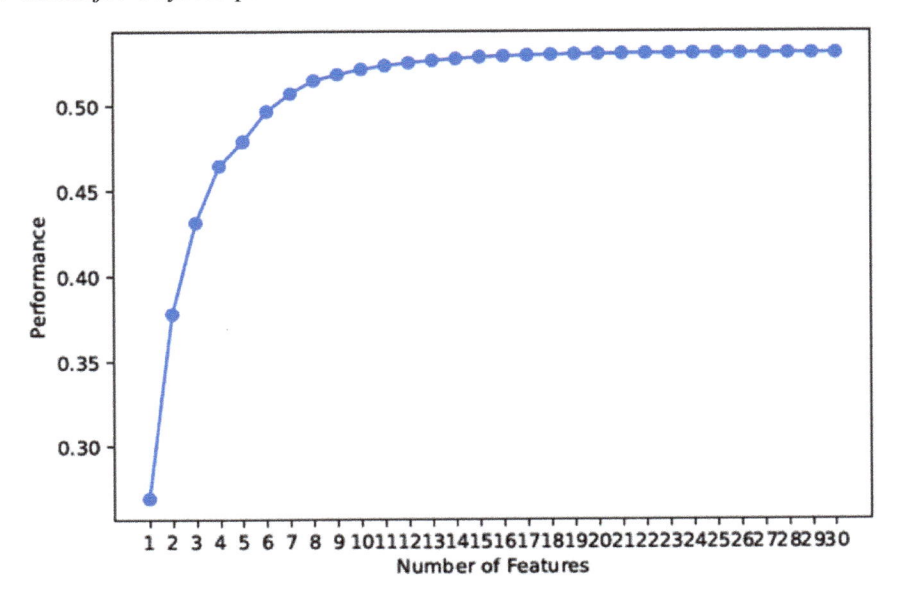

OVERVIEW OF FEW MACHINE LEARNING ALGORITHMS

Table 4 represents an overview of Machine Learning algorithms used for Thyroid prediction in CDSS by several researchers.

Table 4. Overview of machine learning algorithms in CDSS

Algorithm	Equation	Use Cases	Advantages	Limitations
Logistic Regression	$\hat{p}(y=1) = \frac{1}{1+e^{-\theta^T x}}$ Where θ are the weights	Binary classification, probability estimation, medical diagnosis	Simple and interpretable, outputs probabilities, works well with linear decision boundaries	Assumes linear relationship between features and log-odds, not suitable for non-linear problems
Support Vector Machine (SVM)	min $\|w^2\|$ subject to $y_i(w.x_i+b) \geq 1$	Classification tasks, especially with small to medium datasets	Effective in high-dimensional spaces, robust to overfitting, kernel trick for non-linear problems	Computationally expensive, sensitive to the choice of kernel and hyperparameters
Random Forest	Combination of multiple decision trees (bagging)	Both classification and regression tasks, handling large datasets	Reduces overfitting, handles large datasets, can capture complex patterns	Computationally intensive, less interpretable compared to single decision trees
Naive Bayes Classifier	$\hat{y} = argmax_y P(y) \prod_{i=1}^{n} P(x_i/y)$	Text classification, spam filtering, document categorization	Simple and fast, works well with small datasets, handles categorical data well	Assumes feature independence, performs poorly with correlated features or small sample sizes
Decision Tree	Recursive partitioning based on feature values, with decisions at nodes and predictions at leaves	Classification and regression, interpretable models	Easy to interpret, handles both categorical and continuous data, no need for feature scaling	Prone to overfitting, sensitive to noisy data, can create complex trees that are hard to prune

continued on following page

Table 4. Continued

Algorithm	Equation	Use Cases	Advantages	Limitations
XGBoost	Gradient boosting of decision trees: $$\hat{y} = \sum_{m=1}^{M} \gamma_m T_m(x)$$ Where $T_m(x)$ is tree γ_m is learning rate	High-performance tasks, Kaggle competitions, complex datasets	Highly accurate, handles missing data, robust to over fitting with regularization, supports parallel processing	Complex to implement, requires careful tuning, computationally expensive
AdaBoost	Weighted ensemble of weak learners (typically decision trees): $$\hat{y} = sign\left(\sum_{m=1}^{M} \propto_m T_m(x)\right)$$ Where $T_m(x)$ is tree $\propto_m$ is learning rate	Binary classification, improving weak learners	Boosts weak learners to achieve higher accuracy, simple to implement	Sensitive to noisy data and outliers, less effective on complex datasets without sufficient tuning

DISCUSSIONS ON COMPARATIVE ANALYSIS IN LITERATURE

Evaluation Metrics Used for Performance Evaluation of Thyroid Disease Detection and Classification

The most common metrics used for detection and classification of thyroid disease are Accuracy, Precision, Recall and F1-Scores. Table 5 presents an overview of the evaluation metrics used along with its definition and strengths.

Table 5. Overview of evaluation metrics used in machine learning approach for model evaluation

Metric	Equation	Definition	Strengths
Accuracy	$\frac{TP + TN}{TP + TN + FP + FN}$	Part of exact predictions (both true positives and true negatives) out of all predictions	Useful when class distribution is balanced
Precision	$\frac{TP}{TP + FP}$	Part of true positive predictions out of all positive predictions.	Useful when the cost of false positives is high
Recall	$\frac{TP}{TP + FN}$	Part of actual positives correctly identified. (Also known as Sensitivity or True Positive Rate)	Useful when the cost of false negatives is high
F1-Score	$\frac{Precision * Recall}{2 * Precision + Recall}$	Harmonic mean of Precision and Recall. Balances the two metrics.	Useful when balance is needed between Precision and Recall, especially with imbalanced classes.

Comparative Analysis with Various Machine Learning Models Presented in Literature

Most of the approaches in literature use various machine learning models to classify thyroid disease for detection based on various datasets. A few approaches in literature use feature selection or feature engineering to select best features and then train the model to obtain better accuracy for classification.

The section presents results of various machine learning algorithms that are trained without feature selection along with the discussion. The section also discusses results of various machine learning approaches that use feature selection techniques and then train the ML model.

The Table6 presents performance evaluation of a few different ML models performed without feature selection along with the evaluation metrics proposed by researchers.

Table 6. Performance evaluation of different ML algorithms without feature selection

ML/DL Model	Dataset	Target Classes	Evaluation Metrics and Results (%)
Logistic Regression (LR), Random Forest (RF), Support Vector Machine (SVM), XGBoost (XGB) ANN as in Lomana et al. (2020)	ToxCast	2	F1-score for XGB is 83 and Random Forest (RF) is 81
Multiple Linear Regression (MLR), Support Vector Machines (SVM), Naïve's Bayes (NB) and Decision Trees (DT) as in Razia and Rao, (2016)	UCI	2	Accuracy for MLR is 91.59 SVM is 96.04 Naive Bayes is 6.31 Decision Trees is 99.23
multi-kernel SVM as in Shankar et al. (2022)	UCI	3	Accuracy is 97.49, Sensitivity is 99.05and Specificity is 94.5
Decision Trees (DT), K-Nearest Neighbor (KNN), Random Forest (RF), and Support Vector Machine (SVM) as in Das et al. (2021)	UCI	4	Accuracy for KNN is 98.3, SVM is 96.1, DT is 99.5 and RF is 99.81
Support Vector Machine (SVM), Random Forest (RF), Decision Tree (DT), Naïve's Bayes (NB), Logistic Regression (LR), K-Nearest Neighbor (KNN), Multiple Layer Perceptron (MLP), linear discriminant analysis (LDA) and Decision Tree (DT) as in Salman and Sonuc, (2021)	Laboratory and hospitals	3	Accuracy for DT is 90.13, SVM is 92.53, RF is 91.2, NB is 90.67, LR is 91.73, LDA is 83.2, KNN is 91.47 and MLP is 96.4
multiple Multi-Layer Perceptron (MLP) as in Hosseinzadeh et al. (2021)	UCI	3	Accuracy for multiple MLP is 99

continued on following page

Table 6. Continued

ML/DL Model	Dataset	Target Classes	Evaluation Metrics and Results (%)
Decision Tree (DT), Random Forest (RF), K-Nearest Neighbor (KNN), and ANN as in Alyas et al. (2022)	UCI	2	Accuracy for RF is 94.8
Random Forest (RF),GradientBoost Machine (GBM), AdaBoost (ADA),Logistic Regression (LR),Support Vector Machine (SVM) as in Chaganti et al. (2022)	UCI	5	Accuracy for RF is 98, GBM is 97,ADA is 97,LR is 85 and SVM is 85

From the results in Table 6 it is observed that in most of the cases Random Forest (RF) and Multiple Layer Perceptron (MLP) are able to obtain a better accuracy than the other ML models irrespective of the dataset sample size and number of classes. Linear models like Logistic regression (LR) and support vector machine (SVM) demonstrate a poor performance due to size of the dataset and feature performance. The limitation of MLP is that it is computationally complex.

Table 7 illustrates the performance evaluation of various ML algorithms using feature selection methods. From Table 4 it is observed that using feature selection the model performance of Random Forest (RF) algorithm is high when using machine learning feature selection (MLFS). The model performance is greater when using MLFS as feature selection is based on feature correlation with the target class.

Table 7. Performance evaluation of different ML algorithms with feature selection

ML/DL Model	Dataset	Target Class	Results (%)
Combination of Recursive Feature Selection (RFE), Univariate Feature Selection (UFS), PCA and SVM, DT, RF, LR, and NB as in Riajuliislam et al. (2021)	Dhaka, Bangladesh, Diagnostic Center	4	Accuracy of combination of RFE and SVM, DT, RF, LR is 99.35
KNN without feature selection, and KNN using L1-based feature selection, chi-square-based feature Selection as in Abbad et al. (2021)	KEELrepo dataset and hospital	3	Accuracy of KNN is 98
Random Forest, Gradient Boost Machine (GBM), AdaBoost (ADA), Logistic Regression (LR),Support Vector Machine (SVM) using FFS,BFE BDE and MLFS as in Chaganti et al. (2022)	UCI	5	Accuracy RF using MLFS 99%

CASE STUDIES SHOWCASING REAL TIME INTEGRATION OF CDSS FOR THYROID DISEASE DETECTION

In United States, the Mayo clinic and the Cleveland have integrated the CDSS in the Electronic Health Records (EHR). The HER data is analyzed using AI-driven techniques. Such AI driven CDSS derived from HER's assist the health care providers to analyze the patient data including lab results to provide real time diagnostic suggestions for thyroid conditions.

A lot of personalized Mobile applications can be found on various mobile platforms. The parameters like body temperature, sleep conditions, and other health conditions can be input on the app for analysis. Thus, logs of the person's health condition are created which can be sent to the doctor for further analysis of thyroid condition.

Recently wearable devices are playing a crucial role in generating personalized health data for monitoring health conditions and analysis. Such wearable devices are seen to be used for integrating into CDSS for thyroid imbalance condition.

CHALLENGES AND LIMITATIONS IN INTEGRATION OF CDSS

The goal of any clinical decision support system is to achieve transparency and predictions. The first challenge is the integration of the patient's data into the CDSS. Many clinical images, physiological and physiological parameters are needed to be integrated along with the electronic health record (EHR) of the patients for better predictions and accurate diagnosis.

The second challenge is the high imbalance in the real time datasets for positive and negative cases of the diseases. Many other types of target classes of the disease are missed out due to data imbalance or lack of real time data. The machine learning predictions can be accurate for those datasets that have proper data for the number of classes.

The third challenge in thyroid detection CDSS is the number of features to be selected for training the model. Many feature selection techniques are used for training the models. To improve the accuracy, feature selection technique demonstrates enhanced accuracy, at the cost of reduction in size of the data which can be a limitation to the CDSS.

Lastly, the initial findings and assessment of thyroid disease indicators without the participation of a clinician is not easy. Therefore, the CDSS for thyroid disease detection can accurately detect thyroid disease on the condition that the machine learning models are trained for optimized performance. But still further work needs to be done for prediction of thyroid cancer, and other types of thyroid conditions.

CONCLUSION AND FUTURE SCOPE

The role of Thyroid gland in our day-to-day activities is very crucial in functions like digestion and proper working of vital internal organs. Thyroid hormone is released by pituitary gland in the blood. The increase or decrease of this hormone may cause health issues. Early symptoms of thyroid function imbalance can be detected using blood tests. If not detected in early stages, thyroid imbalance can cause cancer and few other critical health conditions.

The proposed work explores clinical decision support system (CDSS) for early and accurate diagnosis of Thyroid disease. The work discusses the pipeline of the CDSS from data gathering to machine and deep learning approach for Thyroid disease detection. The work also explores the various approaches implemented by researchers for accurate evaluation along with the comparison. It also discusses few real-time case studies implemented for thyroid disease detection in early stages.

The work discusses the limitations and challenges in the integration of the CDSS system in real world scenarios. In conclusion in the real world there is a tremendous amount of scope for the implementation of CDSS system for Thyroid detection by working on the integration and data gathering challenges. In conclusion it can be said that no CDSS system can be successful without the involvement of clinicians.

REFERENCES

Gitto, S., Grassi, G., DeAngelis, C., Monaco, C. G., Sdao, S., Sardanelli, F., Sconfienza, L. M., & Mauri, G. (2019). A computer-aided diagnosis system for the assessment and characterization of low-to-high suspicion thyroid nodules on ultrasound. *La Radiologia Medica*, 124(2), 118–125. DOI: 10.1007/s11547-018-0942-z PMID: 30244368

Abbad Ur Rehman, , HLin, , C. YMushtaq, , Z. (2021). Effective K-Nearest Neighbor algorithms performance analysis of thyroid disease. *Zhongguo Gongcheng Xuekan*, 44(1), 77–87. DOI: 10.1080/02533839.2020.1831967

Adebisi, , O. AOjo, , J. ABello, , T. O. (2020). Computer-aided diagnosis system for classification of abnormalities in thyroid nodules ultrasound images using deep learning. *Journal of Computational Engineering*, 22, 60–66.

Akter, , Ferdib-Al-Islam, , Islam, M. M., Al-Rakhami, M. S., & Haque, M. R. (2021). Prediction of Cervical Cancer from Behavior Risk Using Machine Learning Techniques. *SN Computer Science*, 2(3), 177. https://doi.org/. DOI: 10.1007/s42979-021-00551-6

Akter, L., & Islam, M. M. (2021, January). Hepatocellular carcinoma patient's survival prediction using oversampling and machine learning techniques. In *2021 2nd International Conference on Robotics, Electrical and Signal Processing Techniques (ICREST)* (pp. 445-450). IEEE.

Alyas, , THamid, , MAlissa, , KFaiz, , TTabassum, , NAhmad, , A. (2022). Empirical method for thyroid disease classification using a machine learning approach. *BioMed Research International*. Advance online publication. DOI: 10.1155/2022/9809932

Aversano, , LBernardi, , M. LCimitile, , MIammarino, , MMacchia, , P. ENettore, , I. CVerdone, , C. (2021). Thyroid disease treatment prediction with machine learning approaches. *Procedia Computer Science*, 192, 1031–1040. DOI: 10.1016/j.procs.2021.08.106

Ayon, , S. IIslam, , M. M. (2019). Diabetes prediction: A deep learning approach. *International Journal of Information Engineering and Electronic Business*, 11(2), 21–27. DOI: 10.5815/ijieeb.2019.02.03

Cai, , JLuo, , JWang, , SYang, , S. (2018). Feature selection in machine learning: A new perspective. *Neurocomputing*, 300, 70–79. DOI: 10.1016/j.neucom.2017.11.077

Chaganti, , RRustam, , FDe La Torre Díez, , IMazón, , J. L. VRodríguez, , C. LAshraf, , I. (2022). Thyroid disease prediction using selective features and machine learning techniques. *Cancers (Basel)*, 14(16), 3914. DOI: 10.3390/cancers14163914 PMID: 36010907

Chu, , CZheng, , JZhou, , Y. (2021). Ultrasonic thyroid nodule detection method based on U-Net network. *Computer Methods and Programs in Biomedicine*, 199, 105906. DOI: 10.1016/j.cmpb.2020.105906 PMID: 33360682

Das, , RSaraswat, , SChandel, , DKaran, , S. (2021). An AI-driven approach for multiclass hypothyroidism classification. In *International Conference on Advanced Network Technologies and Intelligent Computing* (pp. 319–327).

Elam, , J. JKonsynski, , B. (1987). Using artificial intelligence techniques to enhance the capabilities of model management systems. *Decision Sciences*, 18(3), 487–502. DOI: 10.1111/j.1540-5915.1987.tb01537.x

Garcia de Lomana, , MWeber, , A. GBirk, , BLandsiedel, , RAchenbach, , JSchleifer, , K. JMathea, , MKirchmair, , J. (2020). In silico models to predict the perturbation of molecular initiating events related to thyroid hormone homeostasis. *Chemical Research in Toxicology*, 34(2), 396–411. DOI: 10.1021/acs.chemrestox.0c00304 PMID: 33185102

Gottinger, , H. WWeimann, , P. (1992). Intelligent decision support systems. *Decision Support Systems*, 8(4), 317–332. DOI: 10.1016/0167-9236(92)90053-R

Guan, , QWang, , YDu, , JQin, , YLu, , HXiang, , JWang, , F. (2019). Deep learning based classification of ultrasound images for thyroid nodules: A large scale pilot study. *Annals of Translational Medicine*, 7(7), 137. DOI: 10.21037/atm.2019.04.34 PMID: 31157258

Gupta, , J. NForgionne, , G. AMora, , M. (2007). *Intelligent decision-making support systems: Foundations, applications and challenges*. Springer Science & Business Media.

Gupta, , PRustam, , FKanwal, , KAljedaani, , WAlfarhood, , SSafran, , MAshraf, , I. (2024). Detecting thyroid disease using optimized machine learning model based on differential evolution. *International Journal of Computational Intelligence Systems*, 17(3), 3. Advance online publication. DOI: 10.1007/s44196-023-00388-2

Hosseinzadeh, , Ahmed, O. H., Ghafour, M. Y., Safara, F., hama, H., Ali, S., Vo, B., & Chiang, H.-S. (2021). A multiple multilayer perceptron neural network with an adaptive learning algorithm for thyroid disease diagnosis in the internet of medical things. *The Journal of Supercomputing*, 77(4), 3616–3637. DOI: 10.1007/s11227-020-03404-w

Idarraga, , A. JLuong, , GHsiao, , VSchneider, , D. F. (2021). False negative rates in benign thyroid nodule diagnosis: Machine learning for detecting malignancy. *The Journal of Surgical Research*, 268, 562–569. DOI: 10.1016/j.jss.2021.06.076 PMID: 34464894

Islam, , S. SHaque, , M. SMiah, , M. S. USarwar, , T. BNugraha, , R. (2022). Application of machine learning algorithms to predict the thyroid disease risk: An experimental comparative study. *PeerJ. Computer Science*, 8, 898. DOI: 10.7717/peerj-cs.898

Islam, , Haque, M. R., Iqbal, H., Hasan, M. M., Hasan, M., & Kabir, M. N. (2020). Breast Cancer Prediction: A Comparative Study Using Machine Learning Techniques. *SN Computer Science*, 1(5), 290. https://doi.org/. DOI: 10.1007/s42979-020-00305-w

Jha, , RBhattacharjee, , VMustafi, , A. (2022). Increasing the prediction accuracy for thyroid disease: A step towards better health for society. *Wireless Personal Communications*, 122(2), 1921–1938. DOI: 10.1007/s11277-021-08974-3

Kaggle projects, (2023) https://www.kaggle.com/code/sumitnayek/sudeshna-project

Liang, , XYu, , JLiao, , JChen, , Z. (2020). Convolutional neural network for breast and thyroid nodules diagnosis in ultrasound imaging. *BioMed Research International*.

Lomana, , MWeber, , A. GBirk, , BLandsiedel, , RAchenbach, , JSchleifer, , K.-JMathea, , MKirchmair, , J. (2020). In silico models to predict the perturbation of molecular initiating events related to thyroid hormone homeostasis. *Chemical Research in Toxicology*, 34(2), 396–411. DOI: 10.1021/acs.chemrestox.0c00304 PMID: 33185102

Merkert, J., Mueller, M., & Hubl, M. (2015). A survey of the application of machine learning in decision support systems.

(NHS) National Health Service. (NHS), (2021). Underactive thyroid (hypothyroidism). Retrieved from https://www.nhs.uk/conditions/underactive-thyroid-hypothyroidism/

Ouartani, S., & Taleb, N. (2024). Decision support system for thyroid disease prediction using decision tree algorithm and ontology. *International Journal of Artificial Intelligence Tools and Applications*.

Pavithra, , GYamuna, , & Arunkumar, , R. (2022). Deep learning method for classifying thyroid nodules using ultrasound images. In *2022 International Conference on Smart Technologies and Systems for Next Generation Computing (ICSTSN)* (pp. 1–6).

Pombo, , NAraújo, , PViana, , J. (2014). Knowledge discovery in clinical decision support systems for pain management: A systematic review. *Artificial Intelligence in Medicine*, 60(1), 1–11. DOI: 10.1016/j.artmed.2013.11.005 PMID: 24370382

Prathibha, , SDahiya, , DRobin, , CNishkala, , C. V. (2023). A novel technique for detecting various thyroid diseases using deep learning. *Intelligent Automation & Soft Computing*, 35(1), 199–214. DOI: 10.32604/iasc.2023.025819

Proudlove, N. C., Vaderá, S., & Kobbacy, K A H. (1998). Intelligent management systems in operations: A review. *The Journal of the Operational Research Society*, 49(7), 682–699. DOI: 10.1057/palgrave.jors.2600519

Quinlan, R. (1987). Thyroid disease. *UCI Machine Learning Repository*. https://doi.org/DOI: 10.24432/C5D010

Razia, , SRao, , M. N. (2016). Machine learning techniques for thyroid disease diagnosis—A review. *Indian Journal of Science and Technology*, 9(28), 1–9. DOI: 10.17485/ijst/2016/v9i28/97853

Razia, S., Kumar, P. S., & Rao, A. S. (2020). Machine learning techniques for thyroid disease diagnosis: A systematic review. In *Modern Approaches in Machine Learning and Cognitive Science: A Walkthrough* (pp. 203–212).

Riajuliislam, , MRahim, , K. ZMahmud, , A. (2021). Prediction of thyroid disease (hypothyroid) in early stage using feature selection and classification techniques. In *2021 International Conference on Information and Communication Technology for Sustainable Development (ICICT4SD)* (pp. 60–64). DOI: 10.1109/ICICT4SD50815.2021.9397052

Salman, , KSonuç, , E. (2021). Thyroid disease classification using machine learning algorithms. *Journal of Physics: Conference Series*, 1963(1), 012140. DOI: 10.1088/1742-6596/1963/1/012140

Sankar, , SPotti, , AChandrika, , G. NRamasubbareddy, , S. (2022). Thyroid disease prediction using XGBoost algorithms. *Journal of Mobile Multimedia*, 18(3), 1–18.

Shankar, , KLakshmanaprabu, , SGupta, , DMaseleno, , ADe Albuquerque, , V. H. C. (2020). Optimal feature-based multi-kernel SVM approach for thyroid disease classification. *The Journal of Supercomputing*, 76(2), 1128–1143. DOI: 10.1007/s11227-018-2469-4

Sharma, , K. AArya, , RMehta, , RSharma, , RSharma, , K. A. (2013). Hypothyroidism and cardiovascular disease: Factors, mechanism, and future perspectives. *Current Medicinal Chemistry*, 20(35), 4411–4418. DOI: 10.2174/09298673113206660255 PMID: 24152286

Sundar, K. S., Rajamani, K. T., & Sai, S. S. S. (2018). Exploring image classification of thyroid ultrasound images using deep learning. In *International Conference on ISMAC in Computational Vision and Bio-Engineering* (pp. 1635–1641). Springer.

Zhang, , XLee, , V. C. S. (2024). Deep learning empowered decision support systems for thyroid cancer detection and management. *Procedia Computer Science*, 237, 945–954. DOI: 10.1016/j.procs.2024.05.183

Zhao, , ZYang, , CWang, , QZhang, , HShi, , LZhang, , Z. (2021). A deep learning-based method for detecting and classifying the ultrasound images of suspicious thyroid nodules. *Medical Physics*, 48(12), 7959–7970. DOI: 10.1002/mp.15319 PMID: 34719057

Chapter 6
Machine Learning in Health:
A Study on Heart Disease Prediction

Gönül Kara
https://orcid.org/0009-0002-0524-244X
Pamukkale University, Turkey

Leyla Özgür Polat
https://orcid.org/0000-0002-5143-359X
Pamukkale University, Turkey

ABSTRACT

The rapid increase in the amount of data in the healthcare sector has increased the importance of machine learning and data analysis techniques based on artificial intelligence in disease prediction and risk identification. n this context, heart disease prediction is one of the most frequently addressed problems. In this section, classification algorithms used in health are discussed and a sample application in heart disease prediction is performed to demonstrate the accuracy and reliability of the algorithms. Using a dataset of 1025 samples from the UCI data repository, heart disease prediction was performed with supervised machine learning models such as Logistic Regression, Decision Trees, Support Vector Machines, K-Nearest Neighbor and Naive Bayes over 14 attributes and the results were interpreted. The study tries to show how different algorithms process the features in the dataset and which model performs better. As a result, it is shown how algorithms can be used in heart disease prediction with practical application and how the results can be interpreted.

DOI: 10.4018/979-8-3693-7277-7.ch006

INTRODUCTION

Heart disease is one of the most important health problems worldwide and causes high mortality rates worldwide. According to World Health Organization (WHO) data, 32% of all deaths worldwide in 2019 were due to cardiovascular diseases (WHO, 2023). Early diagnosis and planned management of cardiovascular diseases are critical to improve people's quality of life and reduce mortality rates. Socio-demographic factors, genetic predisposition, lifestyle factors (smoking, alcohol, physical activity, nutrition, etc.), clinical findings (blood pressure, cholesterol levels, blood sugar, etc.) and diagnostic tests (ECG, echocardiography, stress tests, etc.) are critical factors in the identification of heart disease. In addition, risk scoring systems (Framingham, Atherosclerotic Cardiovascular Disease Risk Scoring System, etc.), prevention strategies (lifestyle changes, medication, etc.), education and awareness, clinical guidelines and psychosocial factors (stress, social support, etc.) play an important role (Visseren et al., 2021). While traditional medical methods can diagnose symptoms when they occur, prediction studies in diagnosis and treatment processes in health can be made more efficient and effective with methods such as machine learning technologies. Machine learning (ML) is defined as a technological process that reveals meaningful relationships and structures among large data sets and enables systems to learn using this information (Hastie, 2009; Pulat & Kocakoç, 2021). By analyzing large data sets and detecting relationships between data sets, ML can detect heart diseases in the early stages and develop personalized treatment and preventive strategies. Machine learning algorithms create models to improve performance on a specific task by recognizing and learning patterns in data (Jordan & Mitchell, 2015). This model enables the system to make better predictions and decisions about future data and situations by improving data analysis and decision-making capabilities, resulting in more effective and predictable results.

ML is also perceived as a technology that brings innovations to many different sectors. In the financial sector, it plays an important role in optimizing risk management and investment decisions, providing personalized services by predicting customer behavior (Dixon et al., 2020). In the retail industry, it provides targeted campaigns and product recommendations by analyzing customer preferences and shopping habits (Ngai & Wu, 2022). In the automotive industry, it has a critical role in developing autonomous vehicle technologies and increasing traffic safety (Kar et al., 2021). In the healthcare sector, it has a major impact on the diagnosis and treatment of diseases; by analyzing medical imaging data, early diagnosis of diseases can be made and personalized treatment plans can be created from genetic and clinical data (Oyebode et al., 2023). It is also being used to improve the effectiveness of healthcare and make disease management more efficient. This wide range of uses demonstrates the potential of ML to provide solutions to various challenges of the modern world.

A review of studies on the application of machine learning in heart disease prediction and management shows that there are many studies investigating the effectiveness of machine learning techniques. These studies compare the performance of various algorithms and demonstrate the potential of machine learning in healthcare. Jothi et al., (2021) tried to predict the risk level of heart disease using 1025 data samples. In their study, they used K-nearest neighbor algorithm and decision tree algorithm from machine learning algorithms. They achieved 67% accuracy rate with the k-nearest neighbor algorithm and 81% accuracy rate with the decision tree algorithm. Nikhar & Karandikar (2016) analyzed the Cleveland Heart Disease dataset consisting of 1025 data samples and 76 variables using naive bayes and decision tree algorithms for heart disease prediction. They divided the dataset equally as training set and test dataset. As a result of their analysis, they observed that the decision tree gave better results. Shorewala (2021) analyzed the coronary heart disease dataset for 70 thousand data samples from the Kaggle data center using logistic regression, support vector machines, k-nearest neighbor algorithm, decision tree, naive bayes and neural network algorithms from machine learning algorithms for heart disease prediction. As a result of the study, it was observed that the decision tree algorithm had the highest performance with an accuracy rate of 74.8%. Sevli (2019) analyzed the University of Wisconsin breast cancer dataset consisting of 569 samples with support vector machine, naive bayes, random forest, K-nearest neighbor and logistic regression methods from machine learning algorithms. When the success values of each method are compared, it is concluded that logistic regression is the most successful method with an accuracy rate of 98.24%. Yıldız & Hasan (2019) aimed to implement an algorithm that is useful for classifying 3240 phonocardiogram heart sound recordings without separating them into sub-heart sounds using a collection of support vector machine, K- nearest neighbor and ensemble methods of classification. The study conducted by Chandrasekhar and Peddakrishna (2023) aims to enhance the effectiveness of machine learning techniques in predicting heart disease. In this context, six different algorithms, including random forest, K-nearest neighbor, logistic regression, naive bayes, gradient boosting and AdaBoost classifier, were applied using data obtained from the Cleveland and IEEE Dataport datasets. The comparative analysis of the models revealed that both the AdaBoost and logistic regression models demonstrated high performance.

Hossain et al. (2023) aimed to analyze various components of patient data for heart disease prediction. The feature selection process was carried out using the correlation-based feature subset selection technique in conjunction with best first search. A comparison of artificial intelligence models revealed that logistic regression, naive bayes, K-nearest neighbor, support vector machines, decision trees, random forest, and multilayer perceptron were examined, with the random forest model demonstrating the highest accuracy rate.

When we examine the studies in the literature in general, it is observed that mostly classification algorithms are tested on similar data sets and the algorithm that produces the best result is selected.

Within the scope of this study, it is tried to give information about the use of machine learning algorithms in the field of health and to explain how algorithms can be evaluated through an application. In addition, an application similar to the studies in the literature was considered and heart disease prediction was performed with supervised machine learning models such as logistic regression, decision trees, support vector machines, K-nearest neighbor and naive bayes with 14 attributes in the dataset including 1025 samples in the Kaggle data warehouse and the results were interpreted.

IMPORTANCE OF MACHINE LEARNING IN HEALTH

Machine learning algorithms are used in the effectiveness and efficiency of management and clinical processes in healthcare. Many different data about patients and diseases are kept in systems in the field of health with the digital transformation. The use of disease prediction and artificial intelligence-supported applications and machines in the field of healthcare has also increased according to this diversity of data. In this way, the analysis capability of machine learning algorithms comes to the forefront in improving service quality and accelerating diagnosis and treatment processes. Machine learning algorithms have advantages in the field of health, especially in the diagnosis and management of heart diseases, such as early diagnosis, creation of personalized risk profiles, big data analysis and creation of clinical decision support systems. Diagnosis of heart diseases with manpower can be inefficient in terms of cost and time. Machine learning algorithms provide a much faster and more effective solution than manpower in the diagnosis of the disease and the management of the process after the disease is diagnosed (Mathur et al., 2020). Machine learning algorithms have been developed on the logic of "if this happens, do this" (Berner et al., 1994). It can be difficult to analyze individuals by considering factors such as their genetic structure, health history, lifestyle and family history with manpower. The same diseases may show different symptoms in different patients. For example, dizziness and chest pain in a 60-year-old Asian woman may have a completely different cause than a 30-year-old Latino man presenting with similar symptoms. Moreover, factors such as the patient's gender, geography, genetic makeup, family history and dietary habits can play an important role in determining the true cause behind these symptoms. Likewise, the same symptoms in different individuals may manifest as signs of different diseases due to the influence of various environmental and biological factors. Such complexities complicate the development of clinical decision support systems (Szolovits, Patil, & Schwartz (1988); Murathan & Devecioğlu (2018). By creating personalized risk profiles using machine learning algorithms, more planned, systematic and effective treatment plans can be created in such complexities. At the same time, this can help health authorities to take quick action during the treatment period.

The development of information communication technologies has provided faster and easier access to data. This has led to the emergence of big data (Emre & Erol, 2017). However, the large and complex structure of the data makes it difficult to reach the right result in a short time in terms of cost and time (Köse & Köse, 2022). With the development of technology, the increase in the amount of data, limitations in the capacity of manpower to analyze data accurately and quickly, and the use of machines in data analysis and prediction processes have made it mandatory. Machine learning is an important tool in identifying health trends and risk factors by analyzing large data sets. These analyses can help healthcare professionals make more informed decisions. Decision support systems are software that analyze large and complex data sets and produce meaningful results that can be used after certain processes (Ragab et al., 2022). Machine learning-supported clinical decision support systems minimize the elements that may be overlooked when healthcare professionals manually interpret data. By providing solution-oriented recommendations using data, it enables healthcare professionals to make faster and more accurate decisions. This shortens the diagnosis time of the disease. It also reduces the cost of health activities and enables more patients to benefit from health services. According to the literature, when the uses of decision support systems in the field of health are examined, it is seen that they are mostly used in the diagnosis of cancer, heart disease, infectious diseases and diabetes (Sahu et al., 2020; Gharehbaghi et al., 2020; Paul et al., 2016; Deperlıoğlu & Köse, 2018; Saleh & Eswaran, 2012).

The Most Used Machine Learning Algorithms in Healthcare

Machine learning algorithms are generally divided into supervised and unsupervised learning models. Supervised learning; the model is first trained by giving inputs and outputs at the same time through the data set. In this training process, the output value corresponding to each input is known. When the model completes the training process, it makes predictions on new and unclassified data (Hastie et al., 2001; Çınar, 2019). The model goes through two separate processes: training and testing. In the training process, the model analyzes the relationship between inputs and outputs. As a result of this analysis, it is enabled to decide on "what to do if what happens". In the testing process, the model is confronted with data it has not seen before. The correct output indicates the performance of the model on accuracy and generalizability. For example, supervised learning models are used in various fields such as email filtering, disease diagnosis, electrocardiogram (ECG) analysis, interpretation of X-ray images and credit risk analysis.

Unsupervised learning, on the other hand, only knows the inputs of the model during the training process and the model does not have any information about the outputs. This model analyzes and learns the relationship, pattern and meaning between the data in the data set. Unlike supervised learning, unsupervised learning does not label the data beforehand. In unsupervised learning, classes are determined by the model after the relationship between data is learned (Koyuncugil & Özgülbaş, 2009; Cunningham et al., 2008). For example, it is used in various fields such as customer segmentation, gene expression, and medical imaging analysis.

Within the scope of the study, classification methods used to separate data into specific classes are one of the most widely used types of supervised learning. This model allows the categorization of data of unknown class by means of a test data with known characteristics. For example, take a heart disease diagnosis where we have a large training dataset. This dataset contains feature values such as different patient records, demographic information, medical history and clinical test results. For each instance, there is a class label indicating whether it is a heart disease or not. The training data is used to predict the risk of heart disease for a given set of feature attributes. In other words, based on the features of the data in the training set, the test samples are classified according to whether they have heart disease or not.

When the literature is examined, the most commonly used models among classification algorithms are as follows (Kıran, 2010):

- K-Nearest Neighbors (KNN)
- Decision Tree (DT)
- Artificial Neural Networks (ANN)
- Logistic Regression (LR)
- Random Forest (RF)
- Support Vector Machines (SVM)
- Naive Bayes (NB)
- Genetic Algorithms

In this section, K-NN, DT, LR, SVM, NB algorithms will be discussed and analyzed as applications in heart disease prediction.

K-Nearest Neighbors (KNN)

KNN is an algorithm for classification based on a distance function that measures the difference or similarity between two samples (Jiang et al., 2007). Therefore, how the distance function is defined is extremely important (Guo et al., 2003). In this method, a value of *k* and a metric must be chosen to select other samples that are closest to the data. The success of classification is highly dependent on the chosen value and metric (Wang, 2002). The KNN algorithm is one of the most widely used machine learning algorithms. This algorithm uses the distance between a feature and the feature closest to it for classification. When the functioning of the KNN algorithm is examined, the *k* value is first checked for an object that needs to be defined according to the data whose class is known. Here, *k* is usually chosen as an odd number to avoid equality. Formulas such as cosine, euclidean or manhattan distances are used to calculate the distances between the new sample and the samples with known classes (Kılınç et al., 2016; Dudani, 1976). The KNN algorithm is clear and relatively easy to implement compared to other classification algorithms. Its performance against noisy training data is high. However, there is an inverse relationship between the size of the data, the number of attributes and the processing capacity.

This causes the model to run slowly on large datasets (Bhatia & Vandana, 2010; Liu & Zhang (2012). The number of neighbors, weight and metric parameters affect the performance of the algorithm.

N_neighbors: The number of nearest neighbors that the model considers when making predictions. Model performance should be examined according to different neighbor numbers and the neighbor value that provides the highest success should be selected (Saygın & Baykara, 2021).

Weight: The distance between nearest neighbors that the model considers when making predictions. The 'uniform' parameter should be used if the distances between neighbors are equal, and the 'distance' parameter should be used if closer neighbors are given more weight.

Metric: Specifies the metric used to measure the distance between neighbors. Examples of metrics are minkowski, manhattan, euclidean, chebyshev (maximum norm) (Zhang et al., 2017; Qin et al., 2007).

These parameters are critical to the precision, accuracy and performance of the KNN model. Hyperparameter search methods such as GridSearchCV can be used to find the most accurate performance value of the model. Finding the best combination of these parameters is important for the performance of the model.

Decision Tree (DT)

Decision trees are a classification and regression method used to classify each record in the data set or to predict the target variable. This method creates a series of decision-making steps using the variables in the data set and divides the data into small groups. With each correct division, the test sample is included in the appropriate class (Güner, 2014).

Decision trees start with a root node that covers all the data in the data set and are divided into branches according to the answers given to the questions. This process is repeated for each question until the best split is found. The parsing process is terminated when no statistically significant difference is found. In this way, the decision tree divides the data into smaller groups and gathers records with similar characteristics in the same group (Thomas, 2000; Kotsiantis, 2013). Each internode in the tree structure starting from the root and extending towards the branches is called a node, heterogeneous nodes in the structured tree are called child nodes and homogeneous nodes are called terminal nodes. Three methods are used to find the risk indicating misclassifications in the tree. These are replacement prediction, test sample prediction and cross-validation test (Pehlivan, 2006). The path from the root node to the target leaf node is called a "rule" for the prediction of the target variable. These rules are usually expressed in an "if-then" structure. For example, in a decision tree, a rule might be created such as "If gender=female and cholesterol> 200", the risk of heart disease is high". These rules represent the decisions made as a result of the tests performed at each node of the tree and provide a clear structure for how the model classifies the data. Decision trees organize the data and perform classification or prediction using a combination of these rules (Tosun, 2007). The decision tree technique is one of the most widely preferred classification techniques because it is compatible with other classification methods, the results are reliable and easy to interpret, and its use is cost-effective (Ayık, et al, 2007; Kotsiantis, 2013). However, decision trees can lead to the problem of overfitting, which can reduce the generalization ability of the model. This can cause the model to overfit the training data and thus perform poorly against new, unseen data (Rokach & Maimon, 2008). Decision trees can be used in areas such as categorizing a retail chain's customers into "Young Trend Followers", "Family Oriented Buyers" and "Luxury Goods Consumers" based on demographic characteristics, buying habits and product preferences to develop customized campaigns for each group; in health research institute to predict future disease spread by using weather conditions, population mobility and health data to predict infection rates in specific geographical areas; in educational research to understand the effects of different experience levels on students by analyzing the relationship between student achievement and teacher experience levels. Decision trees are performance-impacted by the parameters maximum depth, criterion, minimum number of sample splits and minimum number of sample leaves.

Max_depth: The maximum depth in the tree determines how far the tree structure branches and manages the risk of overfitting.

Criterion: A criterion used to evaluate the quality of the split at each node. For example, criteria such as Gini purity and entropy (information gain) are often used in classification tasks (Kavzoğlu & Çölkesen, 2010).

Min_samples_split: This parameter is used to prevent over-splitting and over-fitting of trees and is the minimum number of samples a node should be split into (Taşkın, 2005).

Min_samples_leaf: This parameter is the minimum number of samples that a leaf node should have. This parameter can improve the generalization ability of the model by limiting the number of samples in leaf nodes (Taşkın, 2005).

Naive Bayes (NB)

Naive Bayes classification works by using samples with predetermined classes. The probability values calculated over these samples are used for new test samples and the system tries to determine to which class the test samples belong. Böylece, sistem test örneğinin sınıfını tahmin etmek için olasılık hesaplamalarını kullanır (Taşcı & Şamlı, 2020). Thus, the system uses probability calculations to predict the class of the test sample (Taşcı & Şamlı, 2020). The algorithm performs better on categorical data compared to numerical data in the training set (Vembandasamy et al., 2015). A model developed for diagnosing heart disease using the Naive Bayes algorithm may have information such as the patient's age, blood pressure, cholesterol level as variables. The algorithm independently evaluates the impact of the patient's age, blood pressure or cholesterol level on the probability of developing heart disease. This simple approach calculates how each characteristic plays a role in the diagnosis of the disease independently of the others (Metlek & Kayaalp, 2020). The var_smoothing parameter affects the performance of the naive bayes algorithm.

var_smoothing: This parameter can increase the accuracy of the model by better generalizing the model and reducing the risk of overfitting. This parameter smooths the variances of the features by a small amount (Kaur & Oberai, 2014).

Support Vector Machines (SVM)

SVM first move the data to a higher dimension to separate the data, while linear classification problems usually use a linear equation to separate data points. This equation is expressed as $ax+b=0$, where the parameters a and b define the line that best separates the classes (Metlek & Kayaalp, 2020; Qi et al., 2013). For example, when we want to classify two different types of fruit (apples and oranges), a linear dividing line is determined by considering the characteristics of each fruit (such as weight and color). This line is positioned to provide the widest gap between the two types of fruit, so that each type of fruit is divided into classes determined by this linear line. That is, the line formed by the linear equation serves as the boundary that most effectively separates the different classes in the data set (Lin & Wang, 2002). The parameters that affect the performance of the SVM algorithm are the kernel functions, C (Regularization Parameter), gamma and degree.

Kernel: Determines the kernel function that transforms data points in the feature space. Common kernel functions are:

linear: Provides direct linear discrimination.

poly: Polynomial kernel provides a polynomial transformation of features.

rbf (Radial Basis Function): Transforms the data into a higher dimensional space and makes the boundaries more flexible.

sigmoid: Provides feature transformation using a sigmoid function.

C (Regularization Parameter): Determines the level of fit of the support vector machine model to the training data. A high value of C may cause overfitting.

Gamma: Determines the effect of the kernel function. It is especially used in rbf, poly and sigmoid kernels. Gamma value is inversely proportional to the area it affects.

Degree: When used for polynomial kernel, it indicates the polynomial degree. Increasing the degree causes the complexity of the model (Tolun, 2008; Ayhan & Erdoğan, 2014; Güran et al., 2014).

Logistic Regression (LR)

It is a model that defines and predicts the relationship between the independent variable and the dependent variable (Tabakan & Avcı, 2021; Sevli, 2019). It is formulated as Y=a+bx. While it expresses the point where the line crosses the *y*-axis, the value shown as "*b*" indicates the regression coefficient.

Logistic regression analysis is a method that allows new observations to be assigned to classes based on the known number of classes by obtaining a classification model using existing data. Using this model, it becomes possible to classify new observations added to the data (Hosmer Jr et al., 2013). Logistic regression analysis (LRA) is a method that allows us to create a regression model without the need for normal distribution, linearity and equivariance assumptions required in linear regression analysis (Tabachnick et al., 2013). LR is suitable for models that focus on binary outcomes in classification, such as pass-fail, yes-no, patient-healthy. For this reason, it is widely used in studies in the field of health sciences (Boateng & Abaye, 2019). However, it may not perform adequately for more complex data. According to the structure of the dependent variable, LRA is divided into three as Binary Logistic Regression Model, Multinominal Logistic Regression Model and Ordinal Logistic Regression Model (Stephenson et al., 2008). The parameters that affect the performance of the logistic regression model are C (Regularization parameter), penalty and solver.

C (Regularization parameter): Controls how well the model fits the training data.

penalty: Determines the type of regularization. Usually l1: Lasso regularization, l2: Ridge regularization or elasticnet, which is a combination of l1 and l2.

solver: Determines the optimizer algorithm. Common solvers are liblinear which is suitable for small data sets, newton-cg which is suitable for large data sets, lbfgs which is suitable for large data sets and multiple classes, and saga which is suitable for large data sets and high dimensional data (Özcan et al, 2023; Uğurlu et al, 2023).

Evaluation Criteria for Model Performance

The main criteria used to calculate the success of machine learning algorithms in obtaining accurate results in prediction are designed to measure the accuracy, generalizability and errors of the model.

After using machine learning models in data analysis, it is necessary to evaluate the findings obtained to find the model that gives the most accurate result (Ikonomakis et al., 2005; Saygın & Baykara, 2021).

The most commonly used metrics to evaluate the performance of machine learning models are; accuracy, recall, precision, F1 score, Roc Curve and specificity (Laishram & Padmanabhan, 2019).

Accuracy: The ratio of the number of correct predictions made by machine learning algorithms to the total number of predictions. It is used to see the overall success of the model. However, imbalance in classes can affect the accuracy (Tantuğ, 2012; Saygın & Baykara, 2021). It is calculated as in Equation 1.

$$\text{Accuracy} = \frac{\text{True Positives} + \text{True Negatives}}{\text{True Positives} + \text{True Negatives} + \text{False Posivitives} + \text{False Negatives}} \quad (1)$$

Figure 1. Confusion Matrix Example

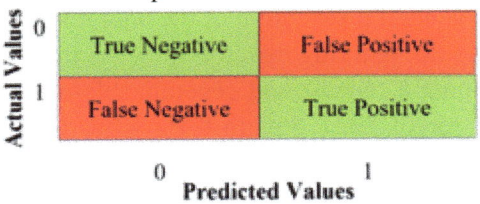

The structure of the confusion matrix is an important tool used to evaluate the classification performance of the model. The columns of the matrix in Figure 1 represent the real classes and show the classes in the real data. For example, it determines whether a patient really "has heart failure" or not. On the other hand, the rows of the matrix represent the classes predicted by the model and show the predictions made by the model on the data (Karakurt & Karcı, 2023). This helps us understand whether the model predicts a patient as "having heart failure" or not. Thanks to this structure, we can analyze in detail in which classes the model makes correct predictions and in which cases it makes mistakes. If the numbers of true positives and true negatives are high, we can say that the model performs well overall. False positive and false negative rates are important to understand where the model falls short.

Precision: It is a criterion that indicates how much of the data classified as positive in the data set predicted using a model is actually positive. It is important in situations where false positives are critical in terms of money and time (Tantuğ, 2012; Saygın & Baykara, 2021).

Recall: It is the criterion that shows how many of the truly positive examples in the data set are correctly predicted (Ikonomakis et al., 2005; Tantuğ, 2012; Saygın & Baykara, 2021). The calculation method is given in Equation 2.

$$\text{Recall} = \frac{\text{True Positives}}{\text{True positives} + \text{False Negatives}} \qquad (2)$$

It is widely used in situations where false negatives are time and cost critical.

F1 Score: As seen in Equation 3, it gives the harmonic mean of the recall and precision values.

$$\text{F1 Score} = 2 * \frac{\text{Recall} * \text{Precision}}{\text{Recall} + \text{Precision}} \qquad (3)$$

Careful examination and evaluation of all data points is important to consider outliers. Extreme cases can negatively affect the performance of the model because they deviate from the general distribution of the data set and have potentially important information, so not ignoring extreme values is the most important part of the process of developing a reliable and generalizable model (Ikonomakis et al., 2005; Uslu & Özmen-Akyol, 2021; Saygın & Baykara, 2021).

Receiver Operating Characteristic (ROC) Curve and Area Under Curve (AUC): As seen in Figure 2, the ROC curve obtained using the KNN model for the application discussed in this book chapter shows the true positive rate against the false positive rate.

Figure 2. ROC Curve of the K-Nearest Neighbors Model

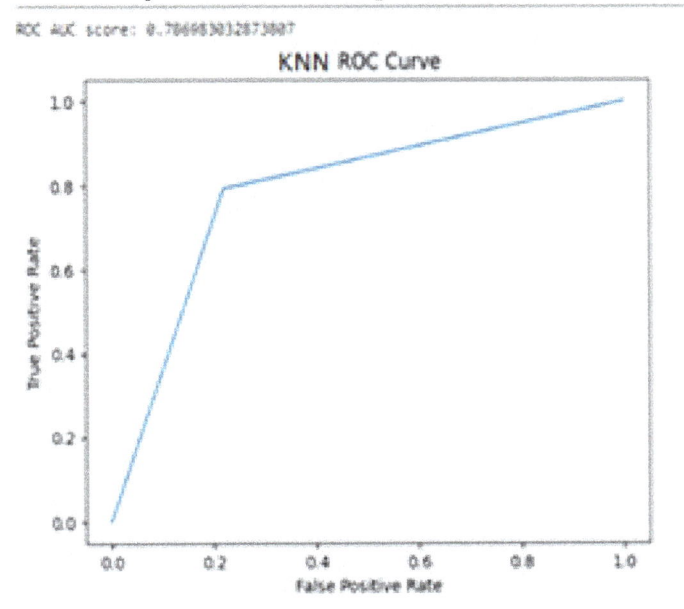

AUC Value: It refers to the area under the ROC curve. As the curve approaches 1, it indicates that the model is close to perfect (Ikonomakis et al., 2005; Uslu & Özmen-Akyol, 2021; Saygın & Baykara, 2021).

Specificity or True Negative Rate: The rate at which true negative instances are correctly detected in the dataset after applying the machine learning model (Ikonomakis et al., 2005; Uslu & Özmen-Akyol, 2021; Saygın & Baykara, 2021).

$$\text{Specificity} = \frac{\text{False Negatives}}{\text{False Negatives} + \text{False Posivitives}} \quad (4)$$

Confusion Matrix: It shows the model's performance in four basic prediction categories (True Positive, False Positive, True Negative, False Negative). It is used to examine the performance of the model in general.

Figure 3. Confusion Matrix of the Decision Tree Model

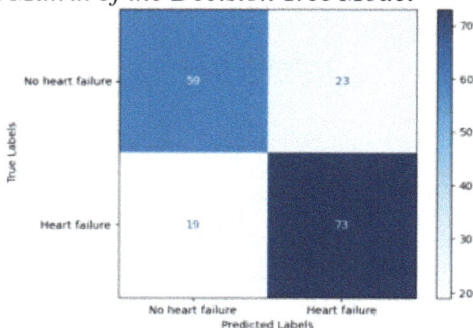

Figure 3 shows the confusion matrix showing the results obtained using the decision tree model for the application discussed in this book chapter. Top left corner (True Negative - TN): The number of data that the model correctly predicts and tests as no heart failure is 59. Upper right corner (False Positive - FP): The number of instances where the model incorrectly predicts heart failure when there is actually none is 23. Bottom left corner (False Negative - FN): The number of instances where the model classifies heart failure as absent when it should have predicted heart failure as present is 19. Bottom right corner (True Positive - TP): The number of instances where the model correctly predicts patients with heart failure is 73. While the model correctly identified 59 people without heart failure, it misclassified 23 people as having heart failure. It correctly identified 73 people with heart failure and misclassified 19 people as not having heart failure. The accuracy, overall performance and generalizability of the model can be assessed by comparing both the false positive and false negative rates. It is very effective to use a confusion matrix to analyze in which cases the model is successful and in which cases it is inadequate.

HEART DISEASE PREDICTION APPLICATION

The flowchart of the study considered in the application is given in Figure 4.

Figure 4. The flowchart of the Application

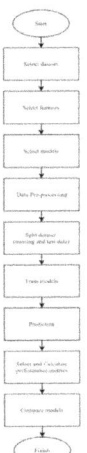

When Figure 4 is analyzed, firstly, the selection of the data set, selection of the features and selection of the models were carried out in the study. Then, after the data preprocessing processes, the data was divided into training and set data. After training the models with the training data, the prediction of the test data was performed. After calculating the appropriate performance metrics, the models were compared. Detailed information about the steps is given below.

Datasets used in heart disease prediction face several challenges in accessing real patient data. Ethical and privacy concerns limit access to real patient information, negatively impacting the timeliness and reliability of these datasets. As a result, researchers often turn to repositories such as Kaggle and UCI, which offer well-organized datasets that meet ethical standards while maintaining data integrity. These repositories allow researchers to conduct analyses and develop predictive models without being affected by restrictions related to direct access to sensitive patient information. The heart disease dataset used in this study was collected by the Cleveland Clinic Foundation in 1988 and enriched with data from hospitals in Hungary, Switzerland and Long Beach (Almustafa, 2020). The dataset includes demographic information, clinical test results and symptoms observed after exercise, and the coronary artery status of the patients was assessed using medical imaging techniques and supported by physicians' observations (Ahmad et al., 2022). The dataset consists of a total of 1025 cases with 14 features, including both sick and healthy individuals, obtained from the Kaggle dataset repository. These features are age, gender, type of chest pain, resting blood pressure, serum cholestoral, fasting blood glucose, resting electrocardiographic results, maximum heart rate achieved, exercise-induced angina, exercise-induced ST depression compared to rest, slope of peak exercise ST segment, number of large vessels colored by fluoroscopy for peak exercise, type of defect (talamus), and whether the decision variable is heart disease. A total of five different machine learning methods were applied to this data. The factors affecting the performance of the model are detailed Table 1.

Table 1. Distribution of Variables in the Data Set

Variable Name	Variable	Values
Age	age	Numeric values between 29 and 77
Gender	sex	1 = Male; 0 = Female
Type of Chest Pain	cp	0 = Typical; 1 = Atypical; 2 = Non-anginal; 3 = Asymptomatic
Resting Blood Pressure	trestbps	Numeric values between 94 and 200 mg/dl
Serum Cholesterol	chol	Numeric values between 126 and 564 mg/dl
Fasting Blood Glucose> 120 mg/dl	fbs	1 = Present; 0 = Absent
Resting Electrocardiographic Results	restecg	0 = Normal; 1 = ST-T wave abnormality; 2 = Left ventricular hypertrophy observed
Maximum Heart Rate	thalac	Numeric values between 71 and 202 bpm
Exercise-Induced Angina	exang	1 = Yes; 0 = No
Exercise Induced ST Depression (relative to rest)	oldpeak	Numeric values between 0 and 6.2
Slope of Peak Exercise ST Segment	slope	0 = Up-sloping; 1 = Flat; 2 = Down-sloping
Number of Major Vessels Visible by Fluoroscopy	ca	0, 1, 2, 3
Talamus: Thallium Stress Test Results	thal	0 = Normal; 1 = Fixed defect; 2 = Reversible defect

Data preprocessing for machine learning models is the most critical and important process that affects the performance of the models. This step is applied to ensure that the raw data is evaluated and made suitable for the use of the machine learning model. Data preprocessing includes processes such as correcting missing, erroneous or incompatible information in the data set, standardizing the data, converting categorical variables into numerical format and creating new features that will improve model performance. This stage provides the basis for improving the generalization ability and accuracy of the model (Uyanık & Kasapbaşı, 2021; Jayalakshmi & Santhakumaran, 2011; Abadi et al., 2016; Ganti & Sarma, 2013).

Machine learning models can use various types of data to analyze data and make predictions. Categorical data is one of these data types. However, machine learning models usually work with numerical data. Therefore, it is necessary to convert categorical data into numerical data. Different methods are used in the literature to convert categorical data into numerical data. One of these methods is the one-hot encoding method. The method first creates a separate binary column for each category. One column is added for each category and the observation belonging to the category is marked as 1 in this column, the other columns are 0. This method prevents the model from making mistakes between categories (Uyanık & Kasapbaşı, 2021; Potdar et al., 2017). Detection of outliers is an important step to assess data quality in statistical analysis. The quartiles and interquartile range (IQR) method are commonly used techniques in this process.

Quartiles divides the data set into four equal parts when sorted and defines three main points, the first quartile (Q1), the median (Q2) and the third quartile (Q3). The interquartile range refers to the difference between Q1 and Q3 and measures the spread of the middle 50% of the data set. Generally, the analysis process is performed to detect outliers within the limits determined using Q1 and Q3. As a result of the calculations, the parts of the values in the data set that fall outside these limits are considered outliers. The quartiles and IQR method identify anomalous observations during data analysis and identifies potential distortions in the data set (Ovla & Taşdelen, 2012; Keskin et al., 2019). In the application, five different machine learning models (K-Nearest Neighbor, Logistic Regression, Decision Tree, Support Vector Machine and Naive Bayes) from supervised learning models were applied on the dataset containing 1025 records and 14 attributes taken from the Kaggle data center and the performance metrics of these models in predicting whether patients have heart disease were examined. Python programming language was used to build the models. NumPy and Pandas libraries were used effectively in data preprocessing and model development processes. In the data analysis and profiling stages, the pandas_profiling library contributed to the evaluation of data quality by providing detailed reporting of the data set. Math and random libraries were used for mathematical calculations and randomization. The powerful and flexible tools provided by seaborn and matplotlib libraries were used to visualize the data sets and analysis results. These libraries have a critical role in data processing, modeling, analysis and reporting of results in Python programming language. There are no null values in the data set considered in the application. However, 3 outliers were observed in the cholesterol variable and 153 outliers were observed in the fasting blood glucose variable. It was decided to remove these values from the dataset as they would negatively affect the performance of the model. The distribution of variables in the dataset is shown in Figure 5.

Figure 5. Distribution of variables in the data set

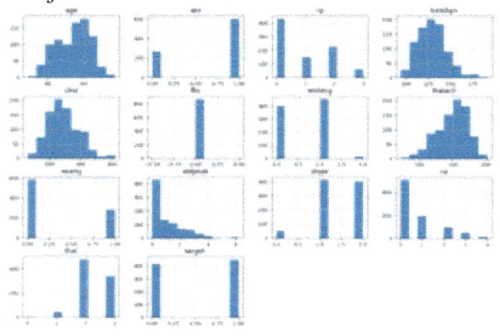

When the distribution of variables in the dataset is examined, it is observed that the patients seen in Figure 5 are mostly between the ages of 40 and 60. According to the gender variable, men are more common. Chest pain type consists of 4 categories and the most common pain type is 0 (typical). Resting blood pressure (trestbps) and cholesterol (chol) variables were close to normal distribution, with values concentrated in the range of 120-140 mmHg and 200-300 mg/dL, respectively. Fasting blood glucose (fbs) and exercise angina (exang) are binary variables; both are dominated by a value of 0, indicating that most individuals have normal fasting blood glucose and do not experience exercise angina. Resting ECG results (restecg) and ST segment slope (slope) were categorical and concentrated in the lower categories. The maximum heart rate (thalach) variable shows a normal distribution with the majority between 140 and 160. Variables such as ST depression (oldpeak) and number of main vessels detected by fluoroscopy (ca) show a wider distribution, but are concentrated in low values. The thalassemia type (thal) variable is concentrated in categories 2 and 3. Finally, the target variable (target) has approximately equal numbers of 0 and 1 values, indicating a balanced distribution across classes. Understanding the statistical properties of the data set before applying machine learning models enables more effective and accurate application of the models. Therefore, examining the basic statistics of the variables in the dataset provides information about possible imbalances or errors that may be encountered in the modeling process. For example, the age variable (age) has a mean of 53.93 with 869 observations and a standard deviation of 9.31, with a relatively narrow distribution from 29 to 77 years old. The gender variable (sex) had a mean of 0.69, indicating that the majority of individuals in the dataset were male. Chest pain type (cp) was concentrated in the lower categories with a mean of 0.90, while resting blood pressure (trestbps) averaged 130.33 mmHg with a large standard deviation (16.64 mmHg). Cholesterol (chol) level averaged 244.31 mg/dL with a high standard deviation (48.47), showing significant differences between individuals. Fasting blood glucose (fbs) averaged 0.55, indicating that approximately 55% of individuals had high fasting blood glucose. After examining the data set, it is necessary to perform the procedures for the application. Accordingly, the values of the variables in the data set were drawn to the range of 0- 1 using the min-max scaler scale. Min-max scaler is a normalization technique created by pulling the variables to a certain range. This process was performed to provide better performance of the models.

80% of the dataset was used as training data and 20% as test data. In the dataset, 695 of the data were used as training data and 174 were used as test data. For each model, various evaluation criteria such as precision, recall, F1 score, macro mean values, accuracy, ROC and AUC curve were found. The results for these values are given in Table 2.

Table 2. Performance Metrics of the Models

MODEL	CATEGORY	PRECISION	RECALL	F1-SCORE	SUPPORT
SVM	0	0.81	0.79	0.80	82
	1	0.82	0.84	0.83	92
KNN	0	0.76	0.83	0.80	82
	1	0.84	0.77	0.80	92
LR	0	0.81	0.78	0.80	82
	1	0.81	0.84	0.82	92
NB	0	0.79	0.78	0.79	82
	1	0.81	0.82	0.81	92
DT	0	0.76	0.72	0.74	82
	1	0.76	0.79	0.78	92

Table 2 shows that SVM and KNN models are more reliable in predicting heart disease based on the precion metric, while the DT model has a lower value than the other models. According to the analysis based on recall values, the KNN model is the most successful model in predicting individuals without heart disease in the dataset. This suggests that the KNN model has a higher competence in correctly identifying negative samples (without heart disease) compared to other models. LR and SVM perform better than other models in predicting patients with heart disease. Considering the F1 score value, it is possible to say that the LR model performs a more balanced analysis. When we examine the evaluations according to the complexity matrix metric, Figures 6, 7, 8, 9 and 10 show the results of DT, KNN, SVM, LR and NB models, respectively.

Figure 6. Confusion Matrix of the DT Model

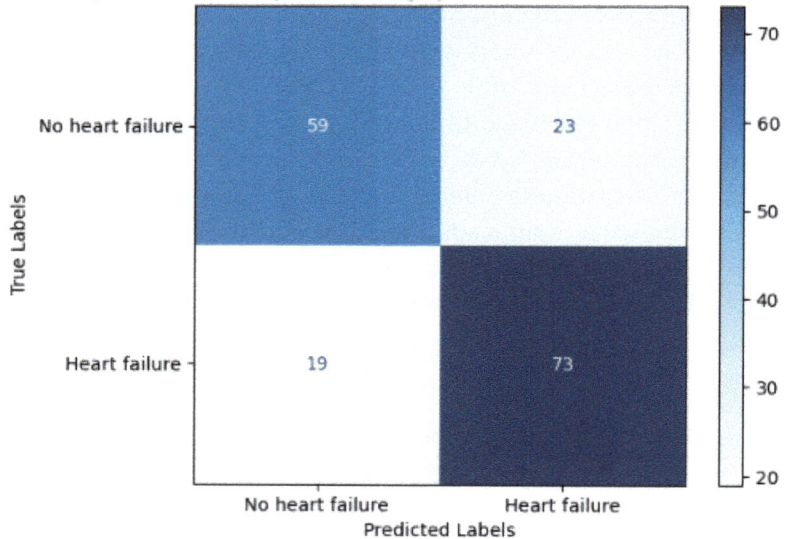

Figure 6 shows that while the DT model correctly identified 59 people without heart failure, but misclassified 23 people as having heart failure. While it correctly detected 73 people with heart failure, it misclassified 19 people as not having heart failure.

Figure 7. Confusion Matrix of the KNN Model

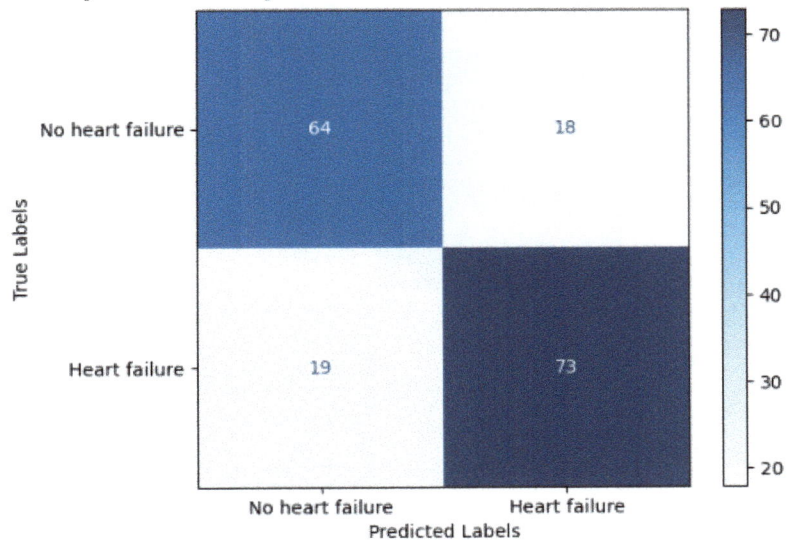

According to Figure 7, the KNN model correctly detected 64 people without heart failure and misclassified 18 people as having heart failure. At the same time, while it correctly detected 73 people with heart failure, it misclassified 19 people as not having heart failure.

Figure 8. Confusion Matrix of the SVM Model

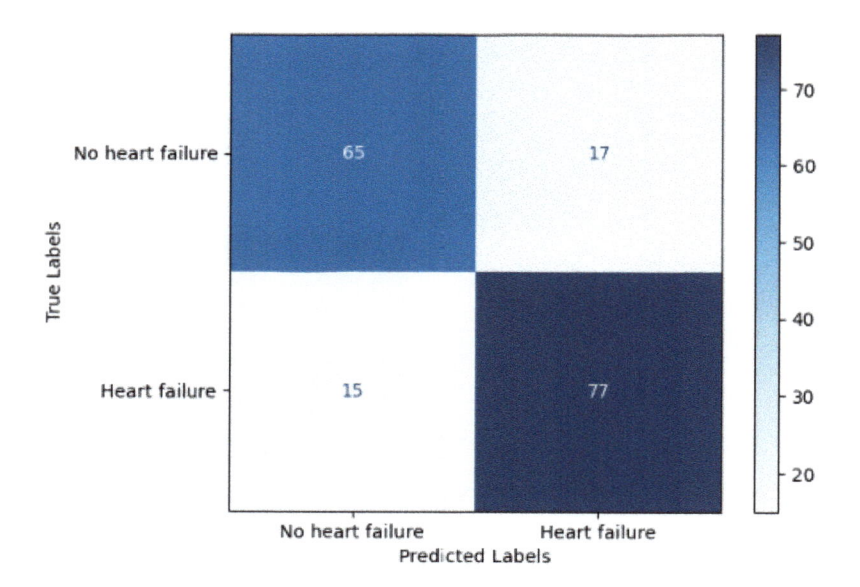

The SVM model in Figure 8 correctly detected 65 people without heart failure and misclassified 17 people as having heart failure. While it correctly detected 77 people with heart failure, it misclassified 15 people as not having heart failure.

Figure 9. Confusion Matrix of the LR Model

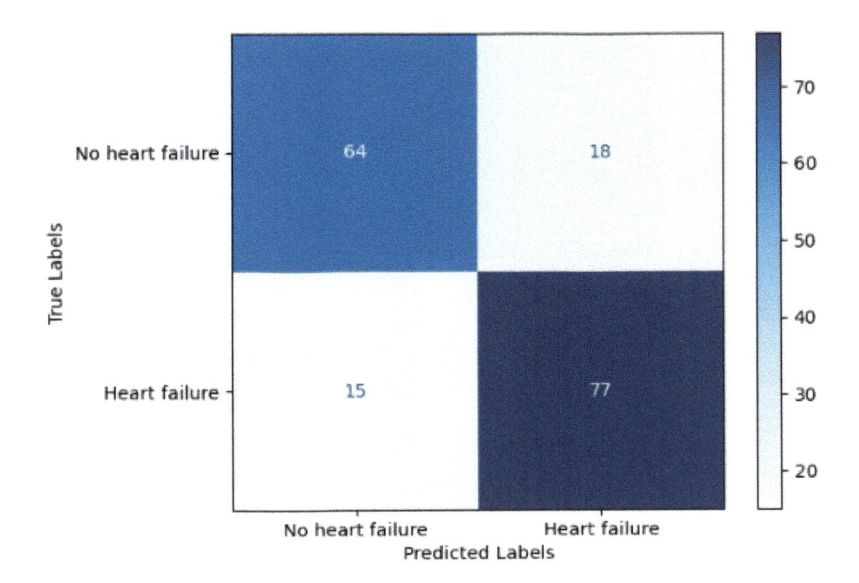

In Figure 9, the LR model correctly identified 64 people without heart failure, but misclassified 18 people as having heart failure. While it correctly detected 77 people with heart failure, it misclassified 15 people as not having heart failure.

Figure 10. Confusion Matrix of the NB Model

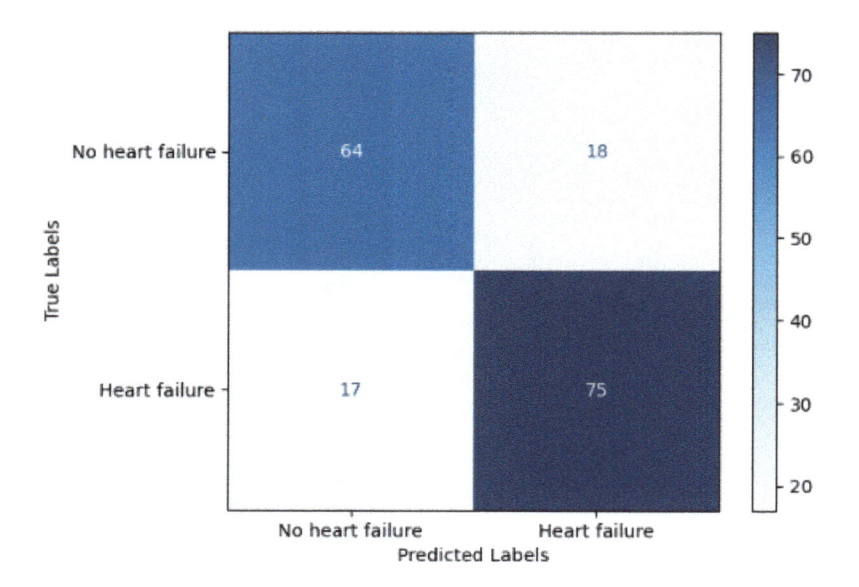

The model in Figure 10 correctly identified 64 people without heart failure, but misclassified 18 people as having heart failure. While it correctly detected 75 people with heart failure, it misclassified 17 people as not having heart failure. The ROC curve graph obtained according to the five machine learning algorithms considered in this study and the evaluation results according to the AUC value are shown in Figure 11. When the ROC Curve and AUC values are analyzed in Figure 11, it can be concluded that the SVM model generally performs well and can effectively distinguish between positive and negative classes. This can be interpreted as both a high ability of the model to predict the number of true positives and a low rate of false positive prediction. Figure 12 shows the accuracy results of all models.

Figure 11. ROC Curve Plot of the Models Considered in This Study

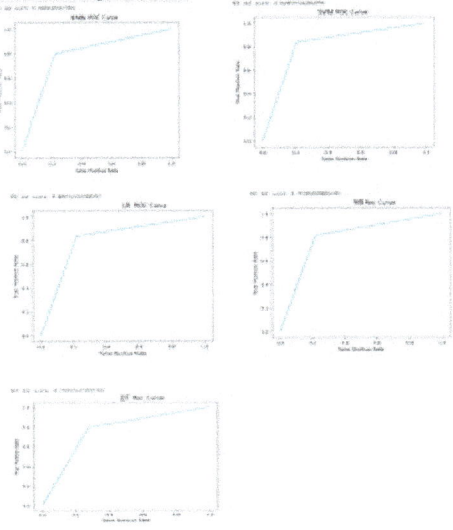

Figure 12. Comparison of Models According to Accuracy Values

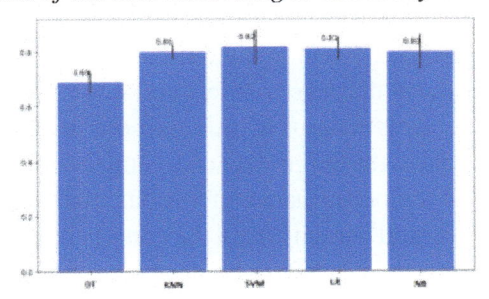

When the accuracy values in Figure 12 are analyzed, it can be interpreted that the SVM provides the highest overall accuracy rate on the given dataset and performs better than other models on the classification task. Although the SVM model seems to perform the best in the classification task for this dataset, the results with the other models are quite close. Therefore, it is recommended to investigate whether there is a significant difference between the models with statistical tests.

When we examine some other studies working on the same dataset as this study, it is seen that there are differences in the results. Almustafa (2020) compared various classifiers including KNN, NB, DT J48, JRip, SVM, AdaBoost, Stochastic Gradient Descent (SGD) and DT for the classification of heart disease dataset.

In terms of classification performance, the model with the highest accuracy was KNN (K=1), which achieved 99.7073% accuracy. In contrast, Absar et al. (2022) compared the performance of four classification methods based on KNN, DT, AB and RF algorithms and the results showed that the KNN algorithm achieved 100% accuracy. This indicates a higher performance for KNN compared to the models evaluated by Almustafa (2020). Furthermore, Ali et al. (2021) performed modeling on a dataset using AdaBoostM1, Multilayer Perceptron (MLP), KNN, DT and RF algorithms. The results of this study reported that the success rates of KNN, DT and RF models were 100%. The analysis of the differences in the results of the studies working on the same data set shows that differences in parameter settings in classification models, data preprocessing methods, cross-validation strategies and hyperparameter optimization are involved. Furthermore, differences in factors such as training and test dataset partitioning ratios, feature selection methods and model evaluation metrics also have the potential to explain the variations in results. As a result, it can be said that these factors play a decisive role in the performance of the models, even when the same dataset is used.

CONCLUSION

Today, technological innovations and the rapid increase in population have led to massive amounts of data collected in the field of health. However, manpower is insufficient to analyze these massive datasets and draw meaningful conclusions. When analyzing these datasets in terms of time and cost, machine learning technologies play an important role in the diagnosis and treatment of diseases. Studies in the literature have evaluated the performance of various machine learning algorithms in heart disease prediction and demonstrated the potential of these techniques in the healthcare field. The opportunities offered by machine learning make a significant contribution to the management of complex health problems such as heart disease. The promising opportunities that these technologies offer for future health research and applications represent an important step towards improving the quality of healthcare.

When we look at the literature, it is seen that traditional methods lag behind machine learning methods in the diagnosis and treatment of heart disease. Early diagnosis of the disease can increase the patient's quality of life and the percentage of positive results of the treatment while reducing treatment costs. In this context, this study provides information on how to use and interpret 5 different machine learning models (K-Nearest Neighbor, Logistic Regression, Decision Tree, Support Vector Machine, Naive Bayes) that are widely used in the literature for diagnosing heart disease. In addition, the accuracy, precision, recall, F1 score values that can be used in the performance evaluations of the machine learning models used are examined and interpreted. When the performance results of all models were analyzed, the decision trees model is the model with the lowest performance in terms of diagnosing heart disease in this dataset. However, due to the close proximity of the obtained accuracy values, statistical tests can be used for a more comprehensive assessment of model performance. In future studies, statistical analyses such as the McNemar test or Wilcoxon test can be effectively used to determine the significance of performance differences between different models. Such tests can improve the reliability of the results of the models and provide a more robust basis for model comparisons.

When we examine the future of machine learning and artificial intelligence-based classification algorithms in the healthcare sector, data integration and increasing data quality in the transformation of healthcare services will enable algorithms to produce more accurate and comprehensive results. In addition, by increasing the transparency and explainability of algorithms, clinical decision-making processes can be accelerated by ensuring the trust of healthcare professionals and patients. The development of personalized health solutions can improve decision-making processes based on individual patient data by making disease prediction and treatment recommendations more effective. In addition, designing algorithms in accordance with ethical and privacy standards will protect the security and privacy of patient data and ensure that they have a wider acceptance rate in society.

As a result, these innovative approaches are critical for enhancing the quality of healthcare and improving patient outcomes. The effective application of machine learning and artificial intelligence-based classification algorithms will be able to lay a solid foundation for future advances in the healthcare sector.

REFERENCES

Abadi, M., Barham, P., Chen, J., Chen, Z., Davis, A., Dean, J., . . . Zheng, X. (2016, November). TensorFlow: A system for large-scale machine learning. In OSDI (Vol. 16, No. 2016, pp. 265-283).

Absar, N., Das, E. K., Shoma, S. N., Khandaker, M. U., Miraz, M. H., Faruque, M. R. I., & Pathan, R. K. (2022, June). The efficacy of machine-learning-supported smart system for heart disease prediction. []. MDPI.]. *Health Care*, 10(6), 1137. PMID: 35742188

Ahmad, G. N., Fatima, H., Ullah, S., & Saidi, A. S. (2022). Efficient medical diagnosis of human heart diseases using machine learning techniques with and without GridSearchCV. *IEEE Access : Practical Innovations, Open Solutions*, 10, 80151–80173. DOI: 10.1109/ACCESS.2022.3165792

Ali, M. M., Paul, B. K., Ahmed, K., Bui, F. M., Quinn, J. M. W., & Moni, M. A. (2021). Heart disease prediction using supervised machine learning algorithms: Performance analysis and comparison. *Computers in Biology and Medicine*, 136, 104672. DOI: 10.1016/j.compbiomed.2021.104672 PMID: 34315030

Almustafa, K. M. (2020). Prediction of heart disease and classifiers' sensitivity analysis. *BMC Bioinformatics*, 21(1), 1–18. DOI: 10.1186/s12859-020-03626-y PMID: 32615980

Ayhan, S., & Erdoğan, Ş. (2014). Destek vektör makineleriyle sınıflandırma problemlerinin çözümü için çekirdek fonksiyonu seçimi. *Eskişehir Osmangazi Üniversitesi İktisadi ve İdari Bilimler Dergisi*, 9(1), 175–201.

Ayık, Y. Z., Özdemir, A., & Yavuz, U. (2007). Lise türü ve lise mezuniyet başarısının, kazanılan fakülte ile ilişkisinin veri madenciliği tekniği ile analizi. *Atatürk Üniversitesi Sosyal Bilimler Enstitüsü Dergisi*, 10(2), 441–454.

Berner, E. S., Webster, G. D., Shugerman, A. A., & Fenton, S. H. (1994). Performance of four computer-based diagnostic systems. *The New England Journal of Medicine*, 330(26), 1792–1796. DOI: 10.1056/NEJM199406233302506 PMID: 8190157

Bhatia, N., & Vandana. (2010). Survey of nearest neighbor techniques. [IJCSIS]. *International Journal of Computer Science and Information Security*, 8(2).

Boateng, E. Y., & Abaye, D. A. (2019). A review of the logistic regression model with emphasis on medical research. *Journal of Data Analysis and Information Processing*, 7(4), 190–207. DOI: 10.4236/jdaip.2019.74012

Chandrasekhar, N., & Peddakrishna, S. (2023). Enhancing heart disease prediction accuracy through machine learning techniques and optimization. *Processes (Basel, Switzerland)*, 11(4), 1210. DOI: 10.3390/pr11041210

Çınar, A. (2019). Veri madenciliğinde sınıflandırma algoritmalarının performans değerlendirmesi ve R dili ile bir uygulama. Öneri Dergisi, 14(51), 90-111. https://doi.org/DOI: 10.14783/maruoneri.vi.522168

Cunningham, P., Cord, M., & Delany, S. J. (2008). Supervised learning. In *Machine learning techniques for multimedia* (pp. 21–49). Springer., DOI: 10.1007/978-3-540-75171-7_2

Deperlıoğlu, Ö., & Köse, U. (2018). Diagnosis of diabetic retinopathy by using image processing and convolutional neural network. In 2018 2nd International Symposium on Multidisciplinary Studies and Innovative Technologies (ISMSIT) (pp. 1-5). IEEE. https://doi.org/DOI: 10.1109/ISMSIT.2018.8567055

Dixon, M. F., Halperin, I., & Bilokon, P. (2020). *Machine learning in finance* (Vol. 1170). Springer International Publishing., DOI: 10.1007/978-3-030-41068-1

Dudani, S. A. (1976). The distance-weighted k-nearest-neighbor rule. *IEEE Transactions on Systems, Man, and Cybernetics*, SMC-6(4), 325–327. DOI: 10.1109/TSMC.1976.5408784

Emre, İ. E., & Erol, Ç. S. (2017). Veri analizinde istatistik mi veri madenciliği mi? *Bilişim Teknolojileri Dergisi*, 10(2), 161–167. DOI: 10.17671/gazibtd.309297

Ganti, V., & Sarma, A. D. (2013). Data cleaning: A practical perspective. *Synthesis Lectures on Data Management*, 5(3), 1–85. DOI: 10.1007/978-3-031-01897-8

Gharehbaghi, A., Linden, M., & Babic, A. (2017). A decision support system for cardiac disease diagnosis based on machine learning methods. *Studies in Health Technology and Informatics*, 235, 43–47. DOI: 10.3233/978-1-61499-753-5-43 PMID: 28423752

Güner, Z. (2014). Veri madenciliğinde CART ve lojistik regresyon analizinin yeri: İlaç provizyon sistemi verileri üzerinde örnek bir uygulama. *Sosyal Güvence*, (6), 53–99. DOI: 10.21441/sguz.2014617906

Guo, G., Wang, H., Bell, D., Bi, Y., & Greer, K. (2003). KNN model-based approach in classification. In On The Move to Meaningful Internet Systems 2003: CoopIS, DOA, and ODBASE (pp. 986-996). Springer. https://doi.org/DOI: 10.1007/978-3-540-39964-3_62

Güran, A., Uysal, M., & Doğrusöz, Ö. (2014). Destek vektör makineleri parametre optimizasyonunun duygu analizi üzerindeki etkisi. *Dokuz Eylül Üniversitesi Mühendislik Fakültesi Fen ve Mühendislik Dergisi*, 16(48), 86–93.

Hastie, T. (2009). *The elements of statistical learning: Data mining, inference, and prediction* (2nd ed.). Springer., DOI: 10.1007/978-0-387-84858-7

Hastie, T., Tibshirani, R., & Friedman, J. (2001). *The elements of statistical learning: Data mining, inference, and prediction.* Springer Series in Statistics., DOI: 10.1007/978-0-387-21606-5

Heart Disease Dataset. Available online: https://www.kaggle.com/johnsmith88/heart-disease-dataset (accessed on 1 April 2024).

Hosmer, D. W., Jr., Lemeshow, S., & Sturdivant, R. X. (2013). Applied logistic regression (Vol. 398). John Wiley & Sons. https://doi.org//arXiv.1007.0085 DOI: 10.48550

Hossain, M. I., Maruf, M. H., Khan, M. A. R., Prity, F. S., Fatema, S., Ejaz, M. S., & Khan, M. A. S. (2023). Heart disease prediction using distinct artificial intelligence techniques: Performance analysis and comparison. *Iran Journal of Computer Science*, 6(4), 397–417. DOI: 10.1007/s42044-023-00148-7

Ikonomakis, M., Kotsiantis, S., & Tampakas, V. (2005). Text classification using machine learning techniques. *WSEAS Transactions on Computers*, 4(8), 966–974.

Jayalakshmi, T., & Santhakumaran, A. (2011). Statistical normalization and back propagation for classification. *International Journal of Computer Theory and Engineering*, 3(1), 89–93. DOI: 10.7763/IJCTE.2011.V3.288

Jiang, L., Cai, Z., Wang, D., & Jiang, S. (2007, August). Survey of improving k-nearest-neighbor for classification. In *Fourth international conference on fuzzy systems and knowledge discovery (FSKD 2007)* (Vol. 1, pp. 679-683). IEEE. https://doi.org/DOI: 10.1109/FSKD.2007.552

Jordan, M. I., & Mitchell, T. M. (2015). Machine learning: Trends, perspectives, and prospects. *Science*, 349(6245), 255–260. DOI: 10.1126/science.aaa8415 PMID: 26185243

Jothi, K. A., Subburam, S., Umadevi, V., & Hemavathy, K. (2021). WITHDRAWN: Heart disease prediction system using machine learning. *Materials Today: Proceedings*. Advance online publication. DOI: 10.1016/j.matpr.2020.12.901

Kar, Y. E., Basgumus, A., & Namdar, M. (2021, October). Machine learning assisted autonomous vehicle design and control. In 2021 5th International Symposium on Multidisciplinary Studies and Innovative Technologies (ISMSIT) (pp. 462-466). IEEE. DOI: 10.1109/ISMSIT52890.2021.9604621

Kaur, G., & Oberai, E. N. (2014). A review article on Naive Bayes classifier with various smoothing techniques. *International Journal of Computer Science and Mobile Computing*, 3(10), 864–868.

Kavzoğlu, T., & Çölkesen, İ. (2010). Karar ağaçları ile uydu görüntülerinin sınıflandırılması. *Harita Teknolojileri Elektronik Dergisi*, 2(1), 36–45.

Keskin, S., Aydın, F., & Yurdugül, H. (2019). Eğitsel veri madenciliği ve öğrenme analitikleri bağlamında e-öğrenme verilerinde aykırı gözlemlerin belirlenmesi. *Eğitim Teknolojisi Kuram ve Uygulama*, 9(1), 292–309. DOI: 10.17943/etku.475149

Kılınç, D., Borandağ, E., Yücala, F., Tunalı, V., Şimşek, M., & Özçift, A. (2016). KNN algoritması ve R dili ile metin madenciliği kullanılarak bilimsel makale tasnifi. *Marmara Fen Bilimleri Dergisi*, 28(3), 89–94. DOI: 10.7240/mufbed.69674

Kıran, Z. B. (2010). *Lojistik regresyon ve CART analizi teknikleriyle sosyal güvenlik kurumu ilaç provizyon sistemi verileri üzerinde bir uygulama* [An application on pharmacy provision system data of social security institution by logistic regression and CART analysis techniques]. Gazi Üniversitesi Fen Bilimleri Enstitüsü.

Köse, G., & Köse, U. (2022). Sağlıkta zeki karar destek sistemleri: Günümüz ve gelecek.

Kotsiantis, S. B. (2013). Decision trees: A recent overview. *Artificial Intelligence Review*, 39(4), 261–283. DOI: 10.1007/s10462-011-9272-4

Koyuncugil, A., & Özgülbaş, N. (2009). Veri madenciliği: Tıp ve sağlık hizmetlerinde kullanımı ve uygulamaları. Bilişim Teknolojileri Dergisi, 2(2).

Laishram, A., & Padmanabhan, V. (2019). Discovery of user-item subgroups via genetic algorithm for effective prediction of ratings in collaborative filtering. *Applied Intelligence*, 49(11), 3990–4006. DOI: 10.1007/s10489-019-01495-4

Lin, C. F., & Wang, S. D. (2002). Fuzzy Support Vector Machines. *IEEE Transactions on Neural Networks*, 13(2), 464–471. DOI: 10.1109/72.991432 PMID: 18244447

Liu, H., & Zhang, S. (2012). Noisy data elimination using mutual k-nearest neighbor for classification mining. *Journal of Systems and Software*, 85(5), 1067–1074. DOI: 10.1016/j.jss.2011.12.019

Mathur, P., Srivastava, S., Xu, X., & Mehta, J. L. (2020). Artificial intelligence, machine learning, and cardiovascular disease. *Clinical Medicine Insights. Cardiology*, 14, 1179546820927404. DOI: 10.1177/1179546820927404 PMID: 32952403

Metlek, S., & Kayaalp, K. (2020). Derin öğrenme ve destek vektör makineleri ile görüntüden cinsiyet tahmini. *Düzce Üniversitesi Bilim ve Teknoloji Dergisi*, 8(3), 2208–2228. DOI: 10.29130/dubited.707316

Murathan, T., & Devecioğlu, S. (2018). Veri madenciliği ve spor alanındaki uygulamaları. *Spor Bilimleri Dergisi*, 29(3), 147–156. DOI: 10.17644/sbd.371590

Ngai, E. W., & Wu, Y. (2022). Machine learning in marketing: A literature review, conceptual framework, and research agenda. *Journal of Business Research*, 145, 35–48. DOI: 10.1016/j.jbusres.2022.02.049

Nikhar, S., & Karandikar, A. M. (2016). Prediction of heart disease using machine learning algorithms. International Journal of Advanced Engineering. *Management Science*, 2(6), 239–484.

Ovla, H. D., & Taşdelen, B. (2012). Aykırı değer yönetimi. *Mersin Üniversitesi Saglik Bilimleri Dergisi*, 5(3).

Oyebode, O., Fowles, J., Steeves, D., & Orji, R. (2023). Machine learning techniques in adaptive and personalized systems for health and wellness. *International Journal of Human-Computer Interaction*, 39(9), 1938–1962. DOI: 10.1080/10447318.2022.2089085

Özcan, B., Kayapınar, K., & Adem, K. (2023). Gelişen teknoloji ile bankacılık sektöründe veri analitiği: Müşteri kaybı tahmini için makine öğrenmesi yaklaşımları. *Uluslararası Sivas Bilim ve Teknoloji Üniversitesi Dergisi*, 2(1), 74–84.

Paul, A. K., Shill, P. C., Rabin, M. R. I., & Akhand, M. A. H. (2016). Genetic algorithm based fuzzy decision support system for the diagnosis of heart disease. In 2016 5th International Conference on Informatics, Electronics and Vision (ICIEV) (pp. 145-150). IEEE. DOI: 10.1109/ICIEV.2016.7759984

Pehlivan, G. (2006). CHAID analizi ve bir uygulama. Yayınlanmamış Yüksek Lisans Tezi. İstanbul: Yıldız Teknik Üniversitesi, FBE.

Potdar, K., Pardawala, T., & Pai, C. (2017). A comparative study of categorical variable encoding techniques for neural network classifiers. *International Journal of Computer Applications*, 175(4), 7–9. DOI: 10.5120/ijca2017915495

Pulat, M., & Deveci Kocakoç, İ. (2021). Türkiye'de Makine Öğrenmesi ve Karar Ağaçları Alanında Yayınlanmış Tezlerin Bibliyometrik Analizi. *Yönetim Ve Ekonomi Dergisi*, 28(2), 287–308. DOI: 10.18657/yonveek.870190

Qi, Z., Tian, Y., & Shi, Y. (2013). Robust twin support vector machine for pattern classification. *Pattern Recognition*, 46(1), 305–316. DOI: 10.1016/j.patcog.2012.06.019

Qin, Y., Zhang, S., Zhu, X., Zhang, J., & Zhang, C. (2007). Semi-parametric optimization for missing data imputation. *Applied Intelligence*, 27(1), 79–88. DOI: 10.1007/s10489-006-0032-0

Ragab, M., Albukhari, A., Alyami, J., & Mansour, R. F. (2022). Ensemble deep-learning-enabled clinical decision support system for breast cancer diagnosis and classification on ultrasound images. *Biology (Basel)*, 11(3), 439. DOI: 10.3390/biology11030439 PMID: 35336813

Rokach, L., & Maimon, O. Z. (2008). *Data mining with decision trees: Theory and applications* (Vol. 69). World Scientific.

Sahu, B., Panigrahi, A., Sukla, S., & Biswal, B. B. (2020). MRMR-BAT-HS: A clinical decision support system for cancer diagnosis. *Leukemia*, 7129(73), 48. DOI: 10.1038/s41375-020-0724-0

Saleh, M. D., & Eswaran, C. (2012). An automated decision-support system for non-proliferative diabetic retinopathy disease based on MAs and HAs detection. *Computer Methods and Programs in Biomedicine*, 108(1), 186–196. DOI: 10.1016/j.cmpb.2012.03.004 PMID: 22551841

Saygın, E., & Baykara, M. (2021). Karaciğer yetmezliği teşhisinde özellik seçimi kullanarak makine öğrenmesi yöntemlerinin başarılarının ölçülmesi. *Fırat Üniversitesi Mühendislik Bilimleri Dergisi*, 33(2), 367–377. DOI: 10.35234/fumbd.832264

Sevli, O. (2019). Göğüs kanseri teşhisinde farklı makine öğrenmesi tekniklerinin performans karşılaştırması. *Avrupa Bilim ve Teknoloji Dergisi*, (16), 176–185. DOI: 10.31590/ejosat.553549

Shorewala, V. (2021). Early detection of coronary heart disease using ensemble techniques. *Informatics in Medicine Unlocked*, 26, 100655. DOI: 10.1016/j.imu.2021.100655

Stephenson, B., Cook, D., Dixon, P., Duckworth, W., Kaiser, M., Koehler, K., & Meeker, W. (2008). Binary response and logistic regression analysis. Available from https://www.example.com

Szolovits, P., Patil, R. S., & Schwartz, W. B. (1988). Artificial intelligence in medical diagnosis. *Annals of Internal Medicine*, 108(1), 80–87. DOI: 10.7326/0003-4819-108-1-80 PMID: 3276267

Tabachnick, B. G., Fidell, L. S., & Ullman, J. B. (2013). *Using multivariate statistics* (Vol. 6). Pearson.

Tabakan, G., & Avcı, O. (2021). Vergiye gönüllü uyumu etkileyen faktörlerin lojistik regresyon analizi ile belirlenmesi. *Sosyoekonomi*, 29(48), 541–561. DOI: 10.17233/sosyoekonomi.2021.02.25

Tantuğ, A. C. (2012). Metin sınıflandırma (Text Classification). Türkiye Bilişim Vakfı Bilgi, Bilim ve Mühendisliği Dergisi, 5(2).

Taşcı, M. E., & Şamlı, R. (2020). Veri madenciliği ile kalp hastalığı teşhisi. Avrupa Bilim ve Teknoloji Dergisi, 88-95. https://doi.org/DOI: 10.31590/ejosat.araconf12

Taşkın, G. G. E. V. Ç. (2005). Veri madenciliğinde karar ağaçları ve bir satış analizi uygulaması. *Eskişehir Osmangazi Üniversitesi Sosyal Bilimler Dergisi*, 6(2), 221–239.

Thomas, L. C. (2000). A survey of credit and behavioral scoring: Forecasting financial risk of lending to consumers. *International Journal of Forecasting*, 16(2), 149–172. DOI: 10.1016/S0169-2070(00)00034-0

Tolun, S. (2008). *Destek vektör makineleri: Banka başarısızlığının tahmini üzerine bir uygulama*. İktisadî Araştırmalar Vakfı.

Tosun, S. (2007). Sınıflandırmada yapay sinir ağları ve karar ağaçları karşılaştırması: Öğrenci başarıları üzerine bir uygulama [Doctoral dissertation, Fen Bilimleri Enstitüsü].

Tushar, A. M., Wazed, A., Shawon, E., Rahman, M., Hossen, M. I., & Jesmeen, M. Z. H. (2022). A review of commonly used machine learning classifiers in heart disease prediction. In 2022 IEEE 10th Conference on Systems, Process & Control (ICSPC), pp. 319-323. https://doi.org/DOI: 10.1109/ICSPC55597.2022.10001742

Uğurlu, M., Doğru, İ., & Arslan, R. S. (2023). Karanlık ağ trafiğinin makine öğrenmesi yöntemleri kullanılarak tespiti ve sınıflandırılması. *Gazi Üniversitesi Mühendislik Mimarlık Fakültesi Dergisi*, 38(3), 1737–1746. DOI: 10.17341/gazimmfd.1023147

Uslu, O., & Özmen-Akyol, S. (2021). Türkçe haber metinlerinin makine öğrenmesi yöntemleri kullanılarak sınıflandırılması. *Eskişehir Türk Dünyası Uygulama ve Araştırma Merkezi Bilişim Dergisi*, 2(1), 15–20.

Uyanık, F., & Kasapbaşı, M. C. (2021). Telekomünikasyon sektörü için veri madenciliği ve makine öğrenmesi teknikleri ile ayrılan müşteri analizi. *Düzce Üniversitesi Bilim ve Teknoloji Dergisi*, 9(3), 172–191. DOI: 10.29130/dubited.807922

Vembandasamy, K., Sasipriya, R., & Deepa, E. (2015). Heart diseases detection using Naive Bayes algorithm. International Journal of Innovative Science. *Engineering & Technology*, 2(9), 441–444.

Visseren, F. L. J., Mach, F., Smulders, Y. M., Carballo, D., Koskinas, K. C., Back, M., Benetos, A., Biffi, A., Boavida, J.-M., Capodanno, D., Cosyns, B., Crawford, C., Davos, C. H., Desormais, I., Di Angelantonio, E., Franco, O. H., Halvorsen, S., Hobbs, F. D. R., Hollander, M., & Williams, B. (2021). ESC guidelines on cardiovascular disease prevention in clinical practice. *European Heart Journal*, 42(34), 3227–3337. DOI: 10.1093/eurheartj/ehab484 PMID: 34458905

Wang, H. (2002). *Nearest neighbours without k: A classification formalism based on probability*. Faculty of Informatics, University of Ulster.

WHO. 2023. Cardiovascular diseases. Retrieved from https://www.who.int/health-topics/cardiovascular-diseases#tab=tab_1 (Accessed 01/09/2024)

Yıldız, A., & Hasan, Z. A. N. (2019). Segmantasyon yapmadan patolojik kalp sesi kayıtlarının tespiti için bir örüntü sınıflandırma algoritması. *Dicle Üniversitesi Mühendislik Fakültesi Mühendislik Dergisi*, 10(1), 77–91.

Zhang, S., Li, X., Zong, M., Zhu, X., & Cheng, D. (2017). Learning k for KNN classification. [TIST]. *ACM Transactions on Intelligent Systems and Technology*, 8(3), 1–19. DOI: 10.1145/2990508

Chapter 7
COVID Detection Model Using X-Ray Images:
Role of Data Science and Machine Learning in Digital Medical System

Vasima Khan
 https://orcid.org/0000-0002-6903-9910
Sagar Institute of Science and Technology, Bhopal, India

Komal Tahiliani
 https://orcid.org/0009-0006-1872-7314
Sagar Institute of Science and Technology, Bhopal, India

ABSTRACT

The global COVID-19 pandemic has posed unprecedented problems to healthcare institutions across the globe. Ensuring timely and precise identification of the virus is crucial to efficiently manage its transmission. In the context of the metaverse, the implementation of a non-contact detection method has possible advantages by replacing the necessity of a physical COVID-19 test with a digital challenge. The present chapter explores the utilisation of machine learning and deep learning methodologies in the creation of a COVID-19 detection model through the analysis of X-ray pictures. The main aim of this approach is to augment the foundational notion of the metaverse. The primary objective of this model is to precisely ascertain the existence of COVID-19, regardless of its positive or negative status, and to identify instances of viral pneumonia by the analysis of X-ray pictures. The present investigation is grounded upon recent research that indicates a correlation between the presence of COVID-19 and detectable findings in chest X-ray pictures.

DOI: 10.4018/979-8-3693-7277-7.ch007

INTRODUCTION

The COVID-19 pandemic exhibits a daily mortality rate of thousands of individuals on a global scale. In many instances, the transmission of COVID-19 occurs through direct contact between humans and other organisms. Early identification and intervention are the most effective approach for interrupting the transmission of infection (Gopatoti & Vijayalakshmi, 2022). The COVID-19 pandemic has overwhelmed several nations' healthcare systems. A viral disease known for its single stranded RNA genomes; the rapid spread of SARS-CoV2 is largely to blame for the current global health crisis. The virus was first discovered in Wuhan, China, in December 2019, and its rapid global spread is due to this (Yan et al., 2020). The virus eventually spread to countries worldwide, including Russia, Turkey, Brazil, France, and India. Coronaviruses are known to cause a diverse range of disorders, with "Middle East respiratory syndrome" (MERS-CoV) and "severe acute respiratory syndrome" (SARS- CoV) being two notable examples. A novel strain of coronavirus was discovered in 2019. The virus was subsequently renamed as SARS-CoV-2. The general population was oblivious of the virus's transmissibility to humans prior to the Commencement of the COVID-19 epidemic. Initial research has demonstrated that a substantial number of individuals diagnosed with COVID-19 experience milder symptoms; however, a small number may experience more severe or incapacitating symptoms (Narin et al., 2021). In March of 2020, the announcement of a pandemic was officially made by the World Health Organisation (WHO). A comprehensive global quarantine was implemented, which required the confinement of billions of individuals indoors.

Globally, chest X-rays often referred to as radiography are quite well-known as indispensable diagnostic tools for pneumonia. Clinically, chest radiography is a fast, reasonably priced, and often used modality for imaging. A chest X-ray exposes a patient to less radiation than other imaging techniques, including MRI and CT scan. Thus, accurate diagnosis calls for specialized knowledge and training in X-ray picture analysis. When comparing a chest X-ray to more advanced imaging modalities like CT or MRI, the diagnostic value is much diminished (Narin et al., 2021).

Highly qualified healthcare professionals use chest radiography. Compared to general practitioners, the number of experts qualified to carry out this diagnosis is rather low. Many countries still lack medical experts to sufficiently service their populations, even under ideal conditions. With a doctor-to-population ratio of 607 doctors per 100,000 people, Greece ranked 1 in the world according to 2017 data. Other countries, on the other hand, have significantly lower statistics. Crises like the COVID-19 epidemic, which call for the simultaneous supply of healthcare services, have the potential to cause the health system to collapse from a lack of hospital beds and medical experts. Moreover, medical professionals including doctors, nurses, and care givers have a higher vulnerability to picking up the quite contagious COVID-19 virus. Early detection of pneumonia allows one to apply patient isolation strategies, accelerating their recovery and preventing wider epidemic transmission. The integration of computer-assisted diagnosis (CAD), particularly in chest X-ray technologies, has significantly enhanced the precision and efficacy of pneumonia diagnosis in medical settings. AI approaches are increasingly used in the medical services sector because they have the potential to manage far larger datasets than human capacity. While simultaneously increasing dependability and quantitative analytic capacities, the application of computer-aided design (CAD) techniques in radiologist diagnostic systems has greatly reduced doctors' workload. Computer-aided design (CAD) systems using deep learning methods and computer-aided medical imaging constitute emerging fields of academic study (Roopashree & Anitha, 2021).

Academic researchers have employed X-ray imaging techniques to devise various approaches for subject identification in the context of the COVID-19 disease inquiry (Gupta et al., 2024). By using the capabilities of machine learning, deep learning, and computer vision technologies, and other methodologies, the field of intelligent healthcare can effectively facilitate the identification and diagnosis of diverse diseases (Khan et al., 2020). The utilisation of deep learning is of great significance across various domains, particularly in the precise detection and classification of skin lesions, the partitioning of the heart and prostate, and the suppression of bone structures in coronary CT scans. The main aim of this research is to demonstrate the effectiveness of a deep learning network in independently detecting COVID-19 in chest X-ray images. The current study utilises a total of nine pretrained transfer learning models to achieve the intended objective. An advantage of employing pretrained transfer learning models lies in their ability to facilitate expedited training processes and enhance performance on tasks characterised by restricted data availability. By leveraging knowledge from large datasets on which the model was initially trained, these models can generalize better and require fewer labeled examples to achieve high accuracy, especially in complex tasks like image classification (Meenai & Khan, 2020).

Deep learning has emerged as a prominent methodology in recent years for developing networks that can replicate complex systems and achieve performance levels comparable to humans. Fatima A. & Associates (2020) offers a deep learning solution for the accurate detection of COVID-19 in chest X-ray images. The objective is to develop a new object detection system that is trained and assessed using a publicly available dataset consisting of 1500 photos of healthy individuals and those afflicted with COVID-19 and pneumonia. In their study, Mangal et al. (2020) proposed the utilisation of modern AI techniques to automatically detect COVID-19 cases by analysing X-ray medical pictures. This strategy is especially useful in cases when radiologists are not accessible since it seeks to increase the scalability of the suggested testing method. This work presents CovidAID, a novel method based on deep neural networks that ranks patients effectively depending on the necessity of specific tests. Using various powerful pre-trained convolutional neural networks, in their study, Makris et al. (2020) assessed their capacity to accurately identify individuals with illness based on CXR images. Using publicly accessible X-ray images of people who have been diagnosed with confirmed cases of COVID-19, a comprehensive dataset was created, individuals with cases of common bacterial pneumonia, and individuals who have not been impacted by the disease. They used transfer learning, a method that helps knowledge from past taught models to be transferred to the model under training, to get over the limited sample size. Emtiaz Hussain et al.'s (2021) original convolutional neural network (CNN) model CoroDet is provided in this work with an aim of automatically detecting Covid-19. This model exclusively utilises raw CT and chest X-ray images. The purpose of CoroDet is to establish a reliable diagnostic instrument that encompasses many classifications.

The study conducted by Ismael et al. (2021) utilised deep learning methodologies to distinguish between persons who had been confirmed to have COVID-19 versus those who were in a state of adequate medical health, as evidenced by CXR images. Several techniques were employed, including end-to-end convolutional neural network training, feature extraction, and CNN microtuning. In the current study, pre-trained iterations of deep convolutional neural networks, were utilised to acquire deep features. Rahman et al. (2021) investigate an old U-Net model against a brand new one when it came time to partition the lungs. This work evaluated the performance of a shallow CNN model comprising six pre-trained CNNs using normal and segmented lung CXR images: ResNet18, ResNet50, ResNet101, InceptionV3, DenseNet 201, and ChexNet. Narin et al. (2021) study comprises three binary categories that can be categorised into four unique groups. The authors achieved this by employing the five-fold cross-validation method. Daniel and colleagues (2021) Pulmonary segmentation is a crucial element of the preprocessing phase in the proposed approach. At this stage, eliminate areas unrelated to the present work and might produce biassed results. The categorisation model then undergoes transfer learning training. The study conducted by Pedro R. et al. (2021) employed image classifiers utilising Dense Convolutional Networks and techniques for transfer learning. The primary aim of this study was to classify chest X-ray pictures into three unique categories. Following training on the ImageNet dataset, the neural networks underwent a fine-tuning phase. The National Institutes of Health dataset was employed in conjunction with a twice transfer learning methodology. Das et al. (2021) developed a method for the automatic identification of COVID-19 positive individuals using chest X-rays. The suggested methodology employs a Deep Convolutional Neural Network as its basis. The present investigation employed the DenseNet 201, ResNet 50V2, and InceptionV3 convolutional neural network models.

The reference Tarun A., et al. (2022) is cited in this document. In the event of a collapse in the medical infrastructure, through the application of AI, it may be possible to identify COVID-19 with little human intervention. In order to identify COVID- 19 from chest imaging, this study aims to present a new architecture. The system's architecture is founded on deep CNNs. Anandbabu Gopatoti et al. (2021) collaborated with other individuals, as documented in their publication. The objective of this study is to employ semantic segmentation networks for the precise identification and classification of lung lobes in CXR images. Gupta et al. (2022) intend to create an artificial intelligence (AI) system capable of accurately classifying chest X-rays into three categories: healthy, virus-infected, or COVID-19 positive. The researchers employed four pretrained DNNs to evaluate the most appropriate model for the specific domain, given the small sample size of the Chest X-ray database for COVID-19 positive patients. The study was conducted by Mousavi and their collaborators. A specialised structure, the CNN- LSTM model is built to hierarchically extract properties from raw input information. The suggested methodology entails the integration of white Gaussian noise into raw CXR images to improve their realism and practicality. Furthermore, in conjunction with the six aforementioned databases, the suggested network undergoes testing and evaluation utilising two supplementary datasets (Mousavi et al., 2022). In their article, Bhattacharyya et al. (2022) propose a new method for diagnosing pneumonia and COVID-19 by applying a C-GAN for splitting unprocessed X-ray pictures is the first stage in the process of obtaining lung images. In the second stage, a specialised pipeline is used for obtaining distinctive characteristics from the segmented lung images. The aim is reached by using DNN and applying important point extracting methods. The penultimate phase is classifying COVID-19, pneumonia, and normal lung tissue in images using many ML models. The investigation carried out by Huang et al. (2022) the aim of the present study was to enhance the effectiveness of seven convolutional neural networks for COVID-19 identification.

Ayalew et al. (2023) establish a robust approach for categorizing chest X-ray pictures into two distinct groups: those showing symptoms of COVID-19 infection and those displaying normal anatomical traits. The model is developed using Convolutional Neural Networks in concert with activation functions, dropout filtering, batch normalisation, and Keras parameters. Using widely available open-source software technologies, Python and OpenCV, were developed the classification technique. George et al. (2023) the study's authors, the current work presents a fresh method based on CXR imaging for the COVID-19 detection. The technique investigates the pixel data inside images using a homomorphic transformation filter and Contrast Limited Adaptive Histogram Equalisation (CLAHE) to derive features from the CXRs by means of relevance. Alaa S. et al (2023) wrote the paper Using a hybrid deep learning architecture, the objective of the COVID-CheXNet system is to improve the diagnostic capacity of chest X-ray pictures. Redie et al. (2023) conducted research. This work aims mostly to create a mathematical model using chest X-ray data that can independently identify COVID-19 events. This objective was accomplished by implementing necessary modifications to the DarkCovidNet model, which employed a CNN. The research conducted by Kumar et al. (2023) sought to develop an ensemble model for the detection of early signs of COVID-19 infection through the processing of chest X-ray images. The suggested approach employs ensemble learning techniques by combining various transfer learning models.

A hybrid deep learning model, COVIDet, was created by Gupta et al. (2022). This methodology integrates the capabilities of CNN with the efficacy of the SURF extraction technique to attain expedited and more dependable feature extraction. The model examines chest x-ray pictures to diagnose COVID-19. A research team, directed by K. Srinivas et al. (2024), performed a study on the effects of COVID-19, researchers have created a novel composite model, termed "Inception V3 with VGG16," that employs data from chest X-ray imaging to forecast the development of COVID-19. This study presents a publicly accessible and user-friendly modelling system for the precise detection of chest infections by radiographic imaging techniques, as noted by Singh et al.(2024). The present study employs a deep convolutional neural network architecture founded on ResNet50. The proposed methodology effectively provides current information on the health status of persons affected by COVID-19, demonstrating a high degree of accuracy in detecting coronavirus infections through the analysis of CT scan images. Talukder et al. (2024) investigated the notion of empowerment in their study. This project seeks to evaluate the viability of employing deep learning algorithms alongside radiographic imaging for the swift and precise diagnosis of COVID-19 patients.

Deep learning techniques are increasingly employed to detect and categorise COVID-19 from chest X-rays. These methods are very important in the fight against the outbreak. Experts have made big steps forward in improving the accuracy and usefulness of COVID-19 diagnosis by using a mix of CNNs, transfer learning methods, and ensemble models. New studies have shown that pre- trained models, new architectures, and hybrid approaches can accurately distinguish between COVID-19, other pulmonary disorders such as pneumonia, and a healthy state. In addition to giving doctors and nurses useful new tools, these changes also make diagnostic solutions easier to use in places with limited resources.

Research Gap

Despite the significant potential of deep learning models to identify COVID-19 from chest X-ray images, there still exists a critical gap in the existing literature. Many research nowadays mostly focus on reaching great accuracy with pre-trained models such DenseNet, VGG, and ResNet. However, there is a particular focus on issues like data bias, interpretability, and their practical applications. Furthermore, there are few studies comparing the effectiveness of these deep learning models with traditional diagnostic techniques and a comprehensive comparison can reveal how deep learning enhances the effectiveness of standard diagnostics, as well as the potential drawbacks that may accompany it. Thirdly, while many studies focus on binary classification, there is a lack of interest in multi-class classification and the recognition of other respiratory diseases (for example, bacterial pneumonia). Ultimately, the quality and accessibility of data remain significant obstacles, as many models are developed using relatively limited or imbalanced datasets. Addressing these shortcomings by introducing larger and more diverse datasets, exploring alternative architectures, and integrating explainability and bias mitigation techniques is crucial for this field.

Classification of the Coronavirus

There are four separate subgroups of coronaviruses, which are members of the family Coronaviridae. Coronaviruses come in four different types: namely Delta Coronavirus (δ-CoV), gamma Coronavirus (γ-CoV), beta Coronavirus (β-CoV), and alpha Coronavirus (α-CoV) (Srinivas et al., 2024). Figure 1 offers a detailed depiction of the different subgroups within the Coronaviridae family. Individuals of both human and animal species are vulnerable to the human coronavirus, which is alternatively referred to as the alpha coronavirus (Korneenko et al., 2024). This viral pathogen is classified as a positive sense one stranded RNA virus. Children exhibit a higher vulnerability to respiratory infections that impact the upper and lower respiratory tract (ARST) in comparison to adults, with a high frequency of association observed between these illnesses and the alpha coronavirus. The primary etiology of gastrointestinal and respiratory ailments in humans and most other animal species is the beta coronavirus (Dai et al., 2020).

The prevailing consensus suggests that mice and bats serve as the principal natural reservoirs for the beta coronavirus. Figure 2 depicts the transmission method of SARS-CoV-2, a newly identified virus capable of infecting humans, exclusively through bats. The presence of saliva or exhalation facilitates the process of viral transmission. Unfortunately, the present prevalence of severe symptoms among infected patients stands at a mere 5 percent. According to reports, the survival rate among them stands around 95%. In the event of a deterioration in the infection, it might lead to enduring angina, impaired organ function, respiratory distress, and in severe cases, mortality. The virus strains "BtCoV-HKU4", "BtCoV-HKU5", and "BtCoV-HKU9" are often known as" bat coronaviruses" among those residing in Hong Kong (Hu et al., 2015). Delta coronaviruses, which are known to infect particular animal species and avian species, are hypothesised to have evolved from genes derived from livestock (Guo et al., 2024), (Wang et al., 2014). In contrast, it has been postulated that gamma coronaviruses originate from avian diseases that predominantly infect birds (Testa et al., 2024). Table 1 presents a synopsis of each coronavirus subgroup, detailing their characteristics, major reservoirs, and modes of transmission.

Figure 1. Categories of coronavirus

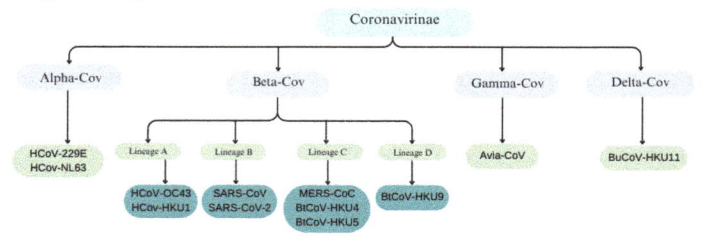

Figure 2. Transmission modalities of SARS-CoV-2

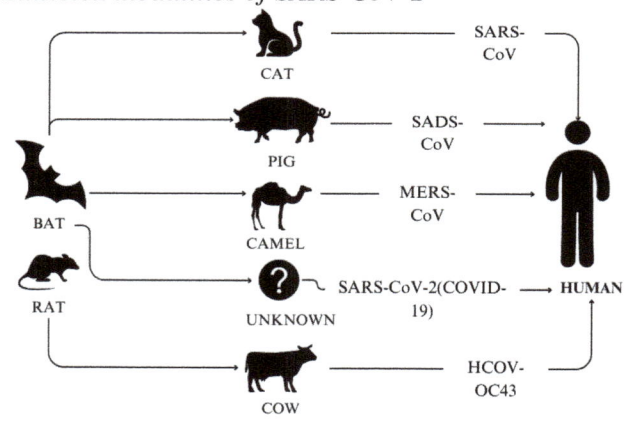

Table 1. List of every coronavirus subgroup together with their unique traits, main animal reservoirs, and known human and other species transmission routes.

Coronavirus Type	Subgroup	Characteristics	Primary Reservoirs	Transmission
Delta Coronavirus	δ-CoV	Infects specific animal and avian species	Hypothesized to have evolved from genes derived from livestock	Saliva or exhalation
Gamma Coronavirus	γ-CoV	Originates from avian diseases, primarily infects birds	Birds	Saliva or exhalation
Beta Coronavirus	β-CoV	Causes gastrointestinal and respiratory ailments in humans and animals	Mice and bats	Saliva or exhalation
Alpha Coronavirus	α-CoV	Known as human coronavirus; affects upper and lower respiratory tract	Humans	Saliva or exhalation

Diagnoses for COVID-19 Types

The primary diagnostic approaches for COVID-19 encompass conventional techniques and AI-based deep learning methodologies. Figure 3 is a visual representation that provides a concise overview of the information pertaining to the COVID-19 epidemic.

Traditional Approach

- Genetic analysis via RT-PCR: Experts believe that RT-PCR, is the most effective way to identify coronaviruses (Wang et al., 2020). The method's capacity to accurately discover and identify a virus is demonstrated even in the early stages of infection. This test is primarily designed to determine the current level of infection in the individual with the detected virus.
- Serological testing for antibody detection: As part of the COVID-19 investigative process, human serum, plasma, or blood samples can be used for qualitative testing to detect IgG and/or IgM antibodies (Spicuzza et al., 2020). This test can detect prior infection history and provide valuable insights into the patient's immunological response to the illness.
- Antigen-based testing: The aforementioned technique is comparable to RT-PCR, a diagnostic tool for detecting coronavirus infections that uses nasal probes to collect samples. This specific test shows better time and cost reductions than other tests when considering alternative ones.

- CT scan: CT scans are a crucial diagnostic tool and are very important for the detection of COVID-19. We provide detailed images of the lungs, identify abnormalities, and assess the severity of the issues. CT scans consume a lot of resources, expose patients to radiation, and require interpretation by specialized staff, making them unsuitable for routine screening.
- Chest X-Ray: A chest X-ray is a straightforward and cost-effective technique for diagnosing COVID-19 by identifying lung abnormalities. CT scans are highly effective for tracking illness development, but due to insufficient detail, it can become difficult to identify early infections and to distinguish COVID-19 from other respiratory illnesses.

Figure 3: Traditional Covid-19 Testing Methods.

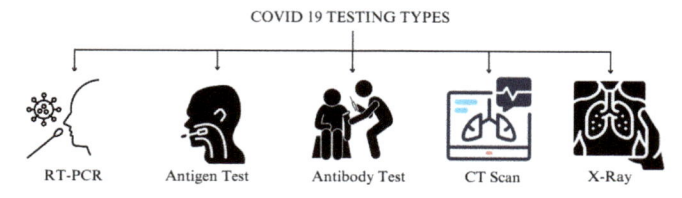

AI Based Deep learning Approach

A complex computational framework that employs artificial intelligence to identify patterns and features from immense datasets is referred to as artificial intelligence-driven deep learning technology. Explicit medical diagnosis, specifically the identification of COVID-19 by CXR and CT scans, is particularly relevant to this. Visual features are analysed using deep learning techniques, predominantly CNNs.

Comparison Between Traditional and AI based Approach

Table 2 presents a comparison between AI-driven deep learning methodologies for COVID-19 detection with traditional techniques.

Table 2. Comparison between Traditional and AI based approach.

Aspects	Traditional Approach	AI based Approach
Speed	Generally slower, requiring manual interpretation and lab processing.	Fast, especially for image-based detection once trained.
Accuracy	Typically, accurate but dependent on the method used and sample quality.	High accuracy with large datasets, but dependent on quality of data.
Cost	Varies depending on method, often higher due to operational and equipment costs.	Lower cost after deployment; initial setup can be expensive.
Resource requirement	Requires specialized equipment and trained personnel for accurate results.	Requires advanced computational resources for training and deployment.
Scalability	Limited scalability due to resource and personnel constraints.	Highly scalable for large-scale, automated screening.
Early Detection	Can be effective for early detection depending on the method.	Effectiveness depends on the availability of early-stage data.

Machine Learning in COVID-19: Case Studies and Predictive Insights

Machine learning's impact on COVID-19 diagnosis and prediction

The utilisation of machine learning has produced significant progress in the identification and management of Covid-19 in various essential areas. Machine learning algorithms, particularly deep learning models, have advanced the diagnostic sector by effectively analysing medical pictures, including CT scans and chest X-rays. Artificial intelligence (AI) models improve diagnostic accuracy by correctly identifying patterns and abnormalities associated with Covid-19 and often provide more accurate and fast results than more traditional methods. In addition, seeing small signs of infectious diseases that can be missed by people with X-ray experience, machine learning (ML) has greatly helped in early virus diagnosis.

Machine learning (ML) is an important component of predictive modeling, and it is possible to predict the development of disease in individual patients by analyzing data on common symptoms and diseases. This, on the contrary, facilitates the development of rapid intervention. Machine learning models can also predict future epidemics by examining patterns of infection rate. Machine learning algorithms are important in pharmaceutical research because they can predict the effectiveness of existing viral infections treatments. In addition, this algorithm helps to optimize the treatment approach to increase its effectiveness (Khan et al., 2024).

Case studies utilising Machine Learning for COVID-19

Numerous significant case studies illustrate the utilisation of machine learning for the identification and management of COVID-19. COVID-Net is an open-source deep learning model developed for the detection of COVID-19 through the analysis of chest X-ray images, employing a convolutional neural network architecture. This methodology categorizes X-ray images as indicative of COVID-19, pneumonia, or normal, achieving notable accuracy (Wang et al., 2020). DeepCOVID-XR is a notable initiative that has created a model designed to assist in the diagnosis of COVID-19 through the analysis of chest X-rays. This model demonstrates an accuracy exceeding 90% through the utilisation of a pre-trained convolutional neural network (CNN), underscoring the efficacy of deep learning in expedited diagnostic processes (Wehbe et al., 2021).

CoroDet is a convolutional neural network designed for the automated detection of COVID-19 in chest X-ray (CXR) and computed tomography (CT) images (Hussain et al., 2021). This model has undergone training utilising a comprehensive dataset that includes a variety of positive and negative instances. An autonomous research initiative focuses on utilising deep learning techniques to predict COVID-19 infections from CT images, employing the U-Net architecture for segmentation purposes. This method achieves high accuracy and demonstrates the capabilities of machine learning in the early detection and assessment of COVID-19 severity (Zheng et al., 2020).

METHODS AND MATERIAL

In the following section, a comprehensive description of the COVID-QU-Ex dataset and the pretrained model employed in this study will be provided.

Dataset overview

The COVID-QU-Ex dataset has made substantial contributions to research on chest X-ray (CXR) imaging (Tahir, 2022). It was carefully chosen by Qatar University scholars. As shown in Table 3, the collection comprised of 33,920 chest X-ray (CXR) photos that have been classified into three groups: The dataset includes 11,956 pictures of persons infected with COVID-19. In addition, there are 11,263 photos of people suffering from non-COVID ailments, such as viral or bacterial pneumonia. Finally, the collection contains 10,701 photos of people who are healthy. Figure 4 depicts a selection of image samples comprising the COVID-QU-Ex Dataset.

Figure 4. Sample images from the dataset with three labels covid-19, Healthy and non-covid infection.

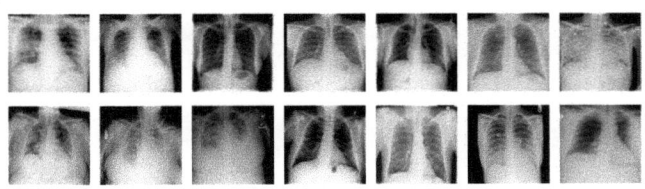

Table 3. Summary of Image Categories in the COVID-QU-Ex Dataset

Category	Number of Images
COVID-19 Infected	11,956
Non-COVID Infections (e.g., Viral or Bacterial Pneumonia)	11,263
Healthy Individuals	10,701
Total Images	33,920

Transfer Learning Models

This section allows one to thoroughly review the several transfer learning techniques applied in the research.

DenseNet201

Convolutional Neural Networks exhibit superior performance across a range of computer vision applications, such as image classification and object detection. With the help of this concept, our goal is ultimately to eliminate the vanishing gradient. In DenseNet architecture, each layer passes its features to the next layer, integrating information from the previous layer (Muhammad & Alrikabi, 2024). Every level has a close association with the next level. As a result, the concept of characteristic reuse is achieved when a strong link is formed between the various levels, hence decreasing the overall number of network parameters. The DenseNet design consists of many dense blocks and transition blocks interspersed between two extremely dense blocks. Every level takes all of the previous characteristic maps as input. Figure 5 depicts the DenseNet-201 structural representation.

Figure 5. Layer Architecture of DenseNet201.

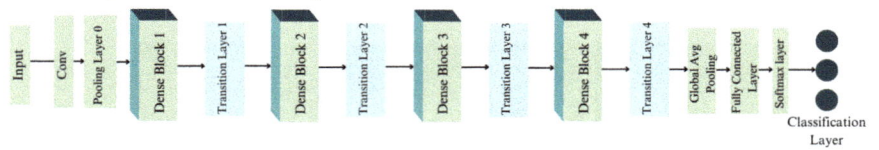

DenseNet121

DenseNet121 is characterized by a variety of modifications and unique architectural components that enhance identification and visual analysis. DenseNet121 starts with a solid foundation of functions collected by pre-trained models extracted from huge datasets like ImageNet and then applies a transfer learning mechanism. DenseNet 121 architectural design consists of dense blocks containing each level that is precisely connected to the next level of the block (Khan & Meenai, 2021). This phenomenon creates a complex network of links that send the output to the next level after each level has received input from the previous level. Wide network connection actively encourages efficient transfer and reuse of functions, significantly improving the network's ability to learn and extract relevant functions from input. Transition layer play an important role in managing network complexity by filling the gaps between the packaged segments. The architectural design of Densenet121 is presented in figure 6.

Figure 6. Densenet121 structural Design.

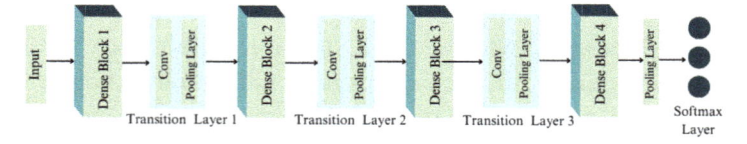

Xception

Xception is an enhanced iteration of the Inception model specifically developed to maximize the effectiveness and energy efficiency of deep learning tasks. The Xception uses depthwise separable convolutions that is better than the normal convolutions used in previous versions, which distinguishes it from the earlier iterations of the Inception model. The ultimate achievement of Xception design is its depthwise separable convolutions that effectively divides the convolution process into two different levels. At the depthwise convolution level, for each input channel, a convolutional filter is implemented, and a pointwise convolution (1 x 1 convolution) is used to spread the filtered output across several channels.

In addition, before applying the special convolutions layer, the 1x1 layer in the Xception architecture is employed for the extraction of the function. The special combination layer of Xception, unlike previous Inception models, offers a combination of 3x3 size and depthwise separable that enhances learning and functional expression (Gupta et al., 2024). Figure 7 shows the structural design of Xception model.

Figure 7. The architectural design of Xception Model.

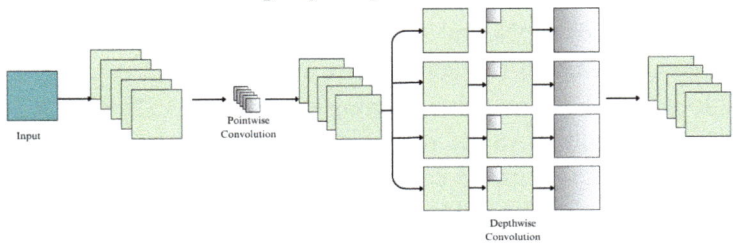

EfficientNet B7

The artificial intelligence team at Google developed EffcientNet B7, a novel deep neural network design by Mingxing Tan and Quoc V. in 2019. This model is meant to be a component of the EfficientNet family to lower the number of parameters and processing resources needed while nevertheless improving accuracy in image classification tasks. In many different computer vision applications, including object detection, semantic segmentation, picture recognition, and others, this method has constantly shown amazing performance. EfficientNet B7's effectiveness may result from its original compound scaling technique, which balances depth, width, and resolution to improve network performance (Sathishkumar et al., 2023). Figure 8 depicts the graphical visual depiction of the EfficientNet B7 model architecture.

Figure 8. The model architecture of EfficientNet B7.

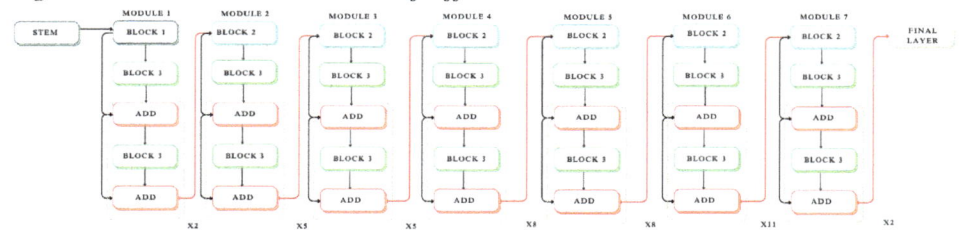

NASNetLarge

NASNet Large stands for Neural Architecture Search Network Large, is a deep learning architecture created by Google that utilizes Neural Architecture search (Nas) technology, which is a machine learning approach. NASNet Large is the most complete iteration of the NASNet model, specifically developed to exceptional performance in the field of image category. The present model consists of iterative components found using the NAS methodology, which finds its ideal neural network structure. NASNet Large models are known for their incredible accuracy and efficiency, consistently surpassing traditional architectures designed by hand in test datasets such as ImageNet (Saber et al., 2024). The NASNetlarge model configuration is shown in Figure 9.

Figure 9. The NASNetlarge Model architecture.

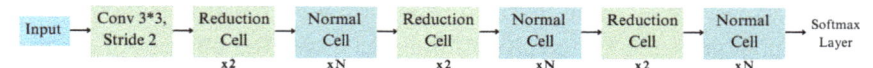

InceptionResNetV2

The InceptionResNetV2 model represents a deep CNN developed by Christian Segedi et al. in 2016. The present methodology combines the functionalities of the Inception architecture with residual connections. It belongs to the Inception family of models, known for its competence in managing wide ranging image recognition needs (Demir & Yilmaz, 2020). InceptionResNetV2 is an extension of the inception architecture, which includes several inception modules and allows models to obtain data of different sizes through the integration of residual connections. These interconnections facilitate the formation of more complex networks, mitigating the problem of lost gradients, thus ensuring smooth transmission of information and gradient throughout the network. InceptionResNetV2's main goals are high degree of accuracy achieved concurrently with optimization of processing efficiency. The model architecture of InceptionResNetV2 is presented in Figure 10.

Figure 10. The architectural framework of InceptionResNetV2.

VGG19

The VGG19 model is an adapted iteration of the VGG architecture, consisting of nineteen distinct layers. The architectural structure of the model consists of sixteen convolutional layers, five Maxpool layers, three fully linked layers, and one Softmax layer. The cumulative count of levels amounts to 19. The VGG model has demonstrated remarkable efficacy as a robust substitute for the AlexNet model. The VGG Convolutional Neural Network consists of six primary components, namely the fully connected layers and many interconnected convolutional layers. The mean number of layers ranged from sixteen to nineteen. The VGG19 method employs an alternating pattern between activation layers and convolutional layers. The model utilises Max pooling layers for the purpose of feature extraction, employed in conjunction with the ReLU activation function (Meenai & Khan, 2020). Figure 11 shows the visual representation of VGG19 model architecture.

Figure 11. Layer architecture of VGG19.

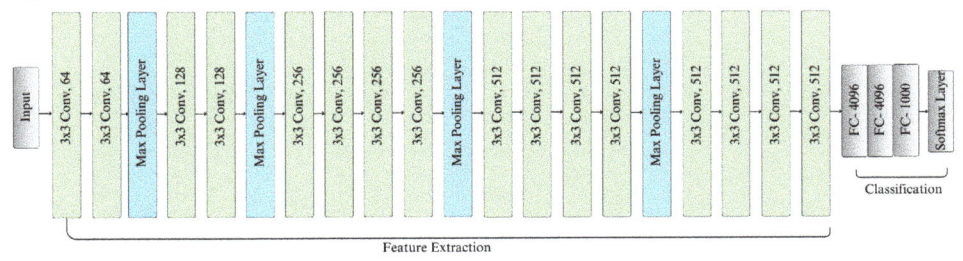

VGG16

The VGG16 neural network was originally built under the direction of the Visual Geography Group (VGG) at the University of Oxford. The 16 layers that comprise this network have parameters that can be learned. Thirteen convolutional layers perform the real classification job, with three more fully linked layers added at the end. One of the notable features of the VGG16 is its sequential architecture, each convolutional layer uses the same 3*3 filter size with step 1 value. This sequence enables the network to accurately capture intricate elements within the image. Following each convolutional layer, a maximum pooling layer is utilised to reduce the dimensionality of the feature map. Thus, diminishing the computational burden and the quantity of parameters. A fully connected layer in the end integrates features from the convolutional layer and does the final classification (Simonyan & Zisserman, 2015). Figure 12 illustrates the architectural configuration of the VGG16 model.

ResNet101

ResNet101, also known as Residual Network with 101 Layers, is an architectural project for convolutional neural networks that aims to solve the difficulties involved in building networks of significant depth. Instead of the ResNet architecture, K. He et al. (2016) introduced the 2015 ResNet101 model. The idea of residual learning is integrated, that is, the formation of short circuit connections that occupy one or more levels and allow a gradient to spread directly across the network. The present architectural design effectively addresses the prevalent issue of vanishing gradient in deep networks, therefore facilitating the effective training of networks comprising several hundred layers. With the 101 levels of ResNet101 architecture, it balances depth with processing efficiency. In a more basic model, this approach maximizes accuracy by minimizing calculation costs. The ResNet101 model configuration is shown in Figure 13.

Figure 12. Layered Configuration of VGG16 model.

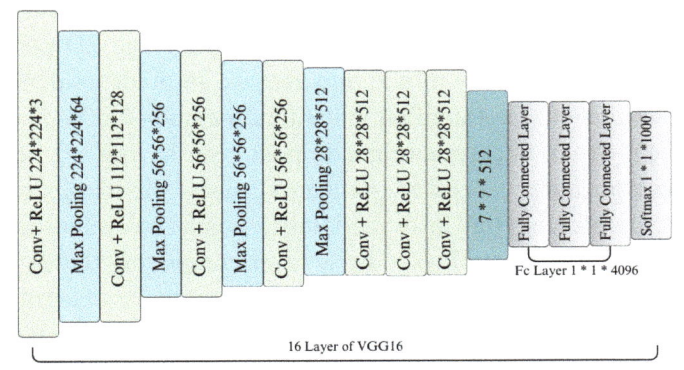

Figure 13. Architectural design of ResNet101.

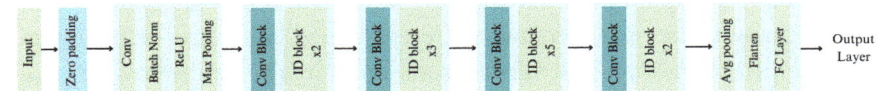

EXPERIMENTS

The methods used for preprocessing and training, as well as the transfer learning models studied, are described below.

Proposed Methodology

The initial step involves preparing CXR images from the COVID-QU-Ex dataset using the preprocessing module of the keras library package. Presented in Table 3, the dataset is categorized into three distinct tags: Covid-19, Healthy, and Non-Covid Infection. This experiment employs nine pre-trained transfer learning models for multi-class categorization: DenseNet201, DenseNET121, Xception, EfficientNetB7, NASNetLarge, InceptionResNetV2, VGG19, VGG16 and ResNet101. In the classification work, the target labels are as follows: zero for Covid-19, one for healthy and two for non-Covid infection and pre-trained models of our study process inputs of 224*224 pixels and three-color channels. These models skip the first few layers of their architecture to assemble the characteristics. After the extraction procedure is completed, the characteristics maps lose their spatial dimensions. However, important properties remain unchanged when using average 2D pooling. These combined feature maps are then turned into vectors. In order to identify intricate models for classification, the Rectified linear unit method (ReLU) is employed to activate a dense layer. By incorporating a dropout layer having a 0.1 dropout rate, the model's generalization capability is enhanced while the likelihood of overlap is reduced. During training, this layer randomly assigns zero values to some input units. The proposed model employs a dense layer comprising three units and implements a Softmax activation function to facilitate multiclass classification. The above configuration produces multiple targets: class Covid19 is represented by value 0, class Healthy value 1 and class non-Covid infection value 2. The model's layer structure is illustrated in diagram 14.

We utilized the ImageDataGenerator module from Keras to implement many picture augmentation methods in order to enhance the variety and length of our learning data. Employing these tactics is essential for enhancing the overall efficacy of machine learning models, particularly in medical imaging applications. The study used many tactics to reproduce different image collection sizes, including random magnification of photos, vertical rotation of images to improve orientation diversity, and horizontal image movement to better represent more points of view and perspectives. In addition, the model was able to deal effectively with the various distortions that are commonly found in the real medical picture by introducing image distortion through cutting transformations. The diversity of the data set has been expanded with the addition of mirror and inverted photos to the training set through horizontal and vertical turns respectively. The changes described above have given priority to consistency, ensuring that new pixels are always formed using the" nearest" filling mode. The parameter settings and descriptions of the augmentation techniques used can be found in Table 4.

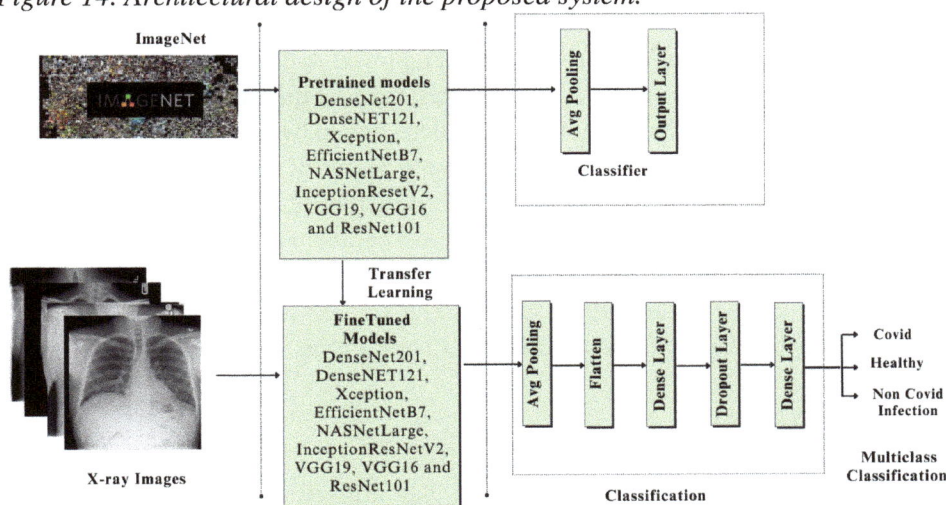

Figure 14. Architectural design of the proposed system.

Table 4: Provide augmentation technique, parameter values, and description.

Augmentation Technique	Parameter Value	Description
Rotation Range	±20 degrees	Perform image rotation within a range of ±20 degrees.
Zoom Range	0.15	Perform random zooming on photos up to 15%.
Width Shift Range	0.20	Vertically reposition photos by up to 20%.
Height Shift Range	0.20	Move the photos vertically by a maximum of 20%.
Shear Range	0.15	Up to 15% shear changes can be applied.
Horizontal Flip	True	Invert the photos horizontally.
Vertical Flip	True	Invert the photos vertically.
Fill Mode	Nearest	Fill recently generated pixels with their closest neighbours.

The X-ray images of the chest are trained and customised using multiclass classification tasks that include COVID-19, healthy, and non-COVID infection conditions. To behave well during training, a number of critical prerequisites must be fulfilled. Pre-prepared models using information from datasets such as ImageNet have shown that they improve task performance and accelerate the convergence process. The selection of image size significantly impacts the efficiency and accuracy of characterization. Model learning cannot work without the use of softmax or ReLU activation functions, which generate nonlinearity. The learning rate is a crucial determinant that directly influences the speed and sequence of the model's convergence. This, in turn, affects the step size in the gradient descent process. The appropriate number of epochs, or iterations, employed to process the learning data set determines the iterative approach for enhancing the quality of the model. The amount of data processed in each iteration is determined by the batch sizes selected during the training, ensuring a balance between memory efficiency and resource use. Optimisers improve training speed and convergence efficiency by adjusting model weights based on gradient data. The hyperparameters have been thoroughly examined to guarantee that the model is appropriate for a variety of classification situations and achieves maximum accuracy. The Table 5 summarizes the hyperparameter values for the 9 models used in this investigation.

Training Strategy

The training set comprises the subset of data utilised for model training. This study employed a dataset comprising 21,715 X-ray images sourced from the COVID-QU-Ex collection, which is available through the Kaggle repository, to facilitate the training process. The validation set comprises 5,417 photos utilised for fine-tuning the model's hyperparameters and evaluating its performance during the training phase. The test set consisted of 6788 X-ray pictures and was used to accurately identify instances of overfitting or underfitting in the model. All proposed transfer learning models resize the input image to 224 by 224 pixels, considering the learning and storage time. All hyperparameters in Table 5 are trained using an optimizer based on the stochastic descent gradient known as ADAM (Adaptive moment estimation). The loss metric employed in this study is softmax cross-entropy with logits, which quantifies the performance of the classification model. The probability assigned to each of the three labels, namely Covid-19, healthy, and non-Covid infection, ranges from 0 to 1.

Table 5: Hyperparameter values for all the proposed pretrained models.

Proposed Models	Hyperparameters
DenseNet201	Image Scale: 224x224 pixels, Activation Function: ReLU, Stepsize: 0.001, Epochs: 50, Batch Volume: 4, Optimizer: Adam
DenseNet121	Image Scale: 224x224 pixels, Activation Function: ReLU, Stepsize: 0.001, Epochs: 50, Batch Volume: 8, Optimizer: Adam
Xception	Image Scale: 224x224 pixels, Activation Function: ReLU, Stepsize: 0.001, Epochs: 50, Batch Volume: 4, Optimizer: Adam
EfficientNetB7	Image Scale: 224x224 pixels, Activation Function: ReLU, Stepsize: 0.001, Epochs: 50, Batch Volume: 16, Optimizer: Adam

continued on following page

Table 5: Hyperparameter values for all the proposed pretrained models. Continued

Proposed Models	Hyperparameters
NATNesLarge	Image Scale: 224x224 pixels, Activation Function: ReLU, Stepsize: 0.001, Epochs: 50, Batch Volume: 16, Optimizer: Adam
InceptionResNetV2	Image Scale: 224x224 pixels, Activation Function: ReLU, Stepsize: 0.001, Epochs: 50, Batch Volume: 16, Optimizer: Adam
VGG19	Image Scale: 224x224 pixels, Activation Function: ReLU, Stepsize: 0.001, Epochs: 50, Batch Volume: 16, Optimizer: Adam
VGG16	Image Scale: 224x224 pixels, Activation Function: ReLU, Stepsize: 0.001, Epochs: 50, Batch Volume: 16, Optimizer: Adam
ResNet101	Image Scale: 224x224 pixels, Activation Function: ReLU, Stepsize: 0.001, Epochs: 50, Batch Volume: 16, Optimizer: Adam

Testing Strategy

As described in training strategy our proposed study uses 6788 X-ray images taken from the COVID-QU-Ex data set. Upon completion of the training and validation phases, the test dataset was employed to assess the model's final performance. The model does not learn from the test set; it is only exposed to this data once training is completed. The performance parameters derived from the test set are utilised to evaluate the model's capacity to generalise predictions. Prior to conducting the tests, all of the photos were downsized to dimensions of 224*224 pixels. All the suggested transfer learning pretrained models are tested for Covid-19 classification with three target labels: class Covid19 is represented by value 0, class Healthy value 1 and class non-Covid infection value 2.

Performance Metrics

The present work investigates the efficacy of nine pre-trained transfer learning models: DenseNet201, DenseNet121, Xception, EfficientNetB7, NASNetLarge, InceptionResNetV2, VGG19, VGG16, and ResNet101. The experimental evaluation was conducted using four widely recognised classification metrics: accuracy, precision, recall, and F1- score. The measurements True positive and True negative were represented by tP and tN, respectively, and the performance measures False positive and False negative by fP and fN. Four widely recognised classification criteria are employed to evaluate the efficacy of all the pretrained networks recommended in this study. The accuracy measure is the ratio of accurate predictions provided by the model across three separate categories, namely COVID-19, Healthy, and Non-COVID Infection, relative to the overall count of predictions generated. This metric can be evaluated via the equation provided below:

$$Accuracy = (tP + tN)/(tP + tN + fP + fN)$$

To find the precision, take the number of positive examples and divide it by the proportion of accurately predicted instances of the targeted class. The following equation can be used to quantify this metric:

$$Precision = tP/(tP + fP)$$

In machine learning, recall is defined as the ratio of successfully predicted positive examples (tP) to the total number of instances in a class (tP + fN). The equation below can be used to evaluate this performance metric.

$$Recall = tP/(tP + fN)$$

One quantitative metric that finds the harmonic mean of recall and precision metrics is the F1-score. This metric may be determined via the subsequent equation:

$$F1\ Score = 2*(Precision*Recall)/(Precision + Recall)$$

RESULT and ANALYSIS

All suggested models including DenseNet201, DenseNET121, Xception, EfficientNetB7, NASNetLarge, InceptionResNetV2, VGG19, VGG16 and ResNet101 have been trained using transfer learning approach. The Training dataset that consists of 3 class labels namely COVID-19, Healthy, and Non-COVID Infection contains wide range of preprocessed CXR images taken from COVID-QU-Ex dataset. The model under goes training for a total of 50 epochs using the Adam optimiser, specifically utilising the Adaptive Moment Estimation variant. The recommended learning rate has been determined to be 0.001. Model validation is performed at the conclusion of each period to verify consistency in performance. The optimum model is selected by observing which one has the least amount of validation loss throughout the training phase.

Analysis of the Proposed Model

The proposed research employs a transfer learning approach for classification, with hyperparameters presented in Table 5. We investigated nine pretrained models on a COVID-QU-Ex dataset in order to classify COVID-19. Visual analysis of the performance indicators is displayed in Figure 15. The DenseNet121 received the highest accuracy of 95.22% among all the tested models. However, it expresses slightly less accuracy and feedback compared to DenseNet201. DenseNet201 demonstrated an exceptional accuracy of 94.56% and a significant F1 score of 94.01%. The Xception model has an accuracy of 91.23% and excellent precision, which is satisfactory. Studies conducted on EfficientNetB7 show that it has the lowest overall accuracy rate of 87.67% and lowest F1 score 87.62%. The NATNesLarge model received a well-deserved F1 rating of 92.67%, demonstrating excellent accuracy and responsiveness. The InceptionResNetV2 shows satisfactory performance with an accuracy of 89.09% and a balanced F1 score of 89.12%. Both models VGG16 and VGG19 showed satisfactory performance: the VGG16, which received the highest score in F1, was 93.61%, and the VGG19. ResNet101, on the other hand, shows uneven performance, with a F1 score of 71.33% and the lowest level of accuracy of 70.34%. Overall, DenseNet121 and Dense Net201 show the highest levels of accuracy and F1 rating, while ResNet101 has significantly lower performance than other models. A comparison of performance metrics between all the models of transfer learning that are displayed and other well-known models can be found in Table 6. The metrics include F1-score, recall, accuracy, and precision measurements.

Table 6. An analysis of performance measures comparing all the presented transfer learning models with other well recognized benchmark models.

Ref.	Input image	Model Employed	Accuracy	Precision	Recall	F1-score
(Wang et al., 2021)	CT scan	InceptionV3	89.50	-	67.00	79.30
(Fan et al., 2020)	CT scan	Semi-Inf-Net	-	-	72.50	73.90
(Gao et al., 2021)	CT scan	DCN	95.99	-	89.14	-
(Yan et al., 2021)	CT scan	COVID-SegNet	-	72.60	75.10	72.60
(Amyar et al., 2020)	CT scan	MTL Architecture	94.67	-	96.00	88.00
(Song et al., 2021)	CT scan	DRE-Net	86.00	79.00	96.00	87.00
(Khan et al., 2020)	CXR	CoroNet	89.60	90.00	89.92	89.80
(Wang et al., 2020)	CXR	COVID-Net	93.30	-	91.00	-
(Sethy et al., 2020)	CXR	ResNet50-SVM	95.33	-	95.33	95.34
Proposed work	CXR	DenseNet201	93.45	94.56	93.25	94.01
		DenseNet121	95.22	96.32	96.54	95.78
		Xception	91.23	92.34	91.63	90.33
		EfficientNetB7	87.67	88.90	87.22	87.62
		NATNesLarge	90.37	93.88	92.55	92.67
		InceptionResNetV2	89.09	90.44	89.43	89.12
		VGG19	93.03	92.63	91.54	91.78
		VGG16	93.55	94.72	93.77	93.61
		ResNet101	70.34	76.67	70.87	71.33

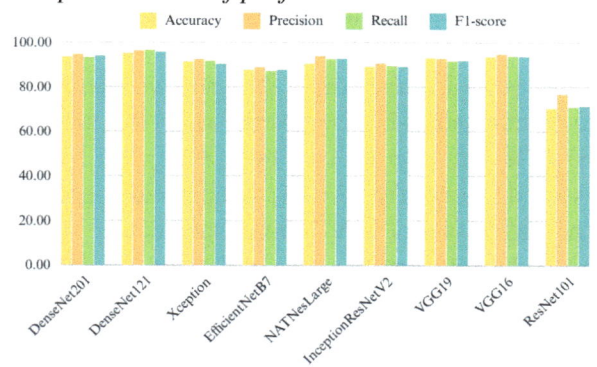

Figure 15. Visual representation of performance metrics.

CONCLUSION

This study investigated the classification of X-ray pictures taken from the COVID QU-Ex dataset into three distinct categories: COVID-19, Healthy, and Non-COVID Infection. The classification was performed using pre-trained transfer learning models. Transfer learning was particularly advantageous, allowing the models to leverage the knowledge gained from large datasets like ImageNet, which improved their ability to accurately diagnose conditions from chest X-rays. By fine-tuning these models for the specific task, the objective of the study was to create a reliable method of diagnosis that could aid healthcare professionals in effectively managing the current pandemic. To enhance the models' performance, the research employed data augmentation techniques and carefully selected hyperparameters. Data augmentation expanded the training dataset by introducing variations in the images, helping the models to learn more generalized features, and reducing the risk of overfitting. As part of the fine-tuning procedure, factors such as learning rate and batch volume were modified to optimize the models for the unique features of the COVID-QU-Ex dataset. Throughout the training, validation sets were used to monitor the models' performance and verify that they preserved their capacity to generalize effectively to novel data.

The efficacy of the models was assessed by four primary measures: accuracy, precision, recall, and F1-score. These identifiers offered a thorough evaluation of the models' capacity to precisely categorise the X-ray photographic images. The findings of the investigation revealed that the pre-trained models exhibited extraordinary efficacy, with certain models attaining notably high levels of accuracy and precision in differentiating among the three categories. This underscores the capacity of transfer learning models in medical imaging, particularly in dynamic situations like as the COVID-19 epidemic, where precise and prompt detection is crucial.

REFERENCE

A. DEMİR and F. YILMAZ. (2020). *"Inception-ResNet-v2 with Leakyrelu and Averagepooling for More Reliable and Accurate Classification of Chest X-ray Images," 2020 Medical Technologies Congress*. TIPTEKNO., DOI: 10.1109/TIPTEKNO50054.2020.9299232

Agrawal, T., & Choudhary, P. (2022). Focus COVID: Automated COVID-19 detection using deep learning with chest x-ray images. *Evolving Systems*, 13(4), 519–533. DOI: 10.1007/s12530-021-09385-2 PMID: 38624806

Al-Waisy, A. S., Al-Fahdawi, S., Mohammed, M. A., Abdulkareem, K. H., Mostafa, S. A., Maashi, M. S., Arif, M., & Garcia-Zapirain, B. (2023). Covid-Chexnet: Hybrid deep learning framework for identifying COVID-19 virus in chest x-rays images. *Soft Computing*, 27(5), 2657–2672. DOI: 10.1007/s00500-020-05424-3 PMID: 33250662

Amyar, A., Modzelewski, R., & Ruan, S. (2020). Multi-task deep learning-based CT imaging analysis. *Computers in Biology and Medicine*, 126, 104037. Advance online publication. DOI: 10.1016/j.compbiomed.2020.104037 PMID: 33065387

Arias-Garzon, D., Alzate-Grisales, J. A., Orozco-Arias, S., Arteaga-Arteaga, H. B., Bravo-Ortiz, M. A., Mora-Rubio, A., Saborit-Torres, J. M., Serrano, J. A. M., Iglesia Vaya, M., & Cardona-Morales, O. (2021). COVID-19 detection in x-ray images using convolutional neural networks. *Machine Learning with Applications*, 6, 100138. DOI: 10.1016/j.mlwa.2021.100138 PMID: 34939042

Ayalew, A. M., Salau, A. O., Tamyalew, Y., Abeje, B. T., & Woreta, N. (2023). X-ray image-based COVID-19 detection using deep learning. *Multimedia Tools and Applications*, 82(28), 44507–44525. DOI: 10.1007/s11042-023-15389-8 PMID: 37362655

Bassi, P. R., & Attux, R. (2021). A deep convolutional neural network for COVID-19 detection using chest x-rays. *Research on Biomedical Engineering*, ●●●, 1–10. DOI: 10.1007/s42600-021-00132-9

Bhattacharyya, A., Bhaik, D., Kumar, S., Thakur, P., Sharma, R., & Pachori, R. B. (2022). A deep learning-based approach for automatic detection of COVID-19 cases using chest x-ray images. *Biomedical Signal Processing and Control*, 71, 103182. DOI: 10.1016/j.bspc.2021.103182 PMID: 34580596

Dai, L., Zheng, T., Xu, K., Han, Y., Xu, L., Huang, E., An, Y., Cheng, Y., Li, S., Liu, M., Yang, M., Li, Y., Cheng, H., Yuan, Y., Zhang, W., Ke, C., Wong, G., Qi, J., Qin, C., & Gao, G. F. (2020). A universal design of betacoronavirus vaccines against COVID-19, MERS, and SARS. *Cell*, 182(3), 722–733. DOI: 10.1016/j.cell.2020.06.035 PMID: 32645327

Das, A. K., Ghosh, S., Thunder, S., Dutta, R., Agarwal, S., & Chakrabarti, A. (2021). Automatic COVID-19 detection from x-ray images using ensemble learning with convolutional neural network. *Pattern Analysis & Applications*, 24(3), 1111–1124. DOI: 10.1007/s10044-021-00970-4

Fan, D. P., Zhou, T., Ji, G. P., Zhou, Y., Chen, G., Fu, H., Shen, J., & Shao, L. (2020). Inf-Net: Automatic COVID-19 lung infection segmentation from CT images. *IEEE Transactions on Medical Imaging*, 39(8), 2626–2637. DOI: 10.1109/TMI.2020.2996645 PMID: 32730213

Gao, K., Jin, Z., & Su, J. (2021). Dual-branch combination network (DCN): Towards accurate diagnosis and lesion segmentation of COVID-19 using CT images. *Medical Image Analysis*, 67, 101836. Advance online publication. DOI: 10.1016/j.media.2020.101836 PMID: 33129141

George, G. S., Mishra, P. R., Sinha, P., & Prusty, M. R. (2023). COVID-19 detection on chest x-ray images using homomorphic transformation and VGG inspired deep convolutional neural network. *Biocybernetics and Biomedical Engineering*, 43(1), 1–16. DOI: 10.1016/j.bbe.2022.11.003 PMID: 36447948

Gopatoti, A., & Vijayalakshmi, P. (2022). Optimized chest x-ray image semantic segmentation networks for COVID-19 early detection. *Journal of X-Ray Science and Technology*, 30(3), 491–512. DOI: 10.3233/XST-211113 PMID: 35213339

Guo, Z., Lu, Q., Jin, Q., Li, P., Xing, G., & Zhang, G. (2024). Phylogenetically evolutionary analysis provides insights into the genetic diversity and adaptive evolution of porcine deltacoronavirus. *BMC Veterinary Research*, 20(1), 22. DOI: 10.1186/s12917-023-03863-2 PMID: 38200538

Gupta, C., Khan, V., Srikanteswara, R., Gill, N. S., Gulia, P., & Menon, S. (2024). A novel secured deep learning model for COVID detection using chest x-rays. *Journal of Cybersecurity and Information Management*, 14(01), 227–244. DOI: 10.54216/JCIM.140116

Gupta, V., Jain, N., Sachdeva, J., Gupta, M., Mohan, S., Bajuri, M. Y., & Ahmadian, A. (2022). Improved COVID-19 detection with chest x-ray images using deep learning. *Multimedia Tools and Applications*, 81(26), 37657–37680. DOI: 10.1007/s11042-022-13509-4 PMID: 35968409

He, K., Zhang, X., Ren, S., & Sun, J. (2016). Deep residual learning for image recognition. In *Proceedings of the IEEE Conference on Computer Vision and Pattern Recognition* (pp. 770–778). https://doi.org/DOI: 10.1109/CVPR.2016.90

Hu, B., Ge, X., Wang, L.-F., & Shi, Z. (2015). Bat origin of human coronaviruses. *Virology Journal*, 12(1), 1–10. DOI: 10.1186/s12985-015-0422-1 PMID: 26689940

Huang, M.-L., & Liao, Y.-C. (2022). A lightweight CNN-based network on COVID-19 detection using x-ray and CT images. *Computers in Biology and Medicine*, 146, 105604. DOI: 10.1016/j.compbiomed.2022.105604 PMID: 35576824

Hussain, E., Hasan, M., Rahman, M. A., Lee, I., Tamanna, T., & Parvez, M. Z. (2021). Corodet: A deep learning-based classification for COVID-19 detection using chest x-ray images. *Chaos, Solitons, and Fractals*, 142, 110495. DOI: 10.1016/j.chaos.2020.110495 PMID: 33250589

Hussain, E., Hasan, M., Rahman, M. A., Lee, I., Tamanna, T., & Parvez, M. Z. (2021). CoroDet: A deep learning based classification for COVID-19 detection using chest X-ray images. *Chaos, Solitons, and Fractals*, 142, 110495. DOI: 10.1016/j.chaos.2020.110495 PMID: 33250589

Ismael, A. M., & Sengur, A. (2021). Deep learning approaches for COVID-19 detection based on chest x-ray images. *Expert Systems with Applications*, 164, 114054. DOI: 10.1016/j.eswa.2020.114054 PMID: 33013005

Khan, A. I., Shah, J. L., & Bhat, M. M. (2020). CoroNet: A deep neural network for detection and diagnosis of COVID-19 from chest X-ray images. *Computer Methods and Programs in Biomedicine*, 196, 105581. Advance online publication. DOI: 10.1016/j.cmpb.2020.105581 PMID: 32534344

Khan, V., & Meenai, T. A. (2021). Pretrained natural language processing model for intent recognition (BERT-IR). *Human Centric Intelligent Systems*, 1(3), 66–74. DOI: 10.2991/hcis.k.211109.001

Khan, V., Patel, D., Azfar Meenai, T., & Shukla, R. (2020). Application of deep learning techniques for automating the detection of diabetic retinopathy in retinal fundus photographs. In *Proceedings of the 2nd International Conference on Data, Engineering and Applications (IDEA)* (pp. 1–7). https://doi.org/DOI: 10.1109/IDEA49133.2020.9170712

Khan, V., Sharma, S., Ramesh, J. V. N., Pareek, P. K., Shukla, P. K., & Pandit, S. V. (2024). Enhancing tomato leaf disease detection through generative adversarial networks and genetic algorithm-based convolutional neural network. Fusion. *Practice and Applications*, 16(2), 147–177. DOI: 10.54216/FPA.160210

Korneenko, E. V., Samoilov, A. E., Chudinov, I. K., Butenko, I. O., Sonets, I. V., Artyushin, I. V., Yusefovich, A. P., Kruskop, S. V., Safonova, M. V., & Sinitsyn, S. O. (2024). Alphacoronaviruses from Pipistrellus bats captured in European Russia in 2015 and 2021 are closely related to those of Northern Europe. *Frontiers in Ecology and Evolution*, 12, 1324605. DOI: 10.3389/fevo.2024.1324605

Kumar, N., Gupta, M., Gupta, D., & Tiwari, S. (2023). Novel deep transfer learning model for COVID-19 patient detection using X-ray chest images. *Journal of Ambient Intelligence and Humanized Computing*, 14(1), 469–478. DOI: 10.1007/s12652-021-03306-6 PMID: 34025813

Makris, A., Kontopoulos, I., & Tserpes, K. (2020). COVID-19 detection from chest x-ray images using deep learning and convolutional neural networks. In *Proceedings of the 11th Hellenic Conference on Artificial Intelligence* (pp. 60–66), https://doi.org/DOI: 10.1145/3411408.3411416

Mangal, A., Kalia, S., Rajgopal, H., Rangarajan, K., Namboodiri, V., Banerjee, S., & Arora, C. (2020). Covidaid: COVID-19 detection using chest x-ray. arXiv preprint arXiv:2004.09803, https://doi.org//arXiv.2004.09803.DOI: 10.48550

Meenai, A., & Khan, V. (2020). Survey of methods applying deep learning to distinguish between computer-generated and natural images. In Shukla, R. K., Agrawal, J., Sharma, S., Chaudhari, N. S., & Shukla, K. K. (Eds.), *Social Networking and Computational Intelligence* (pp. 217–225). Springer., DOI: 10.1007/978-981-15-2071-6_18

Meenai, A., & Khan, V. (2020). Survey of methods applying deep learning to distinguish between computer-generated and natural images. In Shukla, R., Agrawal, J., Sharma, S., Chaudhari, N., & Shukla, K. (Eds.), *Social Networking and Computational Intelligence* (Vol. 100, pp. 97–107). Lecture Notes in Networks and Systems., DOI: 10.1007/978-981-15-2071-6_18

Mousavi, Z., Shahini, N., Sheykhivand, S., Mojtahedi, S., & Arshadi, A. (2022). COVID-19 detection using chest x-ray images based on a developed deep neural network. *SLAS Technology*, 27(1), 63–75. DOI: 10.1016/j.slast.2021.10.011 PMID: 35058196

Muhammad, S. S., & Alrikabi, J. M. (2024). Fire detection by using DenseNet 201 algorithm and surveillance cameras images. *Journal of Al-Qadisiyah for Computer Science and Mathematics*, 16(1), 81–91. DOI: 10.29304/jqcsm.2024.16.11437

Narin, A., Kaya, C., & Pamuk, Z. (2021). Automatic detection of coronavirus disease (COVID-19) using x-ray images and deep convolutional neural networks. *Pattern Analysis & Applications*, 24(4), 1207–1220. DOI: 10.1007/s10044-021-00984-y PMID: 33994847

Rahman, T., Khandakar, A., Qiblawey, Y., Tahir, A., Kiranyaz, S., Kashem, S. B. A., Islam, M. T., Al Maadeed, S., Zughaier, S. M., & Khan, M. S.(2021). Exploring the effect of image enhancement techniques on COVID-19 detection using chest x-ray images. *Computers in Biology and Medicine*, 132, 104319. DOI: 10.1016/j.compbiomed.2021.104319 PMID: 33799220

Redie, D. K., Sirko, A. E., Demissie, T. M., Teferi, S. S., Shrivastava, V. K., Verma, O. P., & Sharma, T. K. (2023). Diagnosis of COVID-19 using chest x-ray images based on modified DarkCovidNet model. *Evolutionary Intelligence*, 16(3), 729–738. DOI: 10.1007/s12065-021-00679-7 PMID: 35281292

Roopashree, S., & Anitha, J. (2021). Deepherb: A vision-based system for medicinal plants using Xception features. *IEEE Access: Practical Innovations, Open Solutions*, 9, 135927–135941. DOI: 10.1109/ACCESS.2021.3116207

Saber, H.-A., Younes, A., Osman, M., & Elkabani, I. (2024). Quran reciter identification using NASNetLarge. *Neural Computing & Applications*, 36(12), 6559–6573. DOI: 10.1007/s00521-023-09392-1

Saiz, F., & Barandiaran, I. (2020). COVID-19 detection in chest x-ray images using a deep learning approach, https://doi.org//arXiv.2004.09803.DOI: 10.48550

Sathishkumar, R., Govindarajan, M., & Dhivyasri, R. (2023). Detection and classification of neurodegenerative disease via EfficientNetB7. In International Conference on Mobile Radio Communications & 5G Networks (pp. 223–234), https://doi.org/ DOI: 10.1007/978-981-97-0700-3_17

Sethy, P. K., & Behera, S. K., & Others. (2020). Detection of coronavirus disease (COVID-19) based on deep features and SVM. International Journal of Mathematical. *Engineering and Management Sciences*, 5(4), 643–651. DOI: 10.47981/ijmems.5.4.181

Simonyan, K., & Zisserman, A. (2015). Very deep convolutional networks for large-scale image recognition. In *Proceedings of the International Conference on Learning Representations (ICLR)*. https://arxiv.org/abs/1409.1556

Singh, A. K., Kumar, A., Kumar, V., & Prakash, S. (2024). COVID-19 detection using adopted convolutional neural networks and high-performance computing. *Multimedia Tools and Applications*, 83(1), 593–608. DOI: 10.1007/s11042-023-15640-2 PMID: 37362712

Song, Y., Zheng, S., Li, L., Zhang, X., Zhang, X., Huang, Z., Chen, J., Wang, R., Zhao, H., Chong, Y., Shen, J., Zha, Y., & Yang, Y. (2021). Deep learning enables accurate diagnosis of novel coronavirus (COVID-19) with CT images. *IEEE/ACM Transactions on Computational Biology and Bioinformatics*, 18(6), 2775–2780. DOI: 10.1109/TCBB.2021.3065361 PMID: 33705321

Spicuzza, L., Montineri, A., Manuele, R., Crimi, C., Pistorio, M. P., Campisi, R., Vancheri, C., & Crimi, N. (2020). Reliability and usefulness of a rapid IgM-IgG antibody test for the diagnosis of SARS-CoV-2 infection: A preliminary report. *The Journal of Infection*, 81(2), 53–59. DOI: 10.1016/j.jinf.2020.04.022 PMID: 32335175

Srinivas, K., Gagana Sri, R., Pravallika, K., Nishitha, K., & Polamuri, S. R. (2024). COVID-19 prediction based on hybrid Inception V3 with VGG16 using chest X-ray images. *Multimedia Tools and Applications*, 83(12), 36665–36682. DOI: 10.1007/s11042-023-15903-y PMID: 37362699

Tahir, A. M. (2022). COVID-QU-Ex [non-COVID infections, and normal chest X-ray images dataset. Kaggle. https://www.kaggle.com/datasets/anasmohammedtahir/covidqu.]. *COVID*, 19, •••.

Talukder, M. A., Layek, M. A., Kazi, M., Uddin, M. A., & Aryal, S. (2024). Empowering COVID-19 detection: Optimizing performance through fine-tuned EfficientNet deep learning architecture. *Computers in Biology and Medicine*, 168, 107789. DOI: 10.1016/j.compbiomed.2023.107789 PMID: 38042105

Testa, C. B., Godoi, L. G., Monroy, N. A. J., Bortolotto, M. R. F. L., Rodrigues, A. S., & Francisco, R. P. V. (2024). Impact of Gamma COVID-19 variant on the prognosis of hospitalized pregnant and postpartum women with cardiovascular disease. *Clinics (São Paulo)*, 79, 100454. DOI: 10.1016/j.clinsp.2024.100454 PMID: 39121513

Wang, L., Byrum, B., & Zhang, Y. (2014). Detection and genetic characterization of delta coronavirus in pigs, Ohio, USA, 2014. *Emerging Infectious Diseases*, 20(7), 1227–1230. DOI: 10.3201/eid2007.140296 PMID: 24964136

Wang, L., Lin, Z. Q., & Wong, A. (2020). COVID-Net: A tailored deep convolutional neural network design for detection of COVID-19 cases from chest X-ray images. arXiv preprint arXiv:2003.09871, https://doi.org//arXiv.2003.09871.DOI: 10.48550

Wang, L., & Wong, A. (2020). COVID-Net: A tailored deep convolutional neural network design for detection of COVID-19 cases from chest X-ray images. *Scientific Reports*, 10(1), 19549. DOI: 10.1038/s41598-020-76550-z PMID: 33177550

Wang, S., Kang, B., & Zhang, J. (2021). A deep learning algorithm using CT images to screen for coronavirus disease (COVID-19). *European Radiology*, 31(8), 6096–6104. DOI: 10.1007/s00330-021-07715-1 PMID: 33629156

Wang, Y., Kang, H., Liu, X., & Tong, Z. (2020). Combination of RT-qPCR testing and clinical features for diagnosis of COVID-19 facilitates management of SARS-CoV-2 outbreak. *Journal of Medical Virology*, 92(6), 538–539. DOI: 10.1002/jmv.25721 PMID: 32096564

Wehbe, R. M., Sheng, J., & Dutta, S. (2021). DeepCOVID-XR: An AI algorithm to detect COVID-19 on chest radiographs. *Radiology*, 299(1). Advance online publication. DOI: 10.1148/radiol.2020203511 PMID: 33231531

Yan, Q., Wang, D. G., & Yang, B. (2021). COVID-19 chest CT image segmentation network by multiscale fusion and enhancement operations. *IEEE Transactions on Big Data*, 7(1), 13–24. DOI: 10.1109/TBDATA.2021.3056564 PMID: 36811064

Yan, Y., Shin, W. I., Pang, Y. X., Meng, Y., Lai, J., You, C., Zhao, H., Lester, E., Wu, T., & Pang, C. H. (2020). The first 75 days of novel coronavirus (SARS-CoV-2) outbreak: Recent advances, prevention, and treatment. *International Journal of Environmental Research and Public Health*, 17(7), 2323. DOI: 10.3390/ijerph17072323 PMID: 32235575

Zheng, C., Deng, X., Fu, Q., Zhou, Q., Feng, J., Ma, H., . . . Wang, X. (2020). Deep learning-based detection for COVID-19 from chest CT using weak label. MedRxiv, 2020-03, https://doi.org/DOI: 10.1101/2020.03.12.20027185

Chapter 8
Optimizing Healthcare Operations With AI Algorithms by Enhancing Skin Cancer Diagnosis Using Advanced Image Processing and Classification Techniques

Abioye Abiodun Oluwasegun
https://orcid.org/0009-0002-0022-5333
Nigerian Defence Academy, Kaduna, Nigeria

Awujoola Joel Olalekan
https://orcid.org/0000-0002-1842-021X
Nigerian Defence Academy, Kaduna, Nigeria

Abraham Evwiekpaefe
https://orcid.org/0000-0002-0279-8410
Nigerian Defence Academy, Kaduna, Nigeria

Anyanwu Obinna Bright
https://orcid.org/0009-0001-8284-1094
Nigerian Defence Academy, Kaduna, Nigeria

Philip Oshiokhaimhele Odion
https://orcid.org/0009-0006-2194-1370
Nigerian Defence Academy, Kaduna, Nigeria

Adelegan Olayinka Racheal
https://orcid.org/0009-0002-2910-8771
Nigerian Defence Academy, Kaduna, Nigeria

DOI: 10.4018/979-8-3693-7277-7.ch008

Uwa Celestine Ozoemenam
 https://orcid.org/0009-0001-1612-0918
Nigerian Defence Academy, Kaduna, Nigeria

Modibbo Gidado Malami
Nigerian Defence Academy, Kaduna, Nigeria

ABSTRACT

Optimizing healthcare through AI algorithms offers significant potential in skin cancer diagnosis. Skin cancer, involving abnormal skin cell growth, includes melanoma, the most dangerous form. Early detection is crucial, but traditional methods like visual inspection and biopsy are time-consuming and subjective. AI provides a more efficient, objective approach. This chapter enhances diagnostic accuracy using advanced image processing and classification on a comprehensive skin cancer dataset with seven classes. Initially imbalanced, data augmentation balanced it, generating 2000 images per class. Gray Level Co-occurrence Matrix (GLCM) and Color Histogram were used for feature extraction, combined with a Random Forest classifier. The best model achieved 97% accuracy, emphasizing balanced data and effective feature extraction in AI-based skin cancer diagnosis.

INTRODUCTION

The American Cancer Society projects that there will be 611,720 cancer-related deaths and 2,001,140 new cancer cases in the US in 2024, based on mortality statistics and cancer registries (Siegel et al., 2024). The incidence of various malignancies, including skin, liver, and prostate cancers, is on the rise. According to the US Skin Cancer Foundation, the number of Americans afflicted with skin cancer each year exceeds the total impacted by all other cancer types combined. The annual expense of treating skin cancer in the United States is estimated at US$8.9 billion. Skin cancer, encompassing both non-melanoma skin cancer (NMSC) and malignant melanoma, remains one of the most prevalent malignancies (Cives et al., 2020).

Early detection of melanoma significantly lowers mortality rates and minimizes treatment complications (Ahmed et al., 2020). Diagnosis typically involves obtaining a biopsy, which a dermatologist analyzes. The accuracy of results depends on the physician's expertise and the diagnostic tools used (Heibel et al., 2020). Visual evaluation alone can often fail to differentiate benign lesions from malignant tumors, making the process intrusive and requiring multiple samples. Non-invasive methods can assist in clinical diagnosis (Owida, 2022). However, challenges like proficiency, cost, and accessibility hinder the widespread use of these tools. Nonetheless, advancements in science and technology have led to several non-invasive imaging techniques for melanoma detection (Soglia et al., 2022).

The healthcare industry benefits significantly from technological innovations, particularly artificial intelligence (AI), which transforms healthcare service, research, and management. This technological revolution promises better quality of care, improved global outpatient flow, and personalized healthcare. AI has transitioned from a theoretical concept to a reality reshaping medical practice (Jutzi et al., 2020). AI can potentially reduce morbidity and mortality linked to skin cancer by aiding in early identification. Although specialists can accurately diagnose cancer, the limited availability of professionals necessitates the development of automated systems that efficiently diagnose diseases, thereby alleviating the financial and health burdens on patients.

The demand for automated solutions is growing to expedite the diagnostic process, reduce turnaround times, and enhance diagnostic accuracy. Significant technological advancements have occurred in deep learning, machine learning, and image processing (El Achi and Khoury, 2020). AI is revolutionizing healthcare by providing quicker, more precise, and personalized treatments. AI algorithms can process large medical datasets at unprecedented speeds, often matching the performance of supercomputers. For instance, in research, AI identifies patterns that predict study outcomes and aids in discovering novel medications or treatments. In administrative roles, AI improves operational efficiency through automation and predictive analytics, lowering costs and enhancing patient management. The potential for further advancements in healthcare is immense as we continue to adopt AI technologies. This ongoing transformation is expected to fundamentally alter how medical issues are addressed and reshape the future of healthcare delivery, ensuring better outcomes and improved quality of life for individuals globally (Alowais et al., 2023).

This chapter aims to provide an overview of AI algorithms designed to enhance healthcare operations, particularly in skin cancer diagnosis and treatment. It focuses on advanced feature extraction methods, such as Color Histograms and the Gray Level Co-occurrence Matrix (GLCM), which are essential for determining the salient features of skin lesions. Additionally, it will examine the classification of these extracted features using Random Forest as a machine learning technique, highlighting the efficacy of these algorithms in improving diagnostic precision and optimizing clinical workflows. The skin cancer dataset called HAM10000, used for this study, was collected from Kaggle. It consists of 10,016 dermatoscopic images, representing all significant diagnostic categories for pigmented lesions: Actinic keratoses and intraepithelial carcinoma/Bowen's disease (akiec), basal cell carcinoma (bcc), benign keratosis-like lesions (solar lentigines/seborrheic keratoses and lichen-planus-like keratoses, bkl), dermatofibroma (df), melanoma (mel), melanocytic nevi (nv), and vascular lesions (angiomas, angiokeratomas, pyogenic granulomas, and hemorrhage, vasc).

Skin Cancer

Skin cancer originates in the epidermis, the outermost skin layer, when abnormal cells grow uncontrollably due to unrepaired DNA damage that causes mutations. These mutations lead to rapid skin cell proliferation, forming cancerous tumors. Skin cancer can appear differently in each individual due to variations in skin tone, type, size, and location on the body. The primary causes of skin cancer are UV radiation from the sun and UV tanning bed use. Normally, new skin cells develop to replace aging and dying ones, but when this process is disrupted such as by UV exposure; cells proliferate abnormally. These cells can be benign, meaning they do not spread or cause harm or are malignant. If skin cancer is not detected early, it can spread to nearby tissue or other parts of the body. Fortunately, most skin cancers are treatable if identified and addressed promptly. It is essential to consult a healthcare professional if you notice any symptoms of skin cancer (Skin Cancer Foundation, n.d.). Skin cancer can affect anyone, at any age, and can occur anywhere on the body. Diagnosing skin cancer can be challenging because it manifests in various sizes and shapes. Common sites for skin cancer include sun-exposed areas such as the scalp, face, lips, ears, neck, chest, arms, hands, and, in women, the legs. However, it can also develop in areas rarely exposed to sunlight, like the palms, under fingernails or toenails, and the genital region. Individuals of all skin tones are susceptible to skin cancer, including those with darker complexions. People with dark skin are more likely to develop melanoma in less sun-exposed areas like the palms and soles of the feet (Mayo Clinic, n.d.).

Changes to the skin are the most typical warning indicator of skin cancer. A new mole, a mole that changes in size, shape, or color, or a mole that bleeds are examples of symptoms. A flat, pink/red, or brown-colored patch or bump; areas on the skin that resemble scars; sores that appear crusty, have a depression in the middle, or bleed frequently; a wound or sore that won't heal or heals but returns; and a rough, scaly lesion that may itch, bleed, and turn crusty are some additional signs. A pearly or waxy bump on the face, ears, or neck is another. The appearance of skin cancer varies according to its type. The most significant sign is evolution. The ABCDE rule can be used to identify the following warning signs: asymmetry (irregular shape), border (blurry or irregular edges), color (mole with multiple colors), diameter (larger than a pencil eraser, 6 millimeters), and evolution (Cleveland Clinic, n.d.). Figure 1 shows Examples of images from the HAM10000 dataset for the following cancer types: (a) Actinic keratosis (b) Basal cell carcinoma (c) Benign keratosis-like lesions (d) dermatofibroma (e) Melanocytic nevi (f) Melanoma (g) Vascular lesions

Figure 1. Visual Examples of Various Skin Lesion Types (a) Actinic keratosis (b) Basal cell carcinoma (c) Benign keratosis-like lesions (d) dermatofibroma (e) Melanocytic nevi (f) Melanoma (g) Vascular lesions (Chaturvedi et al., 2021)

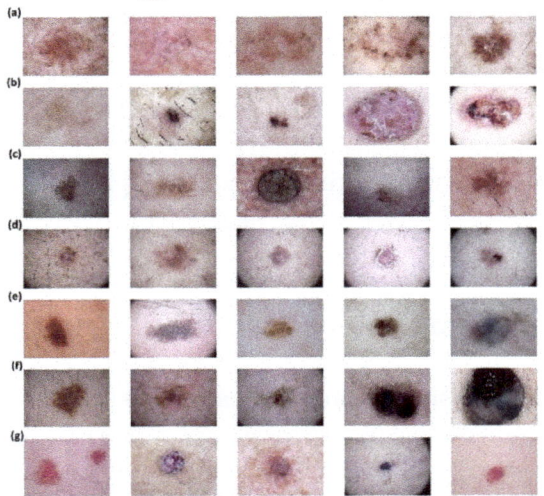

Actinic Keratosis

Actinic keratoses are characterized by the proliferation of keratinocytes in the epidermis that have varied degrees of dysplasia; in other words, they are intraepithelial keratinocytic dysplasias. Actinic keratoses are traditionally classified as preneoplastic lesions; however, some authors propose that, because they originate from clonal DNA alterations in keratinocytes, they should be viewed as in situ neoplasms (Reinehr & Bakos, 2020). Thus, actinic keratoses are regarded as having malignant features from the beginning, from the perspective of the molecularly identical p53 protein mutations that epidermal keratinocytes present, to the cytological changes that mimic those seen in spinocellular carcinomas (SCCs), such as loss of polarity, nuclear pleomorphism, dysregulated maturation, and increased number of mitoses (Winge et al., 2023).

Basal Cell Carcinoma

Basal Cell Carcinoma is a locally invasive, slowly developing malignant epidermal skin tumor that primarily affects Caucasians. Through the uneven proliferation of asymptomatic finger-like outgrowths that stay continuous with the primary tumor mass (Fania et al., 2020). Metastasis is very uncommon and morbidity arises from the invasion and destruction of local tissue, especially on the head, neck, and face. Numerous variations exist in terms of morphology and clinical presentation, such as nodular, cystic, superficial, morphoeic (sclerosing), keratotic, and pigmented forms. Nodular (nBCC), superficial (sBCC), and pigmented forms are common histological subtypes. Morphoeic, micronodular, infiltrative, and basosquamous variants are also common subtypes and are specifically linked to aggressive tissue invasion and destruction (Niculet et al., 2022). Features like perivascular or perineural invasion are linked to the most aggressive tumors.

Benign Keratosis-Like Lesions (seborrheic keratoses)

Benign keratosis-like lesions, commonly called seborrheic keratoses (SK), are non-cancerous skin growths that often appear as people age. It's the most prevalent type of tumor in humans. With advancing age, there might be hundreds of lesions; the prevalence and the median number of lesions rise gradually. It affects both men and women equally. All population groups have seborrheic keratoses, which have a similar occurrence (Jayeb et al., 2022). Any part of the body that bears hair is susceptible to SK. The head, particularly the temples, the neck, the chest, and the back are sites of preference. SK has not been reported on the conjunctiva, but there are isolated cases of it on the palms, soles, or mucous membranes (Barthelmann et al., 2023). The intraepidermal growth of basaloid or squamous epithelial cells is known as seborrheic keratosis. Acanthosis, papillomatosis, (ortho-) hyperkeratosis, keratin cysts, and keratin pseudocysts are the histological diagnostic criteria for SK. While keratin pseudocysts are keratin invasions of the stratum corneum above, keratin cysts are intraepidermal keratin pearls that are expelled transepidermally. Cellular or nuclear atypia is uncommon. Depending on pigmentation, melanin and melanocytes are present in varying amounts.

Dermatofibroma

Dermatofibromas are benign skin growths that typically have a small diameter and are usually pink to light brown on lighter skin or dark brown to black on darker skin. They may appear darker or pinker if irritated, such as during shaving. Many describe dermatofibromas as feeling like small stones beneath the skin. While most are painless, some individuals report itching, discomfort, or tenderness. These growths, also known as benign fibrous histiocytomas, arise from an accumulation of cells in the deeper layers of the skin. The exact cause remains unclear; however, some researchers suggest local trauma, such as a minor injury or insect bite, may trigger their formation. Age may be a risk factor, as dermatofibromas primarily affect adults. Additionally, individuals with immune system suppression or certain underlying conditions, like systemic lupus erythematosus, may be more susceptible to developing multiple dermatofibromas (Medical News Today, 2018)

Melanocytic Nevi

Benign skin cancers are called melanocytic nevi. As mentioned above, they come in a variety of sizes and colors. Benign nevi typically have a uniform tint and a round or oval shape. Nevi are more common in parts of the body exposed to the sun for longer periods, such as the outside arm relative to the inner arm. Melanocytes, or skin cells, are the source of the pigment known as melanin. Melanocytic nevi are tan to dark brown in hue due to this pigment. Along with being the cause of overall skin tone, melanin also darkens skin after exposure to the sun. Environmental factors, namely sun exposure, and genetic ones, including family history, are reflected in melanocytic nevi. Melanocytic nevi are characterized by the following clinical features: round or oval in shape; smooth borders; uniform color throughout; symmetry (when a line is drawn within them, the two sides have identical look); and tan to dark brown, pale pink, and occasionally black (Yale Medicine, n.d.).

Melanoma

Melanocytes, located at the basal level of the epidermis, produce melanin, a pigment that absorbs UV radiation and protects the skin. Although they are a minority cell population, melanocytes are vital for skin protection. In response to UV radiation, keratinocytes release α-melanocyte stimulating hormone (α-MSH), which binds to melanocortin 1 receptor (MC1R) on melanocytes, signaling melanin synthesis. Melanocytes produce two types of melanin: eumelanin (black/brown) and pheomelanin (red/yellow), with their ratio determining skin color. Eumelanin provides better UV protection and reduces skin cancer risk, while pheomelanin offers less protection and can lead to greater DNA damage. Individuals with light skin, blond or red hair, and light eyes are at higher risk for melanoma. Variants of the MC1R gene influence skin, hair, and eye color; certain variants increase the prevalence of pheomelanin and fair skin, resulting in more UV-induced mutations and a higher risk of skin cancers. (Solano, 2020).

Vascular Lesions

The vascular system is the network of vessels that carries blood throughout the body. When compromised, vascular lesions can develop on the skin's surface, beneath the skin, or deep within the vein tissue, appearing as markings, tumors, sores, ulcers, or wounds. These lesions typically start at birth and progress throughout infancy. Treatments for common vascular lesions, such as pyogenic granulomas, vascular malformations, and hemangiomas, vary. Hemangiomas, benign lesions, appear as bright red growths on the skin. While they may leave scars, they usually stop growing after six to twelve months and gradually shrink. Surgery is rarely necessary; laser therapy may be used for sensitive areas like the nose and ears. Abnormal vessel formation can lead to various vascular malformations, including arteriovenous, venous, lymphatic, and capillary abnormalities. Capillary abnormalities, such as birthmarks and port wine stains, can range in color from dark purple to bright red. Some may disappear with age, but persistent lesions can be treated with laser therapy. Venous malformations appear as soft lumps under the skin and can be addressed with sclerotherapy or surgical excision. Sclerotherapy is also effective for lymphatic abnormalities, although severe cases may require surgery. Arteriovenous malformations are rare and can pose serious health risks if untreated. Pyogenic granulomas are quickly growing red lesions that often require conservative surgery, particularly in children and pregnant women. (Piccolo et al., 2018).

RELATED THEORY

Gray-Level Co-occurrence Matrix (GLCM)

The Gray-Level Co-occurrence Matrix (GLCM), also referred to as co-occurrence distributions or matrices, captures the distribution of pixel pairs occurring at specific offsets within an image. This method is crucial for texture analysis, extensively applied in fields such as medical imaging. It serves as a statistical tool to examine spatial relationships between pixels in images by quantifying the frequency of occurrence of pairs of pixels with specific gray-level values. The GLCM is constructed by tallying the occurrences of pixel pairs with defined gray levels and spatial relationships across the image. The co-occurrence matrix can quantify the texture of an image by taking into account its intensity, grayscale values, or different color dimensions. Co-occurrence matrices are often huge and sparse, so to obtain a more relevant collection of features, different matrix metrics are frequently chosen. The features produced by this method are commonly referred to as Haralick features, in honor of Robert Haralick (Haralick et al., 1973). In the Haralick Texture Framework, the Gray-Level Co-occurrence Matrix is computed by evaluating pairs of grayscale pixels i and j across various directional offsets, as illustrated below.

$$P(i,j|d,\theta) = \frac{p(i,j|d,\theta)}{\Sigma i \Sigma j \, p(i,j|d,\theta)} \quad (1)$$

where θ is the direction of the pixel (x_1, y_1), d is the pixel distance that occurs within (x_1, y_1), and $p(i, j)$ is the matrix of relative frequencies. The statistical probability values for transitions between gray levels i and j at a given distance d and angle θ are provided in $p(i, j)$. Textural features extracted from gray-tone spatial dependencies include measures such as Contrast, Entropy, Correlation, and Homogeneity Energy;

- **Contrast**: Measures the intensity contrast between neighboring pixels.

$$Contrast = \sum_{i,j=0}^{N-1} P_{ij}(i-j)^2 \quad (2)$$

Entropy: Represents the randomness or complexity of the image.

$$Entropy = \Sigma_i \Sigma_j P(i,j) \quad (3)$$

- **Correlation**: Measures the correlation between a pixel and its neighboring pixels across the entire image.

$$Correlation = \sum_{i,j} \frac{(i-\mu_i)(j-\mu_j)p(i,j)}{\delta_i \delta_j} \quad (4)$$

- **Energy**: Energy is the GLCM's total squared element and, by default, a permanent image.

$$Energy = \sum_{i,j} (i,j)^2 \quad (5)$$

Color Histogram

One of the key tools in image processing for displaying the distribution of colors is a color histogram. It visually represents color content by indicating the frequency of each color in an image. This technique is beneficial for various applications, such as image identification, segmentation, and retrieval (Gonzalez & Woods, 2008). A color histogram is created by selecting a color space (e.g., RGB, HSV, or LAB) and dividing it into bins for different color ranges. The image is then examined pixel by pixel to determine how many pixels fall into each bin. Normalizing the histogram enhances its usefulness in comparative tasks by making it independent of image size. Color histograms aid in image identification and matching through color distribution. They are used in image segmentation to distinguish areas based on color similarity and enable efficient photo retrieval using color attributes in content-based image retrieval. Additionally, they serve as feature vectors in various machine-learning and image-processing applications (Swain & Ballard, 1991). Despite their simplicity and lower computational intensity compared to more complex feature extraction techniques, color histograms have drawbacks. They are susceptible to variations in lighting and lack spatial information regarding color arrangement. Moreover, the effectiveness of a color histogram can be influenced by the choice of color space and bin size (Forsyth & Ponce, 2003).

Random Forest

The Random Forest classifier is a powerful ensemble tree-based machine learning algorithm composed of multiple decision trees, each built from a randomly selected subset of the training data. By combining the predictions from these trees, the Random Forest algorithm enhances accuracy and robustness. The final class of a test object is determined by aggregating votes from all decision trees, typically through majority voting. This ensemble learning method reduces the risk of overfitting and provides higher accuracy compared to individual decision trees. Ensemble algorithms like Random Forest combine multiple models to improve classification performance. For instance, an ensemble might include Naive Bayes, Support Vector Machines (SVM), and decision trees, with the final prediction based on the majority vote. Random Forest is versatile, applicable for both classification and regression tasks, and can identify important features. There are two types of Random Forest models: one for classification and one for regression. In classification, the prediction is the majority vote of all predicted classes over B trees, expressed as f(x) = majority vote of all predicted classes over B trees. In regression, the prediction is the sum of all subtree predictions divided by B trees, expressed as f(x) = sum of all subtree predictions divided over B trees. Its robustness and flexibility make Random Forest widely applicable in domains such as finance for credit scoring, healthcare for disease prediction, and e-commerce for customer segmentation. Figure 2. shows a random forest classification structure (builtin. n.d.).

Figure 2. The structure of Random Forest

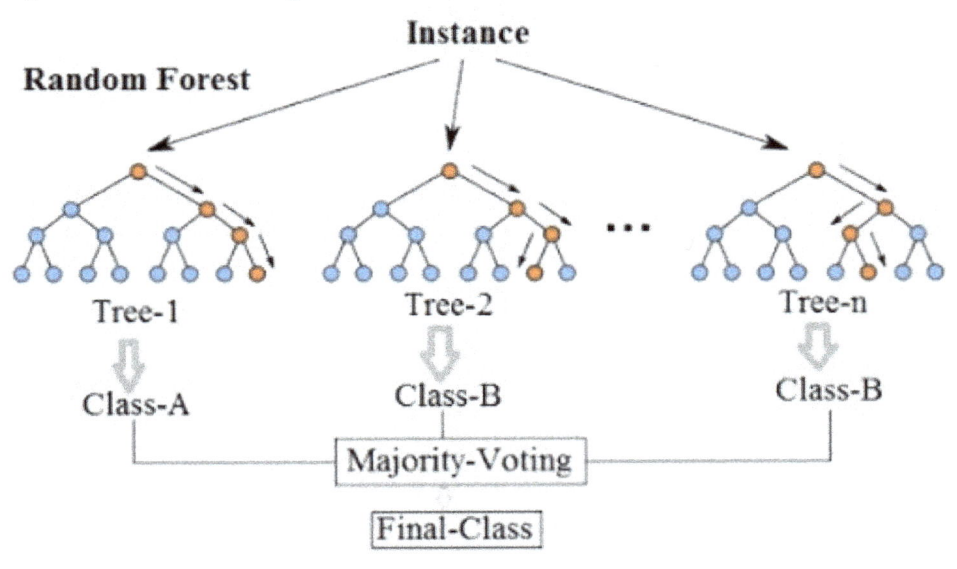

Image Augmentation

Image augmentation is a technique used in computer vision and deep learning to artificially expand the size of a training dataset by creating modified versions of images in the dataset. This is done to improve the performance and robustness of models, especially when the available data is limited. Common augmentation techniques include rotations, translations, scaling, flipping, and adding noise to the images. These modifications help models learn to recognize objects and patterns in a variety of conditions and perspectives, enhancing their generalization capabilities. Image augmentation is a crucial method in computer vision, providing models with a richer set of training data through various transformations such as rotations, translations, and scaling, which helps in improving model robustness and generalization (Shorten & Khoshgoftaar, 2019). The augmented dataset used for this study was created by applying data augmentation techniques, including horizontal flips and 90-degree, -90-degree, and 180-degree rotations, generating 2000 images for each class.

LITERATURE REVIEW

Ismail et al., (2021) proposed a classification framework using the innovations made in deep learning. This can be of great benefit to places where medical resources are minimal. For their diagnosis, it can be of great help to doctors and can give them a better chance in providing the patients with appropriate treatment. This research aims to investigate the efficiency of pre-trained convolutional neural networks and the transfer learning technique for classifying images of skin lesions. In image feature extraction, these neural networks have been demonstrated to be very effective. A dataset of images, with seven different types of skin lesions and a total of 10,015 images, was separated into two classes. Skin lesions of the seven forms were classified as either malignant or benign. By augmenting the number of images, the dataset was balanced. Numerous pre-trained neural networks were trained on this dataset; ResNet50, VGG16, VGG19, MobileNet, DenseNet, Inception V3. A classification framework was proposed based on their results. The framework suggested combining the three best pre-trained networks to enhance the classification accuracy. The combined model was made up of ResNet50, VGG16, and DenseNet. The addition of convolution layers to each model, that were trainable, further improved the classification accuracy. The overall accuracy achieved was 84.01% for this final proposed framework.

Kavitha et al., (2024) used sophisticated image processing techniques to eliminate artifacts from raw datasets techniques at the initial stage of diagnosis. To enable correct analysis, this preparation step makes sure the data input into the classification models is clean and of high quality. After that, they used Convolutional Neural Networks (CNNs) to improve skin cancer detection and classification, leading to higher accuracy rates. The use of region-based Convolutional Neural Network (R-CNN) algorithms, which are extraordinarily efficient at handling massive amounts of data, is highlighted in the study. R-CNN algorithms are excellent at segmenting images into smaller, more manageable chunks, which makes it possible to precisely analyze particular sections of an image. This focused method is very helpful for medical picture analysis, where it's crucial to accurately identify anomalies like skin cancer lesions. Kavitha et al. demonstrated the efficacy of the R-CNN algorithm with an accuracy of 84.32%. The R-CNN is a useful tool in medical diagnostics because of its accuracy and speed while processing big datasets. Its impartiality guarantees regular outcomes, diminishing the possibility of human error, and its usability for extensive application in many healthcare contexts. The study highlights the usefulness of R-CNN algorithms for the categorization and detection of skin cancer. These algorithms enable quicker and more impartial evaluations in addition to increasing diagnostic accuracy. By enabling earlier identification of skin cancer, the use of R-CNN in medical diagnostics can improve patient outcomes by facilitating prompt and effective therapeutic treatments.

Fraiwan et al., (2022) investigated raw deep transfer learning for classifying skin lesions into seven categories using the HAM10000 dataset, a collection of dermoscopy images representing different skin diseases. Their approach bypassed the need for manual feature extraction and preprocessing, streamlining the classification workflow. Thirteen pre-trained deep transfer learning models were utilized, leveraging prior knowledge to improve performance. The results demonstrated the potential of this method, with the best model achieving 82.9% accuracy in identifying specific skin conditions, including some types of skin cancer. However, several challenges were identified. The dataset's imbalance, with some categories having far fewer images than others, impacted the models' ability to generalize across all classes. Models tended to perform better in high-frequency categories but struggled with low-frequency ones. The large number of classes also added complexity to the classification task, as the models had to distinguish between a wide range of conditions. Despite these challenges, the study highlighted the promise of deep transfer learning for skin lesion classification while emphasizing the need for better-balanced datasets and strategies to handle multiple classes effectively.

A revolutionary method of classifying and predicting skin cancer with the application of augmented intelligence was proposed by Kumar et al., in 2023. The deep neural network framework's appended Kaggle Re-Snet50 datasets are used to process the approach. Re-Snet50 datasets are 8 times deeper than VGG net datasets. For the purpose of extracting and clustering cancer regions, the Augmented Deep Neural Networking (AuDNN) technique has retrieved arbitrary features with RoI identification. To increase the prediction ratio, multilayer attribute dependency mapping is synchronized with the extracted datasets. The suggested method uses a dual cross-reference validation mechanism to ensure a trustworthy communication framework for efficient coordination and communication within the global instrumental networking ecosystem. It is built using the nomenclature of Industrial IoT standards. Because of the DNN multi-dimensional mapping based on enhanced intelligence, the technology has demonstrated a clear improvement over earlier methods. Based on logical calculation, the method has achieved 93.26% accuracy in skin cancer categorization and prediction.

Bokori and Mitani (2024) conducted an extensive study to explore the impact of image size and augmentation using perspective transformation on the performance of Convolutional Neural Networks (CNNs) in the context of skin cancer prediction. Their test findings showed that, out of all the sizes they investigated, an image with 64 by 64 pixels had the highest accuracy (82.51%). Subsequent research showed that an augmentation strategy involving perspective modification and the 64×64 image size greatly enhanced model performance. More specifically, when the number of augmented photos was 20 and the k-range was 8, the highest accuracy of 83.91% was attained. This result emphasizes how crucial it is to have a sizable and diverse training sample to improve the CNN model's learning capacity. The research conducted verified that an image size of 64x64 is ideal for this particular use case. It also emphasized the advantages of viewpoint transformation as an augmentation method, which can add more information and variability to the training dataset and enhance the model's capacity to generalize to new, unobserved data. This research provides valuable insights into the best practices for image preprocessing and augmentation in the development of CNN models for skin cancer prediction.

Upadhyay et al., (2023) implemented neural networks to classify segmented skin lesion images as benign or malignant. The process began with image pre-processing to remove noise, followed by segmentation to isolate the lesion from the background. Textural features were extracted from these regions for classification. Perceptron and multilayer perceptron (MLP) architectures were used alongside transfer learning models like ResNet-50, Inception-V3, MobileNet, Inception-ResNet-V2, and DenseNet201. DenseNet201 outperformed the others, achieving an accuracy of 93.24% and an AUC of 0.932. This study demonstrates the effectiveness of advanced neural networks and transfer learning in skin lesion classification, aiding early cancer detection.

Aljohani and Turki (2022) focused on detecting melanoma using deep learning techniques applied to skin images. They tested several convolutional neural network (CNN) architectures, including DenseNet201, MobileNetV2, ResNet50V2, ResNet152V2, Xception, VGG16, VGG19, and GoogleNet, using GPUs for efficient processing. The study utilized a dataset of 7,146 images to train and test the models. The CNN architectures were evaluated based on their accuracy in detecting melanoma, with GoogleNet emerging as the top performer. It achieved an accuracy of 74.91% on the training set and 76.08% on the test set, outperforming the other models. The study highlights GoogleNet's effectiveness for melanoma detection and emphasizes the importance of choosing the right CNN architecture for medical imaging tasks. Their work showcases the potential of deep learning in improving early melanoma diagnosis through automated image analysis.

Bazgir et al., (2024) developed a deep neural network model to classify skin cancer as melanoma or non-melanoma. Their approach optimized the Inception-Net architecture, incorporating data augmentation and additional layers to handle incomplete and inconsistent data, a common issue in medical imaging. The model was trained on 2,637 skin images and evaluated using metrics such as precision, sensitivity, specificity, F1-score, and AUC. The study showed that using the Adam optimizer resulted in 84.39% accuracy, while the Nadam optimizer improved it to 85.94%. Data augmentation significantly enhanced the model's training effectiveness, improving its capacity to distinguish between melanoma and non-melanoma cases.

By increasing accuracy and reliability, this model offers a useful tool for early skin cancer detection, helping medical professionals make timely diagnoses and improve patient outcomes. The study highlights the potential of optimized deep learning models in advancing diagnostic accuracy for skin cancer detection.

Bassel et al., (2022) developed a novel method for classifying melanoma and benign skin cancers using a stacking approach that incorporates multiple classifiers. Their system was trained on a dataset of 1,000 skin images, evenly divided between melanoma and benign categories. The data was split into 70% for training and 30% for testing. They used ResNet50, Xception, and VGG16 for feature extraction due to their ability to capture intricate image details. Classification was carried out using a stacked cross-validation method with various algorithms, including deep learning models, Support Vector Machines (SVM), Random Forests (RF), Neural Networks (NN), k-Nearest Neighbors (KNN), and logistic regression. The system's performance was evaluated using accuracy, F1 score, Area Under the Curve (AUC), and sensitivity. The Xception-based method achieved the highest accuracy at 90.9%, outperforming ResNet50 and VGG16. The study concluded that stacking classifiers with effective feature extraction significantly improved skin cancer detection accuracy. Further optimization and increasing the training dataset size could make this method a reliable tool for skin cancer classification, highlighting the potential of integrating multiple machine learning models to enhance diagnostic accuracy in medical imaging.

Islam and Panta (2024) aimed to enhance binary classification of skin cancer by distinguishing between benign and malignant stages using pre-trained transfer learning models. They fine-tuned various layers and activation functions of five different pre-trained models to better capture nuances in skin cancer images. Using the ISIC dataset, they applied data augmentation techniques to ensure model reliability and effectiveness in diverse scenarios, enhancing the dataset's variability and robustness. Evaluating hyperparameters like batch sizes, epochs, and optimizers, they sought optimal parameters to improve classification performance. The ResNet-50 model performed best, achieving a precision of 0.94, an F1-score of 0.86, and an accuracy of 93.5%. This study underscores the importance of data augmentation and refined pre-trained models in improving skin cancer detection, highlighting the need for robust data preparation and model optimization in medical image classification tasks.

RESEARCH METHODOLOGY AND MATERIALS

This section offers organized methods and materials for carrying out the research work Figure 3 shows the methodology flow of using Color Histogram and Gray-level Co-occurrence Matrix for feature extraction on 2000 Augmented images of Skin Cancer images while Random Forest classifier is utilized for classification.

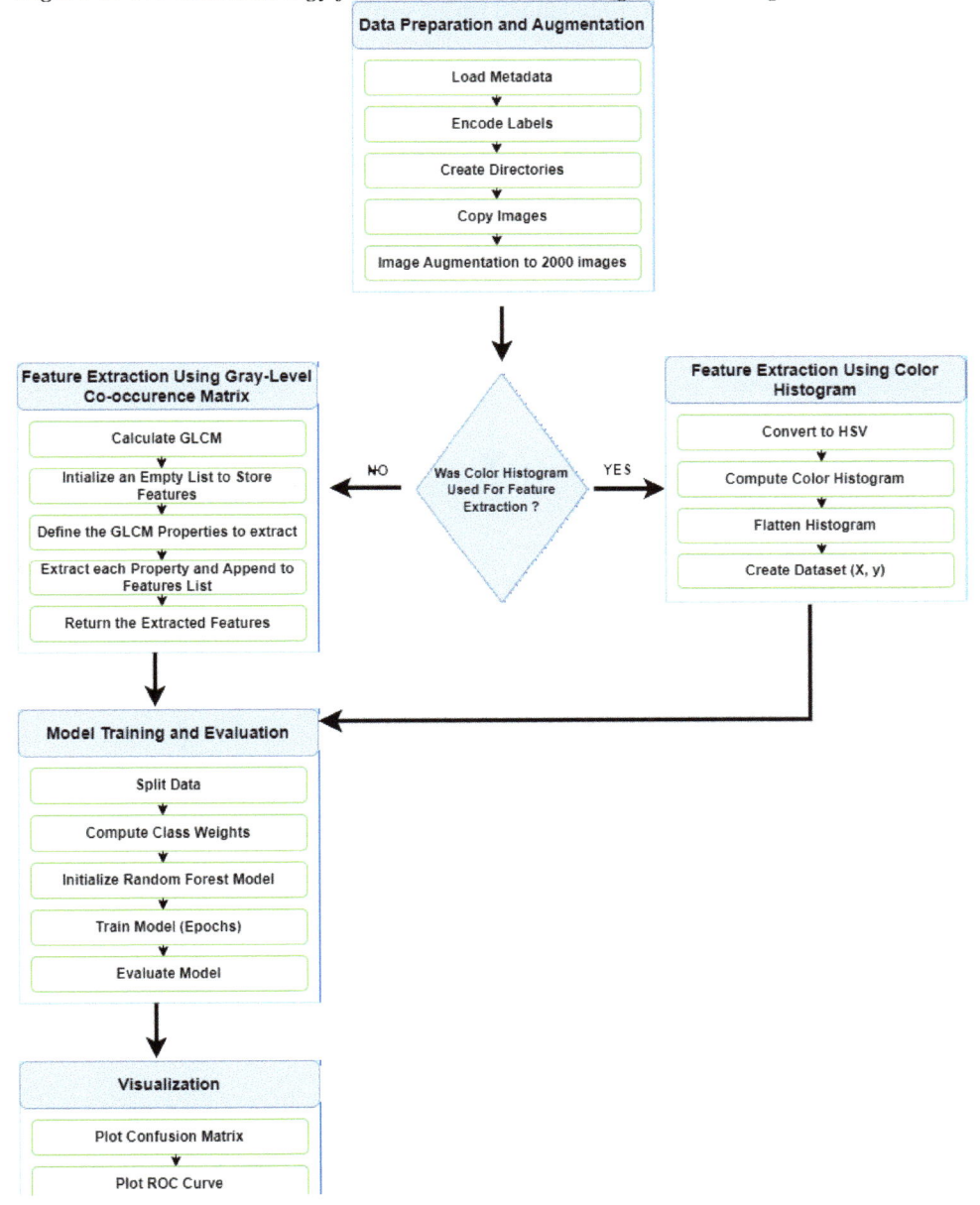

Figure 3. The Methodology flow on Skin Cancer Augmented Images

Figure 4 shows the methodology flow for using a Color Histogram and Gray-level Co-occurrence Matrix for feature extraction on original Skin Cancer images from the HAM10000 dataset, followed by classification using a Random Forest classifier.

Unlike Figure 3, the data preparation section excludes image augmentation in Figure 4, as it only uses the original, imbalanced images from the HAM10000 dataset.

Figure 4. The Methodology flow on Skin Cancer Original HAM10000 Images

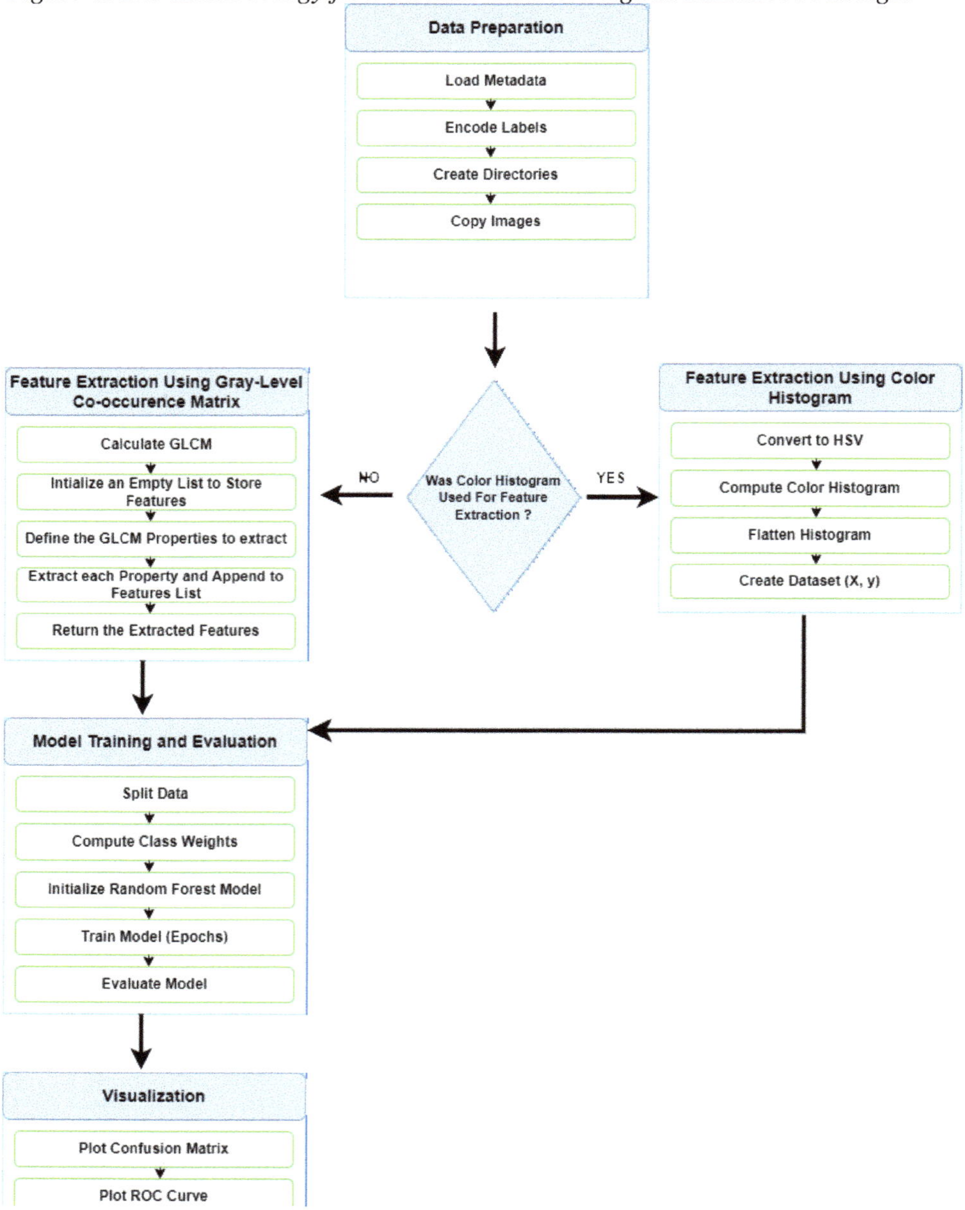

Description of Four Model Architecture

The methodology involves developing and evaluating four distinct model architectures for classifying skin cancer images, utilizing two feature extraction techniques—color histogram and Gray-Level Co-occurrence Matrix (GLCM)—and employing the Random Forest classifier. These models are trained and evaluated on both the original HAM10000 Skin Cancer Dataset and an augmented skin Cancer dataset consisting of 2,000 images per class.

Model 1, as shown in Figure 4, utilizes color histogram feature extraction on the original dataset. The process starts with loading metadata, encoding labels, creating directories, and copying original images without data augmentation. Images are converted to the HSV color space, and color histograms are computed and flattened into feature vectors. The dataset is split into training and testing sets, class weights are computed to handle imbalances, and a Random Forest classifier is trained over multiple epochs. The model's performance is evaluated using accuracy, F1 score, precision, and recall metrics, visualized through confusion matrices, ROC curves, and training and validation metrics.

Model 2, also depicted in Figure 4, employs GLCM feature extraction on the original dataset. Similar to Model 1, metadata is loaded, labels are encoded, directories are created, and original images are copied without data augmentation. GLCM analyzes texture, extracting properties like contrast, dissimilarity, and energy, which are stored in a feature list. The dataset is split, class weights are computed, and a Random Forest classifier is trained and evaluated similarly to **Model 1**, with performance visualizations.

Model 3, illustrated in Figure 3, applies color histogram feature extraction on the augmented dataset. After loading metadata and encoding labels, data augmentation generates 2,000 images per class. The process continues with HSV conversion and feature vector creation. The augmented dataset is split, class weights are computed, and a Random Forest classifier is trained and evaluated, with performance visualizations.

Model 4, also shown in Figure 3, uses GLCM feature extraction on the augmented dataset. After initial processing and data augmentation, GLCM is calculated for texture analysis, with properties stored in a feature list. The classifier is trained and evaluated as in previous models.

In summary, these four models employ various feature extraction techniques and datasets to assess the Random Forest classifier's performance in classifying skin cancer images.

Dataset Description

The HAM10000 Skin Cancer dataset comprises 10,015 dermatoscopic images, offering a valuable training set for academic machine learning. It includes a comprehensive collection of images across significant diagnostic categories for pigmented lesions, such as Actinic keratoses (akiec), Basal cell carcinoma (bcc), Benign keratosis-like lesions (bkl), Dermatofibroma (df), Melanoma (mel), Melanocytic nevi (nv), and Vascular lesions (vasc). The dataset is meticulously labeled and distributed, featuring 6,705 images of Melanocytic nevi, 1,113 of Melanoma, 1,099 of Benign keratosis-like lesions, 514 of Basal cell carcinoma, 327 of Actinic keratoses, 142 of Vascular lesions, and 115 of Dermatofibroma. Despite the substantial number of images in each category, the dataset is notably imbalanced, with Melanocytic nevi dominating and other categories like Dermatofibroma being relatively rare. This imbalance can adversely affect the performance of machine learning models, leading to biases toward more frequent classes and resulting in poor generalization and reduced accuracy for less common lesions.

To counter these issues, data augmentation techniques were employed, including horizontal flips and rotations (90 degrees, -90 degrees, and 180 degrees), which generated an additional 2,000 images for each class. This approach enhances the model's generalization ability and improves its accuracy across all lesion types. This research utilizes both the original and augmented datasets to evaluate and compare their performance. By addressing these challenges, the study aims to develop robust and reliable diagnostic tools for clinical use, ultimately enhancing the accuracy and reliability of skin lesion classification models.

Evaluation metrics are essential for assessing how well classification models work, particularly in significant domains like medical diagnosis where precise diagnosis of diseases like skin cancer is crucial. Patient outcomes can be greatly impacted by how well these models perform in categorizing cases as either indicative of skin cancer or not. Thus, knowing these parameters with the classification of skin cancer offers insights into the diagnostic accuracy and dependability of the model.

1. **Accuracy**: In skin cancer diagnosis, accuracy signifies the proportion of correctly identified instances (both skin cancer and non-skin cancer cases) out of all cases evaluated. Accuracy is important in medical diagnostics because it guarantees that patients receive the right diagnosis and treatment, which is especially important considering the variety of skin cancer types that require different care and treatment approaches.
2. **Sensitivity**: refers to the ability of the diagnostic system to correctly identify patients with skin cancer. It is calculated as the proportion of true positive cases (correctly identified cancer cases) out of all actual cancer cases. To ensure that

patients with skin cancer are correctly recognized and can receive the right therapy, high sensitivity is essential in medical diagnostics. A highly sensitive diagnostic instrument reduces the possibility of false negatives, which could otherwise postpone the necessary medical intervention.

3. **Precision**: relates to the diagnostic system's precision in determining which of all the instances it labels as positive are positive cases of skin cancer. It is the ratio of genuine positive cases—that is, cases of skin cancer that were correctly identified—to all positive cases—that is, both true positives and false positives—that the system was able to identify. To make sure that a medical diagnostic system's indication of skin cancer is extremely likely to be accurate, high precision is essential. By doing this, the likelihood of false positives is decreased, sparing patients from needless worry and needless testing for conditions they do not have.

4. **Recall**: measures the proportion of actual positive skin cancer cases that the diagnostic system correctly identifies. It is calculated by dividing the number of true positive cases (correctly diagnosed skin cancers) by the total number of actual positives (true positives plus false negatives). High recall is crucial in medical diagnostics to ensure that most cases of skin cancer are detected, especially for conditions like actinic keratoses, basal cell carcinoma, and melanoma, where early detection significantly influences treatment outcomes and patient prognosis.

5. **Confusion Matrix**: In the context of skin cancer diagnosis, a confusion matrix is a useful tool to visualize the performance of a classification model. It provides a comprehensive breakdown of the classification outcomes by displaying the number of true positives, true negatives, false positives, and false negatives. Here's what each term means in the context of skin cancer diagnosis:
    a) **True Positives (TP)**: Cases where the model correctly identifies the presence of skin cancer.
    b) **True Negatives (TN)**: Cases where the model correctly identifies the absence of skin cancer.
    c) **False Positives (FP)**: Cases where the model incorrectly identifies the presence of skin cancer (also known as Type I error).
    d) **False Negatives (FN)**: Cases where the model incorrectly identifies the absence of skin cancer (also known as Type II error).

6. **ROC-Curve:** The ROC (Receiver Operating Characteristic) curve is a graphical representation that illustrates the diagnostic ability of a binary classifier system as its discrimination threshold is varied. The ROC curve plots two parameters:
    - **True Positive Rate (TPR)** or **Sensitivity**: The proportion of actual positive cases (skin cancer) that are correctly identified by the model.

- **False Positive Rate (FPR)**: The proportion of actual negative cases (non-cancerous) that are incorrectly identified as positive by the model.

Here's how the ROC curve is interpreted in the context of skin cancer diagnosis:

a) **TPR (Sensitivity)**: This measures how well the model correctly identifies patients with skin cancer. A higher TPR indicates that the model is more effective in detecting skin cancer cases.
b) **FPR**: This measures the rate at which the model incorrectly identifies non-cancerous cases as skin cancer. A lower FPR indicates fewer false alarms, meaning the model is more specific.
c) **Diagonal Line**: An ROC curve that runs along the diagonal line (from the bottom-left corner to the top-right corner) represents a random guess. The closer the ROC curve is to the top-left corner, the better the model's performance.
d) **Area Under the Curve (AUC)**: The AUC provides a single measure of overall model performance. An AUC of 1.0 represents a perfect model, while an AUC of 0.5 represents a model that performs no better than random guessing. For skin cancer diagnosis, a higher AUC indicates a better-performing model.

Healthcare professionals and machine learning practitioners can enhance patient care and treatment decision-making by closely evaluating these measures to gain a better understanding of and improvement in the models' diagnostic performance on skin cancer.

RESULTS AND DISCUSSION

The Results and Discussion section of the study presents experiments, analyses, and conclusions, highlighting key findings and patterns. It critically assesses the study's methodology, examining its strengths and weaknesses. The discussion is divided into two parts: the experiment using original images and the one with augmented images, allowing for a detailed evaluation of how augmentation affects model performance. This approach underscores the importance of using augmented images to address the challenges of an imbalanced original dataset.

Focusing on skin cancer classification, the study reveals that image augmentation significantly enhances the accuracy of classification models. Key strengths include detailed preprocessing and robust training protocols. The findings emphasize the potential of advanced image processing techniques, particularly image augmentation and machine learning algorithms, to improve diagnostic tools for skin cancer.

Overall, the study highlights the effectiveness of these methodologies in enhancing the reliability of skin cancer diagnosis.

Experiment on the Original Skin Cancer Images with Color Histogram

This section displays the classification report that was produced by using Random Forest for classification and Color Histogram for feature extraction on the original Skin Cancer dataset images. A comprehensive overview of these findings is provided in Table 1, and the model's confusion matrix and receiver operating characteristic (ROC) curve are shown visually in Figures 5 and 6, respectively. It is important to note the various abbreviations for the different types of skin cancer which are; Actinic keratoses (akiec), basal cell carcinoma (bcc), benign keratosis lesions (bkl), dermatofibroma (df), melanoma (mel), melanocytic nevi (nv), and vascular lesions (vasc).

Table 1. Classification Report of the Experiment on the Original Skin Cancer Images with Color Histogram

	Precision	Recall	F1-Score	Support
akiec	0.75	0.09	0.16	67
bcc	0.70	0.19	0.30	109
bkl	0.61	0.25	0.35	223
df	0.00	0.00	0.00	20
mel	0.66	0.26	0.37	217
nv	0.74	0.98	0.84	1331
vasc	1.00	0.36	0.53	36
accuracy			0.73	2003
macro avg	0.64	0.31	0.37	2003
Weighted avg	0.71	0.73	0.67	2003

As depicted in Table 1, the model's performance varies across different classes, revealing both strengths and weaknesses. For the akiec (Actinic keratoses) class, the model demonstrates some capability, achieving a precision of 0.75, indicating that 75% of the instances predicted as akiec were correct. However, the recall is notably low at 0.09, meaning that only 9% of the actual akiec cases were correctly identified. The F1-score of 0.16 reflects the imbalance between precision and recall, highlighting that the model missed a substantial portion of the 67 actual akiec instances in the dataset.

In the case of the bcc (Basal cell carcinoma) class, the model exhibits moderate performance. With a precision of 0.70, it correctly predicts 70% of the instances labeled as bcc. However, the recall remains low at 0.19, indicating that the model identified only 19% of the actual bcc cases, resulting in an F1-score of 0.30. There are 109 actual instances of bcc in the dataset, and while the model captures some, it still misses a significant number.

For the bkl (Benign keratosis-like lesions) class, the model shows a precision of 0.61, suggesting that about 61% of the instances predicted as bkl are correct. However, the recall is low at 0.25, meaning the model correctly identified only 25% of the actual bkl cases, leading to an F1-score of 0.35. There are 223 actual bkl instances in the dataset, indicating that the model still overlooks a considerable number.

Performance is particularly poor for the df (Dermatofibroma) class, where the model's precision and recall are both 0.00. This indicates that it failed to correctly predict any of the 20 actual df instances in the dataset, resulting in an F1-score of 0.00.

The mel (Melanoma) class shows a precision of 0.66, indicating that 66% of the instances predicted as mel were correct. However, the recall is only 0.26, showing that the model identified just 26% of the actual mel cases, with an F1-score of 0.37. There are 217 actual instances of mel, and like other classes, many cases go undetected.

In contrast, the model excels with the nv (Melanocytic nevi) class, achieving a precision of 0.74 and a remarkable recall of 0.98. This means that 74% of the instances predicted as nv were correct, and the model accurately identified 98% of the actual nv cases. The F1-score is 0.84, indicating strong overall performance, supported by the 1,331 actual instances of nv in the dataset.

For the vasc (Vascular lesions) class, the model achieves a perfect precision of 1.00, meaning all predictions for this class were correct. However, the recall is lower at 0.36, indicating that the model identified only 36% of the actual vasc cases, resulting in an F1-score of 0.53. With 36 actual vasc instances, the model is accurate but still misses some.

Overall, the model's accuracy is 0.73, indicating that 73% of all instances in the dataset were correctly classified. The macro average precision is 0.64, recall is 0.31, and F1-score is 0.37, reflecting general performance across all types without considering class support. The weighted average precision is 0.71, recall is 0.73, and F1-score is 0.67, taking into account the number of instances in each class. This underscores significant disparities in performance across different classes, highlighting the need to address class imbalance for improved uniformity in the model's performance.

Figure 5. Confusion Matrix of the Experiment on the Original Skin Cancer Images with Color Histogram

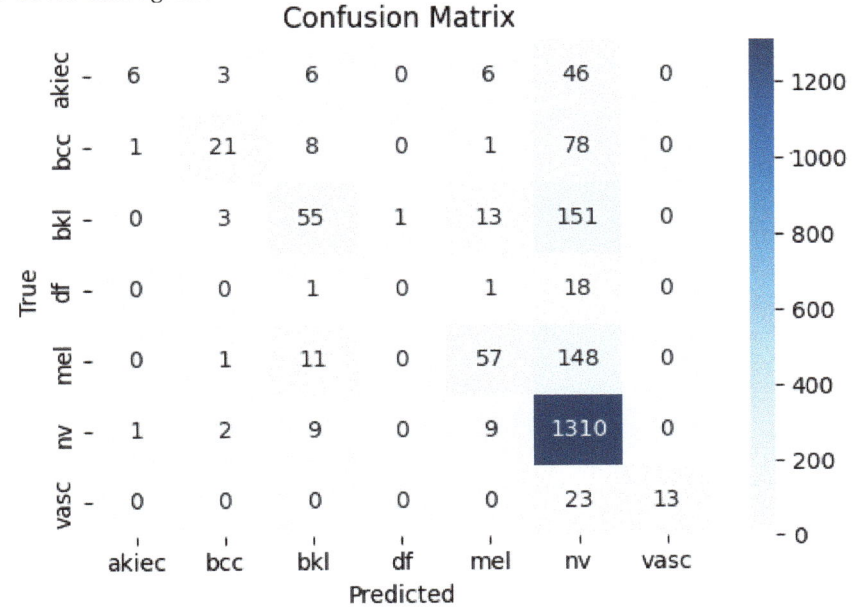

True \ Predicted	akiec	bcc	bkl	df	mel	nv	vasc
akiec	6	3	6	0	6	46	0
bcc	1	21	8	0	1	78	0
bkl	0	3	55	1	13	151	0
df	0	0	1	0	1	18	0
mel	0	1	11	0	57	148	0
nv	1	2	9	0	9	1310	0
vasc	0	0	0	0	0	23	13

The confusion matrix in Figure 5 illustrates the performance of the random forest classifier on a test dataset for various skin lesions: Actinic keratoses (akiec), Basal cell carcinoma (bcc), Benign keratosis-like lesions (bkl), Dermatofibroma (df), Melanoma (mel), Melanocytic nevi (nv), and Vascular lesions (vasc). Rows indicate actual classes (true labels), while columns show predicted classes. Diagonal cells represent correct predictions, while off-diagonal cells denote misclassifications.

The classifier correctly identified 6 instances of akiec, but misclassified others as bcc, bkl, mel, and nv. For bcc, 21 instances were accurately classified, though many were misidentified as nv. The matrix reveals that the classifier performs well on classes with more instances, like nv, with 1,310 correct predictions out of 1,332. However, it struggles with minority classes like akiec and mel, with many misclassified as nv.

This performance highlights a class imbalance, as akiec is misclassified as nv in 46 instances and as bcc in 78 instances. Similar misclassifications occur for bkl and mel. These insights suggest that addressing class imbalance through data augmentation for minority classes may enhance the classifier's performance. Overall, the confusion matrix provides valuable insights into model strengths and weaknesses, guiding further refinement steps.

Figure 6. ROC Curve of the Experiment on the Original Skin Cancer Images with Color Histogram

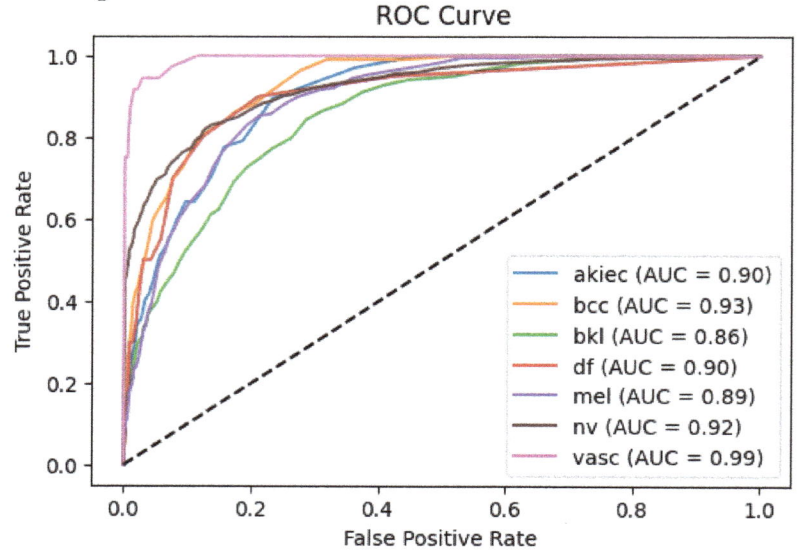

Experiment on the Original Skin Cancer Images with Gray Level Co-occurrence Matrix (GLCM)

This section presents the classification report generated from the original Skin Cancer dataset images using GLCM for feature extraction and Random Forest for classification. Table 2 presents a detailed summary of these results. Figures 7 and 8 visually represent the model's confusion matrix and receiver operating characteristic (ROC) curve, respectively.

Table 2. Classification Report of the Experiment on the Original Skin Cancer Images with Gray Level Co-occurrence Matrix (GLCM)

	Precision	Recall	F1-Score	Support
akiec	0.06	0.01	0.02	70
bcc	0.29	0.09	0.13	104
bkl	0.35	0.15	0.21	224
df	0.00	0.00	0.00	16
mel	0.49	0.17	0.25	221
nv	0.71	0.95	0.82	1332

	Precision	Recall	F1-Score	Support
vasc	0.50	0.06	0.10	36
accuracy			0.68	2003
macro avg	0.34	0.20	0.22	2003
Weighted avg	0.59	0.68	0.60	2003

As shown in Table 2, the model's performance on the akiec class is notably poor, with a precision of 0.06, meaning only 6% of instances predicted as akiec were correct. The recall is even lower at 0.01, indicating the model identified just 1% of actual akiec cases. The F1-score of 0.02 reflects a significant imbalance between precision and recall. There are 70 actual instances of akiec in the dataset, with many missed by the model.

For the bcc class, performance remains limited, with a precision of 0.29, meaning 29% of instances predicted as bcc were correct. The recall is only 0.09, revealing that the model correctly identified just 9% of actual bcc cases. With an F1-score of 0.13, the overall performance for bcc is low, as there are 104 actual instances of bcc, and many were missed.

The model shows low precision of 0.35 for the bkl class, indicating that about 35% of instances predicted as bkl were correct. The recall is 0.15, demonstrating that the model identified 15% of actual bkl cases, leading to an F1-score of 0.21. There are 224 actual instances of bkl in the dataset, with many missed by the model.

Performance for the df class is very poor, with precision and recall at 0.00, indicating the model did not correctly predict any instances of this class. With an F1-score of 0.00, the model's overall performance here is extremely low, as there are 16 actual instances of df, but none were predicted correctly.

The mel class has a precision of 0.49, indicating that 49% of instances predicted as mel were correct. The recall is 0.17, showing that the model identified 17% of actual mel cases. The F1-score of 0.25 reflects poor performance, similar to bkl. There are 221 actual instances of mel, and many cases are missed.

In contrast, the model performs well on the nv class, with a precision of 0.71 and a recall of 0.95. This means 71% of instances predicted as nv were correct, and the model identified 95% of actual nv cases. The F1-score of 0.82 indicates high overall performance, with 1,332 actual instances of nv in the dataset.

For the vasc class, precision is 0.50, indicating that 50% of instances predicted as vasc were correct, while the recall is 0.06, revealing that only 6% of actual vasc cases were identified. The F1-score is 0.10, reflecting poor performance, with 36 actual instances of vasc in the dataset.

Overall, the model achieves an accuracy of 0.68, correctly classifying 68% of all instances. The macro average precision is 0.34, recall is 0.20, and F1-score is 0.22, indicating the need to address class imbalance to enhance uniform performance across all classes.

Figure 7 Confusion Matrix of the Experiment on the Original Skin Cancer Images with Gray Level Co-occurrence Matrix (GLCM)

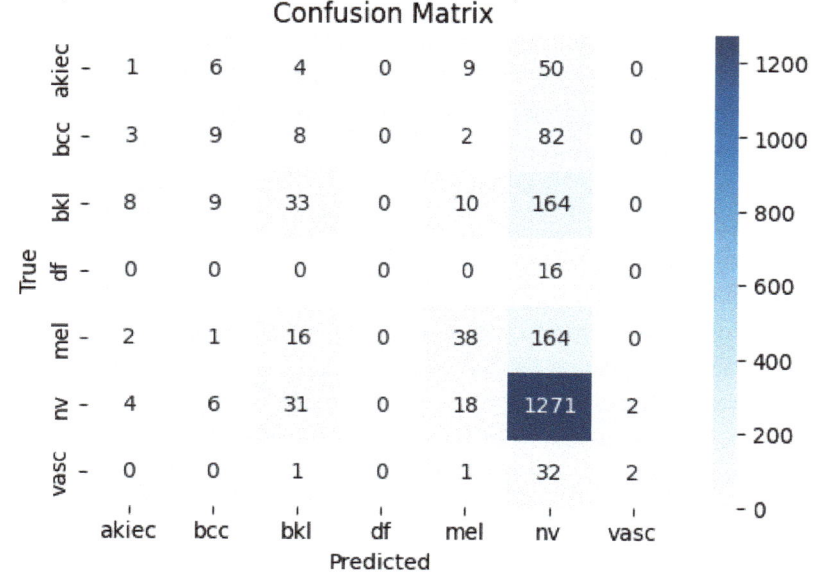

Confusion Matrix

True \ Predicted	akiec	bcc	bkl	df	mel	nv	vasc
akiec	1	6	4	0	9	50	0
bcc	3	9	8	0	2	82	0
bkl	8	9	33	0	10	164	0
df	0	0	0	0	0	16	0
mel	2	1	16	0	38	164	0
nv	4	6	31	0	18	1271	2
vasc	0	0	1	0	1	32	2

The confusion matrix in Figure 7 illustrates the performance of the random forest classifier on a test dataset of skin lesions, including Actinic keratoses (akiec), Basal cell carcinoma (bcc), Benign keratosis-like lesions (bkl), Dermatofibroma (df), Melanoma (mel), Melanocytic nevi (nv), and Vascular lesions (vasc). The matrix shows actual classes in rows and predicted classes in columns, with diagonal cells indicating correct predictions and off-diagonal cells representing misclassifications.

For akiec, the classifier accurately classified 1 instance but misclassified others as bcc, bkl, mel, and nv. The model correctly identified 9 instances of bcc, though many were misclassified as nv. It correctly classified 33 instances of bkl, with some misclassified as akiec, bcc, mel, and nv. The df class had no correct classifications, while the classifier correctly identified 38 mel instances, misclassifying many as nv. It performed well on nv, with 1,271 correct predictions, but struggled with vasc, correctly identifying only 2 instances.

This matrix reveals significant performance issues; the model excels with abundant classes like nv but struggles with minority classes like akiec and mel, indicating class imbalance. For instance, akiec is misclassified as nv in 50 instances. To enhance performance, addressing class imbalance through data augmentation for minority classes is recommended. Overall, the confusion matrix provides valuable insights for refining the classifier.

Figure 8 ROC Curve of the Experiment on the Original Skin Cancer Images with Gray Level Co-occurrence Matrix (GLCM)

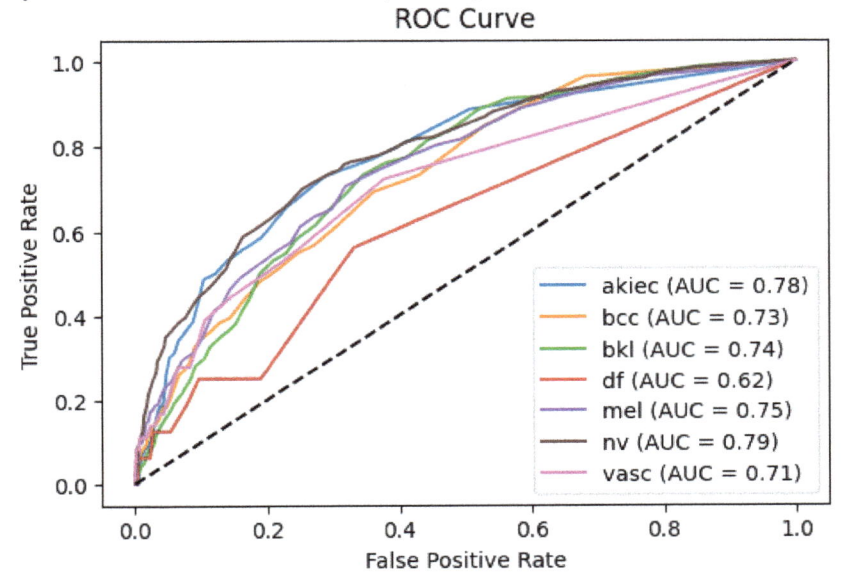

Experiment on the Augmented Skin Cancer Images with Color Histogram

This section displays the classification report from the augmented images in the Skin Cancer dataset. A Random Forest was utilized for image classification, and a Color Histogram was employed to extract features. To address the issue of data imbalance from the original dataset, a set of 2000 images was generated using image augmentation from the original skin cancer images. Table 3 provides a detailed explanation of these findings. Figures 9 and 10 graphically depict the model's receiver operating characteristic (ROC) curve and confusion matrix, respectively.

Table 3. Classification Report of the Experiment on the Augmented Skin Cancer Images with Color Histogram

	Precision	Recall	F1-Score	Support
akiec	0.97	0.98	0.98	400
bcc	0.95	0.96	0.96	400
bkl	0.97	0.94	0.95	400
df	0.99	1.00	1.00	400
mel	0.93	0.94	0.93	400
nv	0.94	0.94	0.94	400
vasc	0.99	0.08	0.99	400
accuracy			0.96	2800
macro avg	0.96	0.96	0.96	2800
Weighted avg	0.96	0.96	0.96	2800

As depicted in Table 3, the model's performance for the akiec class is exceptional, with a precision of 0.97, indicating that 97% of the instances predicted as akiec were correct. The recall is 0.98, meaning the model correctly identified 98% of actual akiec cases, and the F1-score is 0.98, reflecting an excellent balance between precision and recall. With 400 actual instances of akiec in the dataset, the model missed very few.

For the bcc class, the model also shows excellent performance, achieving a precision of 0.95 and a recall of 0.96. The F1-score remains high at 0.96, indicating that the model identified most of the 400 actual instances of bcc correctly.

The model exhibits a high precision of 0.97 for the bkl class, meaning about 97% of the predicted instances were correct, with a recall of 0.94. The F1-score is 0.95, reflecting strong performance, and the model accurately captured most of the 400 actual bkl instances.

For the df class, performance is outstanding, with a precision of 0.99 and a recall of 1.00, indicating almost perfect predictions. The model correctly predicted all 400 actual instances of df, resulting in an F1-score of 1.00.

In the mel class, the precision is 0.93, and the recall is 0.94, showing that the model correctly identified 94% of actual mel cases. With an F1-score of 0.93, the performance remains high, accurately identifying most of the 400 actual instances.

The model performs very well on the nv class, achieving a precision of 0.94 and a recall of 0.94. This means it correctly identified 94% of the 400 actual nv instances, with an F1-score of 0.94.

For the vasc class, the precision is 0.99, indicating that 99% of predicted instances were correct, but the recall is only 0.08, showing the model identified only 8% of actual vasc cases. This results in an F1-score of 0.99, reflecting excellent precision but poor recall.

Overall, the model achieves an accuracy of 0.96, meaning 96% of all instances in the dataset were correctly classified. The macro average precision, recall, and F1-score are all 0.96, indicating strong performance across classes. However, there is still room for improvement, particularly in the vasc class, to achieve more uniform performance across all types.

Figure 9. Confusion Matrix of the Experiment on the Augmented Skin Cancer Images with Color Histogram

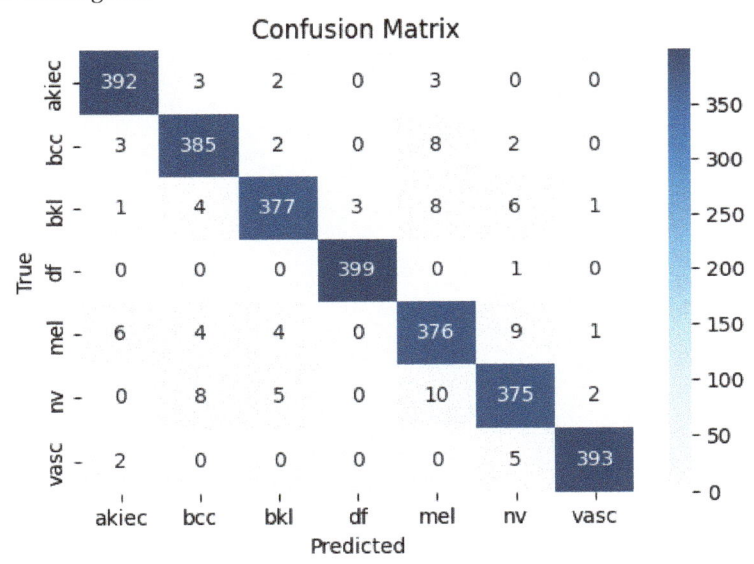

	akiec	bcc	bkl	df	mel	nv	vasc
akiec	392	3	2	0	3	0	0
bcc	3	385	2	0	8	2	0
bkl	1	4	377	3	8	6	1
df	0	0	0	399	0	1	0
mel	6	4	4	0	376	9	1
nv	0	8	5	0	10	375	2
vasc	2	0	0	0	0	5	393

The confusion matrix in Figure 9 details the random forest classifier's performance on a test dataset. The rows represent actual classes (True labels), while the columns represent predicted classes for various skin lesions: Actinic keratoses (akiec), Basal cell carcinoma (bcc), Benign keratosis-like lesions (bkl), Dermatofibroma (df), Melanoma (mel), Melanocytic nevi (nv), and Vascular lesions (vasc).

The classifier correctly classified 392 instances of akiec but misclassified others as bcc, bkl, and mel. For bcc, 385 instances were accurately classified, with some misidentified as nv. The model correctly identified 377 instances of bkl, but a few were misclassified as akiec, bcc, mel, and nv. For df, it classified 399 instances correctly, with only one misclassification as mel. In mel, 376 instances were correctly classified, but some were misidentified as nv. The classifier also performed well on nv with 375 correct predictions, though some were misclassified as bkl and mel. For vasc, 393 instances were accurately classified, with a few misclassifications as bkl and nv.

Overall, while the classifier excels in identifying df and nv, it struggles with classes like akiec and mel, suggesting there are subtle differences not effectively captured. These insights indicate that the classifier is generally effective but still has room for improvement, particularly in refining its identification of certain classes.

Figure 10. ROC Curve of the Experiment on the Augmented Skin Cancer Images with Color Histogram

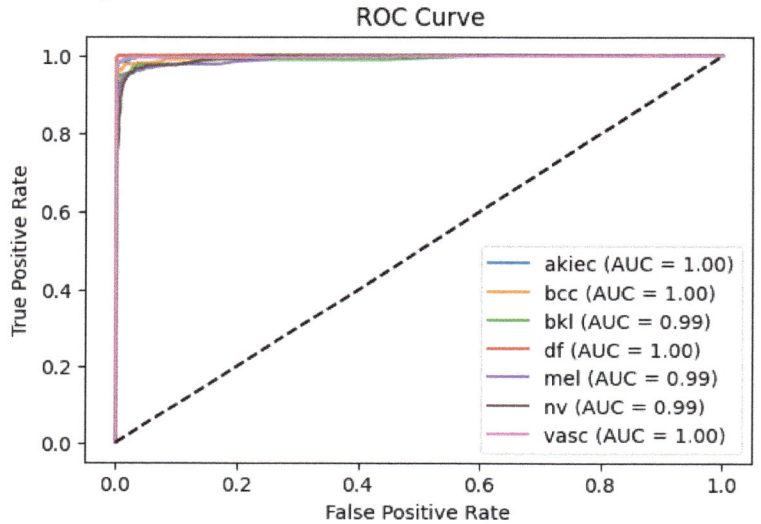

Experiment on the Augmented Skin Cancer Images with Gray Level Co-occurrence Matrix (GLCM)

The Skin Cancer dataset's augmented images' classification report is shown in this section. For image classification, a Random Forest was used, and features were extracted using a Gray Level Co-occurrence Matrix (GLCM). Using image augmentation from the original skin cancer images, a collection of 2000 images was created to address the problem of data imbalance from the original dataset. Table 4 offers a thorough explanation of these results. The receiver operating characteristic (ROC) curve and confusion matrix of the model are shown visually in Figures 11 and 12, respectively.

Table 4. Classification Report of the Experiment on the Augmented Skin Cancer Images with Gray Level Co-occurrence Matrix (GLCM)

	Precision	**Recall**	**F1-Score**	**Support**
akiec	0.96	0.97	0.96	400
bcc	0.95	0.96	0.96	400
bkl	0.97	0.94	0.95	400
df	0.99	1.00	1.00	400
mel	0.96	0.96	0.96	400
nv	0.97	0.96	0.97	400
vasc	0.98	0.09	0.99	400
accuracy			0.97	2800
macro avg	0.97	0.97	0.97	2800
Weighted avg	0.97	0.97	0.97	2800

As depicted in Table 4, the model's performance for the akiec class is exceptional. The precision is 0.96, indicating that 96% of the instances predicted as akiec were correct. The recall is 0.97, meaning the model correctly identified 97% of the actual akiec cases. The F1-score is 0.96, reflecting an excellent balance between precision and recall, with 400 actual instances of akiec in the dataset and very few missed.

For the bcc class, the model also shows excellent performance. The precision is 0.95, meaning that 95% of the instances predicted as bcc were correct. The recall is 0.96, indicating that the model correctly identified 96% of the actual bcc cases. With an F1-score of 0.96, the overall performance for bcc remains high, identifying most of the 400 actual instances accurately.

The model exhibits a high precision of 0.97 for the bkl class, meaning about 97% of the instances predicted as bkl were correct. The recall is 0.94, showing that the model identified 94% of the actual bkl cases. The F1-score is 0.95, reflecting strong performance with 400 actual instances captured accurately.

For the df class, the performance is outstanding, with a precision of 0.99 and a recall of 1.00, indicating the model correctly predicted almost all instances. With an F1-score of 1.00, the model's overall performance is nearly perfect, successfully predicting all 400 actual instances of df.

The mel class has a precision of 0.96, indicating that 96% of the instances predicted as mel were correct. The recall is also 0.96, showing that the model correctly identified 96% of the actual mel cases. The F1-score is 0.96, reflecting high performance similar to other classes, with accurate identification of the 400 instances.

The model performs very well on the nv class, achieving a precision of 0.97 and a recall of 0.96. This means that 97% of the instances predicted as nv were correct, and the model correctly identified 96% of the actual nv cases. The F1-score is 0.97, indicating high overall performance, effectively identifying these 400 instances.

For the vasc class, the precision is 0.98, indicating that 98% of the instances predicted as vasc were correct. However, the recall is low at 0.09, showing that the model identified only 9% of the actual vasc cases. The F1-score is 0.99, reflecting excellent precision but poor recall. With 400 actual instances, the model makes accurate predictions but still misses many.

The overall accuracy of the model is 0.97, indicating that 97% of all instances in the dataset were correctly classified. The macro average precision, recall, and F1-score are all 0.97, reflecting the model's general performance across all classes. The weighted average metrics are also 0.97, illustrating the model's strong performance across the dataset. While the model performs exceptionally well overall, there remains room for improvement in certain classes, particularly the vasc class, to achieve more uniform performance.

Figure 11 Confusion Matrix of the Experiment on the Augmented Skin Cancer Images with Gray level Occurrence Matrix (GLCM)

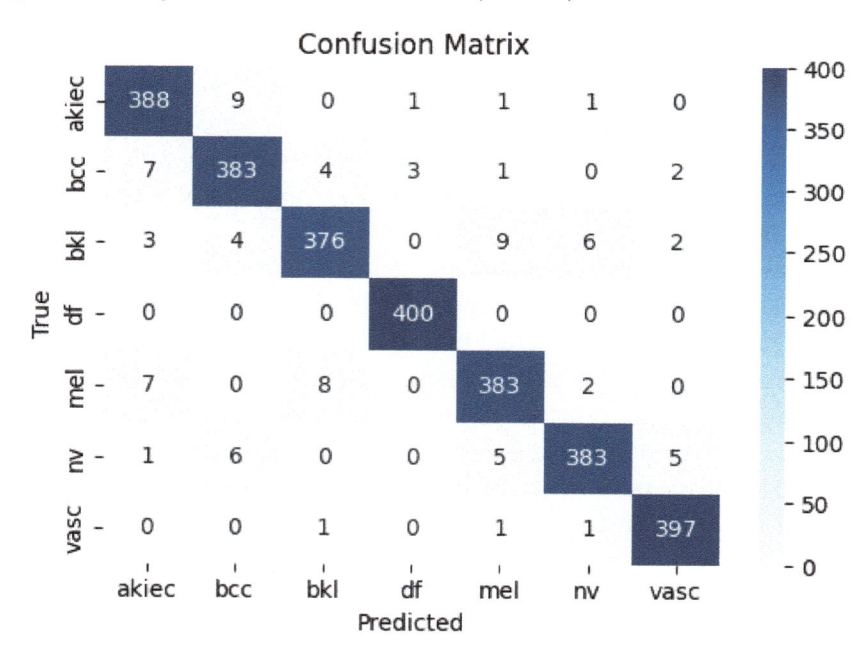

The confusion matrix in Figure 11 provides a detailed overview of the random forest classifier's performance on a test dataset. Rows represent actual classes (true labels), while columns represent predicted classes, which include various skin lesions: Actinic keratoses (akiec), Basal cell carcinoma (bcc), Benign keratosis-like lesions (bkl), Dermatofibroma (df), Melanoma (mel), Melanocytic nevi (nv), and Vascular lesions (vasc). Each cell shows the number of instances predicted for each class, with diagonal cells indicating correct predictions and off-diagonal cells representing misclassifications.

For akiec, the classifier correctly identified 388 instances but misclassified some as bcc, bkl, and mel. The model classified 383 bcc instances accurately but made errors, particularly misclassifying some as nv. It identified 376 bkl instances correctly, with some misclassifications as akiec, bcc, mel, and nv. The model excelled in df classification, correctly identifying all 400 instances without errors. For mel, 383 instances were accurately classified, but some were misclassified as nv. The classifier also performed well on nv, with 383 correct predictions, though some were misidentified as bkl and mel. For vasc, the model correctly classified 397 instances, with minimal misclassifications.

While the classifier performs well on most classes, including df and vasc, it struggles with akiec and mel, suggesting the need for improvements. The confusion matrix offers valuable insights into the model's strengths and areas needing enhancement, guiding future refinements.

Figure 12. ROC Curve of the Experiment on the Augmented Skin Cancer Images with Gray level Occurrence Matrix (GLCM)

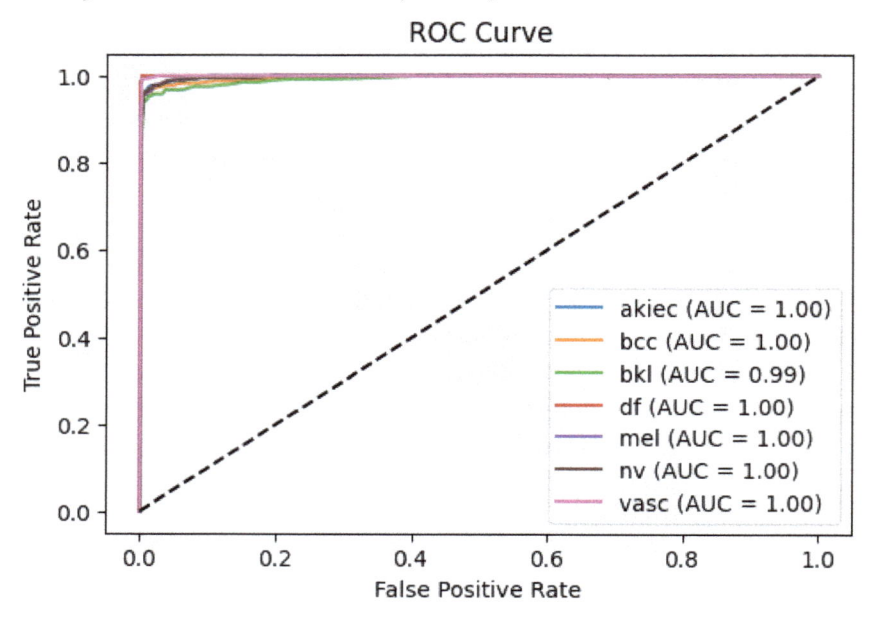

CONCLUSION AND RECOMMENDATION

Based on the evaluation of the four models, distinct performance trends emerge. The model using Original Skin Cancer Images with Color Histogram shows mixed results, particularly struggling with recall for akiec, bcc, bkl, df, and mel classes, while achieving strong precision and recall for nv and vasc classes. Conversely, the Original Skin Cancer Images with Gray Level Co-occurrence Matrix (GLCM) model performs poorly across all classes, indicating significant room for improvement.

The Augmented Skin Cancer Images with Color Histogram model excels, achieving high precision and recall for akiec, bcc, bkl, and mel, resulting in an overall accuracy of 96%. Similarly, the Augmented Skin Cancer Images with GLCM model shows robust performance, with high precision and recall across most classes, achieving an overall accuracy of 97%.

To enhance skin cancer image classification models, several approaches are recommended. First, improving augmentation techniques is crucial for diversifying the dataset, which can help models generalize better. Second, addressing class imbalance through oversampling minority classes or using class weights during training can ensure that all types of skin lesions are accurately classified.

Third, refining algorithms for better feature capture, such as utilizing advanced feature extraction methods tailored to dermatological images, is essential. Lastly, rigorous validation across diverse datasets is vital to assess model robustness and generalizability in real-world clinical settings. In Implementing these recommendations can advance skin cancer detection technology, leading to more accurate and clinically applicable models for healthcare professionals.

REFERENCES

Ahmed, B., Qadir, M. I., & Ghafoor, S. (2020). Malignant melanoma: Skin cancer—diagnosis, prevention, and treatment. *Critical Reviews™ in Eukaryotic Gene Expression, 30*(4).

Aljohani, K., & Turki, T. (2022). Automatic classification of melanoma skin cancer with deep convolutional neural networks. *AI, 3*(2), 512–525. DOI: 10.3390/ai3020029

Alowais, S. A., Alghamdi, S. S., Alsuhebany, N., Alqahtani, T., Alshaya, A. I., Almohareb, S. N., Aldairem, A., Alrashed, M., Bin Saleh, K., Badreldin, H. A., Al Yami, M. S., Al Harbi, S., & Albekairy, A. M. (2023). Revolutionizing healthcare: The role of artificial intelligence in clinical practice. *BMC Medical Education, 23*(1), 689. DOI: 10.1186/s12909-023-04698-z PMID: 37740191

Barthelmann, S., Butsch, F., Lang, B. M., Stege, H., Großmann, B., Schepler, H., & Grabbe, S. (2023). Seborrheic keratosis. *JDDG: Journal der Deutschen Dermatologischen Gesellschaft, 21*(3), 265–277. DOI: 10.1111/1346-8138.16754 PMID: 36892019

Bassel, A., Abdulkareem, A. B., Alyasseri, Z. A. A., Sani, N. S., & Mohammed, H. J. (2022). Automatic malignant and benign skin cancer classification using a hybrid deep learning approach. *Diagnostics (Basel), 12*(10), 2472. DOI: 10.3390/diagnostics12102472 PMID: 36292161

Bazgir, E., Haque, E., Maniruzzaman, M., & Hoque, R. (2024). Skin cancer classification using Inception Network. *World Journal of Advanced Research and Reviews, 21*(2), 839–849. DOI: 10.30574/wjarr.2024.21.2.0500

Bokori, S. A. B. A. J., & Mitani, Y. (2024, January). Skin cancer prediction using convolutional neural network. In *2024 2nd International Conference on Computer Graphics and Image Processing (CGIP)* (pp. 1–5). IEEE. https://doi.org/DOI: 10.1109/CGIP55857.2024.00009

BuiltIn. (n.d.). Random forest classifier in Python. Retrieved July 3, 2024, from https://builtin.com/data-science/random-forest-python-deep-dive

Chaturvedi, S. S., Gupta, K., & Prasad, P. S. (2021). Skin lesion analyser: An efficient seven-way multi-class skin cancer classification using MobileNet. In *Advanced Machine Learning Technologies and Applications: Proceedings of AMLTA 2020* (pp. 165–176). Springer Singapore. https://doi.org/DOI: 10.1007/978-981-16-0186-5_15

Cives, M., Mannavola, F., Lospalluti, L., Sergi, M. C., Cazzato, G., Filoni, E., Cavallo, F., Giudice, G., Stucci, L. S., Porta, C., & Tucci, M. (2020). Non-melanoma skin cancers: Biological and clinical features. *International Journal of Molecular Sciences*, 21(15), 5394. DOI: 10.3390/ijms21155394 PMID: 32751327

Cleveland Clinic. (n.d.). Skin cancer. Retrieved June 29, 2024, from https://my.clevelandclinic.org/health/diseases/15818-skin-cancer

El Achi, H., & Khoury, J. D. (2020). Artificial intelligence and digital microscopy applications in diagnostic hematopathology. *Cancers (Basel)*, 12(4), 797. DOI: 10.3390/cancers12040797 PMID: 32224980

Fania, L., Didona, D., Morese, R., Campana, I., Coco, V., Di Pietro, F. R., Ricci, F., Pallotta, S., Candi, E., Abeni, D., & Dellambra, E. (2020). Basal cell carcinoma: From pathophysiology to novel therapeutic approaches. *Biomedicines*, 8(11), 449. DOI: 10.3390/biomedicines8110449 PMID: 33113965

Forsyth, D. A., & Ponce, J. (2003). *Computer Vision: A Modern Approach*. Prentice Hall.

Fraiwan, M., & Faouri, E. (2022). On the automatic detection and classification of skin cancer using deep transfer learning. *Sensors (Basel)*, 22(13), 4963. DOI: 10.3390/s22134963 PMID: 35808463

Gonzalez, R. C., & Woods, R. E. (2008). *Digital Image Processing* (3rd ed.). Prentice Hall.

Hafner, C., & Vogt, T. (2008). Seborrheic keratosis. *Journal der Deutschen Dermatologischen Gesellschaft*, 6(8), 664–677. DOI: 10.1111/j.1610-0387.2008.06788.x PMID: 18801147

Haralick, R. M., Shanmugam, K., & Dinstein, I. H. (1973). Textural features for image classification. *. IEEE Transactions on Systems, Man, and Cybernetics*, SMC-3(6), 610–621. DOI: 10.1109/TSMC.1973.4309314

Heibel, H. D., Hooey, L., & Cockerell, C. J. (2020). A review of noninvasive techniques for skin cancer detection in dermatology. *American Journal of Clinical Dermatology*, 21(4), 513–524. DOI: 10.1007/s40257-020-00517-z PMID: 32383142

Islam, M. S., & Panta, S. (2024). Skin cancer images classification using transfer learning techniques. *arXiv preprint arXiv:2406.12954*. https://doi.org//arXiv.2406.12954DOI: 10.48550

Ismail, M. A., Hameed, N., & Clos, J. (2021). Deep learning-based algorithm for skin cancer classification. In *Proceedings of International Conference on Trends in Computational and Cognitive Engineering: Proceedings of TCCE 2020* (pp. 709–719). Springer Singapore. DOI: 10.1007/978-981-33-4673-4_58

Janda, M., Cust, A. E., Neale, R. E., & Smith, K. (2015). Cancer epidemiology and prevention. *Australian Family Physician*, 44(1), 16–20. https://www.racgp.org.au

Jayeb, A. W., Hore, A. R., Anjum, R., Sadeque, S. S., & Auqib, S. T. (2022). *Computer vision based skin disease detection using machine learning* (Doctoral dissertation, Brac University).

Jutzi, T. B., Krieghoff-Henning, E. I., Holland-Letz, T., Utikal, J. S., Hauschild, A., Schadendorf, D., Sondermann, W., Fröhling, S., Hekler, A., Schmitt, M., Maron, R. C., & Brinker, T. J. (2020). Artificial intelligence in skin cancer diagnostics: The patients' perspective. *Frontiers in Medicine*, 7, 233. DOI: 10.3389/fmed.2020.00233 PMID: 32671078

Kavitha, C., Priyanka, S., Kumar, M. P., & Kusuma, V. (2024). Skin cancer detection and classification using deep learning techniques. *Procedia Computer Science*, 235, 2793–2802. DOI: 10.1016/j.procs.2024.04.264

Kumar, A., Satheesha, T. Y., Salvador, B. B. L., Mithileysh, S., & Ahmed, S. T. (2023). Augmented intelligence enabled deep neural networking (AuDNN) framework for skin cancer classification and prediction using multi-dimensional datasets on industrial IoT standards. *Microprocessors and Microsystems*, 97, 104755. Advance online publication. DOI: 10.1016/j.micpro.2023.104755

Mayo Clinic. (n.d.). *Skin cancer*. https://www.mayoclinic.org/diseases-conditions/skin-cancer/symptoms-causes/syc-20377605

Medical News Today. (2018, April 17). *What to know about dermatofibromas*. https://www.medicalnewstoday.com/articles/318870

Niculet, E., Craescu, M., Rebegea, L., Bobeica, C., Năstase, F., Lupa teanu, G., & Tatu, A. L. (2022). Basal cell carcinoma: Comprehensive clinical and histopathological aspects, novel imaging tools, and therapeutic approaches. *Experimental and Therapeutic Medicine*, 23(1), 1–8. DOI: 10.3892/etm.2021.11234 PMID: 34917186

Owida, H. A. (2022). Developments and clinical applications of noninvasive optical technologies for skin cancer diagnosis. *Journal of Skin Cancer*, 2022(1), 9218847. Advance online publication. DOI: 10.1155/2022/9218847 PMID: 36437851

Piccolo, V., Russo, T., Moscarella, E., Brancaccio, G., Alfano, R., & Argenziano, G. (2018). Dermatoscopy of vascular lesions. *Dermatologic Clinics*, 36(4), 389–395. DOI: 10.1016/j.det.2018.05.006 PMID: 30201148

Reinehr, C. P. H., & Bakos, R. M. (2020). Actinic keratoses: Review of clinical, dermoscopic, and therapeutic aspects. *Anais Brasileiros de Dermatologia*, 94(6), 637–657. DOI: 10.1016/j.abd.2019.10.004 PMID: 31789244

Shorten, C., & Khoshgoftaar, T. M. (2019). A survey on image data augmentation for deep learning. *Journal of Big Data*, 6(1), 1–48. DOI: 10.1186/s40537-019-0197-0

Siegel, R. L., Giaquinto, A. N., & Jemal, A. (2024). Cancer statistics, 2024. *CA: a Cancer Journal for Clinicians*, 74(1), 1–23. DOI: 10.3322/caac.21820 PMID: 38230766

Skin Cancer Foundation. (n.d.). *Skin cancer 101*. https://www.skincancer.org/skin-cancer-information/

Soglia, S., Pérez-Anker, J., Lobos Guede, N., Giavedoni, P., Puig, S., & Malvehy, J. (2022). Diagnostics using non-invasive technologies in dermatological oncology. *Cancers (Basel)*, 14(23), 5886. Advance online publication. DOI: 10.3390/cancers14235886 PMID: 36497368

Solano, F. (2020). Photoprotection and skin pigmentation: Melanin-related molecules and some other new agents obtained from natural sources. *Molecules (Basel, Switzerland)*, 25(7), 1537. DOI: 10.3390/molecules25071537 PMID: 32230973

Swain, M. J., & Ballard, D. H. (1991). Color indexing. *International Journal of Computer Vision*, 7(1), 11–32. DOI: 10.1007/BF00130487

Upadhyay, M., & Rawat, J. (2023). A review of recent machine learning techniques used for skin lesion image classification. *Advancements in Bio-Medical Image Processing and Authentication in Telemedicine*, 76–90.

Winge, M. C., Kellman, L. N., Guo, K., Tang, J. Y., Swetter, S. M., Aasi, S. Z., Sarin, K. Y., Chang, A. L. S., & Khavari, P. A. (2023). Advances in cutaneous squamous cell carcinoma. *Nature Reviews. Cancer*, 23(7), 430–449. DOI: 10.1038/s41568-023-00583-5 PMID: 37286893

Yale Medicine. (n.d.). *Melanocytic nevi (moles)*. https://www.yalemedicine.org/conditions/melanocytic-nevi-moles

Chapter 9
AI-Driven-IoT(AIIoT)-Based Decision Making in Kidney Diseases Patient Healthcare Monitoring:
KSK Approach for Kidney Monitoring

Kutubuddin Sayyad Liyakat Kazi
https://orcid.org/0000-0001-5623-9211
Brahmdevdada Mane Institute of Technology, Solapur, India

ABSTRACT

As artificial intelligence (AI) and the internet of things (IoT) continue to grow, the KSK approach is poised to revolutionize decision-making processes and make the world a more intelligent and efficient place. To fulfill the requirements of the task that is being proposed, this model was developed expressly for that purpose. During the classification process, these classifiers are utilized in the case of disease datasets, specifically in areas such as those that belong to kidney diseases. When it comes to determining how effectively the classifiers are functioning, there are three basic indicators that are taken into consideration. It is important to note that this is referring to the metrics of accuracy, precision, and recall. It is possible to acquire an accuracy rate that ranges from a minimum of 87% to a maximum of 92.5% for each and every illness by utilizing the proposed KSK approach.

DOI: 10.4018/979-8-3693-7277-7.ch009

INTRODUCTION

Kidney infections are a significant public health issue that affect millions of individuals around the globe. These kidney infections are caused by infectious diseases. According to the World Health Organization (WHO), kidney diseases contribute for around 2.4 million deaths that occur each year. For the purpose of successfully monitoring and managing these conditions, who may have a significant impact on an individual's general wellness and quality of life, it is vital to make use of the appropriate management strategies that have been developed by Pardeshi(2022a),(2022b).

Due to the fact that kidney illnesses affect millions of people worldwide, the healthcare profession is growing increasingly concerned with the particular issue said by Sultanabanu(2024p). There are a few of these diseases that are relatively benign, like urinary tract infections, whereas others can be more severe and have the potential to be fatal, like chronic kidney disease and kidney failure. Infections in the urinary tract are one example of these types of illnesses. In light of this reality, it is of the utmost importance for those who are experiencing kidney difficulties to receive relevant medical monitoring by Pradeepa(2022).

According to Kazi K(2024a), one of the key causes for the rising frequency of renal illnesses is the growing prevalence of risk factors like diabetes, high blood pressure, and obesity. This is one of the primary reasons. There are a number of conditions that can lead to the development of chronic renal disease, which is a condition that can cause damage to the kidneys over time. In the early stages of kidney diseases, it may be challenging to diagnose them since the signs may not be present. This is because kidney diseases might not show any symptoms. Early detection and treatment, on the opposite hand, might prove useful in preventing the progression of the condition if they are supplied with the necessary healthcare monitoring conducted by Priya(2023), Megha(2024), Kutubuddin (2023j)(2023i) and Kutubuddin(2023h).

An approach that incorporates multiple disciplines is applied in the process of monitoring healthcare for renal issues by Kazi K S(2024a), K Sayyad(2022a). Regular checks, blood tests, urine tests, monitoring of blood pressure, and imaging studies, as indicated in Figure 1, are all components of this method. The utilization of these tests allows for the monitoring of the functioning of the kidneys, and they also assist in the identification of any abnormalities that may be present. Patients who have renal disorders that have progressed to a more advanced stage may require additional tests, including glomerular filtration rate (GFR) and kidney biopsies, in order to guarantee that they receive the right monitoring and therapy. These tests are important in order to ensure that patients receive the appropriate care.

Checkups at regular intervals are especially important for patients who are suffering from kidney disease because they allow for the monitoring of the progression of the disease and the change of treatment options in accordance with the findings during the monitoring process. During these examinations, patients are also given the opportunity to convey any worries or symptoms that they may be experiencing. This provides medical professionals with the ability to provide care that is not only timely but also appropriate, as stated by K Sayyad (2023a), and Dixit (2015).

Blood tests are highly significant when it comes to monitoring kidney diseases since they help determine the degree of waste products, electrolytes, and additional substances which accumulate in the blood. This is because blood tests help determine the amounts of these things. The estimated glomerular filtration rate (eGFR), blood urea nitrogen (BUN), and serum creatinine are all tested that fall under this area. Other tests that fall under this category include the serum creatinine test. Because there is a chance that a surge in those levels is suggestive of kidney injury, more testing could be required in order to determine the extent of the damage that has already been done.

The monitoring method for renal health disorders also includes urine tests, which are an essential component of the healthcare monitoring process. The existence of protein, blood, and other abnormal substances in the urine, which may be discovered by these tests, may be an indication of renal damage. This is because these tests are able to discover these abnormal substances. The kidneys may be affected by infections or other conditions that may be contributing to kidney impairment. Urine tests can also be helpful in evaluating the degree to which the kidneys are being damaged by these circumstances.

Figure 1. Kidney Disease Critical Components

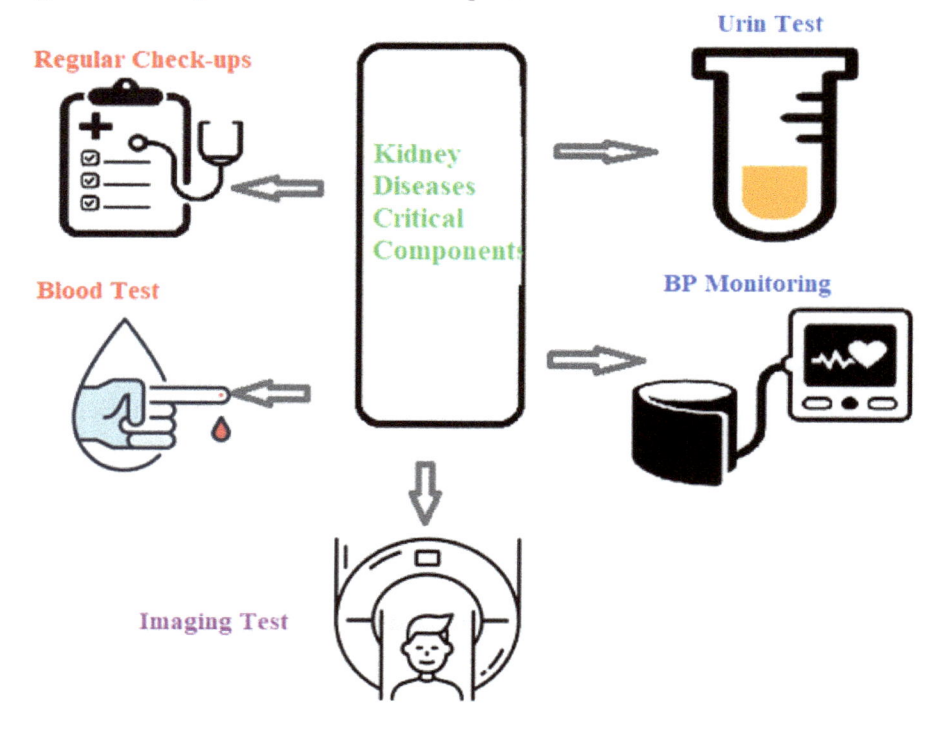

According to Shweta(2014)(2015) & Dixit(2015), the monitoring of blood pressure is of the utmost importance for patients whom are suffering from renal disorders. This is due to the fact that raised blood pressure can result in extra damage to the kidneys. Your healthcare provider will have the opportunity to assist you in controlling your blood pressure by modifying your medications or making improvements to your lifestyle if you check your blood pressure on a frequent basis by Dixit(2014). This will allow your healthcare provider to discover any changes that may occur.

Imaging tests such as computed tomography scans and ultrasounds are examples of the kinds of imaging tests that have utilized in the procedure of examining the anatomy and function of the kidneys. These tests can help in the identification of any abnormalities, like cysts or tumors that may be causing damage to the kidneys. The results of these tests can be particularly helpful in this regard.

In addition to the medical tests that have already been described, a further element of healthcare monitoring for renal illnesses is the education of patients about their condition and the tactics that may be used to manage it. This includes the treatment of pharmaceuticals in the appropriate manner, the modification of one's diet, and the implementation of a variety of lifestyle alterations. In addition, it is suggested that patients maintain an inventory of their ailments and convey any modifications to the medical personnel who are treating them. This recommendation was made by Kasat (2023), Liyakat, Sayyad (2024), Neeraja (2024), and Sayyad Liyakat (2024).

Furthermore, study revealed by Sultanabanu(2023n), with regard to the monitoring of renal disorders in the healthcare industry, technology has been a significant impact. Patients have become allowed to monitor their blood pressure, kidney function, and more vital signs from the comfort of their own homes thanks to the availability of a number of apps and devices. This is a substantial improvement over the previous situation. Not only does this make it feasible to monitor patients on a more regular basis, but it also makes it simpler for patients to have an active role in contributing to their own medical care.

As per K Sayyad(2024b), monitoring renal disorders with the assistance of medical specialists is, consequently, a crucial component in the management and treatment of such illnesses. When it comes to tracking the progression of the condition and making any necessary adjustments to treatment plans, it is essential to undergo imaging tests, blood tests, urine testing, blood pressure monitoring, and regular checks. These are all essential components. If they are monitored in a timely and suitable manner, patients who suffer from renal disorders have the ability to enhance their quality of life and minimize their risk of developing issues. This is because they are able to better manage their medical conditions.

When it comes to the management of renal disease, one of the most essential components is the ability to make judgments for the monitoring of patient healthcare. In order to provide the highest possible level of care and treatment, it is necessary to make decisions which are well-informed and centered on the patient's health, medical history, and any other pertinent concerns, as stated by Veena (2023) and Megha (2024).

There are a number of distinct components that are included in the decision-making process when that comes to the monitoring of patients who have renal problems by Liyakat(2025). These aspects include diagnosis, therapy, and follow-up care by Kutubuddin(2024c). The following is a list of significant parameters that are involved in this process and play a significant role by themselves:

1. *Accurate Diagnosis:* If you want to make judgments that are suitable, the first thing you need to do is make certain the diagnosis is accurate. There is a vast variety of medical problems that could be the cause of kidney diseases, and the symptoms of these conditions can differ from one individual to the next. In order to determine the severity of the problem and, more importantly, the root cause of the disease, it is very required to carry out complete medical assessments. Biopsies, blood tests, urine tests, imaging studies, and other diagnostic procedures must to be included in these examinations. As a result of this information, the decisions that need to be

taken concerning therapy and monitoring are significantly reliant on this information as said by Kutubuddin(2025b).

2. *Having a thorough understanding of the patient's medical history:* Every single patient is a single of a generous, and when it comes to making judgments, the medical history of the individual is an essential component to take into consideration. The medical history of a patient can provide valuable insights about the patient's health by revealing information such as previous treatments, any underlying ailments, and potential risk factors. These are just some of the things that can be gained from the patient's medical history. Another advantage that can be obtained from this is the identification of any patterns or trends which may have an effect on the way the patient reacts to treatment said by Liyakat(2024d).

3. *Collaborative Decision Making:* For the purpose of making decisions that are beneficial in the monitoring of patients who have renal illness, it is vital for healthcare professionals, including nephrologists, primary care physicians, nurses, along with additional specialists, to collaborate with one another. An all-encompassing and well-informed decision-making process is rendered feasible by the reality which every member of the healthcare team offers their own distinct knowledge and point of view to the conversation that is taking place at the table as pr Kutubuddin(2025c) (2025d) & Prasad(2024).

4. *Individualized Treatment Plans:* It is possible for the severity of renal diseases and the progression of the disease to differ significantly from a single patient to the next. Consequently, it is of the utmost importance to develop individualized treatment plans that are based on the state of the patient as well as the requirements that they bring to the table said by Sayyad(2024). It is crucial to take into consideration a number of various criteria in order to choose the most appropriate course of action. Some of these criteria include the age of the patient, their general wellness, and their style of living.

5. *Regular Monitoring:* Monitoring should be carried out on a consistent basis because it is a vital aspect of the management of renal disease. A portion of it is keeping track of the patient's condition, seeing how they are reacting to treatment, and keeping an eye out for any potential complications that may develop by Kutubuddin(2025c). It is possible for medical workers to make the appropriate revisions to the therapy regimen in considering this knowledge to guarantee ensuring the patient receives the greatest possible level of care (Kazi K(2024b).

6. *Education of Patients:* Whenever it pertains to making decisions when it comes to the healthcare monitoring of patients with renal illness, it is necessary to educate patients about their condition, the many treatment options that are available to them, and the necessity of self-management. Patients who have a better awareness of their disease and who actively engage with their care are more likely to adhere to treatment programs and make good lifestyle improvements that can improve

their overall health, according to Kutubuddin (2024e). Patients also have a greater possibility of making positive lifestyle adjustments.

That the process of making decisions on the healthcare monitoring of patients who have kidney disease is one that is complex that requires thorough consideration of a variety of variables is something that we would like to accomplish suggested by K Sayyad(2025). The process includes a variety of key components, some of which include, but are not limited to, the following: an accurate diagnosis, an understanding of the patient's medical history, collaborative decision making, individualized treatment regimens, consistent monitoring, and patient education. When medical professionals are able to successfully control these variables, they're enabled to take decisions which are informed, that can lead to an increase in the quality of life of individuals whom are suffering from problems related to their kidneys.

Incorporating artificial intelligence and the internet of things into the monitoring of patients with renal disease gives a transformative potential to move away from reactive healthcare delivery and toward proactive healthcare delivery. According to Sayyad (2024), Artificial intelligence and the internet of things has the potential to play a crucial role in improving patient outcomes, optimizing resource usage, and eventually contributing to a more sustainable healthcare system if it addresses the issue statement, goals, and objectives that have been outlined. According to Kutubuddin(2024a), & K Sayyad(2024f), Continuous breakthroughs in Internet of Things (IoT) technologies and artificial intelligence analytics are poised to transform the landscape of chronic disease management. This will make it possible for patients suffering from renal disease to get interventions that are both tailored and timely. As this subject continues to develop, it will be essential to involve stakeholders, address ethical concerns, and make certain that the patient continues to be the focal point of all projects pertaining to the Internet of Things (AIIoT).

On a biological level, chronic kidney disease (CKD) often begins with a beginning insult to the kidneys and then proceeds through a series of stages that have been thoroughly characterized. Diabetes mellitus, hypertension, and glomerulonephritis are all common causes of chronic kidney disease (CKD), and they all generate a chain reaction of pathological alterations from one to the next. Podocytes are damaged and glomerulosclerosis develops as a consequence of the insult, which ultimately leads to the loss of nephron function. A process referred to as adaptive nephron hypertrophy occurs when the number of nephrons decreases and the remaining nephrons undertake compensatory hypertrophy. This hypertrophy, which at first appears to be advantageous, ultimately results in the malfunction of the remaining nephrons and eventually leads to their death.

On a molecular level, chronic kidney disease is characterized by the buildup of toxic mediators and the deregulation of a number of different signaling pathways. Renin-angiotensin-aldosterone system (RAAS) is one of the most important elements in the course of chronic kidney disease (CKD). The activation of RAAS is linked to an increase in inflammation, fibrosis, and glomerular hypertension, all of which contribute to an even more severe rise in kidney damage. The activation of immune cells leading to the release of pro-inflammatory cytokines is a significant contributor to the course of chronic kidney disease (CKD), which is characterized by inflammation. This persistent inflammatory state is a contributor to the development of fibrotic alterations in the renal interstitium, which in turn promotes the loss of more nephrons.

The disturbance of the tubuloglomerular feedback mechanism, which results in glomerular hyperfiltration and increased intraglomerular pressure, is another significant mechanism that contributes to the progression of chronic kidney disease (CKD). Because of this, the initial injury is made worse, which results in a feedback loop that hastens the progression of renal impairment.

Apoptosis, fibrosis, and inflammation are all regulated by changes in gene expression, which are part of the molecular profile of chronic kidney disease (CKD). One example is the upregulation of transforming growth factor-beta (TGF-β) signaling in chronic kidney disease (CKD), which leads to the creation of extracellular matrix (ECM) and the development of renal fibrosis. In a similar manner, the activation of matrix metalloproteinases (MMPs) causes abnormalities in the remodeling of extracellular matrix (ECM), which contributes to the gradual scarring of the kidney.

New research also sheds insight on the function that metabolic dysregulation plays in chronic kidney disease (CKD). Increased insulin resistance and the promotion of inflammatory pathways are two of the ways that metabolic syndrome and diseases such as obesity further aggravate chronic kidney disease (CKD). These metabolic changes might result in dyslipidemia and the accumulation of uremic toxin, which ultimately contribute to the development and injury of the kidneys.

When it comes to treating the course of chronic kidney disease (CKD) at the molecular level, the emergence of precision medicine in recent years has opened up new paths. The capacity of certain biomarkers, such as kidney injury molecule-1 (KIM-1) and neutrophil gelatinase-associated lipocalin (NGAL), to predict kidney injury and track the development of disease is currently being investigated.

As a conclusion, chronic kidney disease (CKD) progression is characterized by a complex interaction of biological and molecular processes that ultimately results in irreparable damage to the kidneys. It is essential to take a multi-pronged strategy, with the primary emphasis being placed on early detection, preventative measures, and the development of specialized medicines. It is hoped that as our knowledge expands, novel medicines will be developed that will be able to prevent or even reverse the progression of chronic kidney disease (CKD). This would have a tremendous influence on the quality of life of patients and would reduce the burden on healthcare systems all over the world. The continuation of research in this field is absolutely necessary in order to unravel the complexities of renal disease and realize the possibilities for new therapeutic approaches.

Problem Statement

As the incidence rates of chronic kidney disease (CKD) continue to rise and the morbidity associated with the condition continues to be severe, it poses a significant burden on healthcare systems all over the world. In order to effectively treat complications and prevent the progression of the disease, patients who have chronic kidney disease (CKD) require constant monitoring and appropriate therapies. Reactive care tactics are frequently utilized in traditional approaches to healthcare. These strategies involve actions that are carried out only after the emergence of serious symptoms or problems. This reactive strategy is inefficient, which results in higher rates of hospitalization, higher costs for healthcare, and degraded outcomes for both patients and healthcare providers.

Within the framework of this discussion, the issue statement for deploying AI-Driven Internet of Things (AIIoT) highlights the necessity of adopting a more proactive and predictive approach to the monitoring of healthcare for patients suffering from renal illness. It is not possible for the existing healthcare systems to integrate real-time data collecting with advanced analytics in order to facilitate fast decision-making since they lack the requisite infrastructure. The promise for AIIoT to alter the way healthcare providers interact with patients who have chronic kidney disease is highlighted by this gap.

Goal

In the context of renal disease patient healthcare monitoring, the fundamental objective of artificial intelligence and the internet of things (AIIoT) is to provide a comprehensive framework for continuous patient monitoring and decision assistance. This is making use of the capabilities of Internet of Things devices in order to collect real-time health data from patients. This data may include vital signs, biochemical markers, and statistics regarding lifestyle. The incorporation of algorithms based on artificial intelligence into this data is intended to improve predictive analytics, which will ultimately result in the earlier detection of issues, the development of more individualized treatment regimens, and improved patient outcomes.

To allow prompt treatments, prevent hospital readmissions, and limit problems associated with chronic kidney disease (CKD), the objective is to build a cohesive ecosystem in which patients, healthcare providers, and data analytics all work together.

Objectives

Real-Time Monitoring: The framework for the Internet of Things (IoT) should make it possible to continuously monitor important health indicators that are relevant to kidney illness. These indicators include blood pressure, glucose levels, and electrolyte balance. This monitoring can be accomplished by wearable devices and home monitoring systems.

- To produce a full patient profile, it is necessary to develop a substantial infrastructure that is capable of integrating data from a variety of sources. These sources include electronic health records (EHR), laboratory findings, and data provided by the internet of things (IoT).
- Implementing powerful artificial intelligence algorithms that are able to analyze incoming data streams in order to recognize patterns and forecast unfavorable outcomes, such as acute renal damage or a worsening of chronic kidney disease, is an example of predictive analytics.
- To provide healthcare providers with personalized decision-making tools that make use of artificial intelligence insights to provide recommendations for timely interventions and revisions to treatment plans based on the specific requirements of particular patients, personalized decision support is essential.
- Patient Engagement Encourage patient participation by providing them with interactive interfaces that enable them to take charge of their own health management. These interfaces should include opportunities to receive constant feedback on their health condition, as well as medication reminders and lifestyle coaching.

Determine the impact of artificial intelligence and internet of things interventions on clinical outcomes, patient adherence, quality of life, and healthcare costs. Establish data to support the incorporation of AIIoT into standard care procedures for the management of renal disease.

AI-Driven-IoT Based Decision Making (Ksk Approach)

The introduction of Artificial Intelligence (AI) and the Internet of Things (IoT) has resulted in a There has been a significant change in the way that firms operate. The decision-making process has the potential to be completely transformed by these technologies, which have the capability of delivering information and conclusions in real time. Using artificial intelligence to make judgments based on the Internet of Things has become a game-changer for organizations in a range of industries, including healthcare and manufacturing, according to Mishra (2024)(2024a), Dhanve (2024), and Kutubuddin (2025d).

The term "AI-driven Internet of Things" (IoT) refers to the process of collecting and analyzing data in an instant using Internet of Things (IoT) devices and artificial intelligence (AI) algorithms. Following that, judgments that are based on data and are informed by it are constructed using the data that was originally collected. Through the provision of information that is both precise and prompt, the marriage of artificial intelligence and the internet of things has the potential to revolutionize the decision-making process. The years Liyakat (2023a) and Liyakat (2023b).

The ability to collect and evaluate huge volumes of data is one of the key advantages of decision making that is based on the Internet of Things (IoT) and is powered by artificial intelligence. Devices such as sensors and cameras were instances of Internet of Things products which have the power to collect data from a broad number of sources. These sources include people, autos, and even equipment. Following this, the data is analyzed by artificial intelligence systems, that are capable to identify patterns and provide information that is both insightful and perceptive. The utilization of this information enables firms to arrive at decisions that have been founded upon facts instead of on their instincts, which is a considerable advantage.

This technique has a number of advantages, one of which is the power of AI-driven Internet of Things-based decision making to offer information in real time said by Prashant(2024). The conventional approaches to decision-making typically rely on statistical data from the past, which may or may not be useful in the context of the present situation. As a result of the Internet of Things being powered by artificial intelligence, it is possible to gather and analyze data in real time, which leads to information that is not only accurate but also up to date. This makes it feasible for organizations to react fast to altering conditions and to make decisions which are in conformity with the trends that are now prevalent in the market. The potential outcomes of the AIIoT decision-making approach are depicted in Figure 2.

The healthcare industry is one of the areas that has gained major benefits from AI-driven decision making which relies on the Internet of Things (IoT). With the assistance of Internet of Things devices, data pertaining to patients may prove obtained and monitored over the course of real time. The data is then subjected to an analysis by artificial intelligence systems, which enables them to recognize possible threats to human health and provide early warnings. According to Liyakat (2023a), Kutubuddin (2024d),(2024e) and Sayyad L(2023a), this makes it possible for healthcare practitioners to make decisions in a timely way, which eventually leads to improved outcomes for patients.

A further point to consider is that the industrial industry has been considerably impacted by AI-driven decision making that is founded on the Internet of Things. Utilizing sensors that are connected to the Internet of Things, manufacturers are able to gather information from their machines and equipment. This information gives them insights into the operation of their products as well as any maintenance requirements that may be necessary. In order to identify patterns and anticipate the failure of machines, this data can be analyzed with the use of algorithms that are supported by artificial intelligence. According to Maccha (2022), Shirisha (2022), and Sreenivasulu (2022), this makes it possible for manufacturers to take preemptive measures in order to reduce the amount of downtime they experience and improve their operational efficiency.

The retail industry is yet another sector that has benefited from the advantages that AI-driven decision making based on the Internet of Things has brought about suggested by Kutubuddin(2024v). By making use of devices connected to the Internet of Things and neural network algorithms, retailers are able to collect information regarding the preferences and actions of their customers. After that, this information can be leveraged to improve the management of inventory and to adapt the experiences that clients have with the company. As a direct result of this, better levels of customer satisfaction and increased sales are attained.

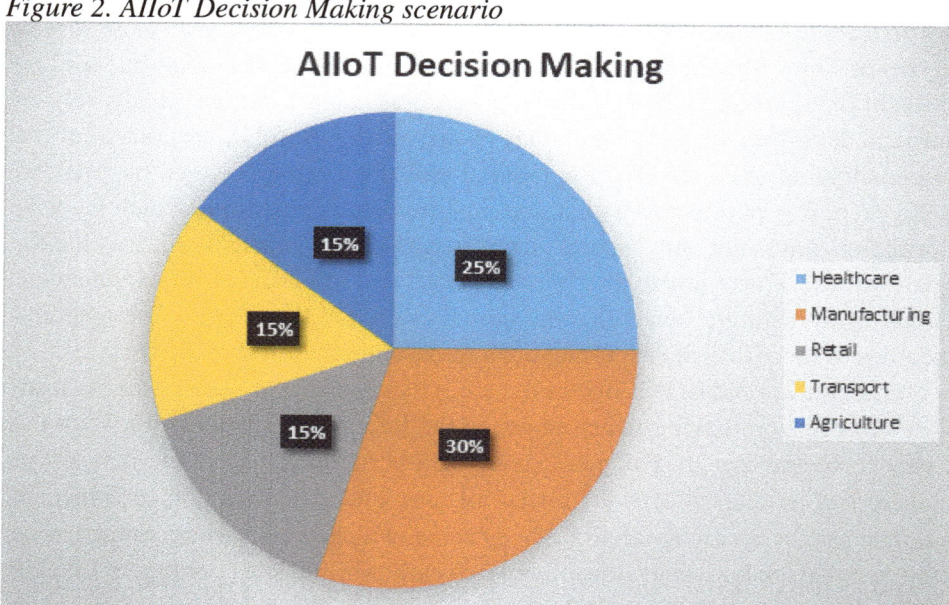

Figure 2. AIIoT Decision Making scenario

On the other side, in response to the increasing use of AI-driven decision making that is based on the Internet of Things (IoT), concerns have been made over the privacy and security of data by Halli(2022). Organizations have a responsibility to ensure that they have proper security procedures in place in order to secure sensitive data from potential cyberattacks. This has the objective of protecting the data from being compromised. In addition to this, they are obligated to adhere to ethical standards when it comes to the collection and utilization of data, and they must also conduct themselves in a transparent manner while utilizing AI and IoT. We suggest the KK strategy for Internet of Things security, which was developed by Halli (2022) and Wale (2019).

To summarize, decision making that is powered by artificial intelligence and is based on the Internet of Things is a powerful tool that has the potential to alter the way in which organizations conduct their decision-making processes. According to K Sayyad(2017)(2018), the collecting and analysis of data in real time is made feasible for businesses, which ultimately results in the production of valuable insights that can be leveraged to influence decision-making processes. To safeguard sensitive data and make ethical utilization of artificial intelligence and the internet of things, however, it is vital for enterprises to install strong security measures. As suggested by Sayyad (2024l), this is because these technologies are becoming increasingly prevalent. Decision making that is driven by artificial intelligence and based on the internet of things has the potential to lead to improved efficiency, increased production, and better outcomes for businesses, provided that the appropriate approach is implemented.

Bringing together the capabilities of artificial intelligence with the internet of things, the KSK approach is a framework that makes it possible to make decisions in real time when they are needed. The abbreviation KSK was selected because the framework is composed of three key components: knowledge, sensing, and knowing. This led to the selection of the acronym. It is Dr. Kutubuddin S. Kazi who is the one who first proposed and presented this method. DT, ANN, and K-NN algorithms are some of the artificial intelligence approaches that are recommended for use in this approach to decision making.

According to Kutubuddin (2022a;2022b)Knowledge is the first component, and it is characterized by the utilization of algorithms that are powered by artificial intelligence in order to analyze data that has been obtained from a wide variety of sources and to generate valuable insights. Following that, these insights are recorded in a knowledge base that is then used as a foundation for making decisions.

The term "sensing" refers to the exploitation of items that are connected to the Internet of Things for the purpose of collecting data in real time from the environment that is surrounding them. In addition to the capacity to collect data on temperature, humidity, and pressure, these devices are also equipped with sensors that are capable of measuring a variety of other variables. Following that, the data is transferred to the knowledge base, wherein it is analyzed with the information which is currently there in the database.

Artificial intelligence algorithms are applied in the third component, which is referred to as Knowledge, to do an evaluation of both the real-time data and the knowledge that's already available in the knowledge base suggested by Ravi(2022), Sunita(2023) & Kutubuddin(2022d). As a result of this, the systems is capable to make decisions which are well-informed, taking into consideration the current situation, data from the past, and analysis of the future.

When it comes to the processes of decision-making, the KSK approach is a game-changer because of the multiple benefits that it provides. According to Vahida(2023) & Karale(2023), to begin, it reduces the necessity of waiting for human data analysis by making it possible to make judgments in real time. This eliminates the importance of waiting. When it comes to industries like as healthcare and transportation, where decisions that are made in a short amount of time have the ability to save lives, this is of utmost importance.

Furthermore, the KSK approach ensures that the data are accurate and reliable, which brings us to the second point. Through the process of combining data from a wide range of sources, the system is capable to recognize anomalies and inconsistencies, thereby ensuring that decisions are founded on information that is reliable and accurate.

LITERATURE SURVEY

As a result of the growth of sensor technologies, Internet of behavioral and physiological monitoring systems, in particular IoT-based pupil medical management systems, have undergone rapid evolution in recent years, as stated by Pradeepa (2022). The monitoring of the health function status of the increasing number of students who live alone and are dispersed across large geographic areas is becoming an integral component of the educational system. This is due to the fact that an increasing number of students are living on their own. One of the goals of this research is to suggest a method for regulating student health that is based on the Internet of Things. This system is intended to continuously monitor the vital signs of pupils and discover changes in both their biological and behavioral states through the application of contemporary medical technologies. The Internet of Things (IoT) module is the one that is accountable for gathering crucial data, and the assessment of that data is done out by utilizing artificial neural network (ANN) models. After that, these models are used to conduct an analysis of the data in order to make an estimation of the potential risks that are connected to the physiological and behavioral changes that occur in children. The results of the trials have shown that the model that was proposed is both effective and accurate in determining the condition of the learners. This has been achieved through the demonstration of the model's efficiency. As a consequence of the evaluation of the suggested model, the support vector machine was able to attain a maximum performance of 99.1%, which is a result that is satisfactory in regard to our objectives. In addition, the results were successful in that they were able to defeat algorithms for decision trees, random forests, and multilayer perceptron neural systems.

This study aims to provide a complete yet condensed analysis of the opportunities and obstacles connected with the program of AI and IoT in the healthcare industry, as stated by Kazi K(2024a). The purpose of this study is to provide this analysis. There is also a brief overview of AI and the IoT, in addition to its relevance, some observations on recent developments, a look at whatever the future may hold, and issues that are currently being addressed by healthcare systems. All of these are mentioned in the document. The web of things can be exploited for an assortment of reasons within the sphere of healthcare firms. Some of these applications include remote monitoring, the integration of medical devices, and the use of advanced sensors. In any event, technology has the ability to assist professionals in sharing ideas with more efficiency whilst simultaneously guaranteeing the security and psychological health of individuals. It is also possible for the Internet of Things to assist human organizations in achieving responsibility and fulfillment by encouraging patients to collaborate more closely with medical professionals. The promise that patients will work more cooperatively alongside medical professionals is what allows this to be realized.

The purpose of this chapter, which was published by Kazi K S (2024a), is to provide an analysis of the expanding applications of deep learning (DL) in the field of ophthalmology. Specifically, it explores the integration of DL systems and the usefulness of these systems in improving patient outcomes, particularly in the diagnosis and management of diseases including as diabetic retinopathy, age-related macular degeneration, and retinopathy of prematurity. Specifically, it focuses on the effectiveness of these systems in improving patient outcomes. Additionally, it explains the employment of deep learning algorithms for the goal of evaluating intricate datasets and retinal images, which ultimately permits early detection, correct diagnosis, and effective treatment alternatives. This is accomplished through the utilization of deep learning. Furthermore, the challenges that are inherent in the process of introducing AI clinical practice are discussed in this chapter as well. Among these challenges are concerns over the bias of the data, the dependability of the algorithm, ethical problems, and the necessity of having various datasets that serve representative of the community. It places an emphasis on the significance of continuous research and development, as well as ethical considerations, and it provides a road map for the proper application of DL in the field of ophthalmology. The objective of this chapter is to put up a vision in which these technologies not only help to the improvement of clinical practice but also to the enhancement of health outcomes in the field of eye care.

According to Priya (2023), this cutting-edge technology makes use of data that has been obtained from previous events in order to create predictions about future patterns and outcomes. The goal of this technology is to assist heart-care firms in arriving at better decisions regarding how to best serve their clients. Forecasting, on the other hand, is a data-driven technology that, just like any other technology, needs to be administered in the appropriate manner in order to guarantee that business operations are both efficient and ethical. The expanding application of AI (Artificial Intelligence) and ML (Machine Learning) has led to an increase in the significance of healthcare forecasting over the course of the previous several years. Forecasting can also help medical personnel provide diagnoses that are more accurate and provided in a timely manner. Within the realm of medicine, forecasting can be of use in this regard. When medical workers are able to foresee possible medical events and take safeguards in accordance with such predictions, they are able to diagnose and treat patients with greater efficiency and precision. It is possible that this will lead to better outcomes for patients, as well as possibly cost reductions associated with the treatment. These systems are able to recognize illnesses and provide effective treatment support because they are able to replicate human cognition capabilities. In addition to this, they have the capability of diagnosing disorders. This study incorporates studies that focus on predicting the heart healthcare system (HHS) by utilizing machine learning algorithms. These papers are included in this study. The K-means Elbow method was applied for the purpose of registration and notification, a decision tree was utilized for the purpose of health and human services, and MySQL was utilized for the purpose of vaccine reminders throughout the deployment of the system.

METHODOLOGY

Through the utilization of the internet, the Internet of Things (IoT) refers to the process of combining millions of different physically distinct means of data collecting and delivery on a global scale. For the Internet of Things to come into existence, it is necessary to have a wide range of sensors and software. Providing connectivity between mobile devices, different physical devices which may be employed, and apparatus that is located in a remote area is performed through the employment of wireless communication protocols. The Internet of Things brings about a significant improvement to the models used in healthcare.

When it comes to the process of gathering information on patients, a wide range of sensors, both internal and external, are deployed. While the eternal sensor is in charge of gathering information about the patient's environment and the environment around them, body-implanted sensors are in charge of gathering information about the patient's internal state. This is done in conjunction with the implantation of the eternal sensor. In order to arrive at estimates regarding the likelihood of disease, the physicians examine the information they were have been given in order to reach their determinations.

During the process of classifying the data which was acquired, the created model makes use of a wide range of different artificial intelligence classification algorithms. As a consequence of this, the model is of the ability to discern between people who are physically healthy versus those who aren't physically healthy. With the help of artificial intelligence, it is possible to obtain disease classification that is both consistent and accurate. By utilizing the Internet of Things, the following three separate categories of patient data items have been obtained in accordance with the methods that have been proposed:

- Information specific to the patients whose are currently being isolated on the premises Those patients who are included in this data group are provided with Internet of Things sensors that do not require a significant financial investment and aren't difficult to acquire. Following the collection of data regarding the health of patients by these sensors that are connected to the Internet of Things, the information is then sent to an Internet of Things assistant for further investigation.

- Data obtained from patients who were either clinically or laboratory-based: In this particular case, the individual visits diagnostic centers and laboratories; yet, despite the reality that they've got access to a wide variety of resources, here are no medical professionals present to answer their problems.

- General information pertaining to the patient who is situated at a different location: In this particular scenario, the patient resides in a neighborhood that is situated in the countryside or in a location that is situated a great distance away from the medical services. The individuals who were responsible for obtaining this information were the staff members who were employed in the medical assistance program. Real-time data collection from sensors which are connected to the Internet of Things (IoT) is transmitted to medical experts. These sensors collect information about patients. Because of this, competent medical personnel are able to provide patients with enhanced care.

The data that is collected can be sent to a cloud server for additional analysis, and it can be collected from any device that is connected to the internet of things. Data analysis is the responsibility of the fog server, which is responsible for using classification algorithms to perform the analysis. For the purpose of providing patients with diagnoses as rapidly as is practically possible, it is essential that the data be received by medical professionals and power storage facilities together. The acceptance of the cloud server is what allows this to be performed. The implementation of artificial intelligence algorithms for classification within the KSK technique for the aim of performing medical model building is the primary focus of the study. The Decision Tree (DT), the Artificial Neural Network (ANN), and the K-Nearest Neighbor (KNN) algorithm designs are few examples of the methodologies that fall under this category.

Figure 3. Suggested KSK approach for Kidney Diseases patient Healthcare Monitoring

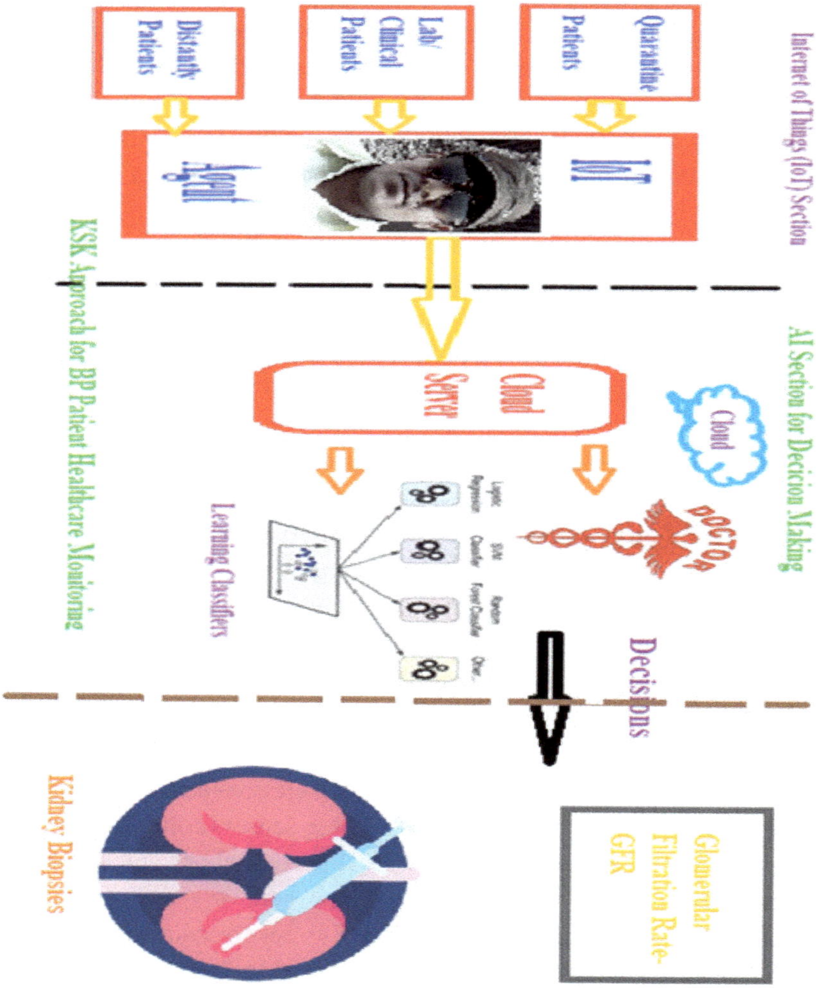

For the purpose of applying these algorithms to the data, a set of data that contains diagnostic information regarding renal problems is applied. The framework which the suggested model incorporates is depicted in Figure 3, which is attached to this sentence. Both artificial intelligence and the internet of things are seen as important components of the paradigm that Kutubuddin (2024a), (2024b), and (2024c) have presented. Simply by making use of the initial parameter, which is generally known as the Internet of Things (IoT), it is feasible to link anything to the internet. During the process of data collection, the information pertaining to patients is gathered and performed analysis in real time. As a consequence of this, it guarantees which the information which had been processed is swiftly communicated to the parties that are responsible for it.

To provide discoveries in a timely manner, artificial intelligence (AI), that is the next parameter, takes advantage of the data that has become accumulated throughout time. With the help of artificial intelligence and internet of things technologies, it is feasible to successfully manage enormous amounts of data.

It's possible that the completion of the work can be broken down into three separate stages. The computation of data, as well as the collection and preliminary processing of data, consists of the second phase in the calculation process. When the third step is complete, the results are kept on a server that can be accessed online, and the ultimate decision is created available to consumers, who may be professionals working in the medical service industry.

1. The collection of information: To achieve this goal, patient data is gathered using a variety of means. These methods include information obtained from people's homes, laboratories, or clinics, which is then added to information collected remotely. To collect data on patients in real time throughout the process, it is necessary to make use of a wide range of sensors and equipment that are connected to the Internet of Things. It has been made available to patients who continue to reside in their current places of residence the required quantity of sensors that have been strategically placed throughout their residences. Once the clinical and analytical data has been provided by the laboratory staff, it is then received by an Internet of Things agent. The patients who live in extremely remote places have a variety of sensors implanted on their bodies with the intention of monitoring their health. It is the responsibility of these sensors to collect the data, which is then sent to an agent involved in the Internet of Things for further processing of the information.
2. The computation and pre-processing of the data both involve the stages of filtering and checking for missing values. These are two of the procedures that are involved in the pre-processing of the data that has been provided.

3. Once the pre-processing stage is complete, the data is transferred to a server located in the cloud so that it can continue to be processed. The data is computed and categorised using three different artificial intelligence classifiers: DT, ANN, and K-NN. These classifiers are also suggested for use in the KSK approach to decision making.

RESULTS AND DISCUSSION

In this part of the article, we are going to take a look at the outcomes of experiments that were carried out using a broad variety of different classification methods. These methods include, amongst others, DT, ANN, and K-NN in the KSK approach. There is additional information regarding these trials that was supplied in the next section. It has been determined that a large variety of disease databases have been deployed, and among these datasets are ones that belong to kidney diseases. A wide range of disorders have been studied using these databases, which have been employed. The dataset that the researchers really used, which included a number of samples, is shown in Table 1 and Figure 4, respectively. the researchers used the dataset.

Table 1. Dataset used

Sr. No.	Dataset	Number of Samples
1	Kidney Diseases	400
2	Training Dataset used	320
3	Testing dataset	80

Figure 4. Dataset used for Experimentation

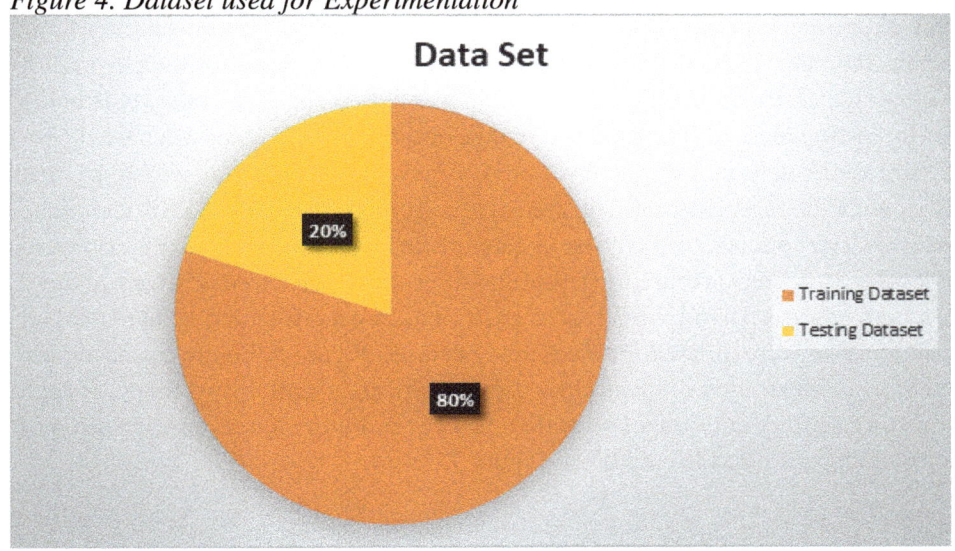

Figure 5. Accuracy of KSK approach methods

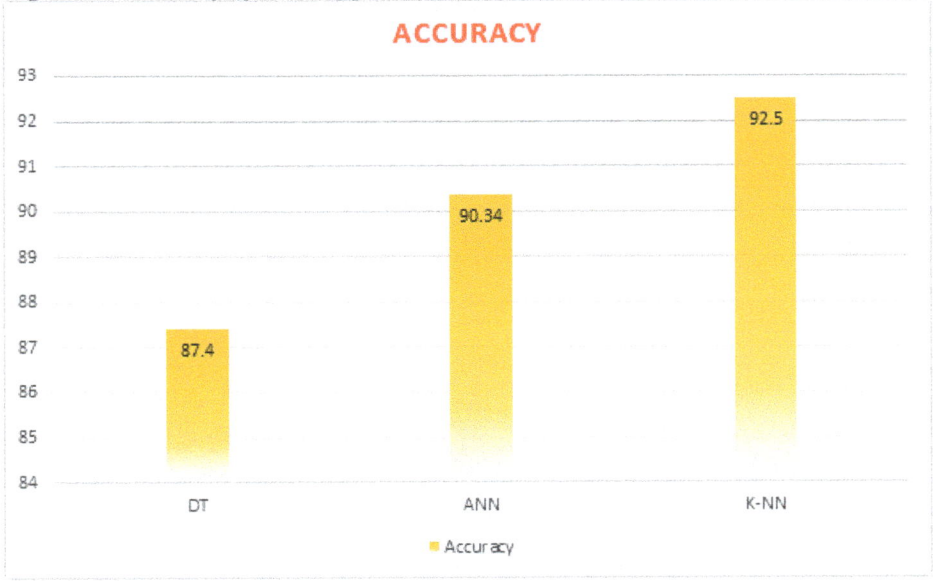

The dataset is divided into two ratios for the aim of the inquiry, which pertains to the experimental study that is being conducted. The ratio in question is 80%, whereas the other is 20%. Eighty percent of the data set is used for the purpose of developing classification algorithms, while twenty percent of the data set is being used for testing reasons. The total percentage of the data set that has been used? For the purpose of determining the level of accuracy, specificity, and sensitivity that every one of the three distinct classifiers that were suggested by the KSK technique possesses, we conduct an analysis on each of them separately. When it comes to kidney diseases, there are three different classifiers that are utilized, and each of these classifiers has its own individual set of performance data. It included three distinct classifiers that were utilized for the Kidney dataset. Figure 5, Figure 6, and Figure 7 provide an illustration of the accuracy, precision, and recall, respectively, of each of those classifiers in the categories that they cover. Figure 5 is a representation of the accuracy as well as Figure 6 and Figure 7.

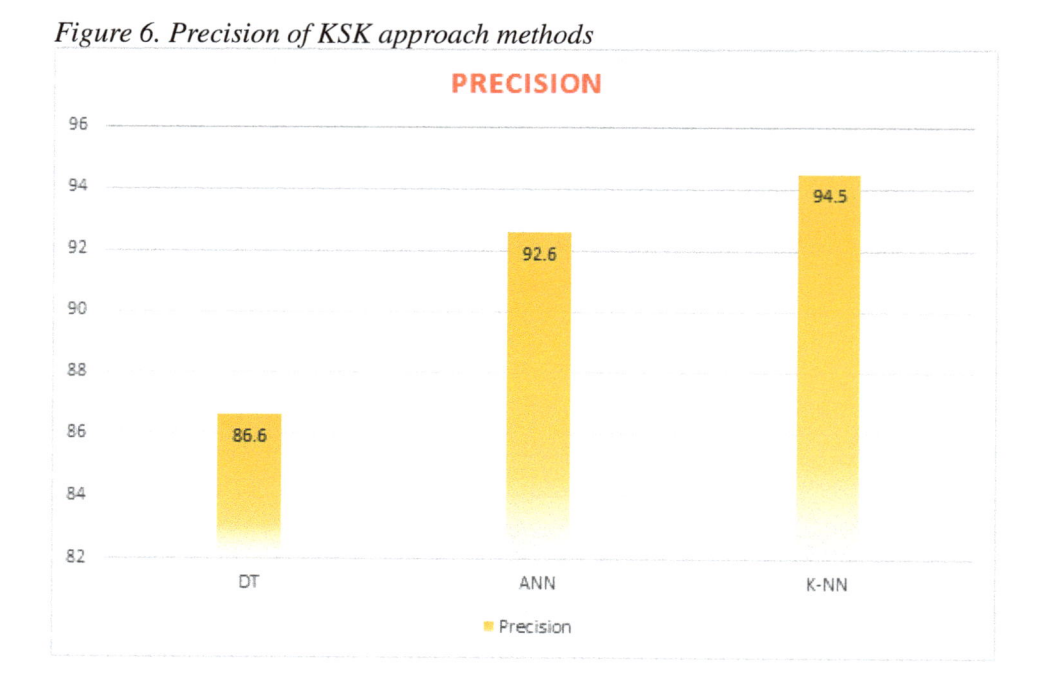

Figure 6. Precision of KSK approach methods

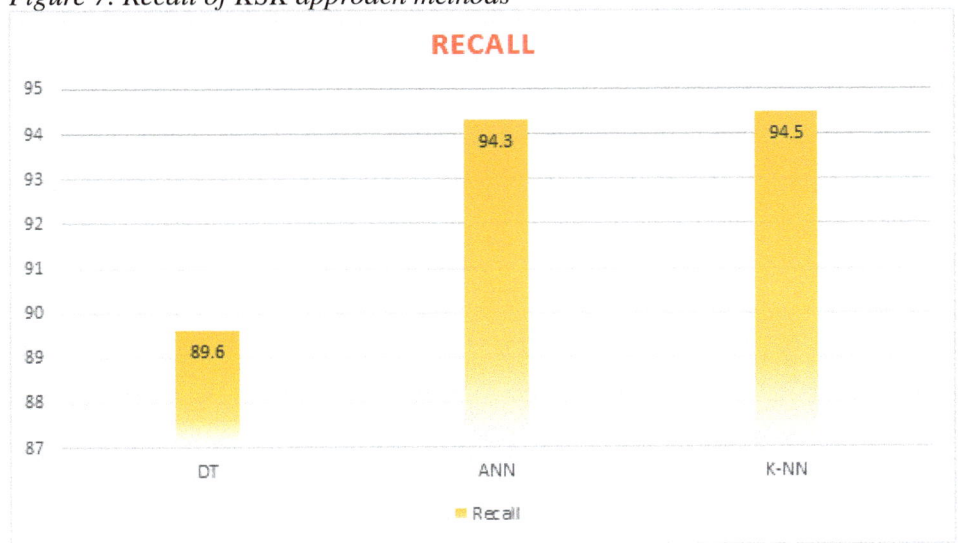

Figure 7. Recall of KSK approach methods

As shown in Figure 5 the accuracy of KSK approach methods are varies from 87 to 92%. For DT, the accuracy is 87.4%, for ANN, it is 90.34% and for K-NN, it is 92.5%. Hence the KSK approach selects the outcome accuracy of 92.5% as output of KSK approach. Hence we say that for Kidney diseases detection, KSK approach has accuracy of 92.5%.

Figure 6 shows the outcome of KSK approach in terms of Precision. The precision is varies from 86 to 94%. For DT, the precision is 86.6%, for ANN, it is 92.6% and for K-NN, it is 94.5%. Hence the KSK approach selects the outcome precision of 94.5% as output of KSK approach. Hence we say that for Kidney diseases detection, KSK approach has precision 94.6%.

Figure 7 shows the outcome of KSK approach in terms of recall. The recall is varies from 89 to 94%. For DT, the recall is 89.6%, for ANN, it is 94.3% and for K-NN, it is 94.5%. Hence the KSK approach selects the outcome recall of 94.5% as output of KSK approach. Hence we say that for Kidney diseases detection, KSK approach has recall 94.6%. Figure 8 shows the KSK approach outcome for accuracy, precision and recall.

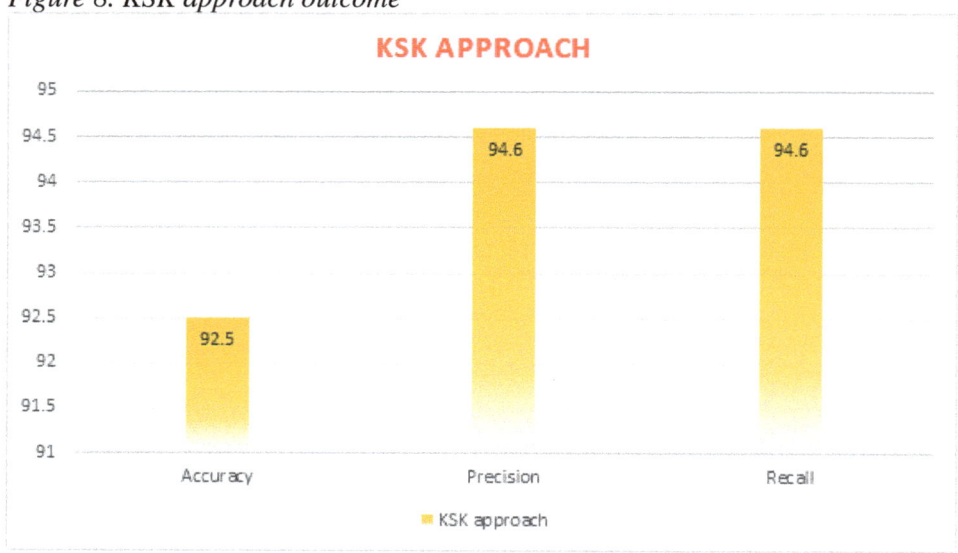

Figure 8. KSK approach outcome

KSK APPROACH

Metric	KSK approach
Accuracy	92.5
Precision	94.6
Recall	94.6

CONCLUSION

At this point in time, the application of artificial intelligence categorization algorithms for the goal of forecasting sickness and illness and making decisions is still in its infancy. It is recommended by the KSK technique that DT, ANN, and K-NN algorithms be utilized for the objective of decision making within the organization. DT, ANN, and K-NN are the three separate artificial intelligence classification algorithms that were utilized in the creation of a healthcare model that was built for the purpose of this proposed research. These algorithms were suggested by the KSK method. To fulfill the requirements of the task specific is being proposed, this model was developed expressly for that purpose. During the classification process, these classifiers are utilized in the instance of disease datasets, specifically in areas such as those that belong to kidney diseases. When it comes to determining how effectively the classifiers are functioning, there are three basic indicators that are taken into consideration. It is important to note that this is referring to the metrics of accuracy, precision, and recall. It is possible to acquire an accuracy rate that ranges from a minimum of 87% to a maximum of 92.5% for each and every illness by utilizing the KSK technique, which is already being utilized in the healthcare industry.

REFERENCES-

Dhanwe, S. S., (2024). AI-driven IoT in Robotics: A Review. *Journal of Mechanisms and Robotics*, 9(1), 41–48.

Halli, U. M. (2022). Nanotechnology in IoT Security, *Journal of Nanoscience. Nanoengineering & Applications*, 12(3), 11–16.

K Sayyad L. (2018). Significance of Projection and Rotation of Image in Color Matching for High-Quality Panoramic Images used for Aquatic study. *International Journal of Aquatic Science*, 9(2), 130–145.

Karale Aishwarya, A., (2023). Smart Billing Cart Using RFID, YOLO and Deep Learning for Mall Administration. *International Journal of Instrumentation and Innovation Sciences*, 8(2).

Kasat, K., Shaikh, N., Rayabharapu, V. K., & Nayak, M. (2023). Implementation and Recognition of Waste Management System with Mobility Solution in Smart Cities using Internet of Things, *2023 Second International Conference on Augmented Intelligence and Sustainable Systems (ICAISS)*, Trichy, India, 2023, pp. 1661-1665, DOI: 10.1109/ICAISS58487.2023.10250690

Kazi, K. (2024a). AI-Driven IoT (AIIoT) in Healthcare Monitoring. In Nguyen, T., & Vo, N. (Eds.), *Using Traditional Design Methods to Enhance AI-Driven Decision Making* (pp. 77–101). IGI Global., available at https://www.igi-global.com/chapter/ai-driven-iot-aiiot-in-healthcare-monitoring/336693, DOI: 10.4018/979-8-3693-0639-0.ch003

Kazi, K. (2024a). Machine Learning (ML)-Based Braille Lippi Characters and Numbers Detection and Announcement System for Blind Children in Learning. In Sart, G. (Ed.), *Social Reflections of Human-Computer Interaction in Education, Management, and Economics*. IGI Global., DOI: 10.4018/979-8-3693-3033-3.ch002

Kazi, K. (2024b). Modelling and Simulation of Electric Vehicle for Performance Analysis: BEV and HEV Electrical Vehicle Implementation Using Simulink for E-Mobility Ecosystems. *In L. D., N. Nagpal, N. Kassarwani, V. Varthanan G., & P. Siano (Eds.), E-Mobility in Electrical Energy Systems for Sustainability (pp. 295-320). IGI Global.* Available at: https://www.igi-global.com/gateway/chapter/full-text-pdf/341172DOI: 10.4018/979-8-3693-2611-4.ch014

Kazi, K. S. L. (2025). IoT Technologies for the Intelligent Dairy Industry: A New Challenge. In *Designing Sustainable Internet of Things Solutions for Smart Industries* (pp. 321-350). IGI Global.

Kazi, K. (2025b). Machine Learning-Driven-Internet of Things(MLIoT) Based Healthcare Monitoring System. In Wickramasinghe, N. (Ed.), *Impact of Digital Solutions for Improved Healthcare Delivery*. IGI Global.

Kazi, K. (2025c). Moonlighting in Carrier. In Tunio, M. N. (Ed.), *Applications of Career Transitions and Entrepreneurship*. IGI Global.

Kazi, K. (2025d). AI-Powered-IoT (AIIoT) based Decision Making System for BP Patient's Healthcare Monitoring: KSK Approach for BP Patient Healthcare Monitoring. *In Sourour Aouadni, Ismahene Aouadni (Eds.), Recent Theories and Applications for Multi-Criteria Decision-Making, IGI Global,* Prasad, Santoshachandra Rao Karanam (2024). AI in public-private partnership for IT infrastructure development, *Journal of High Technology Management Research*, Volume 35, Issue 1, May 2024, 100496. DOI: 10.1016/j.hitech.2024.100496

Kazi, K. (2025d). AI-Driven-IoT (AIIoT) based Decision-Making in Drones for Climate Change: KSK Approach. In Aouadni, S., & Aouadni, I. (Eds.), *Recent Theories and Applications for Multi-Criteria Decision-Making*. IGI Global.

Kazi, K. S. (2024a). Computer-Aided Diagnosis in Ophthalmology: A Technical Review of Deep Learning Applications. In Garcia, M., & de Almeida, R. (Eds.), *Transformative Approaches to Patient Literacy and Healthcare Innovation* (pp. 112–135). IGI Global., Available at https://www.igi-global.com/chapter/computer-aided-diagnosis-in-ophthalmology/342823, DOI: 10.4018/979-8-3693-3661-8.ch006

Kazi, K. S. (2024f). Machine Learning-Based Pomegranate Disease Detection and Treatment. In Zia Ul Haq, M., & Ali, I. (Eds.), *Revolutionizing Pest Management for Sustainable Agriculture* (pp. 469–498). IGI Global., DOI: 10.4018/979-8-3693-3061-6.ch019

Kutubuddin, K. (2022a). Predict the Severity of Diabetes cases, using K-Means and Decision Tree Approach. *Journal of Advances in Shell Programming*, 9(2), 24–31.

Kutubuddin, K. (2022b). A novel Design of IoT based 'Love Representation and Remembrance' System to Loved One's. *Gradiva Review Journal*, 8(12), 377–383.

Kutubuddin, K. (2022d). Detection of Malicious Nodes in IoT Networks based on packet loss using ML, *Journal of Mobile Computing, Communication & mobile. Networks*, 9(3), 9–16.

Kutubuddin, K. (2024c). Vehicle Health Monitoring System (VHMS) by Employing IoT and Sensors, *Grenze International Journal of Engineering and Technology,* Vol 10, Issue 2, pp- 5367-5374. Available at: https://thegrenze.com/index.php?display=page&view=journalabstract&absid=3371&id=8

Kutubuddin, K. (2024e). A Novel Approach on ML based Palmistry, *Grenze International Journal of Engineering and Technology,* Vol 10, Issue 2, pp- 5186-5193. Available at: https://thegrenze.com/index.php?display=page&view=journalabstract&absid=3344&id=8

Kutubuddin, K. (2024e). IoT based Boiler Health Monitoring for Sugar Industries, *Grenze. IACSIT International Journal of Engineering and Technology,* 10(2), 5178–5185. https://thegrenze.com/index.php?display=page&view=journalabstract&absid=3343&id=8

Kutubuddin, S. L. (2023i). Smart Motion Detection System using IoT: A NodeMCU and Blynk Framework. *Journal of Microelectronics and Solid State Devices,* 10(3).

Kutubuddin, (2023h). *IoT based Healthcare Monitoring for COVID- Subvariant JN-1,* Journal of Electronic Design Technology, 4(3).

Kutubuddin (2023j). Nanotechnology in Precision Farming: The Role of Research, *International Journal of Nanomaterials and Nanostructures,* 9(2). https://doi.org/ DOI: 10.37628/ijnn.v9i2.1051

Kutubuddin (2024v). Smart Agriculture based on AI-Driven-IoT(AIIoT): A KSK Approach, *Advance Research in Communication Engineering and its Innovations,* 1(2), 23-32.

Liyakat, K. (2024). Explainable AI in healthcare. *Explainable Artificial Intelligence in Healthcare Systems,* 2024, 271–284.

Liyakat, K. K. S. (2024). Machine Learning Approach Using Artificial Neural Networks to Detect Malicious Nodes in IoT Networks. In Udgata, S. K., Sethi, S., & Gao, X. Z. (Eds.), *Intelligent Systems. ICMIB 2023. Lecture Notes in Networks and Systems* (Vol. 728). Springer., available at https://link.springer.com/chapter/10.1007/978-981-99-3932-9_12, DOI: 10.1007/978-981-99-3932-9_12

Liyakat, S. (2024). Explainable AI in Healthcare. In: Explainable Artificial Intelligence in healthcare System, editors: *A. Anitha Kamaraj, Debi Prasanna Acharjya.* ISBN: 979-8-89113-598-7. doi: https://doi.org/DOI: 10.52305/GOMR8163

Liyakat, S. (2024d). ChatGPT: An Automated Teacher's Guide to Learning. In Bansal, R., Chakir, A., Hafaz Ngah, A., Rabby, F., & Jain, A. (Eds.), *AI Algorithms and ChatGPT for Student Engagement in Online Learning* (pp. 1–20). IGI Global., DOI: 10.4018/979-8-3693-4268-8.ch001

Liyakat, S. (2025). Heart Health Monitoring Using IoT and Machine Learning Methods. In Shaik, A. (Ed.), *AI-Powered Advances in Pharmacology* (pp. 257–282). IGI Global., DOI: 10.4018/979-8-3693-3212-2.ch010

Liyakat, K. K. S. (2023a, March). Detecting Malicious Nodes in IoT Networks Using Machine Learning and Artificial Neural Networks. In *2023 International Conference on Emerging Smart Computing and Informatics (ESCI)* (pp. 1-5). IEEE.

Liyakat, K. K. S. (2023b, March). Machine learning approach using artificial neural networks to detect malicious nodes in IoT networks. In *International Conference on Machine Learning, IoT and Big Data* (pp. 123-134). Singapore: Springer Nature Singapore.

Machha Babitha, C Sushma, et al. (2022). Trends of Artificial Intelligence for online exams in education, *International journal of Early Childhood special. Education*, 14(01), 2457–2463.

Mishra Sunil, B., (2024). Nanotechnology's Importance in Mechanical Engineering. *Journal of Fluid Mechanics and Mechanical Design*, 6(1), 1–9.

Mishra Sunil, B., (2024a). AI-Driven IoT (AI IoT) in Thermodynamic Engineering. *Journal of Modern Thermodynamics in Mechanical System*, 6(1), 1–8.

Dixit, A. J. (2014). A review paper on iris recognition. *Journal GSD International society for green. Sustainable Engineering and Management*, 1(14), 71–81.

Dixit, A. J., & Kazi, M. K. (2015). Iris recognition by daugman's method. *International Journal of Latest Technology in Engineering, Management &. Applied Sciences (Basel, Switzerland)*, 4(6), 90–93.

Nagrale, M., Pol, R. S., Birajadar, G. B., & Mulani, A. O. (2024). Internet of Robotic Things in Cardiac Surgery: An Innovative Approach. *African Journal of Biological Sciences*, 6(6), 709–725. DOI: 10.33472/AFJBS.6.6.2024.709-725

Neeraja, P., Kumar, R. G., & Kumar, M. S. Liyakat and M. S. Vani. (2024), DL-Based Somnolence Detection for Improved Driver Safety and Alertness Monitoring. *2024 IEEE International Conference on Computing, Power and Communication Technologies (IC2PCT)*, Greater Noida, India, 2024, pp. 589-594, . Available at: https://ieeexplore.ieee.org/document/10486714DOI: 10.1109/IC2PCT60090.2024.10486714

Nerkar, P. M., & Dhaware, B. U. (2023). Predictive Data Analytics Framework Based on Heart Healthcare System (HHS) Using Machine Learning, *Journal of Advanced Zoology*, 2023, Volume 44, Special Issue -2. *Page*, 3673, 3686.

Pardeshi, K. P., (2022a). Development of Machine Learning based Epileptic Seizureprediction using Web of Things (WoT). *NeuroQuantology: An Interdisciplinary Journal of Neuroscience and Quantum Physics*, 20(8), 9394–9409.

Pardeshi, K. P., (2022b). Implementation of Fault Detection Framework for Healthcare Monitoring System Using IoT, Sensors in Wireless Environment. *Telematique*, 21(1), 5451–5460.

Pradeepa, M., (2022). Student Health Detection using a Machine Learning Approach and IoT, *2022 IEEE 2nd Mysore sub section International Conference (MysuruCon),* 2022.

Prashant, K. Magadum (2024). Machine Learning for Predicting Wind Turbine Output Power in Wind Energy Conversion Systems, *Grenze International Journal of Engineering and Technology,* Jan Issue, Vol 10, Issue 1, pp. 2074-2080. Grenze ID: 01.GIJET.10.1.4_1 Available at: https://thegrenze.com/index.php?display=page&view=journalabstract&absid=2514&id=8

Ravi, A., (2022). *Pattern Recognition- An Approach towards Machine Learning, Lambert Publications, 2022.* ISBN.

Sayyad, K. (2017). Significance and Usage of Face Recognition System. *Scholarly Journal for Humanity Science and English Language*, 4(20), 4764–4772.

Sayyad, K. (2022a). IoT-Based Healthcare Monitoring for COVID-19 Home Quarantined Patients. *Recent Trends in Sensor Research & Technology*, 9(3), 26–32.

Sayyad, K. (2023a). Detection of Malicious Nodes in IoT Networks based on Throughput and ML. *Journal of Electrical and Power System Engineering*, 9(1), 22–29.

Sayyad, K. (2024b). IoT Driven by Machine Learning (MLIoT) for the Retail Apparel Sector. In Tarnanidis, T., Papachristou, E., Karypidis, M., & Ismyrlis, V. (Eds.), *Driving Green Marketing in Fashion and Retail* (pp. 63–81). IGI Global., DOI: 10.4018/979-8-3693-3049-4.ch004

Sayyad, L. (2023a). IoT-based weather Prototype using WeMos. *Journal of Control and Instrumentation Engineering*, 9(1), 10–22.

Sayyad. (2024). Artificial Intelligence (AI)-Driven IoT (AIIoT)-Based Agriculture Automation. In S. Satapathy & K. Muduli (Eds.), *Advanced Computational Methods for Agri-Business Sustainability* (pp. 72-94). IGI Global. https://doi.org/DOI: 10.4018/979-8-3693-3583-3.ch005

Sunita Sunil Shinde, et al, (2023). Monitoring Fresh Fruit and Food Using IoT and Machine Learning to Improve Food Safety and Quality, *Tuijin Jishu/Journal of Propulsion Technology,* 44(3), pp. 2927 – 2931.

Shweta Nagare, , (2014). Different Segmentation Techniques for brain tumor detection: A Survey, *MM- International society for green. Sustainable Engineering and Management*, 1(14), 29–35.

Shweta Nagare, et al., (2015). An Efficient Algorithm brain tumor detection based on Segmentation and Thresholding, *Journal of Management in Manufacturing and services,* 2(17), pp.19 - 27.

Sirisha Devi, J., Mr. B. Sreedhar, et al. (2022). A path towards child-centric Artificial Intelligence based Education, *International Journal of Early Childhood special. Education*, 14(03), 9915–9922.

Sreenivasulu, D., Dr. J. Sirishadevi, et al. (2022). Implementation of Latest machine learning approaches for students Grade Prediction, *International Journal of Early Childhood special. Education*, 14(03), 9887–9894.

Sayyad(2024l). Nanotechnology in Medical Applications: A Study. *Nano Trends-A Journal of Nano Technology & Its Applications.* 26(02):1-11.

Sultanabanu, (2023n). Nanomedicine as a Potential Therapeutic Approach to COVID-19. *International Journal of Applied Nanotechnology.* 9(2): 27–35p.

(2024). Sultananbanu, (2024p). Polymer Applications in Energy Generation and Storage: A Forward Path. *Journal of Nanoscience. Nanoengineering & Applications.*, 14(2), 31–39p.

Vahida, . (2023). Deep Learning, YOLO and RFID based smart Billing Handcart. *Journal of Communication Engineering & Systems*, 13(1), 1–8.

Veena, C., Sridevi, M., & Liyakat, B. Saha, S. R. Reddy and N. Shirisha,(2023). HEECCNB: An Efficient IoT-Cloud Architecture for Secure Patient Data Transmission and Accurate Disease Prediction in Healthcare Systems, *2023 Seventh International Conference on Image Information Processing (ICIIP)*, Solan, India, 2023, pp. 407-410, . Available at: https://ieeexplore.ieee.org/document/10537627DOI: 10.1109/ICIIP61524.2023.10537627

Wale, A. D., & Dipali, R., (2019). Smart Agriculture System using IoT. *International Journal of Innovative Research in Technology*, 5(10), 493–497.

Chapter 10
Analysis of Insomnia for Old Aged People Using Machine Learning Algorithms

N. T. Renukadevi
https://orcid.org/0000-0002-0010-469X
Kongu Engineering College, India

K. Saraswathi
https://orcid.org/0000-0003-1746-0145
Kongu Engineering College, India

S. Vignesh
Kongu Engineering College, India

ABSTRACT

Sleep plays a crucial role in overall health and well-being, with its significance and being more important in the context of aging. This research explores the application of machine learning algorithms to predict and analyze sleep patterns in older adults. A dataset comprising physiological and lifestyle factors, alongside sleep-related parameters, is collected from a cohort of elderly individuals. Various machine learning models, including but not limited to Random Forest, Support Vector Machines, Decision Tree, KNN are employed to develop predictive models for sleep duration, quality, and disruptions. Insomnia is a sleep disorder characterized by persistent difficulty falling asleep, staying asleep, or experiencing restorative sleep, leading to significant impairment in daily functioning. It can be caused by various factors, including stress, anxiety, depression, or lifestyle choices. Healthcare providers can

DOI: 10.4018/979-8-3693-7277-7.ch010

gain insights into individualized risk factors for sleep disturbances in older adults, facilitating early intervention and personalized sleep management strategies.

INTRODUCTION

Insomnia is a prevalent sleep disorder affecting a substantial portion of the elderly population, leading to a myriad of health challenges and diminishing the overall quality of life in this demography. This research work aims on finding an analysis of this sleep disorder through the magnifying glass of machine learning (ML). The primary objective is to bind the efficiency of ML algorithms to gain deeper insights into the analysis and predictions, potential interventions associated with insomnia among the elder persons.

The scope of this analysis encompasses predictive modelling, feature importance analysis, personalized interventions, and early detection strategies. Leveraging diverse datasets that include demographic information, health records, sleep patterns, and lifestyle factors, ML models are developed to envisage the probability of insomnia in senior people. This predictive capability holds the promise of early identification, enabling timely interventions to prevent the exacerbation of sleep-related complications.

Feature importance analysis is employed to discern the most influential factors contributing to insomnia in older adults. This approach aids in prioritizing interventions by focusing on the key determinants of sleep disturbances in the elderly population. Also, this work explores the potential of ML models to recommend personalized interventions based on individual profiles. These interventions may range from lifestyle modifications to targeted therapeutic approaches, optimizing the efficacy of insomnia management. The analysis also addresses the imperative of early detection by developing ML-based tools capable of identifying insomnia at its nascent stages. This proactive strategy aims to facilitate timely interventions, ultimately improving outcomes and mitigating the potential repercussions of chronic sleep disturbances in older adults.

In conclusion, this study extends the connection between the complex nature of insomnia in old age and the capabilities of machine learning. By incorporating data-driven insights and predictive modelling, the analysis intends to add to the development of smooth methodologies for addressing insomnia in the elderly, thereby promoting healthier aging and enhancing overall well-being.

MACHINE LEARNING

The domain of AI which helps to make the computers to train and develop models, algorithms for classification or predictive analysis based on the experience and data. Dataset is essential for the predictive analysis of ML models. Data pre-processing entails cleaning, organizing and transforming the data to make certain its suitability for analysis. Feature selection and engineering follow, where relevant attributes are chosen or created to represent the problem effectively. Once the data is prepared, machine learning algorithms come into play. The models are trained using historical data, where they learn patterns and relationships that are capable of making decisions on original and concealed data. Model evaluation is a critical aspect, employing various metrics to assess how well the model simplifies to new data. Fine-tuning, or hyper parameter tuning, is often required to optimize model performance, and model selection may involve testing multiple algorithms to determine the most suitable approach for a given problem. The versatility and adaptability of machine learning have found applications in numerous domains, from healthcare and finance to natural language processing and image recognition, empowering organizations to harness data-driven insights for better decision-making and problem-solving (El Naqa & Murphy, 2015).

ML process begins with data collection, varied from structured databases towards unstructured text and images. Data pre-processing is the initial stage, involving data cleaning, transformation, and feature engineering to prepare it for analysis. Feature selection is crucial for identifying the most relevant attributes that influence the problem at hand. These algorithms are classified into supervised learning, where representation of model are trained on labelled data for tasks like classification and regression, and unsupervised learning, which deals with unstructured data and includes clustering and dimensionality reduction techniques. On the other side, one more approach is Reinforcement learning, which concentrates on training the model to have efficient decisions and to produce best possible results. Model training is the core phase, where the algorithms learn from historical data, recognizing patterns and relationships that enable them to make predictions or decisions on new, unseen data. Model evaluation, performed using various metrics, gauges how well the model generalizes followed by hyper parameter tuning and model selection, concerning the options for the most part of appropriate algorithm, rounds out the machine learning process (Habehh & Gohel, 2021).

ML is being an important tool that can examines large volume of data that too exceeding our human thinking and potential, ability to discover patterns and envisage outcomes with accurate results, which shows the enhancement of ML applications by good diagnosis of diseases from data set either as numerical, categorical values or from diversified modal of images like CT scans, MRI images, etc., ML applications helps to predict diseases and outcomes of patients along with suggestions for further medical treatments (Ahsan et al., 2022).

In order to process the large volume of datasets, the data should be pre-processed with methods like data cleaning and reduction. The ultimate objective of data pre-processing is to eradicate errors, missing values and to strengthen quality of data for further processes. Comparing to bench mark datasets, which is of standard and eminent one, the real-time data may contain mistakes, unrelated data, etc. Hence, cleaning of data is an utmost important task in data handling. Data cleaning includes removing noise values such as irrelevant data, dropping the missing data, etc.

Data cleaning is needed for variety of reasons. It may be due to the devices through which data is collected, the samples collected from physicians or data stored in the databases with errors. There are lot of data cleaning processes available in ML which includes removing invalid data by applying filtering methods. The most commonly used approach for removing erroneous data is binning process. The data is divided into equal-sized buckets, followed by statistical techniques like mean or median for smoothing the bins. Related to erroneous data is the missing values, which have to be filled with appropriate values. The effective way is either backward or forward fill method. And, data normalization methods are also used to represent the data in normalized range of values. Normalization methods convert data to common range of values but maintain the actual distribution. Scaling methods focus the data around 0, but depends on standard deviation. Scaling methods such as Linear scaling, Log scaling, and Min-max normalization methods helps to fix data in the ranges from 0 to 1 (Albahra et al., 2023).

In complex applications having data with high volume of dimensions, ML reduction methods are being used. Dimensionality reduction is a technique that ensures the data to be compressed in well-organized manner. Feature selection and extraction methods falls under this category. In feature selection, essential subsets of features are retrieved from dataset. Wrapper and filter methods such as Linear Discriminant Analysis, Chi square methods are used for this purpose (Bharadiya, 2023; Bouchlaghem et al., 2022; Hancer, 2024; Hashim & Yassin, 2023).

Under feature extraction methods, Principal Component Analysis (PCA) is popular one, which converts the data into principal components with reduced dimensions. This helps to avoid overfitting and multicollinearity. The correlation between features will be reduced. Also, backward recursive feature elimination is a method to remove the features one by one according to the iterations. In addition to PCA, discriminant analysis and decomposition techniques also may be implemented (Kabir et al., 2023).

Many times, classes may be imbalanced due to abnormal distribution of data for classification. To rectify this imbalance, the number of data instances for each classes needs to be changed, which is done by sampling methods. These methods may be either undersampling or oversampling. In addition to that, samplings with/

without replacement methods are also applicable for ML process depending on data sets. Synthetic Minority Oversampling Technique (SMOTE) and Random undersampling techniques are being used in more number of imbalanced classes. (Hasanin et al., 2019; Werner de Vargas et al., 2023)

Once feature selection and reduction methods are completed, dataset will be in normalized stage. Various kinds of classification or clustering techniques can be selected based on dataset and problem domain. In order to prepare the classification model, data should be splitted into training and testing data. Usually, 70%-80% of data will be taken into consideration for training the ML model and remaining 30%-20% of data for testing purposes. For validation purposes, sampling and cross validation methods may be applied. K-fold cross validation is the default method in which dataset is splitted into k number of equal folds, where k-1 fold is used for training the data and remaining one fold is for testing. Subsequent to the finishing point of "k" number of iterations, the evaluation results will be averaged. This process is done in order to ensure the powerful performance of evaluation.

There are certain measures needed for the assessment of efficiency of machine learning model. The evaluation metrics are based on parameters like category of dataset, precise problem domain, and the required results. Evaluation metrics includes classification accuracy, specificity, sensitivity etc., (Sarker, 2021)

Thus, machine learning is very successful technology in healthcare ranging from decision support system, predicting disorders such as mental health, diabetes, cancers, and epilepsy diseases, automation of medical records maintenance, investigation of imaging, etc., (Ferdous et al., 2020)(Javaid et al., 2022)(Mian Qaisar & Subasi, 2022; Rajkomar et al., 2019; Saraswathi et al., 2024; Shailaja et al., 2018). And, this research work focus on sleeping disorder of aged people and analyzed the factors that leads to such difficulties.

The remaining section of this research work is detailed as Literature Survey, Dataset Description, and Methodologies of various types of ML algorithms, Results and Discussion and finally conclusion.

LITERATURE SURVEY

Zahra Asghari Varzaneh et.al., has proposed a research work based on Rowe and Kahn's theory and their study aimed to determine the ideal attributes of Successful Aging (SA). Six machine learning (ML) algorithms used these identified variables as inputs in order to build and evaluate predictive models for SA. Pre-processing the raw dataset was the first stage in this retrospective study. Afterwards, five basic machine learning algorithms were trained with a sample size of 983. Various supervised learning algorithms such as Bayes classifier, Artificial Neural Network

(ANN), Support Vector Machine (SVM), and k-Nearest Neighbor(k-NN). Among these, K-NN is considered as weak learner, it works based on ensemble technique. Based on the outputs of each of the different base models, the prediction result was then decided by means of the majority vote method. By applying five-fold cross-validation approach, the experimental outcomes proved that predictive system was successful in forecasting SA, demonstrating high precision (93%), specificity (92.40%), sensitivity (87.80%), F-measure (90.31%), accuracy (89.62%), and a ROC score of 96.10% (Asghari Varzaneh et al., 2022).

A way to measure health status across communities and historical periods are one of the most difficult tasks faced by researchers who studied about aging is proposed by Francisco Félix Caballero and George Soulis (Caballero et al., 2017). In this research work, data from English Longitudinal Study of Aging (ELSA) is taken for implementation. Machine learning and assorted effects multilevel regression are used to find relationships between the generated health score and socio-demographic variables. Subsequent initiatives will apply this technique to a harmonized dataset that includes several longitudinal aging studies. This research offers a foundation for advanced analytical approaches and improves our understanding of the aging process by developing a comprehensive measure of health in an older adult cohort by integrating two data analytical methodologies .If health is understood as a one-dimensional latent construct measured by multiple functional domains, this study shows the psychometric soundness and feasibility of developing a single health metric that includes multiple aspects of functioning, mobility, sensor neural, cognitive, and emotional domains.

The bulk of chronic illnesses and disabilities have aging as a key risk factor is demonstrated and from a biological perspective, SA is characterized by a state of well-being and quality of life, free from illnesses or disabilities that prevent one from engaging in daily activities. At the same time, aging will gives decline of cognitive and physical capacities with aging. The sample was categorized as SA using the Rowe and Kahn Model, which took into account the elements including the ability to engage in daily activities, eminence of life, nutrition, and the presence of two or fewer disorders. ANN shows better performance when compared to other algorithms in predicting SA, giving 100% results in classification accuracy, and true positive rate according to the testing data (Zaccheus et al., 2024).

A system with the assumption that predictive models for SA can improve the Quality of Life (QoL) of senior persons by minimizing substantial and psychological concerns by fostering increased societal involvement is proposed. Social elements have not gotten as much emphasis in prior research on the effects of physical and mental illnesses on quality of life in the elderly. About a count of 975 cases involving older people who were classified as SA or non-SA were examined. By using univariate analysis, it is easy to conclude the main determinants affecting SA. The random forest (RF) model was found to be the most effective in predicting SA, with PPV of 90.96%, NPV of 99.21%, sensitivity of 97.48%, specificity of 97.14%, accuracy of 97.05%, F-score of 97.31%, and AUC of 0.975. Predictive models can be used to improve QoL of the aged, which in turn can reduce financial burdens on both individuals and societies(Ahmadi & Nasiri, 2023).

Netta Mendelson Cohen et al., has proposed in the paper to understand the distinctions between age-related chronic illnesses and natural aging processes. Attaining this difference is difficult, though, because it necessitates fellow people for their whole lives. In this study, we extrapolated from electronic medical records with poor longitudinal coverage to estimate health trajectories spanning adulthood using machine learning approaches. Using a complete score, our algorithm tracked the health state of people who were not known to be at risk for chronic diseases and determined who had a higher or lower potential for longevity. It is proved, that this model and its markers hold true for populations in the US, Britain, and Israel. For example, it is discovered that, independent of the risk for significant chronic diseases; somewhat low neutrophil counts and alkaline phosphates levels could function as early markers of healthy aging. In addition, genetic correlations and heredity of longevity score is also noticed. It is found that parents of patients with high scores typically lived at least a year longer than matched controls. The results of this study demonstrate the value of using healthy individuals in longitudinal modeling to better understand the mechanisms underlying long life and healthy aging(Cohen et al., 2024).

Christopher M. Hatton et al., proposed a study which helps in forecasting determined depression indicators in older persons, using ML algorithms specifically, gradient booting algorithm performs well than related statistical techniques like logistic regression. With mean AUC values of 0.72 versus 0.67, $p < 0.0001$, ML outperformed logistic regression in terms of predictive performance. ML approaches yield somewhat lower mean negative predictive values (45% versus 35%). In conclusion, the experimental results sustain the prospective applications of machine learning to customized, individualized intellectual health care (Hatton et al., 2019).

Soo-Kyoung Lee etal., proposed a study which was two-fold: first, to identify the factors that affect older people with chronic illnesses in terms of their Health-Related Quality of Life (HRQoL); and second, to develop a predictive model based on these factors in order to identify HRQoL risk groups that could benefit from intervention. The study included machine learning (ML) approaches. A total of five statistically significant factors were shown to have an impact on HRQoL of aged people with chronic illnesses. These factors include monthly income, the existence of a diagnosis of a chronic illness, sadness, anxiety, and self-perceived health status. The best results were obtained from the stepwise logistic regression (SLR) analysis, which had an F-score of 0.49 and an accuracy of 0.93. These results provide important information for developing customized health management strategies and intervention plans targeted at improving the HRQoL of older adults with long-term conditions(Lee et al., 2014).

Hong J. Kan et al.,(Kan et al., 2019)were explained Ordinary least squares (OLS) are currently the primary method used by payers and providers to approximate anticipated clinical and economic results for risk adjustment. About 81,106 participants with constant medical prescription and insurance coverage were included for this analysis. The analysis used comorbidity indices from 2009 to 2012 to anticipate the total cost of healthcare in 2013. When compared to other models, Lasso regression constantly yielded forecast ratios that were closer to 1 across a range of projected risk levels. When penalized regression was used on longitudinal data, it performed more accurately in predicting healthcare expenditures than OLS. More specifically, at different anticipated risk levels, lasso regression showed better prediction ratios. Healthcare providers, insurers, and legislators may be able to better manage population health and risk adjustment by implementing penalized regression techniques like lasso regression, which better cater to the unique requirements and hazards of the populations they serve.

Panel Fabrice Mowbray et al. explained on the paper that Emergency Departments (EDs) are the main points of entry into hospitals and have a significant impact on how older persons who are seeking medical assistance navigate the healthcare system. The special requirements and complicated medical histories of older persons make them difficult to prepare for after ED visits. Even if ML methodologies have been used in the past to support in ED disposition decision-making for the general public, their effectiveness and usefulness in anticipating hospital admission among elderly patients in EDs is still a question mark. In this work, ED admission in older persons using a variety of machine learning techniques, and also talked about the possible clinical and policy consequences is also forecasted. Ten-fold cross-validation is utilized for model training, assessment, and analysis while five machine learning methods were implemented. To evaluate the performance of the model, metrics for accuracy, sensitivity, and specificity were also added. Gradient boosted trees were shown to be the most accurate model (AUC = 0.80) for predicting which elderly ED patients will need to be hospitalized. This study is the primary one to exercise a variety of geriatric syndromes and functional tests to predict hospital admission in older ED patients. This predictive capacity may help with ED disposition decision-making, which could speed up admissions and encourage proactive discharge planning (Mowbray et al., 2020).

Sau and Bhakta (Sau & Bhakta, 2017)give emphasis to the relevance of machine learning technology in the field of automated screening for mental health illness among seafarers. Here, two mental health problems such as anxiety and depression were taken for consideration and analyzed using psychometric tool. Ten ML classifiers were implemented and evaluated. Out of them, Random Forest model outperforms with classification accuracy of 91%.

In the proposed work, a framework using electroencephalogram (EEG) signal has been obtained for diagnosing epileptic seizures. Anti-aliasing filters were applied with parameters extraction and the data is processed with 3.3 fold compression and bandwidth is reduced. Appropriate re-sampling and de-noising methods such as adaptive rates would be implemented. Three classes of epilepsy has been analysed and accuracy of 96.4% has been achieved (Mian Qaisar & Subasi, 2022)

ML is used in health care industry for diagnosis and predictive analysis. ML models are used for effective diagnosis of kidney diseases by extracting relevant information from datasets. Various kinds of regression models can be effectively implemented for the diagnosis of disease. Among the various ML classification algorithms such as SVM, KNN, etc., an integrated classification model with Random forest classifier, neural network and logistic regression provides better accuracy of 99.83% with 10-fold cross validation (Qin et al., 2019).

A framework is proposed in this work is about the development of prediction display for Pediatric Intensive Care Unit (PICU). This display gives helping information to guide nurses and physicians. These displays shows less processing works, grouping all the information about the patients, etc., it also favours the interaction of dynamic explanations such as risk factors to physicians (Barda et al., 2020).

Big data analytics, as the name implies, includes data of big volume, heterogeneous collection, veracity, and application of such volume of data in diverse domains. In this research work, an IoT analysis model has been designed in which data is collected from different sources like sensors and networks, ML techniques were applied for analyzing big data. It is proven that big data is applied for IoT applications such as healthcare, monitoring human activities and weather prediction. Here, the architecture enables to implement processing of real-time data, with storage and mining of data for heart disease prediction through three-layered designs(Li et al., 2021).

A consistent system for analysing patient emotions is proposed in this work. Coded transcriptions are implemented to provide suggestions to health care professionals. SVM with Gaussian Kernel, DT with ensemble boosted method and KNN with cosine similarity is evaluated in which SVM shows good accuracy of 83.6% to predict the interactions of professionals with emotional concerns (Barracliffe et al., 2017).

ML algorithms are used for diagnosis of wide variety of diseases including cancers and HIV is also included in this category now. An approach to find the predictors of early HIV diagnosis is proposed in this work based on health records of patients. Poisson LASSO regression model is used for feature selection; data is splitted into 80% for training and 20% for testing. 10-fold cross validations were applied for fine tuning of model's performance. This work compares both missed and non-missed opportunities for detection of HIV infections in a well-timed approach (Weissman et al., 2021).

Access of data for wide range of applications in hospital departments is in demand to improve the decision making pMLrocess by physicians. ML is such a domain which concentrates on all kind of areas such as health records maintenance, imaging, diagnosis, computer vision etc., along with financial aspects in healthcare administration (Anderson et al., 2021; Sun & Wei, 2022).

This proposed work concentrates on services of medical departments in Bangladesh. The application of recent technologies with low cost and investment is in urgent need for patients. Hence, this case study incorporates several domains into a single platform such as databases, mobile and web applications for the discussion of doctors and patients, maintenance of data in databases, etc., ML methods were experimented and about 95% of accuracy were achieved in disease detection and less expensive also(Islam et al., 2019). The comparative analyses of existing techniques with their outcomes are shown in Table 1.

Table 1. Comparative analysis of existing techniques

Author	ML Technique	Dataset	Accuracy
Barracliffe et al. (2017)	Support Vector Machine	Emotions of patients	83.60%
Zahra Asghari Varzaneh et.al., (2022)	K-NN	Successful Aging and Non-successful Aging	89.62%
Ahmadi & Nasiri, (2023)	Random Forest	Successful Aging and Non-successful Aging	97.05%
Soo-Kyoung Lee et al., (2014)	Logistic Regression	Health-Related Quality dataset	93.00%
Sau and Bhakta (2017)	Random Forest	Mental health illness	91.00%

METHODOLOGY

In this research work, we are analyzing the factors that affect the health of elder people, in particular, sleeping disturbance (insomnia) using machine learning algorithms. Even though wide variety of ML algorithms is in recent research work, the most apt algorithms for analysis of insomnia are KNN, DT, SVM and RFC is taken into consideration(Cho et al., 2019).

Based on the various research works, supervised learning methodologies were experimented with mental health prediction of aged people. SVM and RFC provide better results in analysis(Ullas et al., 2020)(Sumathi & B., 2016)(Chung & Teo,

2022).For various disease detection and opinion mining, advancement of machine learning algorithms such as deep learning algorithms were implemented in various research domains (Renukadevi, 2021)(K. Venu, P. Natesan, 2023)(Kuppusamy & Thangavel, 2023)

Dataset Description

Data set is prepared with the data collected from 100 aged persons having sleeping disorders and in need of medication for survival. The system begins by collecting relevant data from sources such as surveys and questionnaires. Dataset description includes features like age, gender, employment, number of doctors visited, stress disturbing their sleep, pain disturbing their sleep, medicine disturbing their sleep, restroom disturbing their sleep which is shown in Table2.

Table 2. Insomnia TECH Dataset

No_of_Doctors_Visited	Age	Gender	Physical_Health	Mental_Health	Dental_Health
0-1 doctors	65-80	Female	Good	Very Good	Good
0-1 doctors	65-80	Male	Good	Good	Poor
0-1 doctors	65-80	Female	Good	Good	Good
0-1 doctors	65-80	Female	Very Good	Excellent	Excellent
0-1 doctors	50-64	Male	Very Good	Very Good	Very Good
2-3 doctors	50-64	Female	Fair	Poor	Good
2-3 doctors	50-64	Male	Very Good	Good	Fair
2-3 doctors	50-64	Male	Very Good	Good	Fair
0-1 doctors	50-64	Female	Fair	Good	Very Good
4 or more doctors	65-80	Female	Fair	Good	Fair
2-3 doctors	50-64	Female	Excellent	Very Good	Very Good
4 or more doctors	65-80	Male	Fair	Good	Fair

continued on following page

Table 2. Continued

No_of_ Doctors_ Visited	Age	Gender	Physical_Health	Mental_Health	Dental_Health
4 or more doctors	50-64	Female	Good	Very Good	Poor
0-1 doctors	50-64	Female	Good	Good	Good
0-1 doctors	50-64	Female	Excellent	Fair	Very Good
0-1 doctors	50-64	Female	Good	Good	Fair

Pre-processing work has been done to convert categorical value to numerical ones for effective implementation of ML algorithms.

The Sleep has been affected by these factors

- Stress disturbing their sleep
- Pain disturbing their sleep
- Medicine disturbing their sleep
- Restroom disturbing their sleep

KNN

KNN is a kind of supervised classification algorithm which is non-parametric, lazy learning and uses closeness distance measure as metric for classifying the data. The data point is envisaged or classified depends on the widely held k-nearest neighbors in the feature vectors. The value of "k" shows the count of neighbors measured for the classification or regression decision. The most commonly used distance metrics option of "k" and requires careful consideration of feature scaling. While simple such as Euclidean distance, is used to compute the distance between data points which is represented in equation (1) where x_1, x_2, y_1, y_2 the attributes of datasets are. The diagrammatic representation of KNN is shown in Figure 1. It is susceptible and intuitive, KNN may be totally pricey for outsized datasets, and its performance be capable of be affected by noisy, and its role extends to areas such as recommendation systems and anomaly detection.

$$\text{dist} = \sqrt{(x_2 - x_1)^2 + (y_2 - y_1)^2} \tag{1}$$

KNN is easy to implement as only the distance metric between data instances needs to be calculated. The results can be easily inferred and the nearest neighbours will be taken into account. KNN do not build any model and hence no training phase in essential for it. It is adaptable to changes and can handle non-linear decision boundaries and complex patterns in the data. It never has strong postulation in relation to the underlying data distribution. Many algorithms requires the dataset to be specific forms like linear, supporting independent, etc.

KNN equally having its demerits also, as it is much sensitive in selecting the choice of hyper parameter "k". It is computationally high-priced for huge datasets, as it entails manipulative distances to all data points. Also, needs storage to processes the entire data. KNN may prone to "curse of dimensionality" where performance deteriorates as the number of features increases. It struggles when the class labels in dataset are imbalanced(Uddin et al., 2022).

Figure 1. KNN Diagram

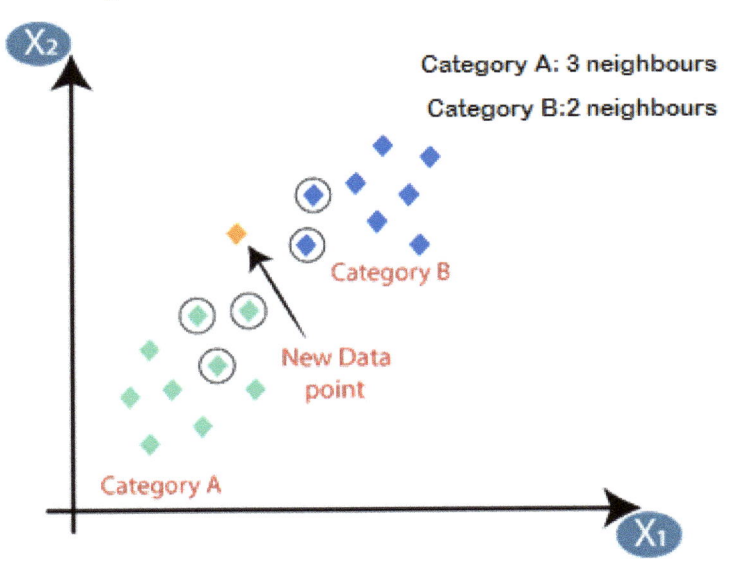

Decision Tree (DT)

The most commonly used supervised algorithm which develops the model based on tree structure is DT. It is implemented for analysis and decision making for multiple classes effectively. DT constructs the tree based on training data called as feature vector and predicts the value of class label.

In DT, a decision node represents a feature vector. Edges from the nodes to children node shows the possible range of values based on the features related with the node. A leaf or terminal node shows the value for output variable and its clear pictorial representation is shown in Figure 2.

The dataset is partitioned recursively on the basis of kinds of attributes and its values. DT algorithm finds the optimal attribute based on splitting criteria such as information gain or gini index and forms a root node. Prior to that, a measure of uncertainty called as Entropy will be calculated as shown in equation (2) to (4).

$$Entropy = \sum -p_i \log p_i \tag{2}$$

where p_i refers to the probability value of an attribute and summation of logarithmic value to base 2 is calculated as Entropy.

$$InformationGain(S, A) = Entropy(S) - \frac{|S_v|}{|S|} . Entropy\left(S_v\right) \tag{3}$$

where S refers to the number of instances, A is an attribute, S_v is a subset of S and v the individual value of A.

$$GiniIndex(S) = 1 - \sum_{i=1}^{c} p_i^2 \tag{4}$$

where c refers to the number of classes.

DT has its advantages as it is transparent and easy to understand, providing human-readable decision rules. It can handle both classification and regression tasks along with numerical and categorical data. Not much pre-processing work is necessary for DT. It is more robust to outliers and can accommodate missing data.

Every algorithm has its own pros and cons. DT also equally faced the equal number of challenges. Once the noise and irrelevant data are more in dataset, the speed of DT deteriorates. Sometimes, few changes in the data also converges the tree to an unusual structure and may leads to unrelated predictions. DT may not perform well with imbalanced datasets. It may subject to over fitting, more than ever when the tree is cavernous and multifarious. DT has its limits in its capability to confine intricate decision limitations compared to ensemble methods. And mostly, greedy search during tree construction may not result in globally optimal solutions.(Bahzad Taha Jijo, Adnan Mohsin Abdulazeez, 2021)

Figure 2. Decision Tree

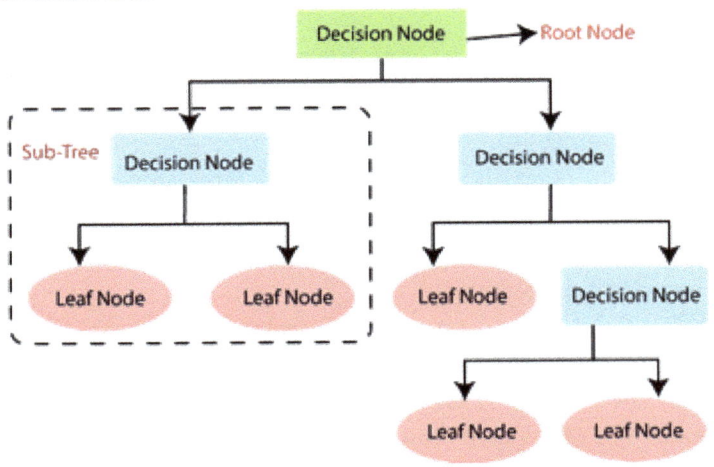

SVM

SVM is one of the most powerful supervised classification algorithms. It works depending on the surface called as hyperplanes that take apart data points as various classes in a high-dimensional space. The data points that are nearer to decision boundary are called as "support vectors" which influences the position along with orientation of the hyperplanes. SVM aims to maximize the boundary between data points and hyperplanes which is shown in Figure 3. SVMs are well-known for their robust performance by handling linear and non-linear data with the help of kernel function and capable to hold complex decision boundaries in various domains.

With vector w, the equation for linear hyper plane written as equation (5) that separates two classes can be mentioned as:

$$w^t x + b = 0 \qquad (5)$$

In binary SVM classifier, the distance between data points and decision boundary will be represented using the equation(6) as

$$d_i = \frac{wt^T x_i + b}{||wt||} \tag{6}$$

where w is weight vector, $||wt||$ is the Euclidean form of normal vector wt, the support vectors will be placed in any of the class labels and the output is given as equation

$$y = \begin{cases} 1 : wt^T x_i + b \geq 0 \\ 0 : wt^T x_i + b < 0 \end{cases} \tag{7}$$

The most commonly used kernel function is Radial Basis Function (RBF) and sigmoid. The maximum-margin hyperplane appropriately splits data into classes exclusive of any misclassifications.

SVM is effective at finding optimal hyper planes for binary and multi-class classification. It can handle both decision boundaries using kernel functions as hard and soft margin classifiers. It is robust to outliers due to the focus on the margin and support vectors. SVM offers high accuracy when properly tuned and is suitable for complex datasets. SVM models are less prone to over-fitting. It works with all kinds of semi and unstructured data like images also. It is non-parametric, it never presume much preceding knowledge about distribution of data.(Pisner & Schnyer, 2020)

SVM is Susceptible to the selection of hyper parameters like the kernel type and regularization parameter. It may not be suitable for large datasets due to computational complexity. Model interpretability can be limited, particularly with non-linear kernels. It is prone to over-fitting if not appropriately regularized. It is difficult to handle datasets with noisy or overlapping classes.(Mall et al., 2022)

Figure 3. Support Vector Classifier

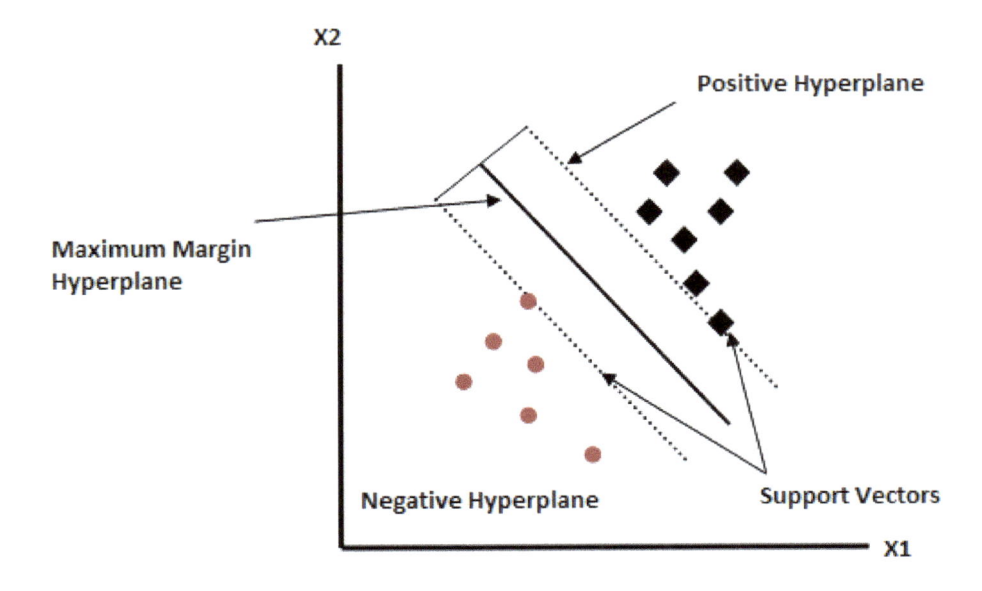

Random Forest Classifier (RFC)

RFC is a collection of learning technique that relies mostly on decision trees. It builds several decision trees through training and produces the output as either classification or regression of the sample trees for more vigorous and precise results. The key idea is to introduce uncertainty in the tree-building procedure by considering a random selection of features and data points for each tree. This assists in ease of over fitting and improves the model's simplification ability. Random Forest is notorious for its high prognostic accurateness, resilience to outliers, and suitability for complex datasets and is shown in Figure 4. It is extensively applied in a range of applications, together with classification, regression, and feature importance analysis in machine learning.

RF helps to improve predictive accuracy through ensemble learning, reducing over-fitting. It is easily adaptable to outliers and noisy data. It can handles both classification and regression tasks. Also, deals with high-dimensional data and large datasets effectively. It provides feature importance scores, aiding in feature selection and interpretation.

RF is less interpretable than a single Decision Tree, especially when many trees are used. It may not perform as well as gradient boosting methods for certain tasks. It requires more memory and computational resources compared to individual Decision Trees.

Figure 4. Random Forest Classifier

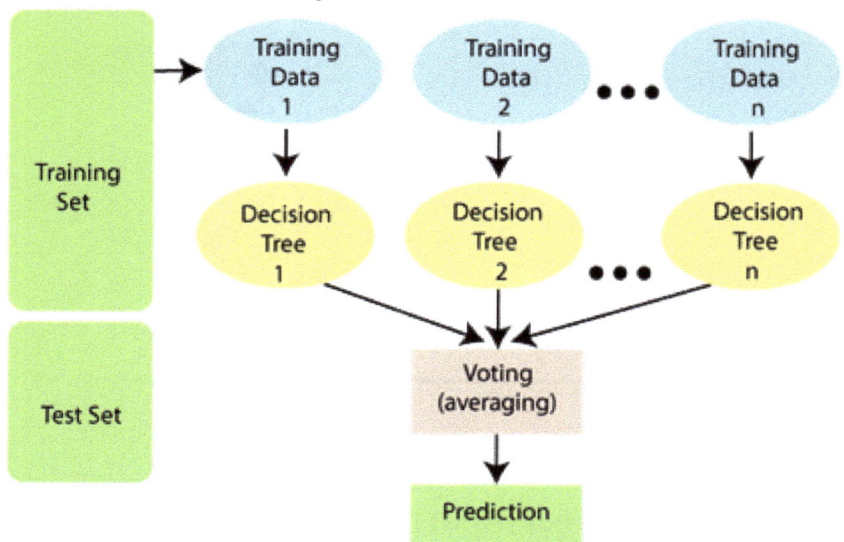

The block diagram of ML Model for the analysis of Insomnia by implementing ML algorithms is shown in Figure 5. Here, the dataset is divided into Training and testing part where 70% of data are splitted for training and 30% for testing. ML Model is built from the given data and the results were analyzed by finding statistical measures such as classification accuracy.

Figure 5. Block Diagram of ML Model

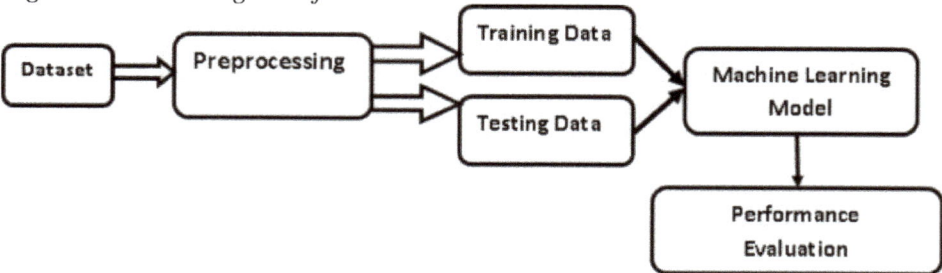

Classification accuracy is evaluated based on the measures such as True Positive (TPs), True Negative (TNs), False Positive (FPs) and False Negative (FNs) which is shown in equation (8).

$$ClassificationAccuracy = \frac{TPs + TNs}{TPs + TNs + FPs + FNs} \quad (8)$$

RESULTS AND DISCUSSION

In this research work, various ML algorithms were implemented for the analysis of certain factors such as stress, pain, medication, frequency of moving to rest rooms for insomnia among the old aged people by collecting reasons from them in the form of tabular data. From that, it is found that more number of people suffered from sleep disorder is due to medicines. Regarding this, ML algorithms such as KNN, DT, SVM and RFC were implemented for analysing the insomnia and it is realized that RFC gives more accurate prediction in finding that sleep disturbance occurred due to stress which gives a result of 85% when compared to other algorithms.

From the results, it is analyzed that in medicinal parameters, RFC shows 90% prediction whereas SVC shows 80% and KNN shows 71%. Hence, it is proved that sleep disturbance happened due to medication is also high. For washroom frequency, RFC and SVC in the ML algorithms shows the accuracy of same prediction of about 71%.And the pain frequency, KNN and RFC in the ML algorithms shows the accuracy of same prediction about 71%. From the above analysis, it is concluded that RFC shows better predictions when compared to other ML algorithms for this research. The factors that affect sleep are analysed using various ML algorithms and are tabulated in Table 3. The comparison of accuracy of four algorithms, the factor stress and medicine in ML algorithms are shown in Figure 6 and Figure 7 respectively.

Table 3. Accuracy Measures of ML algorithms

Factors	DT	KNN	SVC	RFC
Stress	76%	71%	80%	85%
Medicine	66%	71%	80%	90%
Pain	76%	71%	80%	71%
Rest room	66%	61%	71%	71%

Figure 6. Accuracy Comparison for Stress & Medicine in ML Algorithms

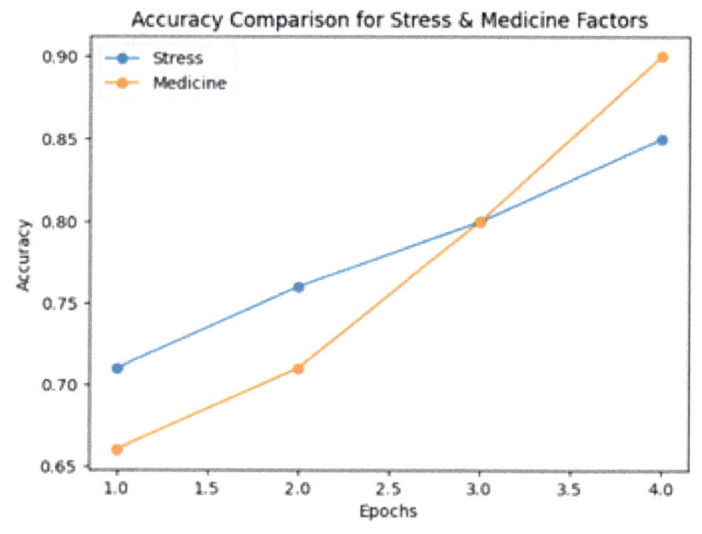

Figure 7. Accuracy Comparison of Four Algorithms in Medicine

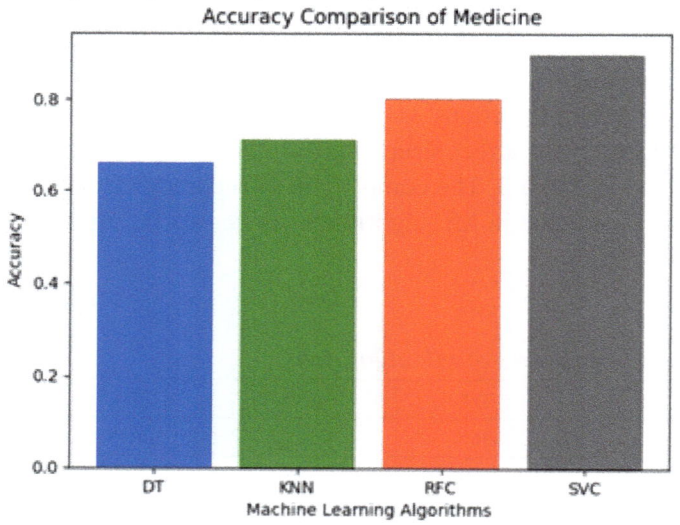

CONCLUSION AND FUTURE ENHANCEMENTS

Every human being is urging to lead a happy life without taking much stress mentally. Pilot study on despair study and analysis will keep many lives safe especially old aged people since they are not able to share their opinions due to their inabilities. In this research work, insomnia is analysed with classifiers such as SVM, RFC, DT, KNN and it is concluded that RFC produces better prediction in the above mention factors. In future work, an interface will be developed for Facial Emotion Recognition (FER) to recognize a individual's recent mental situation by confining their face via a camera or uploading an picture from local storage. Once it is uploaded, it is transformed to greyscale. With the help of Face-APIs, the images are edited. A pre-trained model then processes this collection of values to calculate the results based on its training. By identifying human facial traits, AI can predict human emotions. This prognostic technique will be implemented to accomplish a preliminary assessment of depression and save lives of aged people.

REFERENCES

Ahmadi, M., & Nasiri, S. (2023). Developing a prediction model for successful aging among the elderly using machine learning algorithms. *Digital Health*, 9, 20552076231178425. DOI: 10.1177/20552076231178425 PMID: 37284015

Ahsan, M. M., Luna, S. A., & Siddique, Z. (2022). Machine-learning-based disease diagnosis: A comprehensive review. *Health Care*, 10(3), 541. PMID: 35327018

Albahra, S., Gorbett, T., Robertson, S., D'Aleo, G., Kumar, S. V. S., Ockunzzi, S., Lallo, D., Hu, B., & Rashidi, H. H. (2023). Artificial intelligence and machine learning overview in pathology & laboratory medicine: A general review of data preprocessing and basic supervised concepts. *Seminars in Diagnostic Pathology*, 40(2), 71–87. DOI: 10.1053/j.semdp.2023.02.002 PMID: 36870825

Anderson, D., Bjarnadóttir, M., & Nenova, Z. (2021). *Machine Learning in Health Care: Operational and Financial Impact*. DOI: 10.1007/978-3-030-75729-8_5

Asghari Varzaneh, Z., Shanbehzadeh, M., & Kazemi-Arpanahi, H. (2022). Prediction of successful aging using ensemble machine learning algorithms. *BMC Medical Informatics and Decision Making*, 22(1), 258. DOI: 10.1186/s12911-022-02001-6 PMID: 36192713

Barda, A., Horvat, C., & Hochheiser, H. (2020). A qualitative research framework for the design of user-centered displays of explanations for machine learning model predictions in healthcare. *BMC Medical Informatics and Decision Making*, 20(1), 257. DOI: 10.1186/s12911-020-01276-x PMID: 33032582

Barracliffe, L., Arandjelovic, O., & Humphris, G. (2017, March). *A Pilot Study of Breast Cancer Patients: Can Machine Learning Predict Healthcare Professionals' Responses to Patient Emotions?* Bharadiya, J. P. (2023). A tutorial on principal component analysis for dimensionality reduction in machine learning. *International Journal of Innovative Science and Research Technology*, 8(5), 2028–2032.

Bouchlaghem, Y., Akhiat, Y., & Amjad, S. (2022). Feature Selection: A Review and Comparative Study. *E3S Web of Conferences, 351*, 01046. DOI: 10.1051/e3sconf/202235101046

Caballero, F. F., Soulis, G., Engchuan, W., Sánchez-Niubó, A., Arndt, H., Ayuso-Mateos, J. L., Haro, J. M., Chatterji, S., & Panagiotakos, D. B. (2017). Advanced analytical methodologies for measuring healthy ageing and its determinants, using factor analysis and machine learning techniques: The ATHLOS project. *Scientific Reports*, 7(1), 43955. DOI: 10.1038/srep43955 PMID: 28281663

Cho, G., Yim, J., Choi, Y., Ko, J., & Lee, S.-H. (2019). Review of Machine Learning Algorithms for Diagnosing Mental Illness. *Psychiatry Investigation*, 16(4), 262–269. DOI: 10.30773/pi.2018.12.21.2 PMID: 30947496

Chung, J., & Teo, J. (2022). Mental Health Prediction Using Machine Learning: Taxonomy, Applications, and Challenges. *Applied Computational Intelligence and Soft Computing*, 9970363, 1–19. Advance online publication. DOI: 10.1155/2022/9970363

Cohen, N. M., Lifshitz, A., Jaschek, R., Rinott, E., Balicer, R., Shlush, L. I., Barbash, G. I., & Tanay, A. (2024). Longitudinal machine learning uncouples healthy aging factors from chronic disease risks. *Nature Aging*, 4(1), 129–144. DOI: 10.1038/s43587-023-00536-5 PMID: 38062254

El Naqa, I., & Murphy, M. J. (2015). *What is machine learning?* Springer.

Ferdous, M., Debnath, J., & Chakraborty, N. (2020). *Machine Learning Algorithms in Healthcare: A Literature Survey*. 1–6. DOI: 10.1109/ICCCNT49239.2020.9225642

Habehh, H., & Gohel, S. (2021). Machine Learning in Healthcare. *Current Genomics*, 22(4), 291–300. DOI: 10.2174/1389202922666210705124359 PMID: 35273459

Hancer, E. (2024). An improved evolutionary wrapper-filter feature selection approach with a new initialisation scheme. *Machine Learning*, 113(8), 4977–5000. DOI: 10.1007/s10994-021-05990-z

Hasanin, T., Khoshgoftaar, T. M., Leevy, J. L., & Bauder, R. A. (2019). Severely imbalanced Big Data challenges: Investigating data sampling approaches. *Journal of Big Data*, 6(1), 107. DOI: 10.1186/s40537-019-0274-4

Hashim, M. S., & Yassin, A. A. (2023). Feature Selection Using a Hybrid Approach Depends on Filter and Wrapper Methods for Accurate Breast Cancer Diagnosis. *Journal of Basrah Researches (Sciences)*, 49(1), 45–56. DOI: 10.56714/bjrs.49.1.5

Hatton, C. M., Paton, L. W., McMillan, D., Cussens, J., Gilbody, S., & Tiffin, P. A. (2019). Predicting persistent depressive symptoms in older adults: A machine learning approach to personalised mental healthcare. *Journal of Affective Disorders*, 246, 857–860. DOI: 10.1016/j.jad.2018.12.095 PMID: 30795491

Islam, S., Liu, D., Wang, K., Zhou, P., Yu, L., & Wu, D. (2019). A Case Study of HealthCare Platform using Big Data Analytics and Machine Learning. *HPCCT 2019: Proceedings of the 2019 3rd High Performance Computing and Cluster Technologies Conference*, 139–146. DOI: 10.1145/3341069.3342980

Javaid, M., Haleem, A., Singh, R., Suman, R., & Rab, S. (2022). Significance of machine learning in healthcare: Features, pillars and applications. *International Journal of Intelligent Networks*, 3, 58–73. Advance online publication. DOI: 10.1016/j.ijin.2022.05.002

Jijo, B. T., & Abdulazeez, A. M. (2021).*Journal of Applied Science and Technology Trends*, 2(01), 20–28. DOI: 10.38094/jastt20165

Kabir, M. F., Chen, T., & Ludwig, S. A. (2023). A performance analysis of dimensionality reduction algorithms in machine learning models for cancer prediction. *Healthcare Analytics*, 3, 100125. DOI: 10.1016/j.health.2022.100125

Kan, H., Kharrazi, H., Chang, H.-Y., Bodycombe, D., Lemke, K., & Weiner, J. (2019). Exploring the use of machine learning for risk adjustment: A comparison of standard and penalized linear regression models in predicting health care costs in older adults. *PLoS One*, 14(3), e0213258. DOI: 10.1371/journal.pone.0213258 PMID: 30840682

Kuppusamy, S., & Thangavel, R. (2023). Deep Non-linear and Unbiased Deep Decisive Pooling Learning–Based Opinion Mining of Customer Review. *Cognitive Computation*, 15(2), 1–13. DOI: 10.1007/s12559-022-10089-1

Lee, S.-K., Son, Y.-J., Kim, J., Kim, H.-G., Lee, J.-I., Kang, B.-Y., Cho, H.-S., & Lee, S. (2014). Prediction Model for Health-Related Quality of Life of Elderly with Chronic Diseases using Machine Learning Techniques. *Healthcare Informatics Research*, 20(2), 125–134. DOI: 10.4258/hir.2014.20.2.125 PMID: 24872911

Li, W., Chai, Y., Khan, F., Jan, S., Verma, P., Menon, V. K., & Li, X. (2021). A Comprehensive Survey on Machine Learning-Based Big Data Analytics for IoT-Enabled Smart Healthcare System. *Mobile Networks and Applications*, 26(1), 234–252. Advance online publication. DOI: 10.1007/s11036-020-01700-6

Mall, S., Srivastava, A., Mazumdar, B. D., Mishra, M., Bangare, S. L., & Deepak, A. (2022). Implementation of machine learning techniques for disease diagnosis. *Materials Today: Proceedings*, 51, 2198–2201. DOI: 10.1016/j.matpr.2021.11.274

Mian Qaisar, S., & Subasi, A. (2022). Effective Epileptic Seizure Detection Based on the Event-Driven Processing and Machine Learning for Mobile Healthcare. *Journal of Ambient Intelligence and Humanized Computing*, 13(7), 3619–3631. Advance online publication. DOI: 10.1007/s12652-020-02024-9

Mowbray, F., Zargoush, M., Jones, A., Wit, K., & Costa, A. (2020). Predicting Hospital Admission for Older Emergency Department Patients: Insights from Machine Learning. *International Journal of Medical Informatics*, 140, 104163. DOI: 10.1016/j.ijmedinf.2020.104163 PMID: 32474393

Pisner, D. A., & Schnyer, D. M. (2020). Support vector machine. In Mechelli, A., & Vieira, S. (Eds.), *Machine Learning* (pp. 101–121). Academic Press., DOI: 10.1016/B978-0-12-815739-8.00006-7

Qin, J., Chen, L., Liu, Y., Liu, C., Feng, C., & Chen, B. (2019). A Machine Learning Methodology for Diagnosing Chronic Kidney Disease. *IEEE Access, PP*, 1–1. DOI: 10.1109/ACCESS.2019.2963053

Rajkomar, A., Dean, J., & Kohane, I. (2019). Machine Learning in Medicine. *The New England Journal of Medicine*, 380(14), 1347–1358. DOI: 10.1056/NEJMra1814259 PMID: 30943338

Renukadevi, N. T. (2021). Performance Evaluation of Hybrid Machine Learning Algorithms for Medical Image Classification. In Dash, S., Pani, S. K., Abraham, A., & Liang, Y. (Eds.), *Advanced Soft Computing Techniques in Data Science, IoT and Cloud Computing* (pp. 281–299). Springer International Publishing., DOI: 10.1007/978-3-030-75657-4_12

Saraswathi, K., Renukadevi, N. T., Nandhini, S. S., Sushmitha, E., & Arundhathi, R. (2024). Implementation of Machine Learning Algorithms in Diabetes Prediction. In Asokan, R., Ruiz, D. P., & Piramuthu, S. (Eds.), *Smart Data Intelligence* (pp. 169–186). Springer Nature Singapore. DOI: 10.1007/978-981-97-3191-6_13

Sarker, I. H. (2021). Machine Learning: Algorithms, Real-World Applications and Research Directions. *SN Computer Science*, 2(3), 160. DOI: 10.1007/s42979-021-00592-x PMID: 33778771

Sau, A., & Bhakta, I. (2017). Predicting anxiety and depression in elderly patients using machine learning technology. *Healthcare Technology Letters*, 4(6), 238–243. DOI: 10.1049/htl.2016.0096

Shailaja, K., Seetharamulu, B., & Jabbar, M. (2018). Machine learning in healthcare: A review. *2018 Second International Conference on Electronics, Communication and Aerospace Technology (ICECA)*, 910–914. DOI: 10.1109/ICECA.2018.8474918

Sumathi, M., & B, D. (2016). Prediction of Mental Health Problems Among Children Using Machine Learning Techniques. *International Journal of Advanced Computer Science and Applications*, 7(1). Advance online publication. DOI: 10.14569/IJACSA.2016.070176

Sun, B., & Wei, H.-L. (2022). *Machine Learning for Medical and Healthcare Data Analysis and Modelling: Case Studies and Performance Comparisons of Different Methods.* 1–6. DOI: 10.1109/ICAC55051.2022.9911176

Uddin, S., Haque, I., Lu, H., Moni, M. A., & Gide, E. (2022). Comparative performance analysis of K-nearest neighbour (KNN) algorithm and its different variants for disease prediction. *Scientific Reports*, 12(1), 6256. DOI: 10.1038/s41598-022-10358-x PMID: 35428863

Ullas, T. R., Begom, M., Ahmed, A., & Sultana, R. (2020). A Machine Learning Approach to detect Depression and Anxiety using Supervised Learning. *2020 IEEE Asia-Pacific Conference on Computer Science and Data Engineering (CSDE)*, 1–6.

Venu, K., & Natesan, P. (2023). Optimized Deep Learning Model Using Modified Whale's Optimization Algorithm for EEG Signal Classification. *Information Technology and Control*, 52(3), 744–760. DOI: 10.5755/j01.itc.52.3.33320

Weissman, S., Xueying, Y., Zhang, J., Chen, S., Olatosi, B., & Li, X. (2021). Using a Machine Learning Approach to Explore Predictors of Health Care Visits as Missed Opportunities for HIV Diagnosis. *AIDS (London, England)*, 35(Supplement 1), S7–S18. Advance online publication. DOI: 10.1097/QAD.0000000000002735 PMID: 33867485

Werner de Vargas, V., Schneider Aranda, J. A., dos Santos Costa, R., da Silva Pereira, P. R., & Victória Barbosa, J. L. (2023). Imbalanced data preprocessing techniques for machine learning: A systematic mapping study. *Knowledge and Information Systems*, 65(1), 31–57. DOI: 10.1007/s10115-022-01772-8 PMID: 36405957

Zaccheus, J., Atogwe, V., Oyejide, A., & Salau, A. O. (2024). *Towards successful aging classification using machine learning algorithms..*

Chapter 11
A Contactless Real-Time System to Classify Multi-Class Sitting Posture Using Depth Sensor-Based Data

Huseyin Coskun
https://orcid.org/0000-0002-8380-245X
Kutahya Health Sciences University, Turkey

ABSTRACT

Musculoskeletal disorders are often linked to poor sitting postures, making the assessment of healthy sitting positions crucial. This study develops a system for contactless recognition of office workers' sitting postures, using various classification methods for health applications. Five sitting postures were defined based on medical literature and standards. Thirty subjects held these postures for 30 seconds, with pose data captured via a Kinect device. To overcome challenges like desks and computers, two datasets with different joint points were created. Pose samples were labeled by calculating angles between body parts like legs, hips, and back. Classification methods included Neural Networks, Support Vector Machine (SVM), K-Nearest Neighbors, Naive Bayes, AdaBoost, Decision Tree, Random Forest, and Ensemble Learning (EL). The highest accuracy was achieved by EL and SVM, at 99.8% and 99.7%, respectively. The first and fifth postures were found to be the most comfortable. This system aims to improve sitting behaviors and is useful for health monitoring and robotic vision.

DOI: 10.4018/979-8-3693-7277-7.ch011

INTRODUCTION

In today's modern work environment, prolonged hours in office settings have become a standard for many professionals, leading to an increase in health risks associated with sedentary lifestyles. As technology advances, the time spent sitting at desks has escalated, which, while increasing productivity, also brings about serious health concerns. One of the most pressing issues is the development of musculoskeletal disorders (MSDs) (Bullock et al., 2005; Parry & Straker, 2013), as well as chronic pain, postural abnormalities (Grace et al., 2017; Tremblay et al., 2010), and even circulatory problems. These studies have highlighted how improper sitting postures can exacerbate these conditions, making them prevalent among office workers. These health issues not only diminish the quality of life for affected individuals but also have a detrimental effect on workplace productivity, as noted by these two studies. (Coleman et al., 2009; Ohlendorf et al., 2017). Given the significant impact of these issues, there is a growing need for proactive measures in the workplace. While ergonomic interventions and awareness campaigns are crucial for promoting healthy sitting habits, they are often implemented only after problems have already emerged. This reactive approach is insufficient for the complete prevention of health issues caused by poor posture. As such, there is a compelling case for developing intelligent workplace environments that include automated systems for tracking and correcting sitting postures. These systems could significantly reduce the high costs associated with health problems that arise from incorrect postures by providing real-time feedback and suggestions for improvement. This study introduces an innovative system aimed at proactively reducing the harmful effects of poor sitting postures in office settings. The system is designed as an intelligent solution that continuously monitors and analyzes users' sitting postures, offering ergonomic alerts and corrective suggestions in real-time. The key to this approach is the use of a contactless measurement system, which addresses the challenge of recognizing specified postures as recommended by health institutions and experts. The Kinect v2 device, known for its advanced depth sensor and camera capabilities, was chosen for this purpose. The Kinect can capture detailed information about twenty-five joint positions and can track the skeletal positions of up to six individuals simultaneously, making it ideal for use in a typical office environment. This allows for unobtrusive, contactless monitoring of sitting postures without disrupting employees' work. The core objective of this study is to investigate how different sitting postures can be effectively classified using skeletal position data obtained from depth sensors. By focusing on the minimum and maximum skeletal positions derived from the Kinect's depth-based information, the study aims to explore methods that offer superior performance compared to existing approaches in the literature. The ultimate goal is to help individuals develop and maintain proper sitting habits, thereby preventing the long-term health issues commonly associated with office work and enhancing overall well-being in the workplace. In addition to posture correction, this study also explores the relationship between comfort and correctness in sitting postures. Specifically, it examines the extent to which the postures that users find most comfortable align with the ergonomically correct postures recommended by experts. Understanding this relationship is crucial for designing interventions that are not only effective but also acceptable and comfortable for users. The structure of this paper is organized to guide readers through the various stages of research and development. The section on Related Works provides an overview of previous studies on depth sensor-based sitting posture classification, highlighting the gaps that this study aims to fill. The Materials and Methods section outlines the methodology used to obtain depth sensor-based data with Kinect, label the sitting posture data, and select the appropriate classification methods. Following this, the Results and Discussion section presents the findings from the experimental studies and offers a detailed analysis of these results. Finally, the Conclusion and Future Works section summarizes the key outcomes of the research and suggests possible directions for future studies, including the integration of additional features such as real-time feedback mechanisms and the potential for broader applications in various work environments.

RELATED WORKS

Paliyawan et al. (Paliyawan et al., 2014) developed a system to classify office workers' sitting postures using real-time skeleton data from a Kinect camera in an office environment. They created a dataset with 397,800 poses derived from 10 body skeleton points from 28 subjects. They compared several classification methods, including Decision Tree (DT), Neural Network (NN), Naive Bayes (NB), and k-Nearest Neighbors (KNN), achieving 98% accuracy in classifying a specific posture. The system provided real-time ergonomic feedback based on three health levels.

Ho et al. (Ho et al., 2016) introduced a framework that classifies 3D postures from Kinect data using a max-margin classifier. They also improved the framework's accuracy and robustness by analyzing the reliability of the tracked skeleton points. Using a dataset of 4,323 sitting poses, the framework achieved an accuracy of 80.84% in classifying three different sitting postures. Pal et al. (Pal et al., 2016) studied the occupational hazards of prolonged sitting in specific postures. They used seven similarity measures to recognize sitting postures, classifying two posture types with 94.29% accuracy in 3.83 milliseconds using city-block distance. Their dataset included 6,500 sitting poses from 20 subjects, derived from 16 body skeleton points. Bei et al. (Bei et al., 2018) proposed a method for classifying sitting postures using a Kinect depth sensor. They compiled a dataset with 16,200 poses from six body skeleton points and classified nine postures from 18 subjects, achieving 95.8% accuracy using KNN and body skeleton point features. Yao et al. (Yao et al., 2017) developed a method to separate unhealthy sitting postures from others using neck and torso angle detection with a Kinect sensor. They used 10 body skeleton points to calculate angles, collecting 66,330 sitting postures from 10 subjects across five posture classes. Their method used a threshold-based approach and achieved 86.65% accuracy. However, the angle values calculated by the Kinect device were not validated. Li et al. (B. Li et al., 2017) proposed a backpropagation (BP) neural network method for posture classification using skeleton data from a Kinect depth sensor. They used eight skeleton points to classify sitting postures from 100 subjects, achieving 97.77% accuracy across four posture types. Sun et al. (Sun et al., 2021) introduced a system to recognize sitting postures using the main upper body skeleton points from a Kinect depth sensor. They created a dataset with 513 poses from 20 body skeleton points and used a Convolutional Neural Network to classify two sitting postures with 82.86% accuracy. The system provided real-time feedback when incorrect postures were detected. Ray et al. (Ray & Teizer, 2012) developed an automated approach to classify construction workers' postures as ergonomic or non-ergonomic using 22,226 poses from 12 joint body points. They achieved 94.8% accuracy using linear discriminant analysis (LDA) in real-time. The literature often lacks clear definitions of sitting postures or the medical standards they are based on. Many studies do not define what constitutes a healthy or standard sitting posture. To address this gap, our study reviewed relevant medical and health literature to define standard sitting posture with precise expressions and angle values. We identified four different sitting postures to differentiate a standard sitting posture from others. Additionally, our study revealed the difference between the sitting posture that feels comfortable to subjects and the healthy posture through classification. Some studies mention determining body posture classes by observation. Our study proposes a Kinect-based angular labeling method to overcome the qualitative limitations of observational studies. Unlike many studies that rely on a single classification method, we classified five different sitting postures using data from Kinect and eight different classifiers. We compared the results with those from previous studies and achieved higher accuracy using fewer joint points.

MATERIAL AND METHODS

Sitting Postures

The determination of sitting postures in this study was guided by suggestions from previous research (Canadian Centre for Occupational Health & Safety, 2017; Delleman & Dul, 2007; Elliott, 2020; Fondazione Ergo-MTM Italia, 2021; Kelly, 2014) as well as the definitions provided in the ISO 7250-1:2017 (ISO, 2017). Based on these references, five distinct sitting postures were identified for classifying sitting behaviors. Among these, one posture is considered healthy and standard, as defined by the literature and the ISO 7250-1 standard. Figure 1 presents a sample illustration of the healthy and standard body posture, as determined according to the recommendations from (Canadian Centre for Occupational Health & Safety, 2017; Delleman & Dul, 2007; ISO, 2017).

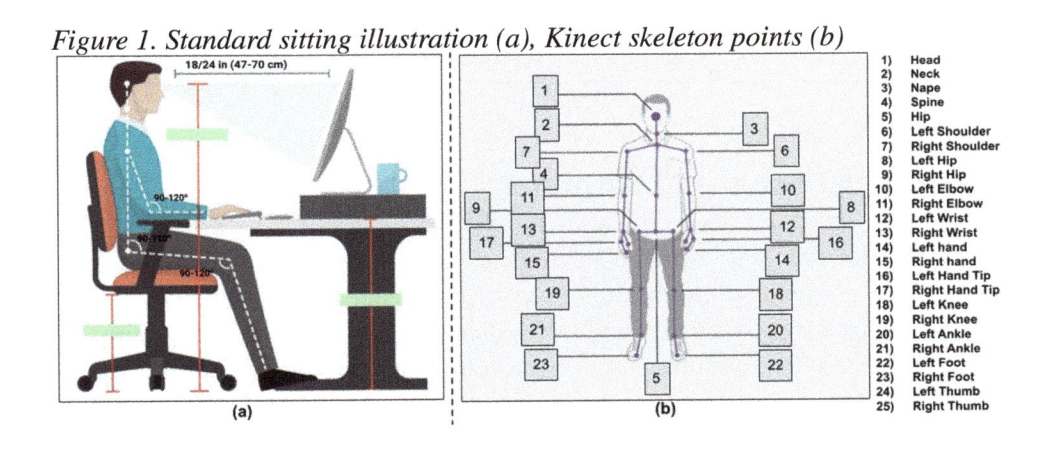

Figure 1. Standard sitting illustration (a), Kinect skeleton points (b)

The five determined sitting positions are presented in Table 1. To ensure that subjects correctly adjusted their sitting postures during the experiment to match the positions outlined in Table 1, they were instructed to monitor and follow their sitting postures throughout the experiment using a provided presentation.

Table 1. Sitting postures explanations

#	Position	Description	Reference
1	Standard sitting	The hands were asked to sit on both armrests with the back fully leaned back, and knees bent 90 degrees straight.	(Canadian Centre for Occupational Health & Safety, 2017; Delleman & Dul, 2007; ISO, 2017)
2	Leaning to the front side	They were asked to sit in such a way that they bent forward as much as possible, avoiding contact with the back.	(Canadian Centre for Occupational Health & Safety, 2017; Delleman & Dul, 2007; Elliott, 2020; Fondazione Ergo-MTM Italia, 2021; ISO, 2017; Kelly, 2014; Kong et al., 2018)
3	Leaning to the left side	It was requested that the body be bent to the left by placing the right foot on the left foot and leaning the left arm on the armrest, and the contact with the right sitting area was cut as much as possible	(Canadian Centre for Occupational Health & Safety, 2017; Delleman & Dul, 2007; Elliott, 2020; Fondazione Ergo-MTM Italia, 2021; ISO, 2017; Kelly, 2014; Kong et al., 2018)
4	Leaning to the right side	It was requested that the body be bent to the right by placing the left foot on the right foot and resting the right arm on the armrest, and the contact with the left sitting area was cut as much as possible.	(Canadian Centre for Occupational Health & Safety, 2017; Delleman & Dul, 2007; Elliott, 2020; Fondazione Ergo-MTM Italia, 2021; ISO, 2017; Kelly, 2014; Kong et al., 2018)
5	Leaning to the backside	They were asked to sit and slide in the seat by creating a triangular gap in this area, in the form of cutting contact with the lower back and sitting back area.	(Canadian Centre for Occupational Health & Safety, 2017; Delleman & Dul, 2007; Elliott, 2020; Fondazione Ergo-MTM Italia, 2021; ISO, 2017; Kelly, 2014; Kong et al., 2018)

Experimental Setup and Software

The data for this study were collected using a Kinect camera, which is part of a depth sensor-based motion tracking system. Such systems, like Microsoft Kinect (v2), have gained popularity in recent years. They work by capturing a depth image using an infrared light and depth sensor, which is then combined with the image from an RGB camera. This process allows for precise tracking of joint positions with both depth and visual information. Other similar depth cameras are available, and selecting the right one for sitting posture classification applications involves considering several key criteria. According to various studies (Guzsvinecz et al., 2019; Ray & Teizer, 2012), these criteria include: (a) depth camera resolution (e.g., 512×424 pixels), (b) noise from mixed pixels at depth discontinuities, (c) frame update rate, and (d) the quality of the color versus signal amplitude display. Once the depth sensor-based database is established, it can be used to recognize human posture by classifying different joints (Keçeli & Can, 2014). A significant advantage of using a depth camera is that monitoring can occur without requiring the user to wear any equipment. To create a depth sensor-based sitting posture database, an experimental setup was arranged where subjects sat on a chair positioned 1.5 meters from the Kinect device. They were asked to perform the postures defined in Table 1. To guide the subjects during the experiment, a presentation was prepared. Multiple versions of this presentation were created, each displaying the sitting postures in six different sequences to ensure variation in the order of the postures. During the experiment, participants were shown one of these randomly selected presentations to help them follow the correct postures.

Figure 2. (a) Data collection software, (b) experimental setup, and (c) guide presentation

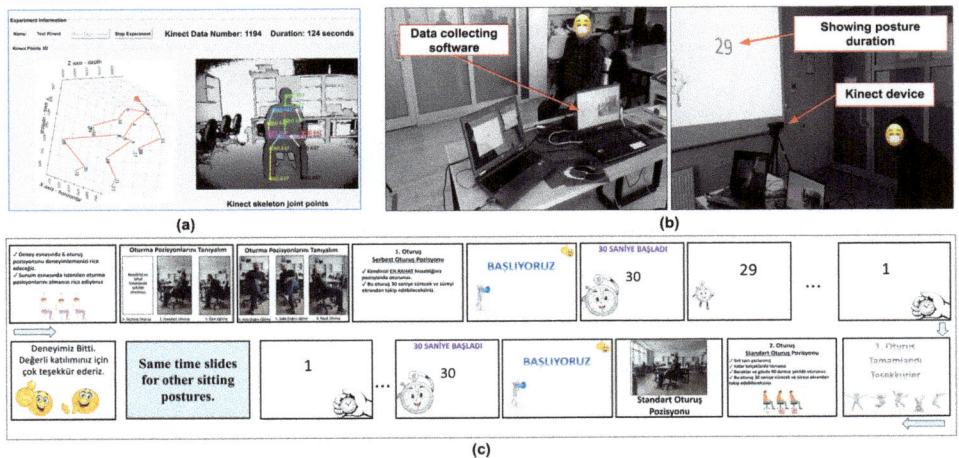

Participants were instructed to maintain each sitting posture for 30 seconds. At the start, they were asked to sit in their most comfortable position for the same duration. This helped identify which sitting posture each participant found most comfortable. Figure 2 shows our setup: (a) the real-time data collection and recognition software developed in Python, (b) the experimental arrangement, and (c) sample presentations. The recognition software uses the TensorFlow machine learning library for classification models. During the experiment, raw data for the x (horizontal), y (vertical), and z (depth) axes of 25 joint points from each subject were collected and stored in a MySQL database. The structure of the database table is shown in Figure 3.

Figure 3. Database structure of depth sensor data

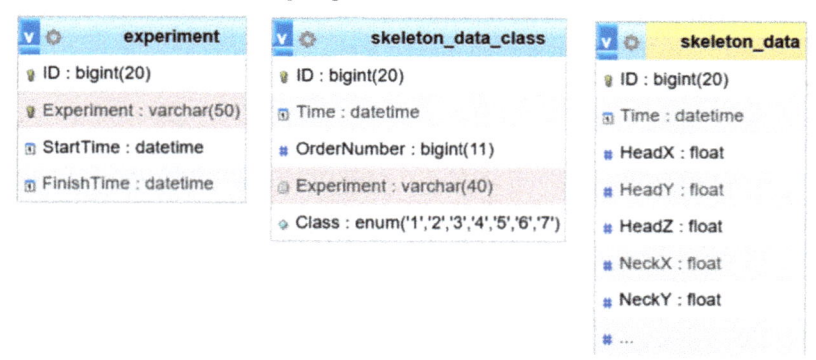

experiment	skeleton_data_class	skeleton_data
ID : bigint(20)	ID : bigint(20)	ID : bigint(20)
Experiment : varchar(50)	Time : datetime	Time : datetime
StartTime : datetime	OrderNumber : bigint(11)	HeadX : float
FinishTime : datetime	Experiment : varchar(40)	HeadY : float
	Class : enum('1','2','3','4','5','6','7')	HeadZ : float
		NeckX : float
		NeckY : float
		...

The database includes experiment table for experiment data such as experiment name (column name: experiment) start time and finish time. All the depth sensor data of skeleton have been stored in skeleton_data table. While there is no common column between the Experiment table and the skeleton_Data table, selection is made according to the common values in terms of time values. When the experiment program runs, it obtains continuous time-stamped data from the Kinect device. When the experiment starts, the start time is recorded in the experiment table, and when it ends, the end time is recorded. While all depth sensor data belonging to this experiment is obtained, the values between the start and end time of the experiment in the skeleton_data table are taken. Angle values are calculated on these values. The codes that enable data acquisition from the Kinect device and saving it to the database using Python are presented in the Figure 4 during sitting experiment.

Figure 4. Python codes for acquiring and storing of depth sensor data

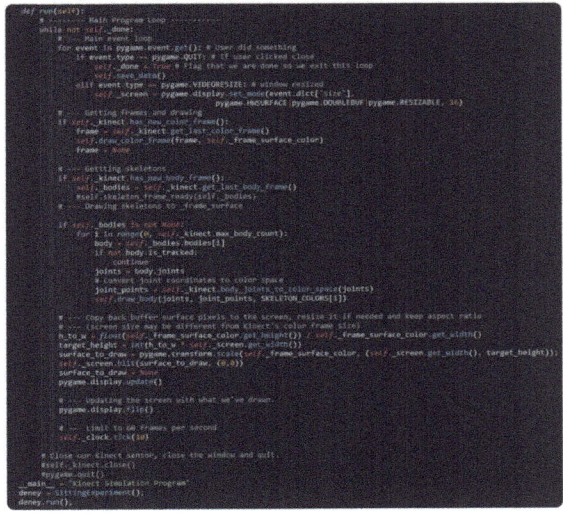

The codes of all methods and other components in the main code can be found in detail at this address (https://drive.google.com/file/d/1DiEOlsLfHTvOcxPukvn2dd PNJ4BPLbN7). The sample raw depth sensor data of a participant during an experiment period and view of the joints pattern are shown in Figure 5.

Figure 5. A subject's Kinect raw data as to sitting postures (between 1 and 2477 of supplementary data)

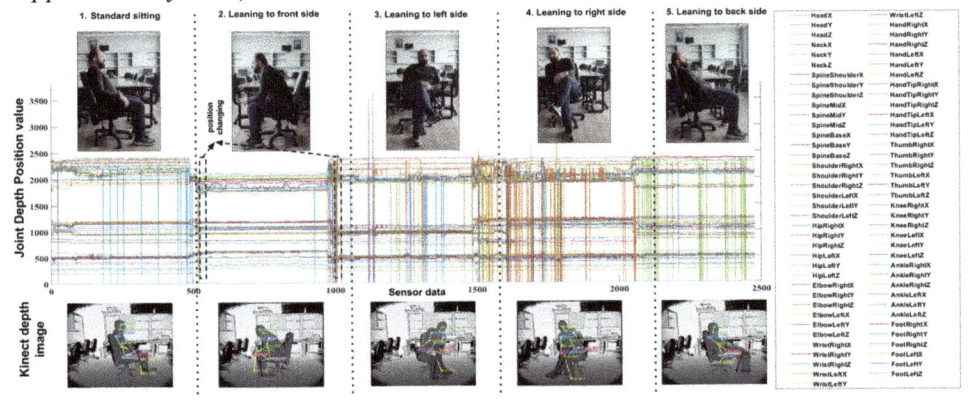

The changes in the period of the joint positions corresponding to the sitting postures for distinct depth sensor values can be observed in Figure 5. It can be observed that depth sensor values suddenly changes because the posture are switched.

Labelling Algorithms

The positions of the skeleton points were utilized to filter out body posture transition values from the dataset and to accurately label the skeleton point data according to the postures defined in Table 1. Figure 6 also includes an example drawing and angle representation of the skeleton point positions for the standard sitting posture. To enhance clarity, these skeleton point position drawings were rotated along the axes, resulting in more comprehensible visuals, as shown in Figure 6. Additionally, specific angle values were chosen for each posture to facilitate the labeling process using the skeleton point data.

Figure 6. The joint points and the specific angles for standard posture

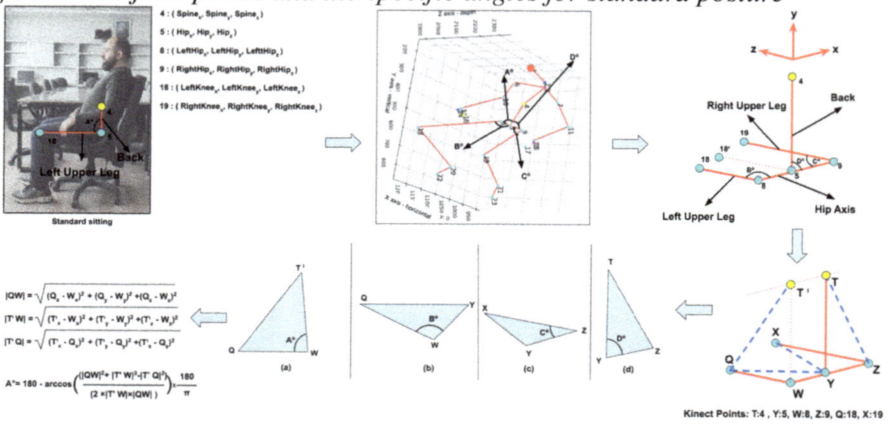

The angles were defined as follows:

- Angle A: The angle between the back and the left upper leg axis in the sitting position.
- Angle B: The angle between the hip axis and the left upper leg.
- Angle C: The angle between the hip axis and the right upper leg.
- Angle D: The angle between the back and the hip axis.

These four angles were determined to be the minimum necessary to effectively represent incorrect sitting postures, based on recommendations from previous studies (Canadian Centre for Occupational Health & Safety, 2017; Delleman & Dul, 2007; ISO, 2017). It is important to note that the joint point coordinate was used as unit lengths rather than actual measurements in meters or inches. To calculate angles A, B, C, and D, four triangles, as illustrated in Figure 6, were constructed, and the lengths of the sides of these triangles were computed. Since the joint point location was obtained from the Kinect device in a 3D space, the edge lengths of the triangles have been computed based on Euclidean distance. Using the example triangle (a) in Figure 6, the value of angle A was determined utilizing the cosine law. Similarly, the cosine law was employed to calculate angles B, C, and D. The edge length and angle values were obtained from the joint region coordinate data recorded in the database.

Figure 7. Angle calculation query of A for standard posture

```
SELECT   ID
FROM     skeleton_data
WHERE
    (SELECT AVG(ACOS((POW(ABS(KneeLeftZ-HipleftZ),2) + POW(ABS(SpineMidY-HipleftY)
,2)-POW(SQRT(POW((KneeLeftX-SpineMidX+ABS(HipLeftX-SpineBaseX)),2)
+POW(ABS(KneeLeftY-SpineMidY),2) + POW(ABS(KneeLeftZ-SpineMidZ),2)),2))
/2*(ABS(KneeLeftZ-HipleftZ)*ABS(SpineMidY-HipleftY) ))*180/PI())  FROM
skeleton_data AS SD,experiment AS E WHERE SD.Time BETWEEN E.StartTime AND
DATE_ADD(E.StartTime,INTERVAL 30 SECOND) OR E.FinishTime BETWEEN
E.FinishTime AND DATE_SUB(E.FinishTime,INTERVAL 30 SECOND))<=95
    AND
    (SELECT AVG(ACOS((POW(ABS(KneeLeftZ-HipleftZ),2) + POW(ABS(SpineMidY-HipleftY)
,2)-POW(SQRT(POW((KneeLeftX-SpineMidX+ABS(HipLeftX-SpineBaseX)),2)
+POW(ABS(KneeLeftY-SpineMidY),2) + POW(ABS(KneeLeftZ-SpineMidZ),2)),2))
/2*(ABS(KneeLeftZ-HipleftZ)*ABS(SpineMidY-HipleftY) ))*180/PI())  FROM
skeleton_data AS SD,experiment AS E WHERE SD.Time BETWEEN E.StartTime AND
DATE_ADD(E.StartTime,INTERVAL 30 SECOND) OR E.FinishTime BETWEEN
E.FinishTime AND DATE_SUB(E.FinishTime,INTERVAL 30 SECOND)) <=105
```

The sample database query regarding the angle value A of the sample standard seating position is given in Figure 7. In Figure 7, the query provides the calculation of the angle values according to Equation 1 and Equation 2 using the joint position values 30 seconds after the experiment start time during the standard sitting position and 30 seconds before the end of the experiment. Angle values calculated in the determined postures were examined, and the average of these values is given in Table 2. When the angle values in Table 2 are analyzed, it is observed that they support the postures in Table 1.

Table 2. Angle values of sitting postures

Posture	Avg. Angle A	Angle A Range	Avg. Angle B	Angle B Range	Avg. Angle C	Angle C Range	Avg. Angle D	Angle D Range
1	104.3	95-105	101.3	95-105	104.2	95-105	92.1	95-105
2	68.8	60-90	121.5	110-125	125.7	105-125	88.2	85-100
3	88.2	80-90	47.1	45-65	44.2	40-55	76.2	95-105
4	80.4	80-90	41.4	40-55	50.5	55-65	72.4	60-80
5	118.2	110-120	115.3	110-125	118.2	110-125	88.4	80-90

"The B and C angles represent the upper legs, so their values should be similar. The values in Table 2 confirm this similarity. Angle A should decrease when leaning forward and increase when leaning backward. The calculated values, especially for the second and fifth sitting postures, accurately reflect this pattern. The D angle values don't change significantly in the second and fifth postures, which is expected since these postures don't involve much sideways bending. We calculated these angle values for each pose in the dataset using the joint points illustrated in Figure 6. Sample participant's data for the angle values calculated for labeling the raw data and sample sitting posture drawings created using the raw data are presented in Figure 8.

Figure 8. Specific angle values and skeleton pattern created from raw data

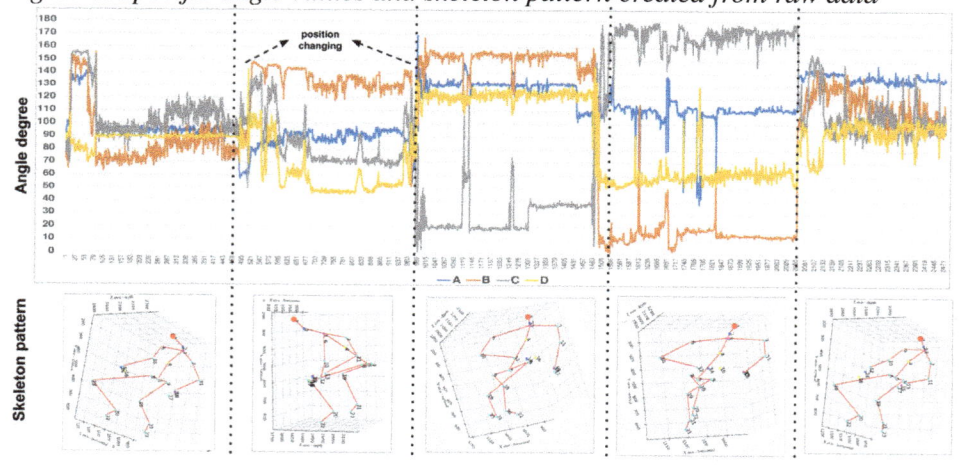

During the sitting experiments, the skeleton point positions of the subjects were obtained in 3 axes with the Kinect device to observe that the sitting angle values in the standard sitting are provided and that the sitting positions are clearly separated from each other. This meaningful observation reveals the necessity of performing a quantitative observation with geometric and mathematical processes instead of qualitative observation in order to distinguish between the identified sitting postures for labeling. The flow diagram of the labeling algorithm is presented in Figure 9. The angle method was used for labeling and then raw joint depth position data was used as input data for the machine learning.

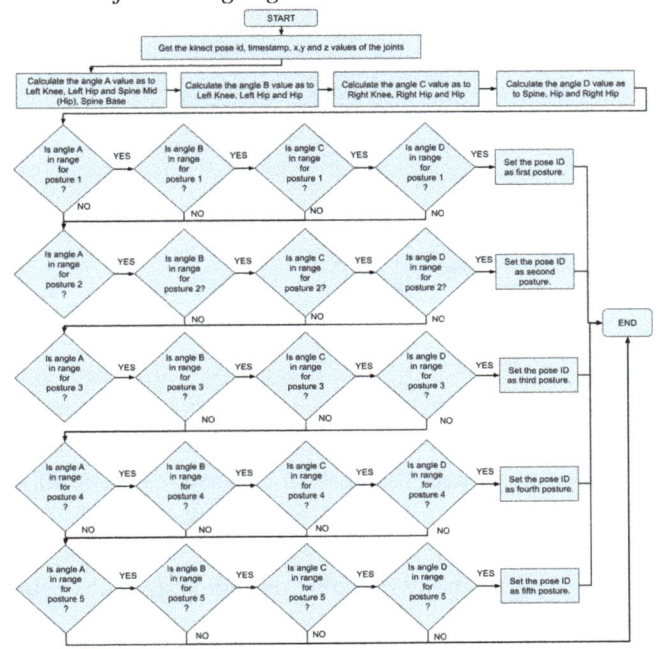

Figure 9. Flow chart of labelling algorithm

Creating the Dataset and Machine Learning Algorithms

After the automatic labeling process, the skeleton joint point data, whose class information was assigned, was classified by different machine learning methods. In the classification process, two different data sets were created according to the selection of joint points. This is because it was difficult for office workers to obtain all joint positions simultaneously due to obstacles such as desks and chairs. For this reason, firstly, a data set (A) containing 75 feature information for all sitting poses with each x, y, and z value belonging to 25 joint points was created. Using the upper joint positions in the more visible areas while working was preferred. In this context, Head (1), Neck (2), right Shoulder (6), and left Shoulder (7) joints were selected, as well as all joint points and another data set (B) containing 12 feature information was created.

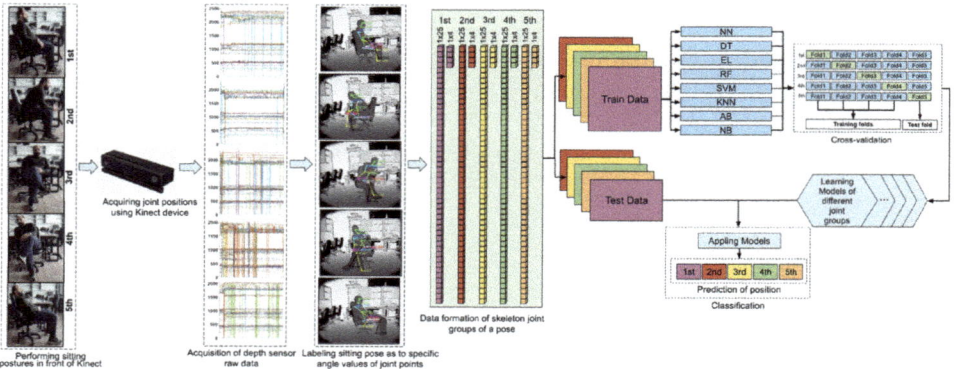

Figure 10. The classification diagram

The depth sensor data of sitting postures were acquired with an average 100 ms (10 Hz), providing a field of view of 84.1 degrees horizontally and 53.8 degrees vertically, with a maximum depth distance of 3 meters. A total of 49,580 sitting body posture poses were recorded from thirty participants across five distinct classes. During the experiment, some subjects adjusted their sitting positions, leading to angle values from the skeleton point data that did not match the desired targets. As a result, angle-based labeling could not accurately categorize these instances for the specified sitting postures. Because the data came from different participants, different numbers of data were acquired for each class. The dataset comprises varying numbers of records for each posture class, specifically:

- First posture: 9,827 samples
- Second posture: 9,617 samples
- Third posture: 9,778 samples
- Fourth posture: 10,553 samples
- Fifth posture: 9,805 samples

For all classifiers used in the study, 15% of the data was allocated for validation and testing purposes. The training model was evaluated using data that had not been included in the training phase, ensuring that the test data was entirely distinct from the training data. Although deep learning methods are becoming increasingly popular, conventional machine learning approach were preferred in this study due to their shorter training times compared to deep learning approaches (Bania, 2022;

Hu et al., 2023; Liu & Zhang, 2020). To classify sitting postures, several classifiers were designed and implemented, including Neural Networks (NN), Decision Trees (DT), Ensemble Learning (EL), Random Forest (RF), Support Vector Machines (SVM), k-Nearest Neighbors (KNN), AdaBoost, and Naive Bayes (NB). Each of these classification models was tested with different parameters to evaluate and identify the configuration that provided the best performance. The evaluation process involved fine-tuning the parameters of each classifier to optimize their performance. This systematic approach allowed for a comprehensive comparison of the classifiers, ensuring that the most effective methods for accurately classifying sitting postures were identified. The results from these classifiers provide valuable insights into which algorithms are best suited for real-time posture monitoring applications. To analyze performance using different sets of skeleton data points, two neural networks (NN) were designed with input sizes of 12 and 75 data points, respectively. Both networks consist of 10 hidden layers and 5 output layers. The following configurations were applied:

- **Data Division**: Random
- **Training Function**: Scaled Conjugate Gradient (SCG)
- **Optimization Method**: Levenberg-Marquardt
- **Loss Function**: Cross-Entropy
- **Activation Function**: Tan-Sigmoid (Tan-Sig)
- **Training Epochs**: 234
- **Error Goal**: Limited to 0.001
- **Weights and Biases Initialization**: Nguyen-Widrow method

These settings were selected to optimize the networks' performance in classifying sitting postures, based on best practices from relevant research (Coskun et al., 2017; Coskun & Yigit, 2018).

For the Decision Tree (DT) classifiers, three levels of flexibility parameters were tested: fine, medium, and coarse. The maximum split parameters were set to 4 for coarse, 20 for medium, and 100 for fine. The hyperparameters for the DT models were configured as follows (Luján et al., 2022):

- **Minimum Number of Instances**: 4 for leaves, 6 for internal nodes
- **Maximum Depth**: 100
- **Splitting Criterion**: Gini Impurity Index
- **Number of Nodes**: 187

After evaluation, the Fine model of the DT method was selected for use, as it demonstrated superior performance compared to the other models across both datasets.

As ensemble learning classifiers, the following models were utilized to classify sitting postures: **Boosted Tree, Bagged Tree, Subspace Discriminant, Subspace KNN,** and **RUSBoosted Tree**.

- **Boosted Tree** is based on the Adaptive Boosting (AdaBoost) classification method, which sequentially adds models that focus on correcting the errors made by previous models.
- **Bagged Tree** and **RUSBoosted Tree** are both derived from the Decision Tree (DT) learner type. For these models, the learning rate was set to 0.1, and the maximum number of splits allowed was 20.
- The boosting process for these models follows the Adaptive Boosting approach for multi-class classification, which involves reweighting the training instances to focus on those that were misclassified in prior iterations (Seiffert et al., 2008).
- **Subspace Discriminant** is based on the Discriminant Analysis learner type, while **Subspace KNN** utilizes the k-Nearest Neighbors (k-NN) learner type. Both of these models operate in a subspace dimension of 24.

For all ensemble learning models, a total of 30 learners were employed. Among these, the **Bagged Tree model** was selected as the most effective classifier, as it demonstrated superior performance across both datasets. This choice reflects its ability to reduce overfitting and improve generalization by aggregating predictions from multiple decision trees.

Random Forest (RF) is an ensemble machine learning technique that constructs multiple classification trees using a bagging strategy. In this approach, a subset of features is randomly selected from the dataset for each tree, and the trees are built on randomly chosen samples. Once the trees are trained, they collectively vote on the class label for a given input vector, allowing for a more robust and accurate classification (T. Li et al., 2016). In this study, the primary parameter adjusted for the Random Forest model was the number of trees in the ensemble, which was set to 10. This configuration helps to balance the model's complexity and performance, ensuring effective classification of sitting postures while minimizing the risk of overfitting. The use of multiple trees allows the Random Forest to leverage the diversity of the individual trees, leading to improved accuracy and reliability in the classification results.

The Support Vector Machine (SVM) was evaluated using various kernel types as model flexibility parameters, including coarse Gaussian (kernel scale, ks = 38), cubic, fine Gaussian (ks = 2.7), medium Gaussian (ks = 7.9), quadratic, and linear kernels. For the cubic, quadratic, and linear kernels, the kernel scale (ks) was set to automatic. To handle multi-class classification, the one-vs-one approach was employed. The hyperparameters (hps) for the SVM were configured as follows:

- **Sigma**: 0.5

- **Cost (C)**: Ranged from 2^{-3} to 2^{15}
- **Gamma**: Ranged from 2^{-15} to 2^{3}
- **Kernel scale (ks)**: Ranged from 0.001 to 1000
- **Numerical tolerance**: 0.001
- **Iteration limit**: 100

Among the various models tested, the Fine model was selected due to its superior classification performance across both datasets. This model's configuration effectively balanced complexity and accuracy, making it well-suited for the task of classifying sitting postures.

For the k-Nearest Neighbors (k-NN) classifier, various model flexibility parameters were tested, including Cubic, Medium, Fine, Coarse, Weighted, and Cosine. Here's a breakdown of the configurations:

- **Number of Neighbors**:
  - Fine: 1 neighbor
  - Medium: 10 neighbors
  - Coarse: 100 neighbors
- **Distance Metric (dm)**:
  - Euclidean: Used for Fine, Medium, Weighted, and Coarse models.
  - Cosine: Used for the Cosine model.
  - Minkowski (Cubic): Used for the Cubic model.
- **Distance Weighting**:
  - Equal weighting: Used for Fine, Medium, Coarse, Cosine, and Cubic models.
  - Squared inverse weighting: Used for the Weighted model.

The Fine model was selected as it achieved the best classification performance for both datasets.

AdaBoost employs a technique that assigns a probability distribution over all training samples. During each iteration, this distribution is updated by incorporating a new weak estimator, which is trained on the data (Sevinç, 2022).

For this study, the key parameters were set as follows:

- Number of Estimators: 50
- Learning Rate: 1
- Classification Algorithms: SAMME and SAMME.R
- Regression Loss Functions: Linear, square, and exponential

After evaluating the performance across both datasets, the SAMME.R classification algorithm combined with the linear loss function was selected, as it provided the best results. For the Naive Bayes (NB) classifier, both Kernel and Gaussian distribution models were tested. It was observed that the Kernel distribution model outperformed the Gaussian distribution model across both datasets. To ensure the predictive ability of all models and to prevent overfitting, a 5-fold cross-validation (CV) process was utilized. This method allows the classifier to operate without bias, as the data is divided into five subsets, and each subset is used once as the validation data while the remaining four subsets are used for training. Importantly, there was no data sharing between the training and validation sets during the CV process, which helped avoid overtraining and ensured the models' robustness.

Figure 11. Python code to design NN model

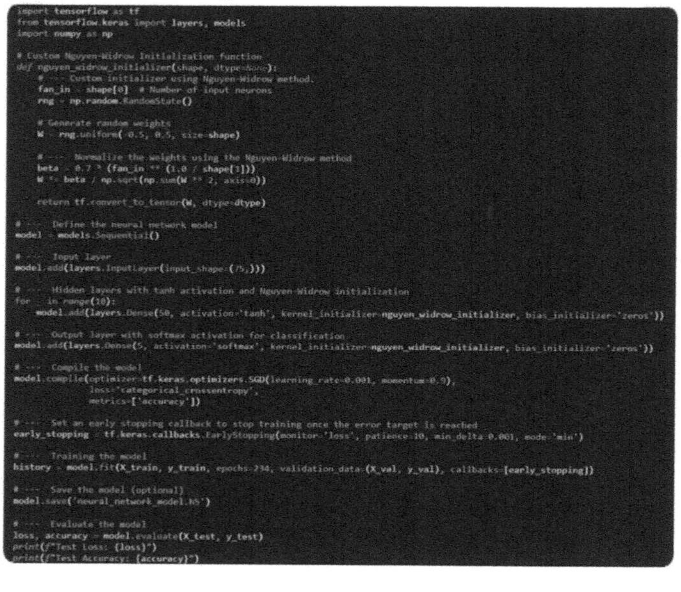

```python
import tensorflow as tf
from tensorflow.keras import layers, models
import numpy as np

# Custom Nguyen-Widrow Initialization function
def nguyen_widrow_initializer(shape, dtype=None):
    # --- Custom initializer using Nguyen-Widrow method.
    fan_in = shape[0]  # Number of input neurons
    rng = np.random.RandomState()

    # Generate random weights
    W = rng.uniform(-0.5, 0.5, size=shape)

    # --- Normalize the weights using the Nguyen-Widrow method
    beta = 0.7 * (fan_in ** (1.0 / shape[1]))
    W *= beta / np.sqrt(np.sum(W ** 2, axis=0))

    return tf.convert_to_tensor(W, dtype=dtype)

# --- Define the neural network model
model = models.Sequential()

# --- Input layer
model.add(layers.InputLayer(input_shape=(75,)))

# --- Hidden layers with tanh activation and Nguyen-Widrow initialization
for _ in range(10):
    model.add(layers.Dense(50, activation='tanh', kernel_initializer=nguyen_widrow_initializer, bias_initializer='zeros'))

# --- Output layer with softmax activation for classification
model.add(layers.Dense(5, activation='softmax', kernel_initializer=nguyen_widrow_initializer, bias_initializer='zeros'))

# --- Compile the model
model.compile(optimizer=tf.keras.optimizers.SGD(learning_rate=0.001, momentum=0.9),
              loss='categorical_crossentropy',
              metrics=['accuracy'])

# --- Set an early stopping callback to stop training once the error target is reached
early_stopping = tf.keras.callbacks.EarlyStopping(monitor='loss', patience=10, min_delta=0.001, mode='min')

# --- Training the model
history = model.fit(X_train, y_train, epochs=234, validation_data=(X_val, y_val), callbacks=[early_stopping])

# --- Save the model (optional)
model.save('neural_network_model.h5')

# --- Evaluate the model
loss, accuracy = model.evaluate(X_test, y_test)
print(f"Test Loss: {loss}")
print(f"Test Accuracy: {accuracy}")
```

The Python codes used to design the NN model are presented in Figure 11. Initialization for Nguyen-Widrow has been manually implemented as TensorFlow/Keras does not provide a built-in initializer. TensorFlow/Keras does not directly support Levenberg-Marquardt optimization. In practice, for large-scale problems, optimizers like Adam or RMSprop are used. Here, the scaled conjugate gradient method has been emulated through the use of SGD with momentum. *X_train, X_val*, and *X_test* variables represent features (input data) of the datasets for training, validation, and testing. They are typically NumPy arrays or pandas DataFrames. *y_train*, *y_val*, and *y_test* variables represent the target labels (output data) associated with each sample in the dataset. They are also typically NumPy arrays or pandas Series/DataFrames. To measure the performance of each model, a multi-class confusion matrix and ROC curve have been generated (Coskun et al., 2022). Python codes in Figure 12 were used for ROC curve plotting and confusion matrix generation.

Figure 12. Python codes for ROC chart and confusion matrix

```python
import numpy as np
import matplotlib.pyplot as plt
from sklearn.metrics import roc_curve, auc

# --- Predict the probabilities for the test data
y_probs = model.predict(X_test)  # --- Predict probabilities

# --- Calculate the ROC curve and AUC for each class
fpr = dict()
tpr = dict()
roc_auc = dict()
n_classes = y_test.shape[1]

for i in range(n_classes):
    fpr[i], tpr[i], _ = roc_curve(y_test[:, i], y_probs[:, i])
    roc_auc[i] = auc(fpr[i], tpr[i])

# --- Plot the ROC curve for each class
plt.figure(figsize=(10, 8))
for i in range(n_classes):
    plt.plot(fpr[i], tpr[i], lw=2, label=f'Class {i+1} (AUC = {roc_auc[i]:0.2f})')

plt.plot([0, 1], [0, 1], color='navy', lw=2, linestyle='--')  # Diagonal line
plt.xlabel('False Positive Rate')
plt.ylabel('True Positive Rate')
plt.title('ROC Curve')
plt.legend(loc="best")
plt.show()

# Convert predicted probabilities to class labels
y_pred_classes = np.argmax(y_probs, axis=1)

# If y_test is one-hot encoded, convert it back to class labels
if y_test.ndim > 1:
    y_test_classes = np.argmax(y_test, axis=1)
else:
    y_test_classes = y_test

# Compute the confusion matrix
cm = confusion_matrix(y_test_classes, y_pred_classes)

# Plot the confusion matrix
disp = ConfusionMatrixDisplay(confusion_matrix=cm)
disp.plot(cmap=plt.cm.Blues)
plt.title("Confusion Matrix")
plt.show()
```

Accuracy (A), Recall (R), precision (P), F1-score (F) and, AUC (Area Under Curve) indicators are computed to evaluate performance (Coskun et al., 2022). In addition to comparing the classification performance of the generated datasets, in order to emphasize the originality of this study, real-time classification of the sitting postures in which the subjects felt most comfortable was performed. Joint position data were acquired in real-time and classified using all trained models. Classification prediction results were recorded and presented in results. The Python code for the NN model for this process is presented in Figure 13.

Figure 13. Real time prediction of depth sensor data

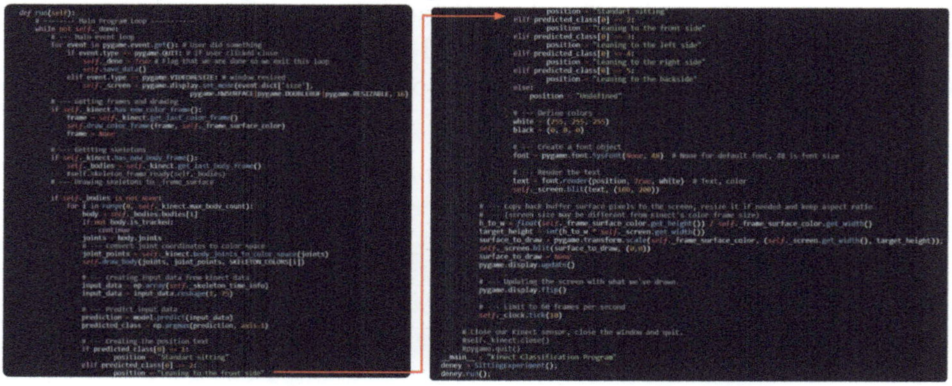

In this python code, the data obtained from the Kinect device is represented by the variable _skeleton_time_info. This data is first plotted using a PyGame object via the *draw_body* method. Then it is predicted with the NN model represented by the designed *model* variable. Since the prediction result is an integer between 1 and 5, the name of the posture is assigned to the *position* variable in a decision control structure. The predicted posture is printed in black color at position (100,200) of the screen.

RESULTS AND DISCUSSION

For the classification of body postures, confusion matrices were generated for the models of the classifiers. These matrices represent the models that achieved the highest accuracy results using the entire dataset, as shown in Figure 14. Both the training and testing processes were conducted on the same computer. Upon examining the confusion matrices, it is evident that the majority of the samples were correctly classified according to their labels, with the exception of the RF classifier, which showed some misclassification in the 5th class. This indicates that most models effectively distinguished between the different body postures, though there was a slight drop in performance for the RF model in one of the posture classes.

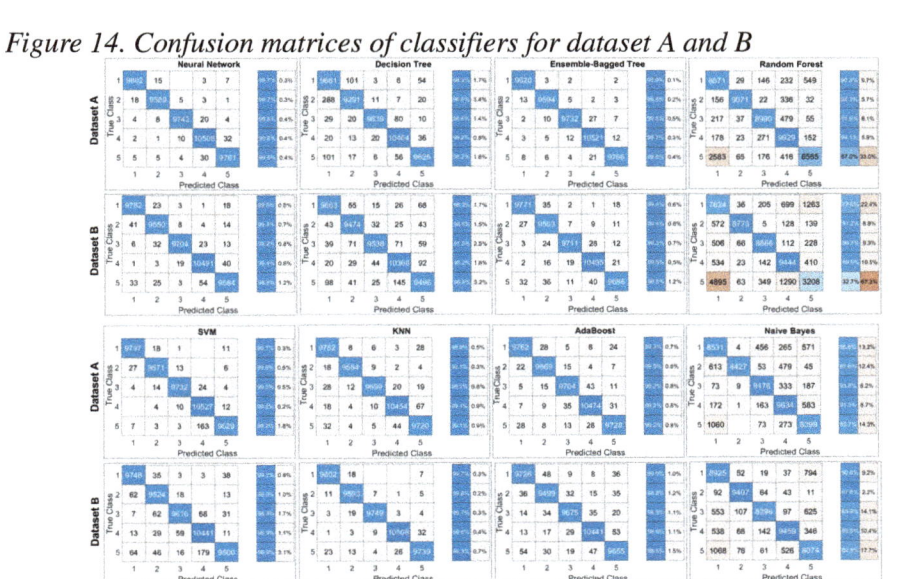

Figure 14. Confusion matrices of classifiers for dataset A and B

The confusion matrices reveal specific patterns of misclassification among the body posture classes. Notably:

- Samples labeled as 1st class are frequently misclassified as 2nd class, and vice versa.
- Samples labeled as 3rd class are often misclassified as 4th class, while those labeled as 4th class are misclassified as 5th class.
- Samples labeled as 5th class are mostly misclassified as either 1st or 4th class.

When evaluating the performance of the classifiers, a comparison of the results in Figure 14 and Figure 15 shows that, for dataset A, the accuracy ranking from highest to lowest is as follows: EL-Bagged Tree, SVM, KNN, Neural Network, AdaBoost, Decision Tree, Naive Bayes, and Random Forest. For dataset B, the ranking is slightly different: KNN, EL-Bagged Tree, SVM, Neural Network, Decision Tree, AdaBoost, Naive Bayes, and Random Forest.

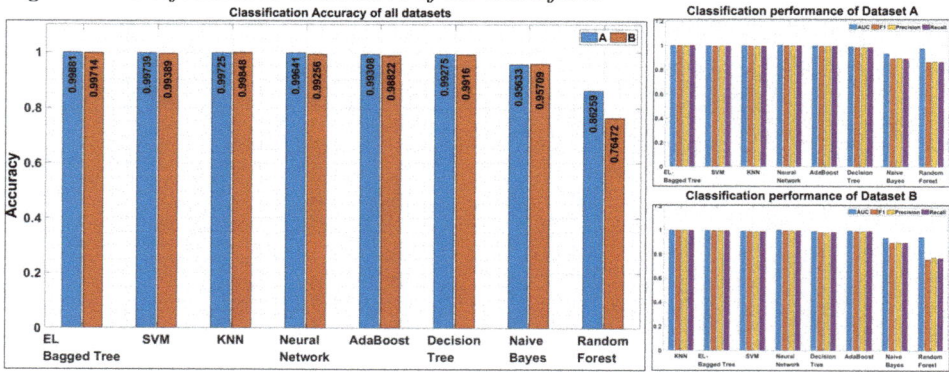

Figure 15. Performance indicators of all classifiers

In both datasets, KNN, EL-Bagged Tree, SVM, and Neural Network classifiers consistently perform well. Conversely, the Random Forest classifier exhibits the poorest performance across both datasets. The classification results also indicate that dataset A generally has higher accuracy values than dataset B. This outcome is expected, as dataset A includes more joint point data, providing richer information for the models to achieve better classification accuracy.

On the other hand, it is seen that the KNN and Naive Bayes models have higher accuracy values for the B data set. Although the dataset contains data for four joint points for B, the fact that these two models have higher accuracy values and very close accuracy values for the other models shows that these joint points represent their classes quite successfully. The ROC curves for the first body posture as defined standard belonging to the models with the highest accuracy values for the interpretation of the accuracy values are presented in Figure 16. When the ROC graphs are examined, it is seen that all models are very close to the upper left corner point (0,1); therefore, the ability of the models to diagnose classes fits quite well.

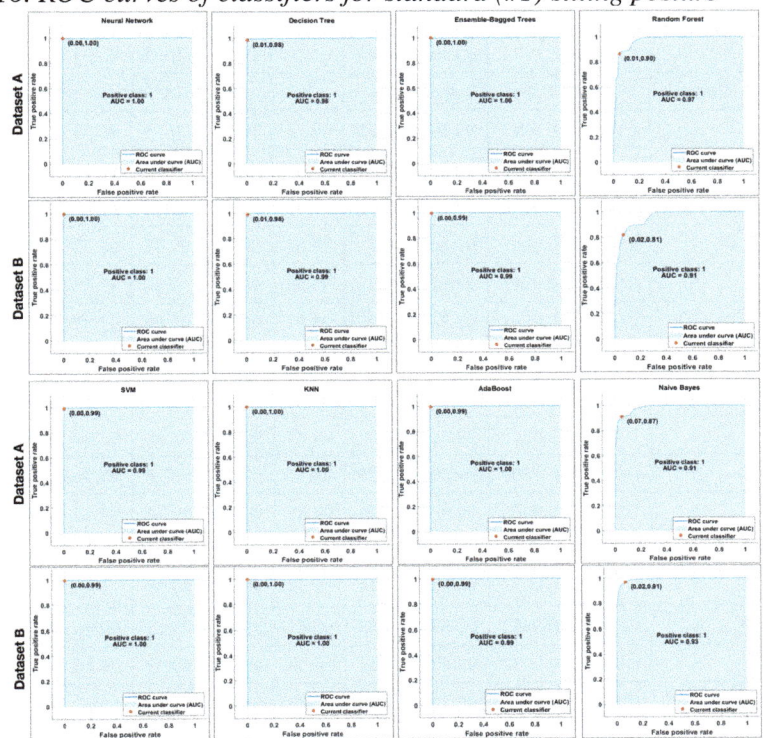

Figure 16. ROC curves of classifiers for standard (#1) sitting posture

In the related literature, various studies have focused on classifying data obtained from different skeleton points. However, these studies typically classify the data from specified skeleton points all at once, rather than separating and classifying data from different skeleton points simultaneously. This approach can lead to differences in classification performance across various body posture classes. When examining the True Positive Rates (TPR) in the confusion matrices from both datasets, as well as the information in Table 3, it becomes evident that the classification performance varies by class. Specifically, the second class shows the highest overall accuracy, while the fifth class has the lowest accuracy. This discrepancy highlights the challenges in accurately classifying certain body postures, particularly when different skeleton points contribute varying levels of information to the classification process. This indicates that the classification performance varies significantly across different classes, highlighting the need for more focused approaches in future studies to improve classification accuracy for all classes.

Table 3. Performances of classification methods for all posture classes with dataset A and B

Model	Posture	AUC A	AUC B	Accuracy (%) A	Accuracy (%) B	F1 (%) A	F1 (%) B	Precision (%) A	Precision (%) B	Recall (%) A	Recall (%) B
Neural Network	1	0.9998	0.9993	99.89	99.75	99.73	99.36	99.71	99.18	99.75	99.54
	2	1.0000	0.9999	99.89	99.70	99.70	99.23	99.70	99.15	99.71	99.30
	3	0.9998	0.9994	99.89	99.77	99.72	99.42	99.81	99.60	99.63	99.24
	4	0.9998	0.9998	99.80	99.71	99.52	99.32	99.47	99.22	99.57	99.41
	5	0.9999	0.9995	99.82	99.58	99.55	98.95	99.54	99.13	99.55	98.77
Decision Tree	1	0.9860	0.9891	98.78	99.27	96.97	98.15	95.66	97.97	98.31	98.33
	2	0.9812	0.9901	99.04	99.32	97.50	98.24	98.41	97.97	96.61	98.51
	3	0.9924	0.9863	99.64	99.28	99.08	98.17	99.59	98.80	98.58	97.55
	4	0.9939	0.9878	99.52	99.09	98.87	97.87	98.58	97.49	99.17	98.25
	5	0.9893	0.9809	99.39	98.85	98.47	97.08	98.77	97.32	98.16	96.85
EL-Bagged Tree	1	0.9993	0.9963	99.93	99.76	99.83	99.39	99.74	99.35	99.93	99.43
	2	0.9985	0.9958	99.91	99.67	99.76	99.14	99.75	98.85	99.76	99.44
	3	0.9974	0.9961	99.86	99.79	99.65	99.46	99.76	99.60	99.53	99.31
	4	0.9978	0.9963	99.83	99.73	99.61	99.36	99.53	99.26	99.70	99.45
	5	0.9977	0.9932	99.87	99.63	99.68	99.07	99.75	99.36	99.60	98.79
Random Forest	1	0.9652	0.9053	90.47	82.43	77.83	63.64	72.21	53.95	84.40	77.58
	2	0.9962	0.9904	98.52	97.92	96.07	94.45	99.15	97.90	93.17	91.22
	3	0.9818	0.9717	96.73	96.75	91.50	91.66	93.86	92.67	89.25	90.67
	4	0.9842	0.9663	95.75	93.27	90.30	84.98	87.91	80.90	92.82	89.49
	5	0.9544	0.8626	91.04	82.58	75.90	42.62	81.13	61.13	71.30	32.72
SVM	1	0.9980	0.9941	99.86	99.55	99.65	98.86	99.61	98.52	99.69	99.20
	2	0.9971	0.9930	99.83	99.47	99.56	98.63	99.59	98.23	99.52	99.03
	3	0.9973	0.9902	99.85	99.47	99.63	98.65	99.72	99.01	99.53	98.28
	4	0.9964	0.9915	99.57	99.27	99.00	98.30	98.25	97.66	99.75	98.94
	5	0.9906	0.9833	99.58	99.20	98.93	97.95	99.66	99.03	98.20	96.89
KNN	1	0.9965	0.9983	99.72	99.87	99.28	99.68	99.03	99.61	99.54	99.75
	2	0.9979	0.9981	99.88	99.84	99.68	99.60	99.71	99.45	99.66	99.75
	3	0.9956	0.9983	99.78	99.90	99.44	99.75	99.69	99.80	99.19	99.70
	4	0.9944	0.9975	99.66	99.85	99.20	99.64	99.34	99.72	99.06	99.57
	5	0.9942	0.9960	99.59	99.77	98.97	99.42	98.80	99.51	99.13	99.33

		AUC		Accuracy (%)		F1 (%)		Precision (%)		Recall (%)	
Model	Posture	A	B	A	B	A	B	A	B	A	B
AdaBoost	1	0.9959	0.9934	99.74	99.56	99.35	98.89	99.37	98.81	99.34	98.97
	2	0.9968	0.9923	99.79	99.50	99.45	98.72	99.41	98.66	99.50	98.77
	3	0.9954	0.9936	99.71	99.61	99.27	99.02	99.30	99.09	99.24	98.95
	4	0.9952	0.9933	99.67	99.56	99.23	98.97	99.21	99.00	99.25	98.94
	5	0.9952	0.9905	99.70	99.41	99.23	98.50	99.26	98.53	99.21	98.47
Naive Bayes	1	0.9099	0.9258	93.52	93.64	84.15	84.99	81.64	79.86	86.81	90.82
	2	0.9380	0.9853	97.57	98.97	93.33	97.35	99.83	96.88	87.63	97.82
	3	0.9599	0.9257	97.28	96.64	93.16	90.96	92.49	96.71	93.84	85.87
	4	0.9392	0.9392	95.42	96.38	89.46	91.33	87.71	93.08	91.29	89.63
	5	0.9109	0.8894	94.37	92.93	85.75	82.16	85.84	81.97	85.66	82.35

In order to visualize the sitting posture data effectively, Figure 17 presents 3D drawings of the data for each sitting class, as well as a sample of the most comfortable sitting posture data. Upon examining these drawings, it is apparent that the True Positive (TP), False Positive (FP), and False Negative (FN) groups differ significantly, highlighting the class in which the most comfortable sitting posture is predicted.

When analyzing the joint points in the 3D drawings, it's clear that the majority of joint points are distinctively aligned with the correct sitting positions for the TP samples. However, joint points 5, 8, and 9, which remain mostly static, appear insufficient in distinguishing between different sitting posture classes. This limitation suggests that these points do not provide enough variability to contribute meaningfully to the classification process. On the other hand, joint points 2, 3, 6, and 7, which were selected for dataset B, demonstrate distinctive characteristics that effectively differentiate the class samples. To improve the classification accuracy of dataset B to match or exceed that of dataset A, incorporating additional distinctive joint points, such as joint point 4, could be beneficial. However, it is important to note that joint point 4, while potentially useful, may be difficult to obtain in an office setting due to constraints related to desk and computer placement, which could limit its practical application in such environments. In summary, while the current selection of joint points provides a solid foundation for classification, exploring additional distinctive points, within the constraints of practical office settings, could further enhance accuracy.

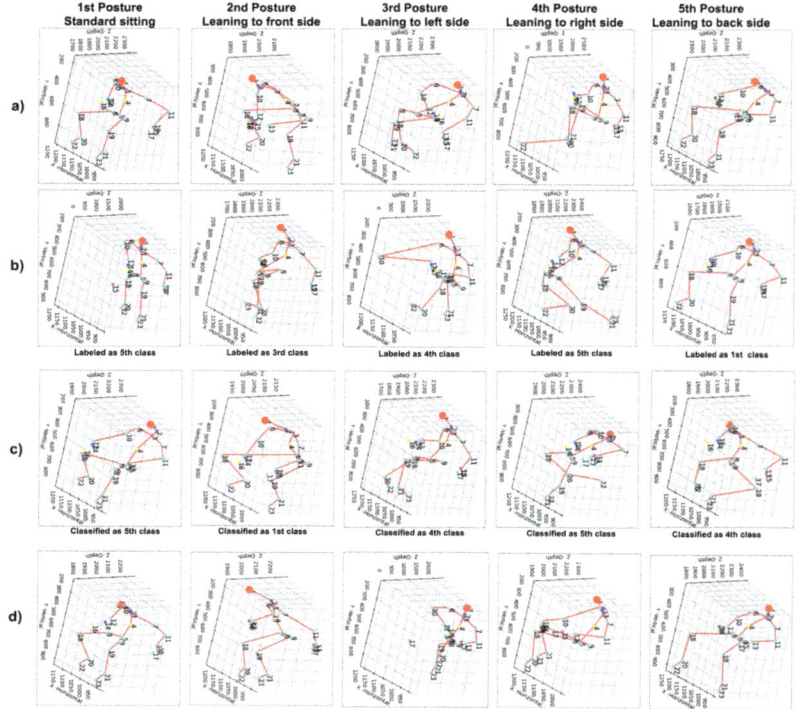

Figure 17. a) TP sitting posture, b) FP sitting posture, c) FN sitting posture, d) prediction of a subject's most comfortable sitting pose

This study achieved a classification accuracy of over 99% for EL-Bagged Tree, SVM, KNN, Neural Network, AdaBoost, and Decision Tree classifiers and over 95% for Naive Bayes.

In this context, the classification accuracy values and other relevant features obtained from the studies in the related literature have been compared with the results of this study. These comparisons are summarized and presented in Table 4. This table highlights the differences and similarities in performance metrics, methodologies, and data sets used in various studies. The purpose of this comparison is to contextualize the findings of this study within the broader body of research on sitting posture classification, offering insights into the relative effectiveness of the techniques employed. By comparing these results, it becomes easier to identify the strengths and potential areas for improvement in this study's approach, as well as to understand how the chosen methods and models perform relative to other studies in the field. The labeling method in Table 4 describes the methods used to distinguish sitting position data from each other. The feature extraction method involves deriving more meaningful data from the raw data, which could simplify the classification process. However, in this study, although angular calculations are employed for labeling sitting poses, the classification itself is done using raw data. This approach is adopted to minimize computational overhead, ensuring the system can operate in real-time without delays. In Table 4, various parameters and results from the classification processes using the datasets in this study are presented. Key aspects include:

- **Dataset Volume:** This refers to the total number of sitting postures recorded and used as training and testing data in the study. A larger dataset volume typically allows for better model training, potentially leading to higher classification accuracy.
- **Number of Subjects:** This indicates the number of participants whose data were collected to create the dataset. A higher number of subjects can improve the generalizability of the classification model.
- **Total Joint Points:** This represents the number of skeleton points considered in the classification of sitting positions. Each joint point corresponds to a specific part of the body, and their coordinates in 3D space are used as features for classification.

By comparing the classification results and features across different datasets in Table 4, the study demonstrates how different parameters influence the accuracy and effectiveness of sitting posture classification. This comparison helps identify the most critical factors that contribute to successful classification, such as the number of joint points used or the volume of data, providing valuable insights for future research and development in this field. When examining Table 4, it is evident that the highest accuracy values for the models used were achieved in this study, both for the A and B datasets. Despite some studies, such as (Paliyawan et al., 2014), (Yao et al., 2017) and (B. Li et al., 2017) utilizing datasets with a larger volume than the one in this study, the models here still managed to attain superior accuracy. In the cases of studies (Paliyawan et al., 2014), (Yao et al., 2017) and (B. Li et al., 2017) which had larger dataset volumes, it is expected that higher accuracy values would be achieved due to the availability of more training data, which typically allows models to generalize better. However, even with the smaller dataset volume used in this study compared to these larger datasets, the models still performed exceptionally well, highlighting the effectiveness of the classification approaches and the quality of the data used. This comparison underscores the robustness of the methodologies employed in this study and suggests that the data quality, feature selection, and model optimization played significant roles in achieving high classification accuracy, even with a relatively smaller dataset.

Table 4. Comparison of studies in the related literature

Study	Accuracy	Labeling Method	Feature Method	Classifier	Total Joint Point	The Number of Position Classes	Dataset Volume (pose number)	The Number of Subjects
Tariq (Tariq et al., 2019)	54.25	Manual	Raw Data	Hidden Markov Model	11	10	16000	40
Ho (Ho et al., 2016)	80.84	Angular calculation	Absent features	Max Margin Classifier	10	3	4323	10
Sun (Sun et al., 2021)	82.86	Cosine distance similarity	Distance to calculate similarity	CNN	10	8	513	several
Yao (Yao et al., 2017)	86.65	Angular calculation	Angular feature	Threshold with Angle Value	10	5	66330	10
Pal (Pal et al., 2016)	94.29	Angular calculation	Angular feature	City-Block Distance	16	2	5600	20
Ray (Ray & Teizer, 2012)	94.80	Angular calculation	Grayscale image	LDA	12	4	22226	8
Bei (Bei et al., 2018)	95.80	Angular calculation	Local contour - topological	KNN	6	9	16200	18
Paliyawan (Paliyawan et al., 2014)	98.19	Automatic Time-based	Statistics features	NB	10	2	397800	28
Li (B. Li et al., 2017)	98.85	Geometric shape calculator	Human body physical features	BP NN	8	2	55080	100
This Study	99.84	Angular calculation	Raw data	KNN	4	5	49580	30
This Study	99.88	Angular calculation	Raw data	EL-Bagged Tree	25	5	49580	30

In comparison to the study (Bei et al., 2018), which utilized the least total joint points in the literature, this study achieved the highest classification accuracy with Dataset B, which has fewer total joint points. Using the same labeling and classification method (KNN), this study (Bei et al., 2018) employed a feature set with more joint points (6) and a dataset with more posture class types (9), resulting in higher accuracy than the other study. Additionally, a higher validation success was noted compared to another study (B. Li et al., 2017) that used the same classification method (NN) but had more total joint points (8) and fewer posture class types (2). When compared to the study (Paliyawan et al., 2014) that utilized the Naive Bayes (NB) method, this study had a feature set with fewer total joint points and a smaller dataset, yet achieved a lower accuracy of 95.7%. This study also includes more sitting posture class types than over half of the studies in the literature (Paliyawan et al., 2014) (Ho et al., 2016) (Pal et al., 2016) (Yao et al., 2017) (B. Li et al., 2017) (Ray & Teizer, 2012), leading to higher accuracy values compared to those with the same or fewer class types. The diversity of subjects in this study, who have different body characteristics, likely contributes to a greater separation among the classes representing sitting posture data, which directly impacts classification success. Although the number of subjects in this study is fewer than in only two studies (B. Li et al., 2017) (Tariq et al., 2019), it is comparable to one study (Paliyawan et al., 2014) and significantly higher than another study (Ray & Teizer, 2012).

It was also investigated that the sitting posture in which the subjects felt most comfortable was labeled as to which class. To that end, all subjects were asked to sit in the most comfortable posture for 30 seconds, and a total of 9747x12 skeleton point data of sitting posture were obtained. The data of this period was classified with the trained models using two datasets.

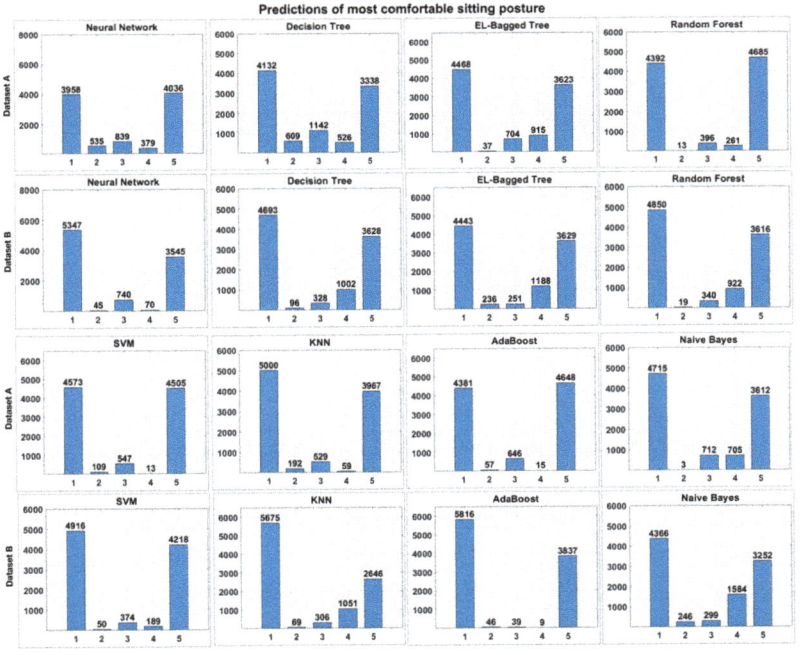

Figure 18. The number of predictions of the most comfortable sitting posture of all subjects

For the prediction process, the models that gave the best results in the training phase of each classifier were used. According to the models, it was desired to determine which body posture class the subject was in during the period when she/he felt most comfortable. The prediction results of the sitting positions in which the subjects felt most comfortable were given in Figure 18, and the percentage chart of the result is shown in Figure 19.

Figure 19. Predicted percentiles of all subjects' most comfortable sitting postures for all classifiers

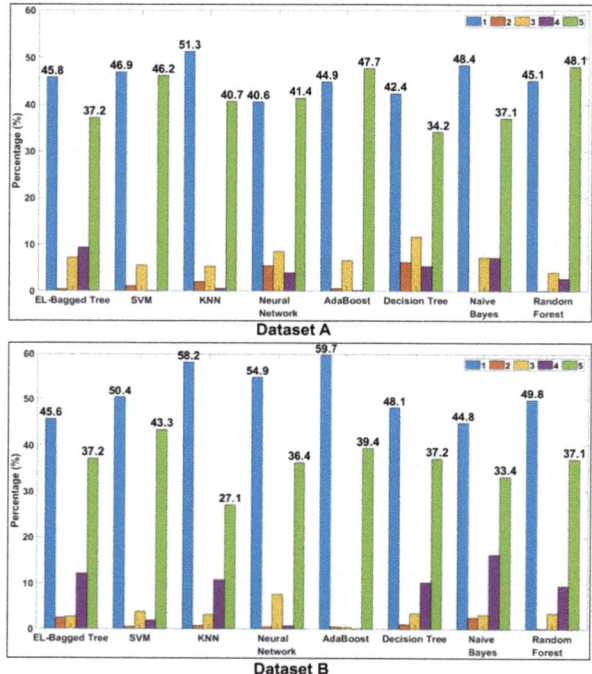

In addition, according to the EL-Bagged Tree, SVM and KNN methods, which have the best accuracy, it is seen that most of the postures in which the users feel comfortable are standard (1) and leaning to the back side (5) postures. When Figure 18 and Figure 19 are examined, it is seen that the most comfortable sitting postures for the A and B data sets have the same and different predictions about which class. In the same direction, the prediction expression is that the most comfortable sitting posture for data sets A and B is estimated chiefly as the standard sitting posture. It is seen that the models with the highest accuracy value have similar estimation results for the A and B data sets. It is also seen that the estimations of the DT and NB models for the A and B data sets are in the same direction. Why the estimation results for NN, RF and AdaBoost models, which have different results for A and B datasets, are obtained in this way is a subject that needs to be investigated. Another remarkable observation is that the EL-Bagged Tree model with the highest classification accuracy has almost the same prediction percentage for both datasets. According to this situation, in the sitting posture where the subjects feel comfortable, at least 45% are sitting in a standard posture, and at least 37% are sitting by leaning to the back side. Screenshots of the software for the classification of the subjects' sitting postures in real time are presented in Figure 20.

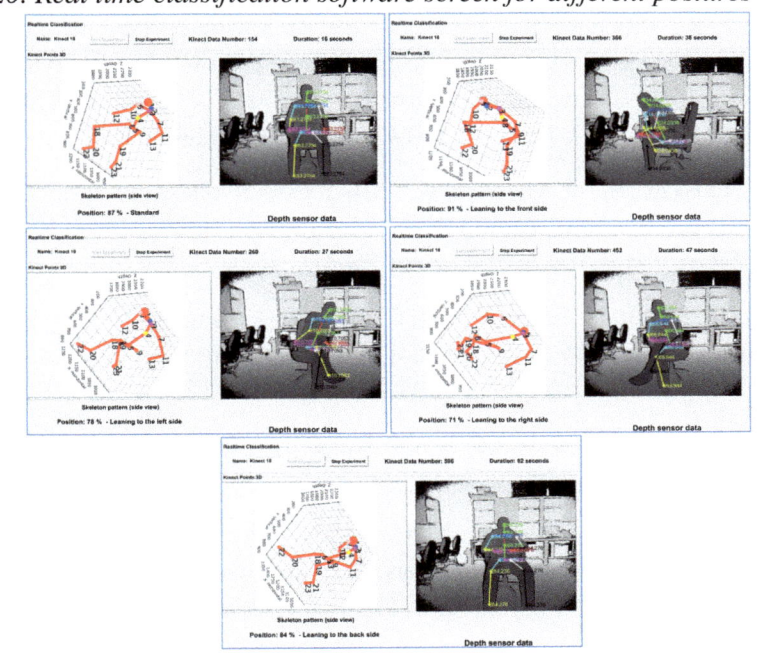

Figure 20. Real time classification software screen for different postures

CONCLUSION AND FUTURE WORKS

The development of affordable and accessible technologies for evaluating sitting postures is crucial, especially for office workers who spend prolonged periods sitting at their desks. Extended sitting has been linked to various musculoskeletal disorders (MSDs), which highlights the importance of monitoring and improving sitting postures to promote health and reduce the risk of such conditions. This study introduces a novel system designed to recognize and classify the sitting postures of

REFERENCES

Aydogan, H., Bozkurt, F., & Coskun, H. (2015). An assessment of brain electrical activities of students toward teacher's specific emotions. *International Journal of Psychology and Behavioral Sciences*, 9(6), 2037–2040.

Bania, R. K. (2022). R-GEFS: Condorcet Rank Aggregation with Graph Theoretic Ensemble Feature Selection Algorithm for Classification. *International Journal of Pattern Recognition and Artificial Intelligence*, 36(9), 2250032. Advance online publication. DOI: 10.1142/S021800142250032X

Bei, S., Xing, Z., Taocheng, L., & Qin, L. (2018). Sitting posture detection using adaptively fused 3D features. Proceedings of the 2017 IEEE 2nd Information Technology, Networking, Electronic and Automation Control Conference, ITNEC 2017, 2018-January, 1073–1077. DOI: 10.1109/ITNEC.2017.8284904

Bozkurt, F., Coskun, H., & Aydogan, H. (2014). Effectiveness of Classroom Lighting Colors Toward Students' Attention and Meditation Extracted From Brainwaves. *Journal of Educational And Instructional Studies*, 4(2), 6–12.

Bullock, M. P., Foster, N. E., & Wright, C. C. (2005). Shoulder impingement: The effect of sitting posture on shoulder pain and range of motion. *Manual Therapy*, 10(1), 28–37. DOI: 10.1016/j.math.2004.07.002 PMID: 15681266

Canadian Centre for Occupational Health & Safety. (2017). Working in a Sitting Position -Good Body Position.

Coleman, J., Straker, L., & Ciccarelli, M. (2009). Why do children think they get discomfort related to daily activities? *Work (Reading, Mass.)*, 32(3), 267–274. DOI: 10.3233/WOR-2009-0825 PMID: 19369719

Coskun, H., Deperlioglu, O., & Yigit, T. (2017). Ekstra Sistol Kalp Seslerinin MFKK Öznitelikleriyle Yapay Sinir A lari Kullanilarak Siniflandirilmasi. 2017 25th Signal Processing and Communications Applications Conference, SIU 2017. DOI: 10.1109/SIU.2017.7960252

Coskun, H., & Yigit, T. (2018). Artificial Intelligence Applications on Classification of Heart Sounds. In Nature-Inspired Intelligent Techniques for Solving Biomedical Engineering Problems (pp. 146–183). IGI Global. DOI: 10.4018/978-1-5225-4769-3.ch007

Coskun, H., Yiğit, T., Üncü, İ. S., Ersoy, M., & Topal, A. (2022). An Industrial Application Towards Classification and Optimization of Multi-Class Tile Surface Defects Based on Geometric and Wavelet Features. *TS. Traitement du Signal*, 39(6), 2011–2022. DOI: 10.18280/ts.390613

Delleman, N. J., & Dul, J. (2007). International standards on working postures and movements ISO 11226 and EN 1005-4. Https://Doi.Org/10.1080/00140130701674430, 50(11), 1809–1819. DOI: 10.1080/00140130701674430

Elliott, J. (2020). How long should I stand at my standing desk? - HealthPostures. https://healthpostures.com/how-long-should-i-stand-at-my-standing-desk/

Fondazione Ergo-MTM Italia. (2021). Ergonomic Assessment Worksheet (V1.3.6). https://www.eaws.it/

Grace, M. S., Climie, R. E. D., & Dunstan, D. W. (2017). Sedentary behavior and mechanisms of cardiovascular disease-getting to the heart of the matter. *Exercise and Sport Sciences Reviews*, 45(2), 55–56. DOI: 10.1249/JES.0000000000000107 PMID: 28306676

Guzsvinecz, T., Szucs, V., & Sik-Lanyi, C. (2019). Suitability of the Kinect sensor and Leap Motion controller—A literature review. *Sensors (Basel)*, 19(5), 1072. DOI: 10.3390/s19051072 PMID: 30832385

Ho, E. S. L., Chan, J. C. P., Chan, D. C. K., Shum, H. P. H., Cheung, Y. M., & Yuen, P. C. (2016). Improving posture classification accuracy for depth sensor-based human activity monitoring in smart environments. *Computer Vision and Image Understanding*, 148, 97–110. DOI: 10.1016/j.cviu.2015.12.011

Hu, T., Chen, Y., Li, D., Long, C., Wen, Z., Hu, R., & Chen, G. (2023). Rice Variety Identification Based on the Leaf Hyperspectral Feature via LPP-SVM. *International Journal of Pattern Recognition and Artificial Intelligence*, 36(15), 2350001. DOI: 10.1142/S0218001423500015

ISO. (2017). ISO 7250-1:2017. Basic Human Body Measurements for Technological Design — Part 1: Body Measurement Definitions and Landmarks. https://www.iso.org/standard/65246.html

Keçeli, A. S., & Can, A. B. (2014). Recognition of Basic Human Actions Using Depth Information. *International Journal of Pattern Recognition and Artificial Intelligence*, 28(2), 1450004. Advance online publication. DOI: 10.1142/S0218001414500049

Kelly, J. (2014). Proper Height For Standing Desks. https://notsitting.com/proper-height/

Kong, Y.-K., Lee, S., Lee, K.-S., & Kim, D.-M. (2018). Comparisons of ergonomic evaluation tools (ALLA, RULA, REBA and OWAS) for farm work. *International Journal of Occupational Safety and Ergonomics*, 24(2), 218–223. DOI: 10.1080/10803548.2017.1306960 PMID: 28301984

Li, B., Bai, B., Han, C., Long, H., & Zhao, L. (2017). Novel hybrid method for human posture recognition based on Kinect V2. *Communications in Computer and Information Science*, 771, 331–342. DOI: 10.1007/978-981-10-7299-4_27

Li, T., Zhou, M., Travieso-González, C. M., & Alonso-Hernández, J. B. (2016). ECG Classification Using Wavelet Packet Entropy and Random Forests. Entropy 2016, Vol. 18, Page 285, 18(8), 285. DOI: 10.3390/e18080285

Liu, J., & Zhang, Y. (2020). An Attribute-Weighted Bayes Classifier Based on Asymmetric Correlation Coefficient. *International Journal of Pattern Recognition and Artificial Intelligence*, 34(10), 2050025. Advance online publication. DOI: 10.1142/S0218001420500251

Luján, M. Á., Sotos, J. M., Santos, J. L., & Borja, A. L. (2022). Accurate neural network classification model for schizophrenia disease based on electroencephalogram data. *International Journal of Machine Learning and Cybernetics*, ●●●, 1–12. DOI: 10.1007/S13042-022-01668-7/TABLES/9

Ohlendorf, D., Wanke, E. M., Filmann, N., Groneberg, D. A., & Gerber, A. (2017). Fit to play: Posture and seating position analysis with professional musicians - a study protocol. *Journal of Occupational Medicine and Toxicology (London, England)*, 12(1), 1–14. DOI: 10.1186/s12995-017-0151-z PMID: 28265296

Pal, M., Saha, S., & Konar, A. (2016). Distance matching based gesture recognition for healthcare using Microsoft's Kinect sensor. *International Conference on Microelectronics, Computing and Communication, MicroCom 2016*. DOI: 10.1109/MicroCom.2016.7522586

Paliyawan, P., Nukoolkit, C., & Mongkolnam, P. (2014). Prolonged sitting detection for office workers syndrome prevention using Kinect. 2014 11th International Conference on Electrical Engineering/Electronics, Computer, Telecommunications and Information Technology, ECTI-CON 2014. DOI: 10.1109/ECTICon.2014.6839785

Parry, S., & Straker, L. (2013). The contribution of office work to sedentary behaviour associated risk. *BMC Public Health*, 13(1), 1–10. DOI: 10.1186/1471-2458-13-296 PMID: 23557495

Ray, S. J., & Teizer, J. (2012). Real-time construction worker posture analysis for ergonomics training. *Advanced Engineering Informatics*, 26(2), 439–455. DOI: 10.1016/j.aei.2012.02.011

Seiffert, C., Khoshgoftaar, T. M., van Hulse, J., & Napolitano, A. (2008). RUSBoost: Improving classification performance when training data is skewed. 2008 19th International Conference on Pattern Recognition, 1–4.

Sevinç, E. (2022). An empowered AdaBoost algorithm implementation: A COVID-19 dataset study. *Computers & Industrial Engineering*, 165, 107912. DOI: 10.1016/j.cie.2021.107912 PMID: 35013637

Sun, H., Zhu, G. A., Cui, X., & Wang, J. X. (2021). Kinect-based intelligent monitoring and warning of students' sitting posture. Proceedings - 2021 6th International Conference on Automation, Control and Robotics Engineering, CACRE 2021, 338–342. DOI: 10.1109/CACRE52464.2021.9501372

Tariq, M., Majeed, H., Beg, M. O., Khan, F. A., & Derhab, A. (2019). Accurate detection of sitting posture activities in a secure IoT based assisted living environment. *Future Generation Computer Systems*, 92, 745–757. DOI: 10.1016/j.future.2018.02.013

Tremblay, M. S., Colley, R. C., Saunders, T. J., Healy, G. N., & Owen, N. (2010). Physiological and health implications of a sedentary lifestyle. Https://Doi.Org/10.1139/H10-079, 35(6), 725–740. DOI: 10.1139/H10-079

Yao, L., Min, W., & Cui, H. (2017). A new Kinect approach to judge unhealthy sitting posture based on neck angle and torso angle. Lecture Notes in Computer Science (Including Subseries Lecture Notes in Artificial Intelligence and Lecture Notes in Bioinformatics), 10666 LNCS, 340–350. DOI: 10.1007/978-3-319-71607-7_30

Ylmaz, Ö., Boz, H., & Arslan, A. (2017). The validity and reliability of depression stress and anxiety scale (DASS-21) Turkish short form. *Research of Financial Economic and Social Studies*, 2(2), 78–91.

Chapter 12
Harnessing Machine Learning and Deep Learning in Healthcare From Early Diagnosis to Personalized Treatment:
Comprehensive Approach of Deep Learning In Healthcare

Ajay Sharma
https://orcid.org/0000-0001-6620-4805
uPGrad Campus, India

Devendra Babu Pesarlanka
https://orcid.org/0009-0001-1052-9210
Lovely Professional Unviersity, India

Shamneesh Sharma
https://orcid.org/0000-0003-3102-0808
uPGrad Campus, India

ABSTRACT

Machine learning (ML) and deep learning (DL) are transforming healthcare by improving patient outcomes, reducing costs, and accelerating drug development. ML algorithms analyze large datasets such as EHRs, medical imaging, and genomics to enable early disease detection and personalized treatments. The current work highlights new approaches in pharmaceutical design and predicts medication side

DOI: 10.4018/979-8-3693-7277-7.ch012

effects. Deep Learning (DL), a branch of AI using neural networks, excels in medical imaging, identifying subtle patterns in MRIs and X-rays. The current manuscript highlights how DL models can identify genetic markers linked to diseases like cancer, Parkinson's, and Alzheimer's. Integrating ML and DL into clinical workflows empowers healthcare professionals with data-driven tools for better decision-making. However, some challenges remain, including ensuring data privacy, and security, addressing biases in algorithms. Collaboration between healthcare providers, researchers, and tech firms is essential for the ethical and effective adoption of these technologies have been discussed in the work.

INTRODUCTION

In recent years, machine learning has significantly transformed the healthcare industry, garnering widespread popularity and recognition. One important aspect of artificial intelligence (AI) is machine learning (ML) leverages models based on statistics and mathematics to empower computer systems to evaluate and learn from large datasets. This capability enables these systems to make accurate predictions, and informed judgments without requiring explicit human intervention. Among the numerous applications of machine learning (ML) in healthcare, medical image analysis stands out as one of the most prominent and important ones as well. Machine learning algorithms can be accurately trained to identify and interpret patterns in medical images produced by MRI, CT scans, and X-rays, which significantly aids in accurate diagnosis and effective treatment planning. Beyond image analysis, machine learning is crucial to the analysis of electronic health records (EHR) encompassing extensive volumes of organized and unorganized data. Through sophisticated algorithms, machine learning can extract crucial insights from EHRs, such as identifying potential risk factors for specific diseases and predicting patient outcomes with a high degree of accuracy.

The development of artificial intelligence (AI) and deep learning (DL) has been transforming and has been a part of the revolution, particularly in the domain of healthcare. These advanced computational techniques, which are the subsets of artificial intelligence (AI), have initiated to transform the way doctors or practitioners understand, diagnose, and treat diseases. By analyzing vast amounts of data far more quickly and accurately than humanly possible, ML and DL have unlocked new possibilities in early diagnosis, personalized treatment, drug discovery, and even in predicting patient outcomes. The integration of these technologies into healthcare is not just a breakthrough in technology but also a paradigm change that offers to make healthcare more efficient, accurate, and accessible (Carbonell et al., 1983b; Fradkov, 2020; Kononenko, 2001).

The journey of integrating computational power into healthcare began several decades ago, with the development of early computing systems in the mid-20th century. The first attempts to apply computational methods to medicine were largely focused on statistical methods, simple algorithms that could aid in medical decision-making. However, these systems were rudimentary(traditional ones) by today's standards, often requiring manual input and being limited to specific tasks. Throughout the 1960s and 1970s, as computers gained power and accessibility, the idea of using them for medical purposes gained traction. One of the earliest examples of this was the development of MYCIN in the 1970s, a rule-based expert system designed to diagnose bacterial infections and recommend antibiotics. The MYCIN tool was never seen and used in clinical studies, but this laid the groundwork for future developments by demonstrating the potential of computers to assist in complex medical decisions(Carbonell et al., 1983; Jordan & Mitchell, 2015). The 1980s and 1990s saw the emergence of more sophisticated medical informatics, driven by advances in computer science and the increasing availability of digital data. During this period, electronic health records (EHRs) began to gain popularity, providing a digital alternative to paper-based medical records and making it easier to store, retrieve, and analyze patient data. One of the disadvantages of these systems was still largely limited to data management rather than data analysis(Bustos et al., 2024; Carbonell et al., 1983; Jordan & Mitchell, 2015; Molnar et al., 2020; Nishat et al., 2024).

It wasn't until the late 1990s and early 2000s, with the rise of machine learning, that significant advancement was made in the application of AI to healthcare. Machine learning algorithms, gain knowledge from data, and develop over time, offered a new approach to diagnosing and predicting diseases. Early applications of ML in healthcare included predictive modeling for disease outbreaks and patient outcomes, in addition to picture analysis for medical imaging. The real turning point, came with the advent of deep learning in 2010. A branch of computer science, deep learning uses neural networks with multiple layers with automatic feature learning from data. This ability to process and learn from vast amounts of unstructured data, such as medical images, genetic sequences, and clinical notes, opened up new possibilities for AI in healthcare (Baiardi & Naghi, 2024; Barbierato et al., 2024; Jin, 2024; Serles & Fensel, 2024).

Machine Learning in Healthcare

Healthcare using machine learning primarily revolves around the analysis of structured data, such as demographic data, blood test results, and electronic health records. ML Models are constructed using algorithms that can predict patient outcomes, identify risk factors for diseases, and assist in decision-making processes.

One of the most significant applications of ML in healthcare is in early diagnosis. By analyzing ML models can identify trends in patient data and disease before they become apparent to human clinicians. By examining a patient's medical history and genetic information, machine-learning algorithms have been used to predict the beginning of diseases like diabetes, heart disease, and cancer. These models can identify understand correlations and trends that human observers would overlook, enabling a faster diagnosis and course of action (Chen et al., 2021; Qayyum et al., 2021; Sabry et al., 2022).

One more significant use of ML in healthcare is in personalized treatment. Examining information from numerous patients in hospitals or medical centers, ML algorithms can identify which treatments are most effective for specific types of patients. This approach, often referred to as precision medicine (Personalised Medicine) pursues to adapt care for each patient based on their unique set of circumstances(disease pattern, Genomic, Genetic and Geological, Morphological). For example, A patient's genetic information can be analyzed using ML models to forecast how they will react to a specific medication, allowing doctors to choose the most effective treatment with the fewest side effects. ML is also being used to optimize clinical workflows and raise the standard of healthcare delivery efficiency. Machine learning algorithms can predict patient with disease showing no symptoms, optimize scheduling, and identify patients at risk of readmission. These applications help healthcare professionals to enhance and manage their resources, and provide more timely care to patients. Machine learning's uses in healthcare extend beyond medical imaging and EHR(Electronic Health Records) analysis to include drug discovery and development, patient monitoring, management, and clinical decision support systems. Due to its vast potential, the implementation of machine learning in healthcare is fraught with significant challenges discussed further in the manuscript. Issues related to data quality and privacy, as well as concerns regarding transparency and biases in algorithmic decision-making, present substantial obstacles. Ensuring that machine learning technologies are employed ethically and efficiently requires ongoing investigation and creation to tackle these issues. The successful integration of machine learning in healthcare promises to revolutionize patient outcomes and propel the medical profession into a new era of innovation and efficiency (Alanazi, 2022; Gabriel et al., 2024; Habehh & Gohel, 2021; Sarker, 2024).

One of the most promising areas where machine learning is making a profound impact is personalized medicine. By enabling physicians to customize treatment plans for each patient according to their genetic makeup, lifestyle, and other unique characteristics, machine learning is revolutionizing the approach to patient care. In the field of precision oncology, the algorithms for machine learning evaluate genomic data to identify specific biomarkers associated with different types of cancers. This analysis facilitates targeted therapies, which can significantly improve patient outcomes. Natural Language Processing (NLP) is a machine learning subfield, that is being utilized to scrutinize unstructured text data from a variety of sources, including medical records, research articles, and clinical notes. NLP techniques can extract pertinent information, recognize intricate patterns, and generate valuable insights that help in making clinical decisions and improving patient care. The algorithms used in machine learning are being employed to analyze data collected from wearable devices and other remote monitoring systems, like glucose meters, heart rate monitor sensors, and sleep trackers. These advanced algorithms can detect anomalies, predict potential health events, and provide personalized recommendations to patients. Figure 1 highlights the machine learning steps involved in the decision-making process for the health care sector. This proactive approach to health management enables better management of chronic conditions and overall well-being, allowing for timely interventions and improved health outcomes. The integration of machine learning in these diverse areas highlights its transformative potential in modern healthcare, emphasizing the need for continuous innovation and ethical considerations to harness its full benefits (Baiardi & Naghi, 2024; Gabriel et al., 2024; Kolasa et al., 2024; Teo et al., 2024).

Figure 1. Image showing the steps involved in building up a Machine Learning model in healthcare for effective decision-making

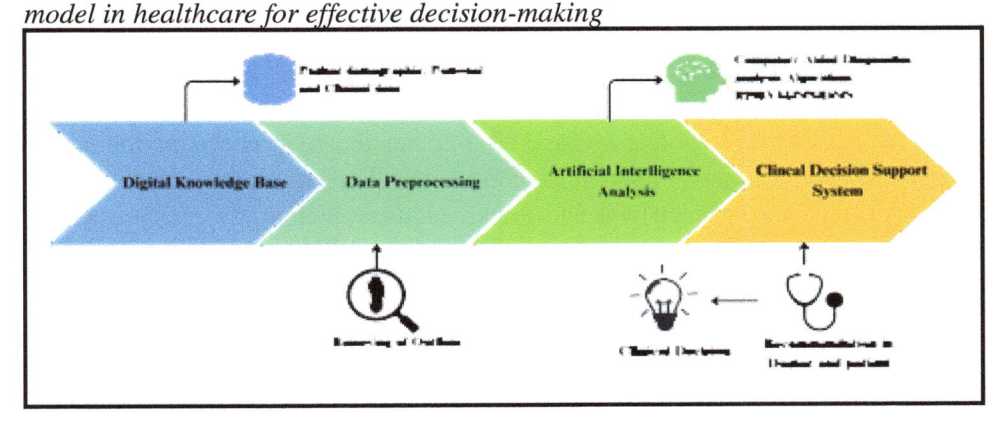

Deep Learning in Healthcare: Deep learning, with its ability to analyze unstructured data, has become particularly valuable in fields like medical imaging, genomics, drug design, healthcare (different dept in hospitals), and natural language processing (NLP). Unlike traditional ML models, which often require manual feature engineering, deep learning models can automatically recognize significant patterns in unprocessed data. This ability makes DL particularly well-suited for complex tasks like image recognition and sequence analysis (Helaly et al., 2023; Loftus et al., 2022).

One of the most prominent uses of DL in healthcare is in medical imaging. Deep learning models, Convolutional neural networks (CNNs), in particular, have shown remarkable success in examining medical imaging data from MRIs X-rays, and CT scans. These models can be trained to recognize patterns and anomalies that are indicative of various diseases, such as tumors, fractures, and infections. In some cases, DL models have been shown to perform on par with or even surpass human radiologists in diagnosing certain conditions (Hussain et al., 2024; Zhou et al., 2024).

In addition to medical imaging, DL is also being used in genomics to analyze genetic data and identify mutations that are associated with diseases. Deep learning models have been used to analyze whole-genome sequences(WGS) to predict an individual's risk of developing certain genetic disorders. This application is particularly important in the field of customized medicine generally called personalized medicine, where understanding an individual's genetic makeup is key to providing tailored treatment (Helaly et al., 2023; Hussain et al., 2024; Loftus et al., 2022; Zhou et al., 2024).

Another area where DL is making significant contributions is in NLP, particularly in the analysis of clinical notes and other unstructured text data. Clinical notes, which contain detailed information about a patient's history, symptoms, and treatment, are a rich source of data but are difficult to analyze using traditional ML techniques. DL models, particularly recurrent neural networks (RNNs) and transformers can be applied to obtain valuable data from these notes, such as identifying mentions of specific symptoms, medications, or conditions. This information can then be used to improve diagnosis, treatment planning, and patient care. From a technological perspective, how to incorporate ML and DL into healthcare has been facilitated by several key advancements. First and foremost is the abundance of readily available data. A lot of data is produced by the healthcare industry, including electronic health records and medical images to genomic sequences and sensor data from wearable devices. The availability of this data is crucial for training the complex models used in ML and DL. One of the important factors is the increase in computational power, particularly with the advent of specialized hardware such as TPUs (Tensor Processing Units) and GPUs (Graphics Processing Units). These advancements have made it possible to train deep-learning models that require significant computational resources. The development of cloud computing has also played a role in optimizing the process for healthcare organizations to access the computational power needed to train and deploy ML and DL models (Helaly et al., 2023; Loftus et al., 2022).

The creation of novel algorithms and techniques has also been crucial. For example, advances in deep learning architectures, such as convolutional neural networks (CNN) for image analysis and transformers for NLP, have significantly improved the performance of these models in healthcare applications. The methods such as transfer learning, in which a model trained on one task is adapted for another, have made it easier to apply deep learning to new healthcare problems. The development of regulatory frameworks and standards for AI in healthcare is playing an increasingly important role. As ML and DL models are integrated into the practice of medicine, it is essential to guarantee that they are safe, effective, and fair. Organizations such as the FDA(Food and Drug Administration), Europe's European Medicines Agency and the United States FDA are beginning to develop strategies for applying AI in healthcare, with an emphasis on issues like transparency, explainability, and bias (Loftus et al., 2022).

Importance of Integration

Machine learning is increasingly being integrated into telemedicine and virtual care platforms to enhance remote consultations and support clinical decision-making. This integration is revolutionizing how healthcare services are delivered, particularly in remote or underserved areas. By leveraging machine learning algorithms, telemedicine platforms can offer more efficient and accurate patient care(Acharjya et al., 2022; Esteva et al., 2019a; Mittal & Hasija, 2020). For instance, AI-powered chatbots are being utilized to triage patient symptoms, provide initial assessments, and direct patients to the proper degree of attention. During virtual consultations, machine learning processes can evaluate patient information instantly, offering treatment suggestions to clinicians, and thereby enhancing the quality and speed of care (Dash et al., 2020; Esteva et al., 2019a; Gerges et al., 2023; Mittal & Hasija, 2020). Machine learning is progressing noticeably in the area of mental health by analyzing behavioral and physiological data collected from patients. This includes speech patterns, facial expressions, and social media usage, which can provide invaluable insights into a patient's mental state. Such data analysis can predict mental health disorders, monitor symptom progression, and assist in developing personalized treatment plans tailored to individual needs. This strategy not only improves patient results but additionally facilitates early intervention, which is crucial in mental health care (Dash et al., 2020; Gerges et al., 2023; Miotto et al., 2018; Mittal & Hasija, 2020; Nayak et al., 2022).

Despite the numerous applications and potential advantages of machine learning in medical fields. Various issues must be resolved to guarantee its ethical and effective deployment. Data privacy is a major concern, as the sensitive nature of health information necessitates stringent security measures. The biases in algorithms can lead to disparities in care, making it imperative to develop fair and unbiased models. Openness and comprehensibility of machine learning models are also critical, as clinicians must recognize, and have faith in the recommendations produced using these systems. Ongoing development and research are essential to overcome these obstacles and completely secure the rewards of machine learning in healthcare (Kaul et al., 2022; Liang et al., 2014).

TYPES OF DATA USED IN MACHINE LEARNING AND HEALTHCARE

The healthcare industry is undergoing a substantial revolution with the advent of various data sources that can transform patient care and treatment options. Among these sources are Electronic Health Records (EHRs), which provide digitized, persistent health information, including diagnoses, medications, and procedures. EHRs consolidate patient history into an easily accessible format, facilitating improved communication and coordination among healthcare providers (Dua et al., 2014; Manogaran & Lopez, 2017). Medical images play a vital part in facilitating the diagnosis and monitoring of diseases through detailed digital images of organs, tissues, and bones. These images are invaluable for detecting abnormalities, guiding surgical procedures, and tracking disease progression. Genomic data is another pivotal resource, offering deep insights into a patient's genetic makeup, which helps identify disease risks and tailor personalized treatment options based on individual genetic profiles (Divya & Kannadasan, 2024; Dua et al., 2014).

Wearable devices, such as fitness trackers and smartwatches, contribute valuable data regarding physical activity, heart rate, and sleep patterns. This continuous monitoring allows for real-time health tracking and early detection of potential health issues. Social determinants of health (SDOH) provide critical insights into non-medical factors that influence health, such as income, education, and social support (Doupe et al., 2019; Dua et al., 2014). Understanding these determinants is essential for developing comprehensive care plans that address the broader context of a patient's life. Clinical trial data are crucial as well, offering proof of the effectiveness and safety of new treatments, drugs, and medical devices. This data is foundational for evidence-based medicine, ensuring that patient care is grounded in the latest scientific research (Dua et al., 2014; Manogaran & Lopez, 2017).

Prescription data offers essential information about medications prescribed to patients, including dosage, duration, and potential side effects. This data is instrumental in monitoring drug utilization patterns, adherence to prescribed treatments, possible drug interactions, and enhancing overall medication safety. Patient-reported outcomes (PROs) are another valuable data source, collecting information directly from patients about their health status, quality of life, and treatment satisfaction. These insights help assess the effectiveness of therapies and inform patient-centered care approaches, ensuring that treatments align with patients' experiences and needs (Doupe et al., 2019; Dua et al., 2014). Health insurance claims data provides a wealth of information on healthcare service utilization, costs, and population health trends. This data helps identify patterns in healthcare delivery and spending, informing policy decisions and resource allocation. Epidemiological data offers vital information on the occurrence, prevalence, distribution of diseases and health conditions within populations. This information supports public health interventions, the identification of vulnerable groups, enabling targeted efforts to improve community health and mitigate risks. Collectively, these diverse data sources are driving a transformation in healthcare, promoting more informed, resourceful, and specified care (Doupe et al., 2019; S. Gupta & Sedamkar, 2020; Kalaiselvi & Deepika, 2020).

ADVANTAGES OF MACHINE LEARNING OVER HEALTHCARE

Machine learning has made tremendous advances in healthcare in recent years. It has changed the way healthcare workers deliver medical care and maintain patient data. ML has the impending to increase diagnostic accuracy, efficiency, and efficacy. The author explored the benefits of adopting machine learning (ML) in healthcare based on research publications (Sharma, 1 C.E.; Sharma, Kala, et al., 2021). Figure 2 depicts certain of the benefits of applying machine learning algorithms to healthcare wellness and related healthcare sectors. A complete overview of some of the advantages of machine learning in healthcare is discussed in the section:

Figure 2. Image showing the Advantages of Machine Learning in Healthcare

Advantage of Machine Learning Over Healthcare
- Advanced Diagnosis
- Personalized Medical Treatment
- Seamless Healthcare Process
- Enhanced Patient Outcomes
- Cost Optimization

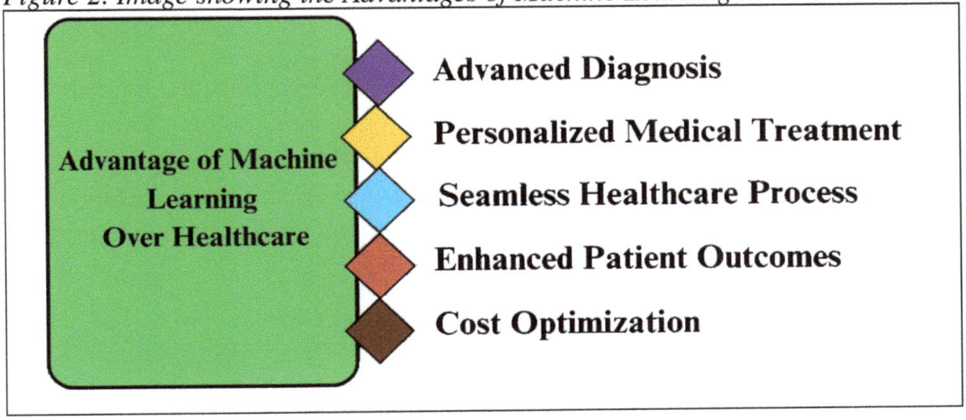

Improved Diagnosis: Among the most prominent benefits of machine learning for medical applications is its ability to improve diagnosis accuracy. Research has shown that machine learning algorithms can scan massive volumes of medical data and reveal patterns that humans find difficult to perceive. ML methods may also find trends across many medical pictures, leading to more accurate diagnoses (Esteva et al., 2019b; Feero et al., 2011; R. Lakshmana. Kumar et al., 2021; Rahmani et al., 2021).

Personalized Treatment: Machine learning algorithms may assess enormous amounts of healthcare data, such as patient history, test results, and medical imaging, to provide personalized therapeutic recommendations. These algorithms may assess patient data and develop individualized remedies based on the individual's needs. Machine learning may also analyze medical information to assist in identifying those at higher risk of developing particular illnesses and suggest preventative treatment recommendations (Sharma, Guleria, Gupta, et al., 2022).

Efficient Healthcare Processes: Machine learning may boost the efficiency of healthcare procedures including medical imaging analysis, clinical reporting, and medication discovery. Machine learning algorithms may automate repetitive procedures, decreasing the strain on healthcare personnel while producing faster and more accurate outcomes. This may result in shorter patient wait times and more efficient use of healthcare resources (Sharma, Guleria, Gupta, et al., 2022; Satti et al., 2024; Lankadasu et al., 2024).

Cost Reduction: The application of artificial intelligence to medicine can also lead to cost reductions. Research has shown that medical imaging costs can be decreased by machine learning analysis by up to 50% of the total healthcare cost. Machine learning algorithms like Support Vector Machine(SVM), Neural Networks (NN), Convolutional Neural Networks (CNN), and Decision Tree(DT) can also identify areas of inefficiency in healthcare processes and provide recommendations for cost-saving measures.

Improved Patient Outcomes: Artificial intelligence's application in medicine can potentially result in cost savings. According to research, machine learning can save up to 50% on medical imaging analysis costs. Machine learning algorithms like Support Vector Machines, and Decision Trees, may also discover inefficiencies in healthcare procedures and provide recommendations for cost-cutting strategies (Awasthi et al., 2024).

CHALLENGES OF DATA IN HEALTHCARE

The difficulties with information in the medical field have been discussed in this section, with special attention paid to four important areas, interoperability, small sample size, data governance bias in the data as well and the data's quality. These difficulties may have a major effect on consistency, and equity, regarding machine learning models' security in medical environments. The author may attempt to resolve these issues and guarantee the successful use of machine learning applications in the healthcare sector by being aware of the possible outcomes and investigating suggested remedies (Esteva et al., 2019b; Feero et al., 2011; R. Lakshmana. Kumar et al., 2021a). Figure 3 illustrates some of the difficulties ML encountered in the healthcare industry.

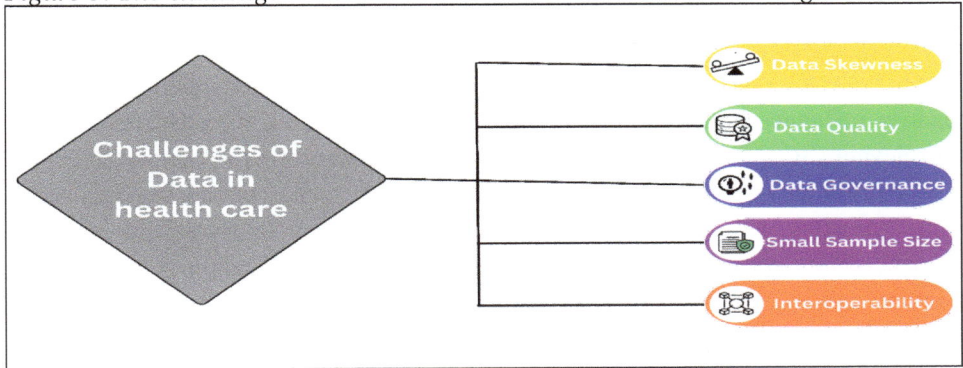

Figure 3. The challenge related to healthcare data Machine Learning Process

Data Biasness: A significant problem with machine learning datasets in the healthcare industry is data bias, which can result in skewed ML models and have a detrimental effect on the diagnosis and care of particular patient populations. Various stages of the data lifecycle, such as data collection, selection, and annotation, can lead to bias in health care data. For instance, a gender bias may be introduced into the ML model, leading to erroneous predictions for female patients, if a dataset has more data on male patients than female patients (Johnson et al., 2016; R. Lakshmana. Kumar et al., 2021b). Biases in healthcare data might have serious repercussions while diagnosing patients suffering from the diseases. A study, on a popular machine learning algorithm for healthcare greatly underestimated the medical needs of black patients in comparison to white patients, which resulted in fewer referrals to crucial healthcare initiatives. The study emphasizes how crucial it is to remove bias in healthcare data to guarantee that machine learning models are impartial and accurate for every patient group (R. Lakshmana. Kumar et al., 2021; Obermeyer et al., 2019). Researchers have put forth several strategies to combat data bias in healthcare, such as enhancing data gathering techniques, integrating a diverse range of patient groups in the dataset, and doing bias audits of machine learning models. The creation of explainable machine learning models can aid in locating and resolving biases in the data, offering perceptions of the elements that influence model predictions (Obermeyer et al., 2019, 2019; Sendak et al., 2019).

Data Quality: A major problem with machine learning datasets in the healthcare industry is data quality, which can impair ML model performance and have a detrimental effect on patient care(Yin, 2022). It can be difficult to create accurate and trustworthy machine-learning models due to the fragmentary, inconsistent, and erroneous nature of healthcare data. Concerns about the quality of information can arise for several reasons, such as incorrect data entry, missing data, or outdated data. Numerous research has demonstrated how data quality affects machine learning models' ability to function in the healthcare industry. An analysis of an ML model's ability to forecast hospital readmission rates using data from electronic health records (EHRs) was conducted (Sharma, Guleria, Gupta, et al., 2022). The study revealed that poor data quality, including missing and inconsistent data, had a major negative influence on the model's performance and produced forecasts result were not relevant (Sendak et al., 2019). Researchers have suggested several approaches to solve problems with data quality in healthcare data, such as enhancing data gathering strategies, creating data cleaning, pre-processing procedures, and carrying out data quality audits of machine learning models. The application of explainable machine learning models can help, categorize issues related to data quality, and offer insights into the elements that influence model predictions (Rao et al., 2015; Sharma, Guleria, Gupta, et al., 2022).

Data Governance: Healthcare machine learning datasets have a significant data governance challenge since poor data governance can lead to privacy violations, data breaches, and legal ramifications (Davenport & Kalakota, 2019; Sendak et al., 2019b). The term "data governance" describes the guidelines, practices, and rules for handling and utilizing medical data. Data ownership, data sharing, and data security are all included under the umbrella of data governance in the context of machine learning. The significance of data governance in healthcare machine-learning applications has been emphasized by numerous studies. Strong data governance frameworks are essential, according to a study that looked at the difficulties of using big data analytics in the healthcare industry (Internet of Things (IoT): A Review of Integration of Precedent, Existing & Inevitable Technologies, n.d.). The study found that to guarantee the successful application of big data analytics in healthcare, some data governance concerns, including data ownership, data quality, and data security, need to be addressed. Some data governance frameworks, including the General Data Protection Regulation (GDPR) in the European Union and the Health Insurance Portability and Accountability Act (HIPAA) in the United States, have been proposed to address data governance issues in healthcare machine learning applications (Davenport & Kalakota, 2019; Ho & Caals, 2021; n.d.; Sukums et al., 2023). These frameworks provide methods for using medical data in ML applications safely and morally.

Small Sample Size: Small sample sizes might cause ML models to overfit, which is a major problem for machine learning datasets in the healthcare industry, particularly for uncommon diseases or conditions. When a prediction model is overly complex, it is said to be overfitting and fits the noise in the training data rather than the underlying patterns. Because of this, the ML job identification algorithm may work well on training data but not well on fresh data. Numerous research works have emphasized the impact of negligible sample sizes on machine learning models' functionality in the medical field. A study that assessed the efficacy of deep learning algorithms in the identification of skin cancer discovered that the models' effectiveness increased with the size of the datasets. A similar type of study that created a deep learning algorithm for the diagnosis of breast cancer discovered that the dataset's short sample size restricted the model's effectiveness (Allugunti, 2022; Singh et al., 2019). Several methods, including transfer learning, data augmentation, and ensemble learning, have been proposed to address the problem of limited sample sizes in healthcare machine-learning applications. Using models learned on large datasets to improve their performance on smaller datasets is known as transfer learning (Sharma, Kumar, et al., 2021; Sharma, Pal, et al., 2022; Shin et al., 2016). The act of generating synthetic data through modifying existing information is known as data augmentation, and it can increase the size of the dataset. To improve a model's performance on fresh data, ensemble learning combines many models ("Ensemble Machine Learning," 2012; Shorten & Khoshgoftaar, 2019).

Interoperability: One major challenge in creating and using machine learning (ML) algorithms in the healthcare industry is interoperability. The fragmentation, compartmentalization, and multiform storage of healthcare data poses a challenge to the sharing and integration of data across many systems and organizations. In research, public health, and patient care, a lack of interoperability can result in serious mistakes, delays, and inefficiencies (Holzinger, Goebel, et al., 2017; Holzinger, Malle, et al., 2017). A study conducted by the Office of the National Coordinator for Health Information Technology (ONC) found that just thirty percent of the institutions could discover, send, receive, and integrate electronic patient data from other organizations. This suggests that most healthcare organizations are having difficulty obtaining interoperability, which is a crucial need for the successful application of ML models in the healthcare industry. The completeness and quality of healthcare data used to train machine learning models might be impacted by a lack of interoperability. An incomplete or erroneous patient medical record, for instance, can have a detrimental effect on the performance of the machine learning model that was trained on that data, leading to incorrect treatment recommendations and diagnoses. Improving the quality and effectiveness of machine learning models in healthcare and guaranteeing the smooth sharing of healthcare data depend on the establishment of standards and frameworks for data transfer and interoperability (Sharma, 2024; Sharma, Guleria, & Jaiswal, 2022a; Sharma & Kumar, 2022).

IMPACT OF MACHINE LEARNING IN HEALTHCARE

Machine learning (ML) has been extremely beneficial to the healthcare industry, especially in the fields of medicine, biology, physical & mental health, and social welfare. ML has revolutionized illness diagnosis and therapy in medicine. To detect, create, and generate precise predictions, machine learning (ML) algorithms may evaluate a vast amount of medical data, including electronic health records (ECH), medical imaging (x-ray, CT scan, ultrasound), and genetics. This aids medical professionals in creating individualized treatment regimens for individuals and making earlier, more accurate diagnoses of illnesses. ML algorithms are used to discover possible adverse effects of current pharmaceuticals as well as to design novel treatments and cures. Machine learning is used in biology to analyse intricate biological systems and comprehend their interactions. Large volumes of genomic and proteomic data may be processed by machine learning algorithms to find biomarkers for various illnesses. This aids in the development of novel diagnostic methods and therapeutic approaches for conditions including heart-related conditions, diabetes, Parkinson's, Alzheimer's, and cancer illnesses. Machine learning is utilized in the field of physical health to track patients and forecast results (Holzinger, Malle, et al., 2017; Thakur et al., 2023). Fitness trackers and smartwatches are examples of wearable technology that can capture data on heart rate, sleeping patterns, and physical activity. Machine learning algorithms may be used to evaluate this data to identify patterns and predict potential health effects, such as the likelihood of getting a chronic illness. In mental health, machine learning (ML) is used to diagnose and treat mental illnesses. ML is used in mental health to identify and treat mental diseases. Speech and language patterns may be analyzed by machine learning algorithms to find indicators of mental health issues including anxiety and depression. This facilitates faster and more accurate diagnosis and treatment of certain ailments by medical specialists. Machine learning (ML) is used to analyse social health determinants about social well-being, including social support, education, and healthcare access. Figure 4 illustrates how machine learning has affected healthcare. The field of human healthcare is severely impacted by machine learning. Algorithms using machine learning (ML) may be used to identify communities that are more likely to suffer from undesirable health consequences and to create interventions aimed at enhancing their social and medical outcomes. All things considered, machine learning has transformed healthcare by enabling more accurate diagnosis, customized drug regimens, and improved patient outcomes (Ho & Caals, 2021; Thakur et al., 2023). The current work highlights a lot more advancements in healthcare as a result of machine learning as technology advances.

Figure 4. Image shows the Impact of Machine Learning on Health care

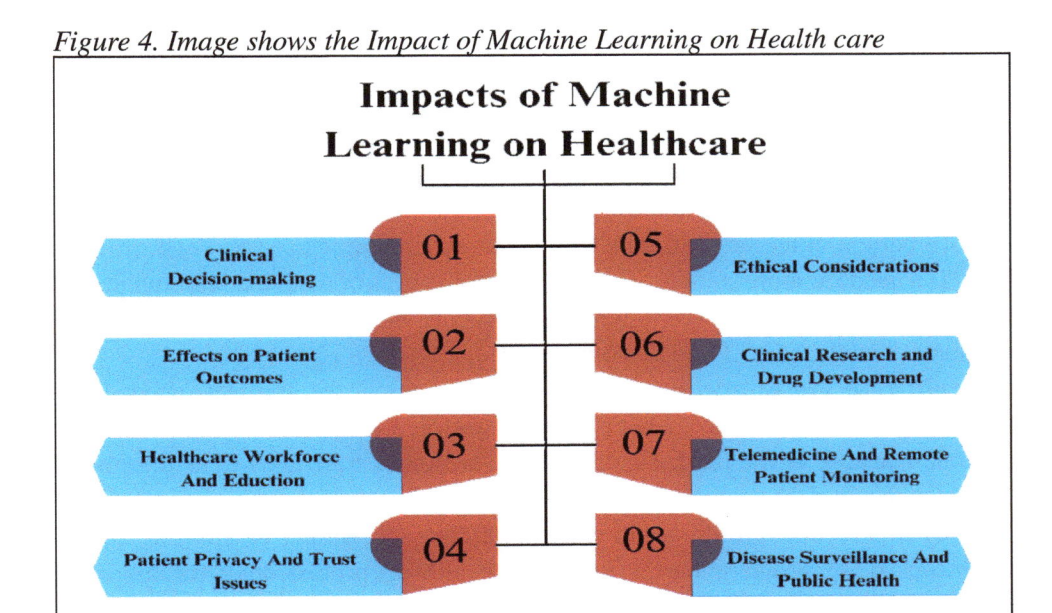

Clinical Decision-Making: Algorithms for machine learning (ML) have demonstrated promise in improving healthcare medical decision-making processes. Better diagnosis and treatment plans can result from using ML models to provide doctors with a more thorough and accurate knowledge of patient data. However, there are issues with applying machine learning models to clinical decision-making, including the algorithms' transparency and interpretability (Kansagara et al., 2011; Sharma, Sameer, et al., 2021; Wiens & Shenoy, 2018).

Patient Outcomes: By identifying high-risk patients, predicting potential health issues, and offering customized treatment plans, machine learning in healthcare might enhance patient outcomes. For instance, ML algorithms may analyze patient data to forecast the course of an illness and spot possible side effects, allowing medical professionals to take action and enhance patient outcomes. To fully understand how machine learning affects medical outcomes, including aspects like patient happiness and quality of life, further study is necessary (Bates et al., 2017; Norgeot et al., 2019).

Effects On Healthcare Costs: The execution of ML in healthcare has the possible to decrease costs through improved efficiency and accuracy in diagnosis, treatment, and resource allocation(Shams et al., 2015). The progress of a machine learning model using medical, and demographic data to predict the likelihood of readmission. By improving diagnosis, treatment, and resource allocation efficiency and accuracy, machine learning (ML) use in the healthcare industry may result in lower costs (M. Gupta et al., 2022). The development of a machine learning algorithm to forecast the chance of readmission within 30 days following hospital discharge by utilizing demographic and medical data (Malik et al., 2024; Shams et al., 2015). The model demonstrated efficacy in identifying patients at high risk, and the study concluded that implementing targeted treatments based on the model's predictions reduced the rate of readmissions to hospitals. Predictive analytics can identify patients at high risk for adverse events and let doctors act before significant issues arise, which might improve patient outcomes and save healthcare expenditures (Lee & Yoon, 2017). There is a need for more studies on the cost-effectiveness of machine learning in the healthcare industry because designing and applying ML models may be expensive (Lankadasu et al., 1 C.E.; Lee & Yoon, 2017).

Healthcare Workforce and Education: Changes in the skill sets needed by healthcare workers and the makeup of the workforce may result from the use of machine learning in the field. Healthcare professionals may need to acquire new competencies in data analysis, algorithm interpretation, and the moral application of AI as ML models proliferate in clinical practice (R. Kumar & Sharma, 2023; McGraw, 2013a). To guarantee that upcoming healthcare professionals are equipped to deal with machine learning models, medical schools and continuing education programs may need to modify their curricular (Sharma, Guleria, & Jaiswal, 2022).

Patient Privacy and Trust: Concerns about patient privacy and trust are raised by the use of machine learning in healthcare. The potential for data breaches and unauthorized use of patient data is a major concern since machine learning algorithms often rely on large datasets that contain personally identifiable information (McGraw, 2013). Sustaining patient trust and safeguarding their privacy requires implementing efficient data security procedures and upholding privacy rules. A patient's confidence in the technology may be impacted by the ML models' interpretability and openness. Creating comprehensible models, proficiently conveying their utilization and possible advantages to patients helps foster confidence in machine learning applications in the healthcare industry (Sharma, Guleria, Gupta, et al., 2022).

On Ethical Considerations: Several ethical issues are brought up by the use of ML in healthcare. These include accountability, transparency, and justice. Healthcare practitioners need to make sure that machine learning (ML) models are applied morally and sensibly, weighing the technology's risks and limits against any potential advantages. This involves eliminating algorithmic bias, protecting the privacy and security of data, and including patients and healthcare providers in the process of development and implementation. The proper application of ML in healthcare contexts can be aided by rules of ethics and guidelines, which include the World Health Organization's (WHO) suggestions for governance and supervision of AI in healthcare (Guleria et al., n.d.; McGraw, 2013).

Clinical Research and Drug Development: By streamlining the process of finding new medications and increasing the efficacy of clinical trials, machine learning has the potential to advance medical research and drug development. Massive amounts of genomic, proteomic, and clinical data may be analyzed using ML models to find potential pharmaceutical targets and biomarkers for certain illnesses. Machine learning can improve patient recruitment and classification in clinical trials, resulting in more productive and economical research. There are drawbacks to employing machine learning (ML) in clinical research, such as the requirement for strong validation and regulatory approval procedures, as well as issues with data uniformity and quality (Guleria et al., n.d.; R. Kumar & Sharma, 2023; Lankadasu et al., 1 C.E.; McGraw, 2013b).

Telemedicine And Remote Patient Monitoring: Particularly for people who reside in underserved or rural areas, the application of machine learning in telemedicine and remote patient tracking has the potential to improve access to healthcare. To anticipate health risks, facilitate prompt treatments, machine learning algorithms can evaluate data from wearable devices, smartphone applications, and other remote monitoring technologies (Steinhubl et al., 2015). Better patient outcomes, lower healthcare costs, and increased patient engagement in their health management are possible benefits. There are issues with data security and confidentiality, in addition to the need for trustworthy, user-friendly technology that is easy to integrate into standard operating procedures in the healthcare industry (Malik et al., 2024) (Sharma, Guleria, & Jaiswal, 2022a, 2022b).

Disease Surveillance and Public Health: By facilitating early outbreak detection, Forecasting the transmission of contagious illnesses, and influencing public health measures, the potential of artificial intelligence is to significantly impact disease observation and public health. Machine learning models can assess data from many sources, such as digital medical records, social media, and environmental data, to identify patterns and trends that can indicate novel health hazards (Broniatowski et al., 2013; Sharma, Kumar, et al., 2021; Sharma, Pal, et al., 2022; Steinhubl et al., 2015). This can help public health experts allocate resources more effectively and make informed judgments. Health risks to stop and manage disease epidemics. Cooperation across various parties, including governmental organizations, healthcare providers, and researchers, is required for the successful application of machine learning (ML) in disease monitoring and public health. The issues with data quality, privacy, and interoperability must be addressed(Lankadasu et al., 2024; Rahmani et al., 2021; Rajkumar et al., 2019).

CONCLUSION

To sum up, the application of machine learning (ML) in the medical field has shown to have enormous promise for enhancing patient outcomes, treatment planning, and diagnosis. To fully utilize ML's potential in this industry, a few challenges must be addressed.

- Data availability and quality are crucial because machine learning (ML) algorithms need a lot of precise, consistent, and varied data to learn and provide correct predictions. Data privacy concerns, and interoperability are challenges that the healthcare sector must deal with that may prevent the efficient application of machine learning.
- It is impossible to overlook the ethical ramifications of ML in healthcare. Ensuring transparency and equity in decision-making algorithms is essential to preventing biases that can worsen already-existing health inequities. Maintaining patient privacy while using their data for machine learning is a problem that needs constant attention.
- To guarantee the security and effectiveness of ML models in healthcare, validation and assessment are essential. To ensure the best possible patient care, ML models must undergo rigorous testing, be implemented by following regulations, and be continuously monitored. Smooth communication between medical technologists and clinicians is necessary for the integration of machine learning into clinical processes. Ensuring that healthcare practitioners possess the necessary abilities and knowledge to decipher and use machine learning-driven insights is crucial for the effective implementation of these technologies.
- Another major problem is the development of reliable, scalable, and affordable machine learning technologies that can be applied in a variety of healthcare contexts. For machine learning to be widely used in healthcare, infrastructural, financing, and computational resource obstacles must be removed.

Discussing these issues is critical to fully realizing the possibilities of machine learning in healthcare and revolutionizing patient care, diagnostics, and treatment planning. By encouraging interdisciplinary collaboration, improving data management procedures, and emphasizing ethical issues, the healthcare industry may continue to progress and harness machine learning's transformative capacity. Diseases on individuals and healthcare systems, and possibly save lives. Machine Learning (ML) in the medical field, various promising areas and uses possess the capacity to transform medical care, analysis, and action planning, while dramatically increasing the effectiveness and efficiency of healthcare systems worldwide.

Personalized Medicine: ML will be crucial to the development of personalized healthcare, enabling individual therapy suggestions determined by a patient's genetic composition, medical record, and other unique characteristics (Gergeset al. 2023, Nishat et al. 2024). This will result in more tailored treatments, fewer side effects, and better healthcare outcomes. Early disease detection and prediction advanced machine learning algorithms will help with disease diagnosis and prediction by recognizing patterns and trends in large datasets. This will allow for timely interventions, decreasing the burden of diseases on patients and healthcare systems, and potentially saving lives.

Drug Discovery and Development: The analysis of extensive genetic data using machine learning, proteomic, and metabolomic data will accelerate drug development by identifying new therapeutic targets and more precisely projecting pharmaceutical effectiveness. This will result in the development of more effective and safe pharmaceuticals at a lower cost and in a shorter time frame.

Telemedicine and Remote Patient Monitoring: The incorporation of machine learning with Remote patient monitoring and telemedicine will improve care delivery outside of traditional healthcare settings. By examining information from wearable technology and other sensors, machine learning algorithms will be able to observe patients' health in real-time, make personalized suggestions, and notify healthcare providers of potential problems.

Medical Imaging and Diagnostics: Machine learning will continue to change medical tomography and diagnostics by automating the assessment of medical pictures such as X-rays, MRIs, and CT scans. This will increase diagnosis accuracy, reduce the time and expense of image interpretation, and help healthcare providers make better judgments (Esteva et al. 2019a). Machine learning algorithms can also detect the patterns form the dataset that may be bypassed by the human eye, enabling earlier and more precise diagnosis of diseases. The integration of AI in medical imaging enhances the consistency of interpretations across different healthcare providers. As a result, patient outcomes can be improved by providing timely and personalized treatment plans.

Healthcare Workflow Optimization: ML algorithms will be increasingly employed to enhance healthcare workflows, including patient scheduling and resource allocation, as well as hospital readmission prediction and prevention. This will lead to reduced costs, better patient experiences, and more efficient healthcare systems. Machine learning can also modernize administrative tasks by automating billing processes and optimizing staff workloads. The optimization can assist in identifying high-risk patients, allowing healthcare providers to allocate resources more effectively. The advancements in healthcare will contribute to faster decision-making and improved overall care quality.

Virtual Health Assistants: Patients will receive tailored support, health information, and help in managing their diseases as virtual health assistants are developed using ML and Natural Language Processing (NLP) technology. This will enhance long-term involvement, self-management, and adherence to treatment regimens (Esteva et al. 2019a).

Mental Health: ML will help to advance mental health care by detecting patterns in behavioural, cognitive, and emotional data, enabling the development of customized therapies and more successful treatments for mental health diseases. Machine learning helps in the enhanced early detection of mental health conditions by analyzing data from wearable devices and digital platforms or online platforms. There is a need and enable continuous monitoring and real-time intervention, offering more proactive care. Personalized recommendations for coping strategies and treatment adjustments can be provided based on individual progress.

Public Health and Epidemiology: ML will play an important role in public health and epidemiology, allowing for the prediction and tracking of disease outbreaks, the identification of at-risk populations, and the optimization of intervention measures to lessen the impact of transmissible illnesses and other public health hazards. In addition, algorithms can analyze vast amounts of public health data to uncover hidden trends and correlations that may not be immediately apparent. This enables more accurate forecasting of disease spread and resource needs. ML-driven models can help adapt public health campaigns and interventions to specific communities, improving overall health outcomes.

Ethical and Regulatory Frameworks: With the increasing integration of machine learning (ML) in the healthcare industry, the creation of rigorous ethical and regulatory frameworks will be important to assure the safety, effectiveness, and fairness of these technologies, while addressing concerns about privacy, data security, and algorithmic bias. The frameworks will need to ensure transparency in how ML algorithms make decisions, promoting trust among both healthcare providers and patients. Ongoing monitoring and evaluation will also be essential to mitigate any unintended consequences. There is a need to develop ethical guidelines that should prioritize patient consent and the equitable distribution of benefits across all populations.

In conclusion, the future of machine learning in healthcare is extremely promising, with multiple applications ready to alter the way care is delivered, diseases are diagnosed, and cures are produced. By tackling the hurdles and developing interdisciplinary collaboration, the healthcare industry can leverage the power of machine learning to better patient outcomes, reduce costs, and modernize healthcare systems globally. Despite the significant progress performed in machine learning and deep learning healthcare, several challenges remain. Among the most difficult tasks is the issue of data privacy and security. Healthcare data is highly sensitive, and ensuring that it is protected while being used for ML and DL applications is a critical concern. Techniques like differential privacy and federated learning, which allow models to be trained on decentralized data without compromising privacy, are being explored as potential solutions.

Another challenge is the need for Clarification and Interpretability. Deep learning models are highly effective, they are often seen as "black boxes," meaning that it is It's challenging to comprehend how they make their predictions. This lack of openness may prevent them from being adopted in clinical settings, where it is essential to comprehend the reasoning behind a decision. Developing methods for explaining the decisions of ML and deep learning models is a field of active research. There is also the challenge of ensuring that ML and DL models are generalizable and unbiased. Healthcare data is often heterogeneous, with variations in how data is collected, labeled, and stored across different institutions. This heterogeneity can lead to biases in the models, which can affect their performance on different populations. Ensuring that models are trained on diverse datasets and are validated across different settings is essential for their widespread adoption.

Looking forward, the future of ML and DL in medical care is bright. As computational techniques continue to evolve and as more data becomes available, the potential for these technologies to transform healthcare will only grow. Emerging domains such as training-based reinforcement learning models' trial-and-error decision-making have the potential to optimize treatment plans and enhance patient outcomes. The integration of ML and DL combined with other cutting-edge technologies, such as wearable devices and the Internet of Things (IoT), also offers exciting possibilities. By combining real-time data from sensors and wearables with predictive models, it may be possible to develop systems that can monitor patients continuously and provide early warnings of potential health issues.

In conclusion, the harnessing of ML and DL in healthcare represents a significant technological and scientific achievement. From early diagnosis to personalized treatment, these technologies have the potential to revolutionize healthcare and improve patient outcomes. However, realizing this potential will require addressing the challenges of data privacy, model interpretability, and bias, as well as continuing to develop new techniques and applications. As we move forward, the successful integration of these technologies into healthcare will depend not only on technological advancements but also on collaboration between clinicians, researchers, and policymakers to guarantee that they are utilized safely, effectively, and equitably.

REFERENCES

Acharjya, D. P., Mitra, A., & Zaman, N. (Eds.). (2022). Deep Learning in Data Analytics. 91. DOI: 10.1007/978-3-030-75855-4

Alanazi, A. (2022). Using machine learning for healthcare challenges and opportunities. *Informatics in Medicine Unlocked*, 30, 100924. DOI: 10.1016/j.imu.2022.100924

Allugunti, V. R. (2022). Breast cancer detection based on thermographic images using machine learning and deep learning algorithms. *International Journal of Engineering in Computer Science*, 4(1), 49–56. DOI: 10.33545/26633582.2022.v4.i1a.68

Awasthi, R., Mishra, S., Grasfield, R., Maslinski, J., Mahapatra, D., Cywinski, J. B., . . . Mathur, P. (2024). Artificial Intelligence in Healthcare: 2023 Year in Review. medRxiv, 2024-02.

Baiardi, A., & Naghi, A. A. (2024). The value added of machine learning to causal inference: Evidence from revisited studies. *The Econometrics Journal*, 27(2), 213–234. DOI: 10.1093/ectj/utae004

Barbierato, E. ;, Gatti, A., Barbierato, E., & Gatti, A. (2024). The Challenges of Machine Learning: A Critical Review. Electronics 2024, Vol. 13, Page 416, 13(2), 416. DOI: 10.3390/electronics13020416

Bates, D. W., Saria, S., Ohno-Machado, L., Shah, A., & Escobar, G. (2017). Big Data In Health Care: Using Analytics To Identify And Manage High-Risk And High-Cost Patients. Https://Doi.Org/10.1377/Hlthaff.2014.0041, 33(7), 1123–1131.

Broniatowski, D. A., Paul, M. J., & Dredze, M. (2013). National and Local Influenza Surveillance through Twitter: An Analysis of the 2012-2013 Influenza Epidemic. *PLoS One*, 8(12), e83672. DOI: 10.1371/journal.pone.0083672 PMID: 24349542

Bustos, D. F., Narváez, D. A., Dewitte, B., Oerder, V., Vidal, M., & Tapia, F. (2024). Revisiting historical trends in the Eastern Boundary Upwelling Systems with a machine learning method. *Frontiers in Marine Science*, 11, 1446766. DOI: 10.3389/fmars.2024.1446766

Carbonell, J. G., Michalski, R. S., & Mitchell, T. M. (1983). An Overview Of Machine Learning. *Machine Learning*, 3–23. DOI: 10.1016/B978-0-08-051054-5.50005-4

Chen, I. Y., Pierson, E., Rose, S., Joshi, S., Ferryman, K., & Ghassemi, M. (2021). Ethical Machine Learning in Healthcare. Annual Review of Biomedical Data Science, 4(Volume 4, 2021), 123–144. https://doi.org/DOI: 10.1146/ANNUREV-BIODATASCI-092820-114757/CITE/REFWORKS

Dash, S., Acharya, B. R., Mittal, M., Abraham, A., & Kelemen, A. (Eds.). (2020). Deep Learning Techniques for Biomedical and Health Informatics. 68. DOI: 10.1007/978-3-030-33966-1

Davenport, T., & Kalakota, R. (2019). The potential for artificial intelligence in healthcare. *Future Healthcare Journal*, 6(2), 94–98. DOI: 10.7861/futurehosp.6-2-94 PMID: 31363513

Divya, K., & Kannadasan, R. (2024). A systematic review and applications of how AI evolved in healthcare. *Optical and Quantum Electronics*, 56(3), 301. Advance online publication. DOI: 10.1007/s11082-023-05798-2

Doupe, P., Faghmous, J., & Basu, S. (2019). Machine Learning for Health Services Researchers. *Value in Health*, 22(7), 808–815. DOI: 10.1016/j.jval.2019.02.012 PMID: 31277828

Dua, S., Acharya, U. R., & Dua, P. (Eds.). (2014). Machine Learning in Healthcare Informatics. 56. DOI: 10.1007/978-3-642-40017-9

Esteva, A., Robicquet, A., Ramsundar, B., Kuleshov, V., DePristo, M., Chou, K., Cui, C., Corrado, G., Thrun, S., & Dean, J. (2019a). A guide to deep learning in healthcare. Nature Medicine 2019 25:1, 25(1), 24–29. DOI: 10.1038/s41591-018-0316-z

Esteva, A., Robicquet, A., Ramsundar, B., Kuleshov, V., DePristo, M., Chou, K., Cui, C., Corrado, G., Thrun, S., & Dean, J. (2019b). A guide to deep learning in healthcare. Nature Medicine 2019 25:1, 25(1), 24–29. DOI: 10.1038/s41591-018-0316-z

Feero, W. G., Guttmacher, A. E., O'Donnell, C. J., & Nabel, E. G. (2011). Genomics of Cardiovascular Disease. *The New England Journal of Medicine*, 365(22), 2098–2109. DOI: 10.1056/NEJMra1105239 PMID: 22129254

Fradkov, A. L. (2020). Early History of Machine Learning. *IFAC-PapersOnLine*, 53(2), 1385–1390. DOI: 10.1016/j.ifacol.2020.12.1888

Gabriel, J., Ramírez, C., Mafiqul Islam, M., Ibnul, A., Even, H., & Islam, M. M. (2024). Machine Learning Applications in Healthcare: Current Trends and Future Prospects. Journal of Artificial Intelligence General Science, 1(1). DOI: 10.60087/jaigs.v1i1.33

Gerges, C. Al, Vessies, M. B., van de Leur, R. R., & van Es, R. (2023). Deep learning-Prediction. Clinical Applications of Artificial Intelligence in Real-World Data, 189–202. DOI: 10.1007/978-3-031-36678-9_12

Guleria, V., Sharma, A., & Gupta, G. (n.d.). Biosensors in bioinformatics, biotechnology, and healthcare. Researchgate.NetA Sharma, V Guleriaresearchgate.Net. DOI: 10.52305/LDXT8191

Gupta, M., Sharma, S., Sakshi, & Sharma, C. (2022). Security and Privacy Issues in Blockchained IoT: Principles, Challenges and Counteracting Actions. Blockchain Technology: Exploring Opportunities, Challenges, and Applications, 27–56. https://doi.org/DOI: 10.1201/9781003138082-3/SECURITY-PRIVACY-ISSUES-BLOCKCHAINED-IOT-MANIK-GUPTA-SHAMNEESH-SHARMA-SAKSHI-CHETAN-SHARMA

Gupta, S., & Sedamkar, R. R. (2020). Machine Learning for Healthcare: Introduction. *Learning and Analytics in Intelligent Systems*, 13, 1–25. DOI: 10.1007/978-3-030-40850-3_1

Habehh, H., & Gohel, S. (2021). Machine Learning in Healthcare. *Current Genomics*, 22(4), 291–300. DOI: 10.2174/1389202922666210705124359 PMID: 35273459

Helaly, H. A., Badawy, M., & Haikal, A. Y. (2023). A review of deep learning approaches in clinical and healthcare systems based on medical image analysis. Multimedia Tools and Applications 2023 83:12, 83(12), 36039–36080. DOI: 10.1007/s11042-023-16605-1

Ho, C. W. L., & Caals, K. (2021). A Call for an Ethics and Governance Action Plan to Harness the Power of Artificial Intelligence and Digitalization in Nephrology. *Seminars in Nephrology*, 41(3), 282–293. DOI: 10.1016/j.semnephrol.2021.05.009 PMID: 34330368

Holzinger, A., Goebel, R., Palade, V., & Ferri, M. (2017). Towards Integrative Machine Learning and Knowledge Extraction. Lecture Notes in Computer Science (Including Subseries Lecture Notes in Artificial Intelligence and Lecture Notes in Bioinformatics), 10344 LNAI, 1–12. DOI: 10.1007/978-3-319-69775-8_1

Holzinger, A., Malle, B., Kieseberg, P., Roth, P. M., Müller, H., Reihs, R., & Zatloukal, K. (2017), 10344 LNAI, 13–50. DOI: 10.1007/978-3-319-69775-8_2

Hussain, I. khan, S., & Nazir, M. Bin. (2024). Empowering Healthcare: AI, ML, and Deep Learning Innovations for Brain and Heart Health. International Journal of Advanced Engineering Technologies and Innovations, 1(4), 167–188. https://ijaeti.com/index.php/Journal/article/view/268

Internet of Things (IoT). A Review of Integration of Precedent, Existing & Inevitable Technologies. (n.d.). Retrieved October 4, 2024, from https://www.researchgate.net/publication/317231159_Internet_of_Things_IoT_A_Review_of_Integration_of_Precedent_Existing_Inevitable_Technologies

Jin, X. (2024). Editorial: Intelligent Systematics: A New Transactions. *IEEE Transactions on Intelligent Systematics*, 1(1), 1–2. DOI: 10.62762/TIS.2024.100001

Johnson, A. E. W., Pollard, T. J., Shen, L., Lehman, L. W. H., Feng, M., Ghassemi, M., Moody, B., Szolovits, P., Anthony Celi, L., & Mark, R. G. (2016). MIMIC-III, a freely accessible critical care database. Scientific Data 2016 3:1, 3(1), 1–9. DOI: 10.1038/sdata.2016.35

Jordan, M. I., & Mitchell, T. M. (2015). Machine learning: Trends, perspectives, and prospects. *Science*, 349(6245), 255–260. DOI: 10.1126/science.aaa8415 PMID: 26185243

Kalaiselvi, K., & Deepika, M. (2020). Machine Learning for Healthcare Diagnostics. *Learning and Analytics in Intelligent Systems*, 13, 91–105. DOI: 10.1007/978-3-030-40850-3_5

Kansagara, D., Englander, H., Salanitro, A., Kagen, D., Theobald, C., Freeman, M., & Kripalani, S. (2011). Risk Prediction Models for Hospital Readmission: A Systematic Review. *Journal of the American Medical Association*, 306(15), 1688–1698. DOI: 10.1001/jama.2011.1515 PMID: 22009101

Kaul, D., Raju, H., & Tripathy, B. K. (2022). Deep Learning in Healthcare. *Studies in Big Data*, 91, 97–115. DOI: 10.1007/978-3-030-75855-4_6

Kolasa, K., Admassu, B., Hołownia-Voloskova, M., Kędzior, K. J., Poirrier, J. E., & Perni, S. (2024). Systematic reviews of machine learning in healthcare: A literature review. *Expert Review of Pharmacoeconomics & Outcomes Research*, 24(1), 63–115. DOI: 10.1080/14737167.2023.2279107 PMID: 37955147

Kononenko, I. (2001). Machine learning for medical diagnosis: History, state of the art and perspective. *Artificial Intelligence in Medicine*, 23(1), 89–109. DOI: 10.1016/S0933-3657(01)00077-X PMID: 11470218

Kumar, R., & Sharma, A. (2023). Computational strategies and tools for protein tertiary structure prediction. Basic Biotechniques for Bioprocess and Bioentrepreneurship, 225–242. DOI: 10.1016/B978-0-12-816109-8.00015-5

Lankadasu, N. V. Y., Pesarlanka, D. B., Sharma, A., Sharma, S., & Gochhait, S. (2024). Skin Cancer Classification Using a Convolutional Neural Network: An Exploration into Deep Learning. *2024 ASU International Conference in Emerging Technologies for Sustainability and Intelligent Systems, ICETSIS 2024*, 1047–1052. DOI: 10.1109/ICETSIS61505.2024.10459368

Learning, E. M. (2012). Ensemble. *Machine Learning*. Advance online publication. DOI: 10.1007/978-1-4419-9326-7

Lee, C. H., & Yoon, H. J. (2017). Medical big data: Promise and challenges. *Kidney Research and Clinical Practice*, 36(1), 3–11. DOI: 10.23876/j.krcp.2017.36.1.3 PMID: 28392994

Liang, Z., Zhang, G., Huang, J. X., & Hu, Q. V. (2014). Deep learning for healthcare decision making with EMRs. Proceedings - 2014 IEEE International Conference on Bioinformatics and Biomedicine, IEEE BIBM 2014, 556–559. DOI: 10.1109/BIBM.2014.6999219

Loftus, T. J., Shickel, B., Ruppert, M. M., Balch, J. A., Ozrazgat-Baslanti, T., Tighe, P. J., Efron, P. A., Hogan, W. R., Rashidi, P., Upchurch, G. R., & Bihorac, A. (2022). Uncertainty-aware deep learning in healthcare: A scoping review. *PLOS Digital Health*, 1(8), e0000085. DOI: 10.1371/journal.pdig.0000085 PMID: 36590140

Malik, A., Sharma, S., Batra, I., Sharma, C., Kaswan, M. S., & Garza-Reyes, J. A. (2024). Industrial revolution and environmental sustainability: An analytical interpretation of research constituents in Industry 4.0. *International Journal of Lean Six Sigma*, 15(1), 22–49. DOI: 10.1108/IJLSS-02-2023-0030

Manogaran, G., & Lopez, D. (2017). A survey of big data architectures and machine learning algorithms in healthcare. *International Journal of Biomedical Engineering and Technology*, 25(2–4), 182–211. DOI: 10.1504/IJBET.2017.087722

McGraw, D. (2013). Building public trust in uses of Health Insurance Portability and Accountability Act de-identified data. *Journal of the American Medical Informatics Association : JAMIA*, 20(1), 29–34. DOI: 10.1136/amiajnl-2012-000936 PMID: 22735615

Miotto, R., Wang, F., Wang, S., Jiang, X., & Dudley, J. T. (2018). Deep learning for healthcare: Review, opportunities and challenges. *Briefings in Bioinformatics*, 19(6), 1236–1246. DOI: 10.1093/bib/bbx044 PMID: 28481991

Mittal, S., & Hasija, Y. (2020). Applications of Deep Learning in Healthcare and Biomedicine. *Studies in Big Data*, 68, 57–77. DOI: 10.1007/978-3-030-33966-1_4

Molnar, C., Casalicchio, G., & Bischl, B. (2020). Interpretable Machine Learning – A Brief History, State-of-the-Art and Challenges. *Communications in Computer and Information Science*, 1323, 417–431. DOI: 10.1007/978-3-030-65965-3_28

Nayak, D. K., Mishra, P., Das, P., Jamader, A. R., & Acharya, B. (2022). Application of Deep Learning in Biomedical Informatics and Healthcare. *Intelligent Systems Reference Library*, 213, 113–132. DOI: 10.1007/978-981-16-5304-9_9

Nishat, N., Raasetti, M. M., Shoaib, A. S., & Ali, B. (2024). Machine learning and the study of language change: A review of methodologies and application. *International Journal of Management Information Systems and Data Science*, 1(2), 48–57. DOI: 10.62304/ijmisds.v1i2.144

Norgeot, B., Glicksberg, B. S., & Butte, A. J. (2019). A call for deep-learning healthcare. Nature Medicine, 25(1), 14–15. DOI: 10.1038/s41591-018-0320-3

Obermeyer, Z., Powers, B., Vogeli, C., & Mullainathan, S. (2019a). Dissecting racial bias in an algorithm used to manage the health of populations. *Science*, 366(6464), 447–453. DOI: 10.1126/science.aax2342 PMID: 31649194

Qayyum, A., Qadir, J., Bilal, M., & Al-Fuqaha, A. (2021). Secure and Robust Machine Learning for Healthcare: A Survey. *IEEE Reviews in Biomedical Engineering*, 14, 156–180. DOI: 10.1109/RBME.2020.3013489 PMID: 32746371

Rahmani, A. M., Yousefpoor, E., Yousefpoor, M. S., Mehmood, Z., Haider, A., Hosseinzadeh, M., & Ali Naqvi, R. (2021). Machine Learning (ML) in Medicine: Review, Applications, and Challenges. Mathematics, 9(22), 2970. DOI: 10.3390/math9222970

Rajkomar, A., Dean, J., & Kohane, I. (2019). Machine Learning in Medicine. *The New England Journal of Medicine*, 380(14), 1347–1358. DOI: 10.1056/NEJMra1814259 PMID: 30943338

Rao, D., Gudivada, V. N., & Raghavan, V. V. (2015). Data quality issues in big data. Proceedings - 2015 IEEE International Conference on Big Data, IEEE. *Big Data*, 2015, 2654–2660. DOI: 10.1109/BigData.2015.7364065

Sabry, F., Eltaras, T., Labda, W., Alzoubi, K., & Malluhi, Q. (2022). Machine Learning for Healthcare Wearable Devices: The Big Picture. *Journal of Healthcare Engineering*, 2022(1), 4653923. DOI: 10.1155/2022/4653923 PMID: 35480146

Sarker, M. (2024). Revolutionizing Healthcare: The Role of Machine Learning in the Health Sector. Journal of Artificial Intelligence General Science, 2(1), 36–61. DOI: 10.60087/jaigs.v2i1.96

Satti, S. R., Lankadasu, J. S. K., Sharma, A., Sharma, S., & Gochhait, S. (2024). Deep Learning in Medical Image Diagnosis for COVID-19. *2024 ASU International Conference in Emerging Technologies for Sustainability and Intelligent Systems, ICETSIS 2024*, 1858–1865. DOI: 10.1109/ICETSIS61505.2024.10459430

Sendak, M., Gao, M., Nichols, M., Lin, A., & Balu, S. (2019a). Machine Learning in Health Care: A Critical Appraisal of Challenges and Opportunities. EGEMs (Generating Evidence & Methods to Improve Patient Outcomes), 7(1), 1. DOI: 10.5334/egems.287

Serles, U., & Fensel, D. (2024). The Five Levels of Representing Knowledge. *An Introduction to Knowledge Graphs*, 93–96, 93–96. Advance online publication. DOI: 10.1007/978-3-031-45256-7_12

Shams, I., Ajorlou, S., & Yang, K. (2015). A predictive analytics approach to reducing 30-day avoidable readmissions among patients with heart failure, acute myocardial infarction, pneumonia, or COPD. *Health Care Management Science*, 18(1), 19–34. DOI: 10.1007/s10729-014-9278-y PMID: 24792081

Sharma, A., Pal, T., & Jaiswal, V. (2021). Decision support algorithms for data analysis (pp. 31–95). Nova Science Publishers, Inc. https://cris.bgu.ac.il/en/publications/decision-support-algorithms-for-data-analysis

Sharma, A. (2024). Artificial Intelligence in Healthcare. 1–25. DOI: 10.4018/979-8-3693-3731-8.ch001

Sharma, A., Guleria, V., & Jaiswal, V. (2022a). The Future of Blockchain Technology, Recent Advancement and Challenges. *Studies in Big Data*, 105, 329–349. DOI: 10.1007/978-3-030-95419-2_15

Sharma, A., Guleria, V., & Jaiswal, V. (2022b). The Future of Blockchain Technology, Recent Advancement and Challenges. *Studies in Big Data*, 105, 329–349. DOI: 10.1007/978-3-030-95419-2_15

Sharma, A., Kala, S., Guleria, V., & Jaiswal, V. (2021). IoT-based data management and systems for public healthcare. Assistive Technology Intervention in Healthcare, 189–224. https://doi.org/DOI: 10.1201/9781003207856-13/IOT-BASED-DATA-MANAGEMENT-SYSTEMS-PUBLIC-HEALTHCARE-AJAY-SHARMA-SHASHI-KALA-VANDANA-GULERIA-VARUN-JAISWAL

Sharma, A., & Kumar, R. (2022). Recent Advancement and Challenges in Deep Learning, Big Data in Bioinformatics. *Studies in Big Data*, 105, 251–284. DOI: 10.1007/978-3-030-95419-2_12

Sharma, A., Kumar, R., & Jaiswal, V. (2021). Classification of Heart Disease from MRI Images Using Convolutional Neural Network. Proceedings of IEEE International Conference on Signal Processing,Computing and Control, 2021-October, 358–363. DOI: 10.1109/ISPCC53510.2021.9609408

Sharma, A., Pal, T., & Jaiswal, V. (2022). Heart disease prediction using convolutional neural network. *Cardiovascular and Coronary Artery Imaging*, 1, 245–272. DOI: 10.1016/B978-0-12-822706-0.00012-3

Shin, H. C., Roth, H. R., Gao, M., Lu, L., Xu, Z., Nogues, I., Yao, J., Mollura, D., & Summers, R. M. (2016). Deep Convolutional Neural Networks for Computer-Aided Detection: CNN Architectures, Dataset Characteristics and Transfer Learning. *IEEE Transactions on Medical Imaging*, 35(5), 1285–1298. DOI: 10.1109/TMI.2016.2528162 PMID: 26886976

Shorten, C., & Khoshgoftaar, T. M. (2019). A survey on Image Data Augmentation for Deep Learning. *Journal of Big Data*, 6(1), 1–48. DOI: 10.1186/s40537-019-0197-0

Singh, P., Singh, S. P., & Singh, D. S. (2019). An introduction and review on machine learning applications in medicine and healthcare. *2019 IEEE Conference on Information and Communication Technology, CICT 2019*. DOI: 10.1109/CICT48419.2019.9066250

Steinhubl, S. R., Muse, E. D., & Topol, E. J. (2015). The emerging field of mobile health. *Science Translational Medicine*, 7(283). Advance online publication. DOI: 10.1126/scitranslmed.aaa3487 PMID: 25877894

Sukums, F., Mzurikwao, D., Sabas, D., Chaula, R., Mbuke, J., Kabika, T., Kaswija, J., Ngowi, B., Noll, J., Winkler, A. S., & Andersson, S. W. (2023). The use of artificial intelligence-based innovations in the health sector in Tanzania: A scoping review. *Health Policy and Technology*, 12(1), 100728. DOI: 10.1016/j.hlpt.2023.100728

Teo, Z. L., Jin, L., Li, S., Miao, D., Zhang, X., Ng, W. Y., Tan, T. F., Lee, D. M., Chua, K. J., Heng, J., Liu, Y., Goh, R. S. M., & Ting, D. S. W. (2024). Federated machine learning in healthcare: A systematic review on clinical applications and technical architecture. *Cell Reports Medicine*, 5(2), 101419. Advance online publication. DOI: 10.1016/j.xcrm.2024.101419 PMID: 38340728

Thakur, A., Sharma, S., & Sharma, T. (2023). Design of Semantic Segmentation Algorithm to Classify Forged Pixels. Proceedings - 2023 12th IEEE International Conference on Communication Systems and Network Technologies, CSNT 2023, 409–413. DOI: 10.1109/CSNT57126.2023.10134649

Wiens, J., & Shenoy, E. S. (2018). Machine Learning for Healthcare: On the Verge of a Major Shift in Healthcare Epidemiology. *Clinical Infectious Diseases*, 66(1), 149–153. DOI: 10.1093/cid/cix731 PMID: 29020316

Yin, R. (2022). Examining the Impact of Design Features of Electronic Health Records Patient Portals on the Usability and Information Communication for Shared Decision Making. All Dissertations. https://open.clemson.edu/all_dissertations/3050

Zhou, X., Leung, C. K., Wang, K. I. K., & Fortino, G. (2024). Editorial Deep Learning-Empowered Big Data Analytics in Biomedical Applications and Digital Healthcare. *IEEE/ACM Transactions on Computational Biology and Bioinformatics*, 21(4), 516–520. DOI: 10.1109/TCBB.2024.3371808

Chapter 13
Harnessing AI for Better Health Outcomes:
Emerging Trends

Ahmad Tasnim Siddiqui
https://orcid.org/0000-0002-1884-9331
Sandip University, Nashik, India

Pawan R. Bhaladhare
Sandip University, Nashik, India

ABSTRACT

Artificial Intelligence (AI) is revolutionizing healthcare by enhancing patient outcomes through innovative applications and emerging trends. AI-driven technologies are transforming diagnostics, treatment planning, and patient management, making healthcare more efficient and personalized. Key trends include the use of machine learning algorithms for early disease detection, predictive analytics to anticipate patient needs for improved clinical documentation and patient communication. AI-powered imaging systems are providing more accurate and faster interpretations of medical scans, while personalized medicine is benefiting from AI's ability to analyze vast amounts of genetic and clinical data. AI is playing a crucial role in managing chronic diseases through continuous monitoring and real-time data analysis, enabling proactive interventions. The integration of AI with telemedicine platforms is expanding access to care, particularly in remote areas. But, the adoption of AI in healthcare also raises ethical concerns, such as privacy and algorithmic bias, which need to be addressed.

DOI: 10.4018/979-8-3693-7277-7.ch013

INTRODUCTION

Artificial Intelligence (AI) is rapidly transforming the healthcare landscape, offering unprecedented opportunities to enhance patient outcomes, streamline operations, and reduce costs. Healthcare systems are complicated and demanding for all participants; nonetheless, artificial intelligence (AI) has revolutionized many sectors, including healthcare, with the capacity to enhance patient care and standard of life (Alowais et al., 2023). The integration of AI into healthcare systems is driven by the need for more efficient, accurate, and personalized care. Recent advances in technology, including artificial intelligence (AI) and machine learning, are revolutionizing various sectors, notably the healthcare industry, which constitutes 11% of global GDP, equating to $9 trillion yearly (Yoon & Amadiegwu, 2023). Emerging trends in AI applications are reshaping various aspects of healthcare, from diagnostics and treatment planning to patient management and administrative tasks. One of the most significant trends is the use of AI in diagnostics (AHA, 2023). Machine learning algorithms are being trained to detect diseases at their earliest stages, often with greater accuracy than traditional methods. For example, AI-powered imaging systems can analyze medical scans to identify anomalies, such as tumors or fractures, with remarkable precision. This early detection capability is crucial for conditions like cancer, where timely intervention can significantly improve survival rates. The AI-assisted diagnosis demonstrated more sensitivity in identifying breast cancer with a mass compared to radiologists, achieving 90% versus 78%, respectively. AI demonstrated superior efficacy in early breast cancer detection at 91%, compared to radiologists' 74% accuracy (Alowais et al., 2023).

According to Bartley, AI refers to a set of techniques that allow machines to sense, reason, act, and adapt in the same way that humans can. AI is made up of several underlying technologies, as shown in Figure 1. Consider these to be a variety of tools for solving different types of data problems. As your AI projects become more complex, you will most likely require multiple of these technologies as part of a complete solution.

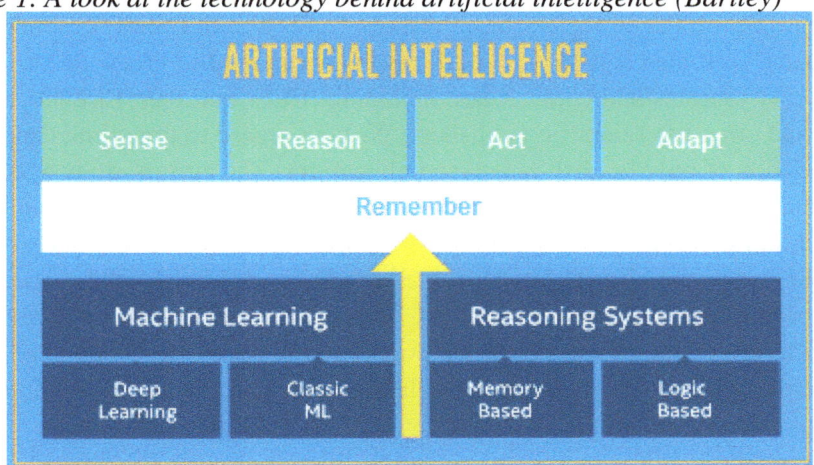

Figure 1. A look at the technology behind artificial intelligence (Bartley)

Predictive analytics is another burgeoning area where AI is making a substantial impact. By analyzing vast amounts of patient data, AI can predict potential health issues before they become critical, allowing for preventive measures and tailored treatment plans. This proactive approach not only enhances patient outcomes but also reduces the burden on healthcare systems by minimizing emergency interventions and hospital readmissions. Medical Imaging, Clinical decision support, Healthcare analytics, Natural Language Processing (NLP), and Robotics are AI applications in Healthcare settings (Yelne et. al., 2023). Natural Language Processing is enhancing clinical documentation and patient communication. NLP algorithms can sift through medical records to extract relevant information, aiding healthcare providers in making informed decisions. Additionally, AI-driven chatbots and virtual assistants are improving patient engagement by providing round-the-clock support and answering queries, thereby increasing patient satisfaction and adherence to treatment protocols.

AI is also revolutionizing personalized medicine. By analyzing genetic, lifestyle, and environmental data, AI can help design individualized treatment plans that maximize efficacy and minimize side effects. This precision medicine approach is particularly beneficial for managing chronic diseases, where tailored interventions can lead to better management and improved quality of life. While the benefits of AI in healthcare are profound, its adoption also brings challenges. Issues such as data privacy, algorithmic bias, and the need for robust regulatory frameworks must be addressed to ensure ethical and equitable use of AI technologies. Despite these challenges, the ongoing advancements in AI hold immense potential for transforming healthcare and achieving better health outcomes for all.

METHODOLOGY

We have presented and published the results of our studies in a wide variety of high-quality journals and conferences, including IEEE, Springer, Elsevier, BMC, MDPI, and other top scientific publishers. Without regard to time limits and with the restriction of only English-language publications. The current study examined the application of AI in the healthcare system by a thorough evaluation of pertinent indexed literature from sources like PubMed/Medline, MDPI, Scopus, and EMBASE. Apart from these databases we have also considered articles and blogs from Hewlett Packard, Foresee medicals, Forbes, Los Angeles Pacific University etc. The targeted study investigates the possible effects and implications of using AI in healthcare environments for better health outcomes. The process of articles inclusion can be given as:

Figure 2. Article inclusion process

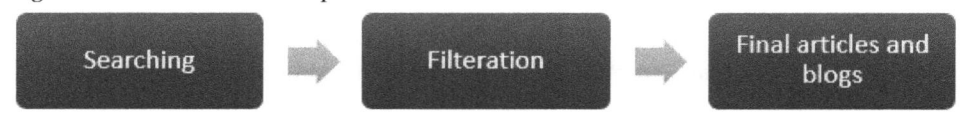

Searching → Filteration → Final articles and blogs

DEFINITION AND SCOPE OF AI IN HEALTHCARE

The use of machine learning (ML), deep learning (DL), natural language processing (NLP), and other AI-enabled tools to support and, ideally, improve the patient experience, including diagnosis, treatment, and results, is known as artificial intelligence (AI) in healthcare. In order to produce more precise diagnosis and treatment plans, artificial intelligence (AI) in healthcare can be a vital tool for evaluating enormous amounts of distinct patient and raw medical data. It has the ability to swiftly evaluate data from numerous sources, spot possible issues, and make recommendations for fixes in a range of situations, including administrative and clinical settings (Hewlett Packard Enterprise). Scope of AI in healthcare is not limited.

Some of important functional areas can be given as (HyScaler, 2024):

- Data analysis for improved diagnosis

AI technology reigns dominant in the field of medical records and healthcare data analysis, processing information at unprecedented speeds and with greater accuracy than humans. This skill considerably speeds up diagnostic procedures, allowing medical personnel to recognize conditions quickly and carry out their obligations more efficiently.

- Enhanced patient care

The potential of AI in healthcare, when properly applied, promises improved patient care. AI provides revolutionary advantages through reducing errors, optimizing resource allocation, and expediting research. By incorporating medical AI into clinician workflows, healthcare providers are empowered to make treatment decisions by receiving critical contextual support.

- Lower medical expenses

AI has far more applications in healthcare than just automation; it enables professionals to better manage resources, streamline processes, and improve patient outcomes. Healthcare organizations may achieve unmatched efficiency, raise care standards, lowering the cost, and lead the sector toward a future characterized by innovation and excellence by adopting AI-driven solutions.

- Real-time and accurate

In the field of health care, prompt and precise diagnosis is critical. Accurate data is essential for healthcare professionals to make well-informed decisions. By utilizing AI to its extent in the healthcare industry, we enable professionals to provide proactive and effective care, which eventually improves patient outcomes.

- Improved workload and reduced staff stress

The implementation of artificial intelligence provides a ray of hope in the harsh world of healthcare, where a lack of personnel and excessive workloads are commonplace. Healthcare institutions can reduce workloads for overworked personnel, reduce stress, and increase productivity by utilizing AI technologies. AI helps healthcare workers focus on their mental health by reducing the workload, which allows them to provide the best possible treatment with compassion and attention.

- Administrative assistance

AI enhances healthcare efficiency by streamlining administrative duties and freeing up medical staff to focus on patient care. AI drastically cuts down on time spent on repetitive tasks by automating data entry, scan processing, and record-keeping. This raises the standard of treatment by enabling healthcare professionals to focus more on important facets of their jobs.

- Health monitoring and digital consultations

In the field of healthcare, artificial intelligence (AI) is transforming patient care by enabling digital consultations on smart devices and wearable technology for ongoing health monitoring. This revolutionary innovation expands the application of artificial intelligence (AI) in healthcare by improving the productivity of medical personnel in collecting and interpreting data.

BENEFITS OF AI IN HEALTHCARE

AI analytics offers a quicker, more thorough analysis of data for healthcare outcomes without the possibility of human error (for example, spotting tumors or precursors for disease). Physicians and surgeons can then use these findings to inform better treatment plans that may lead to better patient outcomes. AI has processing capability that isn't case-by-case; it can gather data from all across the world and produce insights that can be used to develop innovative medical treatments and save lives. AI might be used, for instance, to examine novel strains of the COVID-19 pandemic and develop novel, efficient treatments more quickly than human-based research and evaluation. AI has historically been crucial to groundbreaking genetics research such as gene mapping (Hewlett Packard Enterprise).

Artificial intelligence (AI) can find ways to improve operational efficiencies by streamlining and productivity-boosting procedures, such as surgery. AI, in turn, helps medical and IT managers make better decisions by providing them with increased visibility, which enables them to proactively avoid errors, address problems, and reduce operational expenses. Artificial intelligence (AI) has the potential to enhance patient outcomes and improve the way medical professionals and caregivers provide care. This can be achieved through faster access to more patient records or by identifying more effective ways to manage patient care. AI is even capable of combing through clinical notes, or unstructured data, classifying it, and using it to improve clinical procedures with the use of NLP (Hewlett Packard Enterprise).

Moreover, AI supports medical companies in adhering to increased security and safety standards. AI not only makes it harder for hackers to obtain private health information, but it also makes intelligent video analytics (IVA) possible, allowing staff members to keep an eye on their patients and facilities. Through the use of IVA and smart sensors, smart hospitals are able to match and identify the faces of patients and doctors, detect elevated body temperatures, and distinguish objects like medical equipment and face coverings. These inputs are used to identify people who are at high risk and produce results that can be implemented (Hewlett Packard Enterprise).

PREDICTIVE ANALYTICS IN HEALTHCARE

Global healthcare is experiencing a shift in data collection as it provides patients with a variety of healthcare services, including medical data from computerized physician order entry (CPOE), patient data from electronic health records (EHRs), machine sensor data, and social media posts, driven by rising costs and an aging population (Divyeshkumar, 2024). By 2025, the global population is expected to be 8.1 billion, with 2.1 billion of them aged 50 and up. Multiple sources, including the World Health Organization and the United Nations, predict that chronic conditions will account for more than 70% of all illnesses that year. Place that against the backdrop of rising global healthcare spending, which is anticipated to hit USD 18.3 trillion by 2030, and change becomes clear (Bartley).

These factors have caused global healthcare reform to shift away from volume-driven payment models and toward outcome- or value-based models. This shift necessitates significant changes in the way providers operate. They must prioritize the delivery of personalized medicine tailored to each patient, while also broadening their awareness of population health in order to better recognize and react to patterns. Both goals can only be achieved through implementing advanced analytics to a healthcare provider's data (Bartley).

Technological advancements, data mining, and machine learning tools have made it possible to work with a wide range of predictive analytics models. It is still important to note, however, that some of the top predictive analytics models generally used by developers are not necessarily highly recommended. Top five predictive analytics model are given as (Ariwala, 2023):

1. Classification Model: In comparison to other predictive analytics models, classification models are the simplest and easiest to use. Using the historical data, these models categorize the data based on what they have learned.
2. Clustering Model: Considering that different data collections may have similar attributes and types, the clustering model is used to sort data into different groups. In order to develop effective marketing strategies, this predictive analytics model is the ideal way to segment the data into other datasets according to common characteristics.

3. Forecast Model: In predictive analytics, the metric value is predicted for analyzing future outcomes as part of the forecast model. Predictive analytics is a method used to estimate the numerical value of new data using historical data.
4. Outliers Model: For predictive analytics, the outliers' model is different from the classification and forecast model because it makes use of anomalous entries from a given dataset to predict future outcomes.
5. Time Series Model: If time is taken into consideration as an input parameter in predictive analytics, the time series model is the best choice. Based on the historical data, the numerical metric is developed and future trends can be predicted using this model.

Predictive analytics uses prior information to predict future target events. This shift to proactive analytics is a significant transition for an organization in terms of both technology and business processes. Predictive analytics employs a variety of methods involving machine learning and statistical analysis, which are refined over time with the emergence of new data. Predictive analytics would include using historical data from the hospital's records, as well as outside sources such as climate predictions and social media, to predict increases in ER admissions in order to improve staffing levels (Bartley).

A health organization can benefit greatly from the incorporation of predictive analysis in a number of areas. One such area is clinical assistance, which can be provided in the identification of disease transmission pathways and in the anticipation of events to enable patients to receive better and more precise care. If we consider that improved hospital organization can result in more services being provided to a developing community, then the administrative level of this area's introduction into a healthcare organization's management can have a very high influence (Lopes et al., 2020).

AI-POWERED DECISION SUPPORT SYSTEMS

AI has showed impressive capabilities in clinical decision making, including diagnosis prediction and classification, as well as suggestions and insights. The growing body of empirical research indicates that knowledge-based computerized decision support (CDS), particularly knowledge-based clinical decision support systems, has the potential to improve practitioner performance (Khosravi et al., 2024). Decisions under the medical service delivery system are frequently reliant on clinicians' personal judgments (Ozer et al., 2019). Patients also struggle to plan their future care and grasp resuscitation scenarios, thus they may fail to communicate their preferences or have unreasonable expectations, such as overestimating the success of cardiopulmonary resuscitation (Harari & Macauley, 2020). AI may enhance the quality and efficiency of healthcare decision-making, as well as user satisfaction and engagement. AI is a fast-expanding field with the potential to alter many aspects of healthcare, including diagnosis, medical care, prevention, and management.

Medical capacity for decision-making denotes to an individual's ability to comprehend important medical facts, recognize the implications and repercussions of the proposed therapy, and make an informed decision based on their personal values and preferences. Allowing patients to make decisions for themselves respects their autonomy and self-determination. To safeguard vulnerable people and provide appropriate care, healthcare providers must guarantee that a patient has the ability to make informed decisions (Michael et al., 2023).

The decision-making of healthcare workers improved, which improved clinical management and patient outcomes, according to Fernandes et al. (2020) in their publications where clinical decision support systems were validated in the emergency department. It was discovered, meanwhile, that this implementation phase was absent from more than half of the research. The authors concluded that in order to show how much integrating clinical decision support systems at triage might genuinely improve treatment, it was required for these researches to validate the clinical decision support systems and specify important performance measures.

Organizational Decision Making

According to (Khosravi et al., 2024), study suggests that AI can be employed in organizational decision-making. This primary theme has two subthemes: anticipating administrative and quality indicators, and delivering cost-effective solutions for time and resource management. According to the scholarly literature now in publication, there are a number of subthemes within the main issue of clinical decision-making where artificial intelligence can be used. These subthemes include prognosis and diagnosis facilitation, computerized graph interpretation, and remote monitoring (Khosravi et al., 2024).

Shared Decision-Making

The final main subject is shared decision-making, which is divided into three subthemes: delivering tailored and customized information, facilitating patient self-management, and improving patient medication adherence. The first subtheme is individualized and customized information, the second is facilitating patient self-management, and the final subtheme is improving drug adherence in patients (Khosravi et al., 2024).

Clinical Decision Tools

One of AI's most potential usage is in clinical decision support at the point of care. AI algorithms analyze massive amounts of patient data to help medical professionals make more informed decisions about care, outperforming traditional tools like the Modified Early Warning Score (MEWS), which is commonly used by medical centers to calculate the risk of clinical decay in a patient over the next few hours.

According to Juan Rojas, M.D., a pulmonary and critical care specialist at the University of Chicago and an authority on the application of machine learning to electronic health record data, "MEWS has served its purpose for a long time, and certainly did move the needle further in trying to be proactive with clinical deterioration, but I think it's pretty clear now that most of the tools that are developed using AI methods are more accurate than those bedside calculations."

However, Rojas pointed out that how well AI tools have been integrated into healthcare systems will soon determine how useful they are. These sophisticated instruments necessitate front-line users' desire to interact with these models, an advanced information technology infrastructure to support them, and specialists to oversee their usage and safety.

Any AI technology used for decision-making assessments will face hurdles. AI must be trained, and the data used to train the model determines the quality of the output. As a result, AI has a considerable risk of replicating or even exacerbating biases that already exist in capacity assessments (Garrett et al., 2023).

AI IN REMOTE AND TELEMEDICINE

Since artificial intelligence, specifically generative AI, and virtual care have become increasingly popular, it has become more important to understand how they can be used together to enhance and improve members' experiences and outcomes. The World Health Organization defines telemedicine as the use of information and communication technology to offer healthcare services where distance is a critical consideration. The concept includes various aspects, such as diagnosing, treating, and preventing diseases and injuries, as well as conducting research and providing continuing education to healthcare workers, all with the goal of improving individual and community health. Telemedicine is a healthcare method, not a product; it can be implemented in a variety of ways, including live video consultations and store-and-forward message systems. Although terms like telemedicine and telehealth are frequently used interchangeably, they have distinct technical and regulatory definitions, whereas other phrases such as digital health and mobile health are utilized to provide a deeper and more comprehensive picture of people's health care in the digital age ().

Artificial Intelligence in Telemedicine Has a Bright Future. These days, AI-powered telemedicine instruments that remotely diagnose patients and route them to the appropriate care setting have begun to appear; they are intended to increase accessibility to healthcare services and assist healthcare professionals in making informed decisions, ensuring timely and adequate care (Siwicki, 2023). AI has the power to completely transform telemedicine by improving its efficacy, efficiency, and accessibility. The following are a few examples of current and potential applications of AI in telemedicine (Fouhy et al., 2023):

- AI-powered virtual assistants: These assistants can offer patients round-the-clock access to medical guidance and assistance. These helpers can help patients track their symptoms, provide answers to frequent medical queries, and, if necessary, put them in touch with a physician or other healthcare professional.
- Remote patient monitoring: AI can be used to remotely monitor a patient's health by utilizing wearable technology and sensors. This can lessen the need for in-person visits, identify and manage chronic illnesses early on, and prevent problems.
- Image analysis: AI can be used to evaluate medical pictures, including MRIs, CT scans, and X-rays, in order to find anomalies and diseases. This may lessen the need for invasive treatments and increase the accuracy of diagnoses.
- Triage: AI is useful for triaging patients, setting priorities for their care, and figuring out the best course of action. This can guarantee that patients receive the care they require at the appropriate time and assist to improve the effectiveness of healthcare delivery.
- Personalized medicine: AI can assess medical and genetic data from individuals to create individualized treatment strategies. This may minimize the possibility of adverse effects and increase the efficacy of treatments.

Employers may use AI to its fullest potential to offer real-time decision support, whether it be for scheduling an elective operation using personalized prompts or assisting a member in selecting the best plan during open enrollment. The delivery of benefits and the quality, accessibility, cost, and ultimately value of healthcare could be impacted by generative AI. But until the dangers, obstacles, and intricacies of this technology are well understood, employers might be slow to adopt it (Fouhy et al., 2023).

Case Study of US Telemedicine Industry

According to Healthcare Research Insight, (2024), The U.S. telemedicine industry share, which is expanding quickly, was estimated to be worth USD 38.04 billion in 2022. By 2030, it is projected to have generated revenue and be rising at a pace of 15.1%. Although the data provides an overview, the research explores the hidden aspects of the sector, breaking down its intricate dynamics, charting regional dominance, predicting demand patterns, and spotting prospective innovations that could influence the future business environment. Size, Share, and COVID-19 Impact Analysis of the U.S. Telemedicine Industry by Products and Services, Applications, Modality (Store-and-forward, Real-time, and Others), End User, and Country Forecast, 2023–2030.

Growth Factors for the US Telemedicine Industry:

Surging Demand: As a result of the COVID-19 pandemic, telemedicine has become more popular, and the demand for accessible, convenient healthcare continues to be high.

Regulatory Changes: Although regulations are relaxing to make telemedicine more accessible, reimbursement and provider licensing remain inconsistent from state to state.

Technology Environment: The capabilities and reach of telemedicine services are constantly being enhanced through advances in videoconferencing, remote diagnostics, and wearable technology.

Integration Challenges: The efficient sharing of patient information and management of telemedicine requires ongoing effort to integrate seamlessly into existing healthcare systems.

Reimbursement Policies: There are a variety of reimbursement policies for telemedicine, creating uncertainty for providers and possibly limiting accessibility for patients.

Top players In U.S. Telemedicine Industry are American Well, Encounter Telehealth, MDLIVE Inc., Doctor on Demand Inc., Teladoc Health Inc., MeMD, Global Med, and SnapMD (Healthcare Research Insight, 2024).

ETHICAL CONSIDERATIONS AND CHALLENGES OF AI IN HEALTHCARE

Implementing AI will be challenging mostly because of patient privacy and the need for data analysis. Healthcare businesses must have the right infrastructure in place to store and handle the increasing amount of data that is generated and used. Similarly, for any AI to interpret any data set in a meaningful way, the right algorithms are required. Organizations run the danger of abusing patient medical information or leaving it open to cyber-attacks and other threats if they don't have an efficient infrastructure in place. Additionally, poorly designed algorithms may result in inadvertently biased decisions.

Software that uses machine learning has an inherent relationship between its performance and the caliber of its training dataset. The quality and completeness of the data used to train a model determines how good it can perform. In order to train the model and deal with data efficiently, the AI development team needs to consist of both data scientists and seasoned software developers who can collaborate to provide optimal outcomes. Additionally, there are some ethical questions raised by the use of AI in data processing and diagnosis. AI systems rely largely on large amounts of patient data, including private medical records. Upholding patient confidence and following rules depends critically on protecting the security and privacy of this data. Healthcare providers must put strong security measures in place to guard against abuse, illegal access, and breaches involving patient data (Sulymka, 2023).

Cyber security Risks in the Healthcare Sector: A growing number of ransom ware and phishing attempts that target patient data are directed against the healthcare sector. This damages patient trust and may have an impact on patient care in addition to causing financial losses. Outdated software leaves many medical devices open to assault. Even when gadgets are recently issued, they are frequently outdated due to the protracted FDA certification procedure. Because of this weakness, fraudsters find the healthcare industry to be an attractive target (Jordanabukasis, 2024).

Data Security and Management: Healthcare providers are concentrating on how to handle and derive insights from the growing volume of patient data. But it's crucial to guarantee patient security and privacy. Suppliers that keep data for several healthcare organizations become more complicated, and some of them share data with other suppliers, which leads to more vulnerabilities. To handle these issues, healthcare institutions need professionals with expertise in security and privacy (Jordanabukasis, 2024).

ADVANTAGES AND DISADVANTAGES OF AI IN HEALTHCARE

AI is crucial to healthcare for a variety of reasons (Tomberlin, 2023 & Corn 2023). The primary rationale is that, according to Marketing Director of Foresee Medical (Barth), healthcare systems can become smarter, faster, and more efficient in providing care to millions of people worldwide. This will lower healthcare expenses while simultaneously giving people high-quality care. Healthcare systems may enhance patient outcomes by using AI to optimize and accelerate a variety of operations, from administrative tasks to treatment planning and diagnosis.

While there are numerous advantages of AI in healthcare, there are also possible drawbacks and challenges that could arise. Although AI offers the healthcare industry a plethora of prospects, this revolutionary path is not without obstacles. The following are the main benefits that drive the sector ahead and the innate drawbacks that need to be carefully considered in order to ensure that artificial intelligence (AI) is used in healthcare delivery in a seamless manner in the future.

Advantages

- Early Detection and Diagnosis
- Improved diagnostics and medical precision
- Personalized Treatment Plans
- Streamlined workflow and administrative tasks
- Enhanced research and development
- Telemedicine
- Remote Monitoring
    Disadvantages
- Ethical concerns and data privacy problems
- Possible job displacement and human-AI collaboration challenges
- Diagnostic Accuracy
- Reliability and trust questions in AI-driven decision-making

When discussing the issues surrounding artificial intelligence, it is not enough to limit the discussion to the study of human intellect alone. This is the reason the definition we came up with in strictly philosophical terms is important (Suleimenov et al., 2020).

FUTURE TRENDS AND INNOVATIONS

In recent times, the healthcare industry has encountered various obstacles stemming from global digital revolution, the pandemic, notable changes in the population, and increasing patient expectations. In the era of personalized healthcare, evidence-based treatment, and digital customer service, it is critical for startups, entrepreneurs, and healthcare professionals to remain up to date on the latest developments that are reshaping the sector. However, it's critical to recognize the difference between a truly workable solution and a bright concept with plenty of promise. Here, we've highlighted six technological innovation trends in the healthcare sector that you can start implementing right now and that can result in real business benefits (Sulymka, 2023).

Since technology is advancing so quickly, it is difficult to predict what the future may bring. Although industry-wide security measures are anticipated to improve, the dynamic nature of threats demands a proactive strategy to prevention as opposed to a reactive one (Sulymka, 2023). Technologies like extended reality, machine learning, and artificial intelligence will continue to progress and increase the standard and effectiveness of healthcare. Though it may sound like science fiction, 3D-printed body parts are becoming a reality and have already started clinical trials. Trials for 3D bio printing of organs like ears, corneas, bones, and skin are now underway. Smart pills are another remarkable breakthrough. These tablets serve as medications and give healthcare providers with important patient health information. Even though the FDA approved the first smart pill in 2017, widespread use of this medication is still developing (Sulymka, 2023). Future trends in AI enabled healthcare (Jordanabukasis, 2024):

1. Early Disease Detection: AI may be able to save lives by identifying illnesses in their earliest stages.
2. Personalized Treatment Plans: AI is anticipated to help in creating treatment programs that are specific to each person's need.
3. Drug discoveries and development: By sifting through enormous databases to find promising drug candidates, AI speeds up the drug discovery process. It can practically screen millions of chemical compounds, repurpose already-approved medications, and improve the design of clinical trials. This lowers expenses and speeds up the development of novel treatments.
4. Healthcare Accessibility: By utilizing telehealth and Mhealth technologies, AI may guarantee that healthcare is available in remote locations.
5. Streamlined Operations: AI-driven optimization may lead to operational excellence in hospitals.
6. Data Security: AI is expected to be essential in protecting medical information and averting breaches.

We've emphasized six technological innovation trends in the healthcare sector that can be implemented right now and that may result in real business benefits (Sulymka, 2023):

Trend 1: AI is one of the keys

- Healthcare data management
- AI in diagnosis & drug discovery
- AI in mental health

- Data and privacy

Trend 2: Telemedicine continues to drive the evolution of remote care

- Mobile health
- Complying with regulations
- Webrtc for video conferencing
- Cloud hosting and data storage

Trend 3: Using extended reality in healthcare settings

- Augmented reality and mixed reality in healthcare
- Virtual reality in healthcare

Trend 4: IoT and wearables become more widespread in healthcare
- Wearables
- Other IoT solutions

Trend 5: Upgrading legacy healthcare systems for market demands
- According to a Kaspersky Lab analysis from 2021, 73% of health systems use medical equipment that runs on older operating systems. The increased frequency of security breaches and rising patient expectations over the last two years have hampered healthcare organizations' capacity to innovate. As a result, now is an excellent time to modernize your healthcare software.

Trend 6: Data security as a priority for healthcare providers
- Despite the efficiency and quality of service, privacy and security are significant considerations in the healthcare sector. As reported by IBM, during March 2021 and March 2022, 550 firms throughout the world experienced data breaches. For example, Postmeds, a company that conducts business as Truepill and fills mail-order prescriptions for pharmacies, experienced a large data breach in 2023 that impacted 2,364,359 people.

CONCLUSION

Throughout this chapter, we demonstrate the value of AI systems for a variety of healthcare tasks e.g. decision-making tasks, including clinical, organizational, and shared decisions. During a decision-making process, the brain collects information and chooses alternatives based on the information. A wide range of responses are anticipated as artificial intelligence becomes more integrated into healthcare; a few individuals may be quick to welcome the benefits AI offers, while others might show resistance to collaborating with and embracing AI in their line of work. The future of healthcare will probably be defined by the coexistence of human competence and AI innovation, which will promote a harmonious balance between medical advancement and compassionate care. AI offer a well-organized framework for investigating the various uses and ramifications of artificial intelligence in healthcare, with an emphasis on how these new developments may improve patient outcomes. These points provide a structured outline for exploring the diverse applications and implications of AI in healthcare, focusing on how these emerging trends can lead to better health outcomes.

REFERENCES

AHA. (2023). How AI Is Improving Diagnostics, Decision-Making and Care. Accessed from https://www.aha.org/aha-center-health-innovation-market-scan/2023-05-09-how-ai-improving-diagnostics-decision-making-and-care Accessed on 23/05/2024

Alowais, S. A., Alghamdi, S. S., Alsuhebany, N., Alqahtani, T., Alshaya, A. I., Almohareb, S. N., Aldairem, A., Alrashed, M., Bin Saleh, K., Badreldin, H. A., Al Yami, M. S., Al Harbi, S., & Albekairy, A. M. (2023). Revolutionizing healthcare: The role of artificial intelligence in clinical practice. *BMC Medical Education*, 23(1), 689. DOI: 10.1186/s12909-023-04698-z PMID: 37740191

Ariwala, P. (2023). Deep dive into predictive analytics models and algorithms. Accessed from https://marutitech.com/predictive-analytics-models-algorithms/ Accessed on: 11/06/2024

Barth, S. Artificial intelligence (AI) in healthcare & hospitals. Accessed from https://www.foreseemed.com/artificial-intelligence-in-healthcare. Accessed on: 27/05/2024

Bartley, A. (n.d.). Predictiive Analytics in Healthcare. Intel Corporation. Accessed from https://www.intel.vn/content/dam/www/public/us/en/documents/white-papers/gmc-analytics-healthcare-whitepaper.pdf, Accessed on: 29/05/2024

Corn, J. (2023). Balancing the Pros and Cons of AI in Healthcare. Forbes. Accessed from https://www.forbes.com/sites/forbesbusinesscouncil/2023/12/01/balancing-the-pros-and-cons-of-ai-in-healthcare/?sh=39d91e04752b Accessed on: 27/05/2024

Divyeshkumar, V. (2024). Predictive Analysis for Personalized Machine: Leveraging Patient Data for Enhanced Healthcare. *International Journal of Current Science Research and Review*, 07(05). Advance online publication. DOI: 10.47191/ijcsrr/V7-i5-59

Fernandes, M., Vieira, S. M., Leite, F., Palos, C., Finkelstein, S., & Sousa, J. M. C. (2020). Clinical decision support systems for triage in the emergency department using intelligent systems: A review. *Artificial Intelligence in Medicine*, 2020(102), 101762. DOI: 10.1016/j.artmed.2019.101762 PMID: 31980099

Fouhy, R., Halpert, A., & Rogers, C. (2023). What is the future of AI in telemedicine? US health news. Accessed from https://www.mercer.com/en-us/insights/us-health-news/what-is-the-future-of-ai-in-telemedicine/ Accessed on: 31/05/2024

Garrett, W. S., Verma, A., Thomas, D., Appel, J. M., & Mirza, O. (2023). Racial disparities in psychiatric decisional capacity consultations. *Psychiatric Services (Washington, D.C.)*, 74(1), 10–16. Advance online publication. DOI: 10.1176/appi.ps.202100685 PMID: 36004436

Harari, D. Y., & Macauley, R. C. (2020). Betting on CPR: A modern version of Pascal's wager. *Journal of Medical Ethics*, 46(2), 110–113. DOI: 10.1136/medethics-2019-105558 PMID: 31527140

Healthcare Research Insight. (2024). US telemedicine industry: The AI revolution in remote healthcare. Accessed from https://www.linkedin.com/pulse/us-telemedicine-industry-ai-revolution-hpuqf/ Accessed on: 01/06/2024

Hewlett Packard Enterprise. What is AI Healthcare? Accessed from https://www.hpe.com/in/en/what-is/ai-healthcare.html, Accessed on 26/05/2024

HyScaler. (2024). Scope of AI in healthcare: 7 powerful advantages unlocked. Available at: https://hyscaler.com/insights/scope-of-ai-in-healthcare-7-advantages/ Accessed on: 26/05/2024

Jordanabukasis (2024). The future of AI in healthcare: Trends and innovations. Cprime. CPRIME. Accessed from https://www.cprime.com/resources/blog/the-future-of-ai-in-healthcare-trends-and-innovations/ Accessed on: 05/06/2024

Khosravi, M., Zare, Z., Mojtabaeian, S. M., & Izadi, R. (2024). Artificial Intelligence and Decision-Making in Healthcare: A Thematic Analysis of a Systematic Review of reviews. *Health Services Research and Managerial Epidemiology*, 11, 23333928241234863. Advance online publication. DOI: 10.1177/23333928241234863 PMID: 38449840

Lopes, J., Guimarães, T., & Santos, M. F. (2020). Predictive and Prescriptive Analytics in Healthcare: A Survey, Procedia Computer Science, Volume 170, Pages 1029-1034, ISSN 1877-0509, DOI: 10.1016/j.procs.2020.03.078

Michael, R. MacIntyre, Richard G. Cockerill, Omar F. Mirza, Jacob M. (2023). Appel, Ethical considerations for the use of artificial intelligence in medical decision-making capacity assessments, Psychiatry Research, Volume 328, 115466, ISSN 0165-1781, DOI: 10.1016/j.psychres.2023.115466

Ozer, J., Alon, G., Leykin, D., Varon, J., Aharonson-Daniel, L., & Einav, S. (2019). Culture and personal influences on cardiopulmonary resuscitation—Results of international survey. *BMC Medical Ethics*, 20(1), 102. DOI: 10.1186/s12910-019-0439-x PMID: 31878920

Sharma, S., Rawal, R., & Shah, D. (2023, September 29). Addressing the challenges of AI-based telemedicine: Best practices and lessons learned. *Journal of Education and Health Promotion*, 12(1), 338. DOI: 10.4103/jehp.jehp_402_23 PMID: 38023098

Siwicki, B. (2023). The intersection of Telehealth and AI: How can they reinforce each other? Accessed from https://www.healthcareitnews.com/news/intersection-telehealth-and-ai-how-can-they-reinforce-each-other, Accessed on: 27/09/2024

Suleimenov, I., Vitulyova, Y., Bakirov, A. S., & Gabrielyan, O. A. (2020). Artificial Intelligence: what is it? *ICCTA '20: Proceedings of the 2020 6th International Conference on Computer and Technology Applications.* Association for Computing Machinery, New York, NY, USA, pp. 22-25, DOI: 10.1145/3397125.3397141

Sulymka, A. (2023). Healthcare technology trends and digital innovations in 2023. Accessed from https://mobidev.biz/blog/technology-trends-healthcare-digital-transformation Accessed on 28/05/2024

Tomberlin, C. (2023). Revolutionizing healthcare: How is AI being used in the healthcare industry? Los Angeles Pacific University. Available at: https://www.lapu.edu/ai-health-care-industry/ Accessed on: 27/05/2024

Yelne, S., Chaudhary, M., Dod, K., Sayyad, A., & Sharma, R. (2023, November 22). Harnessing the Power of AI: A Comprehensive Review of Its Impact and Challenges in Nursing Science and Healthcare. *Cureus*, 15(11), e49252. DOI: 10.7759/cureus.49252 PMID: 38143615

Yoon, S., & Amadiegwu, A. (2023). Emerging tech, like AI, is poised to make healthcare more accurate, accessible and sustainable. Accessed from https://www.weforum.org/agenda/2023/06/emerging-tech-like-ai-are-poised-to-make-healthcare-more-accurate-accessible-and-sustainable/, Accessed on: 27/09/2024

Compilation of References

Abadi, M., Barham, P., Chen, J., Chen, Z., Davis, A., Dean, J., . . . Zheng, X. (2016, November). TensorFlow: A system for large-scale machine learning. In OSDI (Vol. 16, No. 2016, pp. 265-283).

Abbad Ur Rehman, , HLin, , C. YMushtaq, , Z. (2021). Effective K-Nearest Neighbor algorithms performance analysis of thyroid disease. *Zhongguo Gongcheng Xuekan*, 44(1), 77–87. DOI: 10.1080/02533839.2020.1831967

Absar, N., Das, E. K., Shoma, S. N., Khandaker, M. U., Miraz, M. H., Faruque, M. R. I., & Pathan, R. K. (2022, June). The efficacy of machine-learning-supported smart system for heart disease prediction. []. MDPI.]. *Health Care*, 10(6), 1137. PMID: 35742188

Acharjya, D. P., Mitra, A., & Zaman, N. (Eds.). (2022). Deep Learning in Data Analytics. 91. DOI: 10.1007/978-3-030-75855-4

Adebisi, , O. AOjo, , J. ABello, , T. O. (2020). Computer-aided diagnosis system for classification of abnormalities in thyroid nodules ultrasound images using deep learning. *Journal of Computational Engineering*, 22, 60–66.

Agrawal, T., & Choudhary, P. (2022). Focus COVID: Automated COVID-19 detection using deep learning with chest x-ray images. *Evolving Systems*, 13(4), 519–533. DOI: 10.1007/s12530-021-09385-2 PMID: 38624806

AHA. (2023). How AI Is Improving Diagnostics, Decision-Making and Care. Accessed from https://www.aha.org/aha-center-health-innovation-market-scan/2023-05-09-how-ai-improving-diagnostics-decision-making-and-care Accessed on 23/05/2024

Ahmad, G. N., Fatima, H., Ullah, S., & Saidi, A. S. (2022). Efficient medical diagnosis of human heart diseases using machine learning techniques with and without GridSearchCV. *IEEE Access : Practical Innovations, Open Solutions*, 10, 80151–80173. DOI: 10.1109/ACCESS.2022.3165792

Ahmadi, M., & Nasiri, S. (2023). Developing a prediction model for successful aging among the elderly using machine learning algorithms. *Digital Health*, 9, 20552076231178425. DOI: 10.1177/20552076231178425 PMID: 37284015

Ahmed, B., Qadir, M. I., & Ghafoor, S. (2020). Malignant melanoma: Skin cancer–diagnosis, prevention, and treatment. *Critical Reviews™ in Eukaryotic Gene Expression, 30*(4).

Ahsan, M. M., Luna, S. A., & Siddique, Z. (2022). Machine-learning-based disease diagnosis: A comprehensive review. *Health Care*, 10(3), 541. PMID: 35327018

Akter, L., & Islam, M. M. (2021, January). Hepatocellular carcinoma patient's survival prediction using oversampling and machine learning techniques. In *2021 2nd International Conference on Robotics, Electrical and Signal Processing Techniques (ICREST)* (pp. 445-450). IEEE.

Akter, , Ferdib-Al-Islam, , Islam, M. M., Al-Rakhami, M. S., & Haque, M. R. (2021). Prediction of Cervical Cancer from Behavior Risk Using Machine Learning Techniques. *SN Computer Science*, 2(3), 177. https://doi.org/. DOI: 10.1007/s42979-021-00551-6

Alanazi, A. (2022). Using machine learning for healthcare challenges and opportunities. *Informatics in Medicine Unlocked*, 30, 100924. DOI: 10.1016/j.imu.2022.100924

Albahra, S., Gorbett, T., Robertson, S., D'Aleo, G., Kumar, S. V. S., Ockunzzi, S., Lallo, D., Hu, B., & Rashidi, H. H. (2023). Artificial intelligence and machine learning overview in pathology & laboratory medicine: A general review of data preprocessing and basic supervised concepts. *Seminars in Diagnostic Pathology*, 40(2), 71–87. DOI: 10.1053/j.semdp.2023.02.002 PMID: 36870825

Ali, M. M., Paul, B. K., Ahmed, K., Bui, F. M., Quinn, J. M. W., & Moni, M. A. (2021). Heart disease prediction using supervised machine learning algorithms: Performance analysis and comparison. *Computers in Biology and Medicine*, 136, 104672. DOI: 10.1016/j.compbiomed.2021.104672 PMID: 34315030

Aljohani, K., & Turki, T. (2022). Automatic classification of melanoma skin cancer with deep convolutional neural networks. *AI*, 3(2), 512–525. DOI: 10.3390/ai3020029

Allugunti, V. R. (2022). Breast cancer detection based on thermographic images using machine learning and deep learning algorithms. *International Journal of Engineering in Computer Science*, 4(1), 49–56. DOI: 10.33545/26633582.2022.v4.i1a.68

Almustafa, K. M. (2020). Prediction of heart disease and classifiers' sensitivity analysis. *BMC Bioinformatics*, 21(1), 1–18. DOI: 10.1186/s12859-020-03626-y PMID: 32615980

Alowais, S. A., Alghamdi, S. S., Alsuhebany, N., Alqahtani, T., Alshaya, A. I., Almohareb, S. N., Aldairem, A., Alrashed, M., Bin Saleh, K., Badreldin, H. A., Al Yami, M. S., Al Harbi, S., & Albekairy, A. M. (2023). Revolutionizing healthcare: The role of artificial intelligence in clinical practice. *BMC Medical Education*, 23(1), 689. DOI: 10.1186/s12909-023-04698-z PMID: 37740191

Al-Waisy, A. S., Al-Fahdawi, S., Mohammed, M. A., Abdulkareem, K. H., Mostafa, S. A., Maashi, M. S., Arif, M., & Garcia-Zapirain, B. (2023). Covid-Chexnet: Hybrid deep learning framework for identifying COVID-19 virus in chest x-rays images. *Soft Computing*, 27(5), 2657–2672. DOI: 10.1007/s00500-020-05424-3 PMID: 33250662

Alyas, , THamid, , MAlissa, , KFaiz, , TTabassum, , NAhmad, , A. (2022). Empirical method for thyroid disease classification using a machine learning approach. *BioMed Research International*. Advance online publication. DOI: 10.1155/2022/9809932

Amyar, A., Modzelewski, R., & Ruan, S. (2020). Multi-task deep learning-based CT imaging analysis. *Computers in Biology and Medicine*, 126, 104037. Advance online publication. DOI: 10.1016/j.compbiomed.2020.104037 PMID: 33065387

Anderson, D., Bjarnadóttir, M., & Nenova, Z. (2021). *Machine Learning in Health Care: Operational and Financial Impact*. DOI: 10.1007/978-3-030-75729-8_5

Anita, M., Ambhika, C., & Anish, T. P. (2024). Exploring the Landscape of Artificial Intelligence in Healthcare Applications. In AI Healthcare Applications and Security, Ethical, and Legal Considerations (pp. 29-48). IGI Global.

Arias-Garzon, D., Alzate-Grisales, J. A., Orozco-Arias, S., Arteaga-Arteaga, H. B., Bravo-Ortiz, M. A., Mora-Rubio, A., Saborit-Torres, J. M., Serrano, J. A. M., Iglesia Vaya, M., & Cardona-Morales, O. (2021). COVID-19 detection in x-ray images using convolutional neural networks. *Machine Learning with Applications*, 6, 100138. DOI: 10.1016/j.mlwa.2021.100138 PMID: 34939042

Ariwala, P. (2023). Deep dive into predictive analytics models and algorithms. Accessed from https://marutitech.com/predictive-analytics-models-algorithms/ Accessed on: 11/06/2024

Asghari Varzaneh, Z., Shanbehzadeh, M., & Kazemi-Arpanahi, H. (2022). Prediction of successful aging using ensemble machine learning algorithms. *BMC Medical Informatics and Decision Making*, 22(1), 258. DOI: 10.1186/s12911-022-02001-6 PMID: 36192713

Aversano, , LBernardi, , M. LCimitile, , MIammarino, , MMacchia, , P. ENettore, , I. CVerdone, , C. (2021). Thyroid disease treatment prediction with machine learning approaches. *Procedia Computer Science*, 192, 1031–1040. DOI: 10.1016/j.procs.2021.08.106

Awasthi, R., Mishra, S., Grasfield, R., Maslinski, J., Mahapatra, D., Cywinski, J. B., . . . Mathur, P. (2024). Artificial Intelligence in Healthcare: 2023 Year in Review. medRxiv, 2024-02.

Ayalew, A. M., Salau, A. O., Tamyalew, Y., Abeje, B. T., & Woreta, N. (2023). X-ray image-based COVID-19 detection using deep learning. *Multimedia Tools and Applications*, 82(28), 44507–44525. DOI: 10.1007/s11042-023-15389-8 PMID: 37362655

Aydogan, H., Bozkurt, F., & Coskun, H. (2015). An assessment of brain electrical activities of students toward teacher's specific emotions. *International Journal of Psychology and Behavioral Sciences*, 9(6), 2037–2040.

Ayhan, S., & Erdoğan, Ş. (2014). Destek vektör makineleriyle sınıflandırma problemlerinin çözümü için çekirdek fonksiyonu seçimi. *Eskişehir Osmangazi Üniversitesi İktisadi ve İdari Bilimler Dergisi*, 9(1), 175–201.

Ayık, Y. Z., Özdemir, A., & Yavuz, U. (2007). Lise türü ve lise mezuniyet başarısının, kazanılan fakülte ile ilişkisinin veri madenciliği tekniği ile analizi. *Atatürk Üniversitesi Sosyal Bilimler Enstitüsü Dergisi*, 10(2), 441–454.

Ayon, , S. IIslam, , M. M. (2019). Diabetes prediction: A deep learning approach. *International Journal of Information Engineering and Electronic Business*, 11(2), 21–27. DOI: 10.5815/ijieeb.2019.02.03

Ay, S., Ak, T., & Yilmaz, I. (2023). Comparative analysis of meta-heuristic algorithms for feature selection in heart disease prediction. *Journal of Computational Biology*, 30(5), 741–754.

Ay, Ş., Ekinci, E., & Garip, Z. (2023). A comparative analysis of meta-heuristic optimization algorithms for feature selection on ML-based classification of heart-related diseases. *The Journal of Supercomputing*, 79(11), 11797–11826. DOI: 10.1007/s11227-023-05132-3 PMID: 37304052

Badiger, M., & Mathew, J. A. (2023). Tomato plant leaf disease segmentation and multiclass disease detection using hybrid optimization enabled deep learning. *Journal of Biotechnology*, 374, 101–113. DOI: 10.1016/j.jbiotec.2023.07.011 PMID: 37543108

Baiardi, A., & Naghi, A. A. (2024). The value added of machine learning to causal inference: Evidence from revisited studies. *The Econometrics Journal*, 27(2), 213–234. DOI: 10.1093/ectj/utae004

Bania, R. K. (2022). R-GEFS: Condorcet Rank Aggregation with Graph Theoretic Ensemble Feature Selection Algorithm for Classification. *International Journal of Pattern Recognition and Artificial Intelligence*, 36(9), 2250032. Advance online publication. DOI: 10.1142/S021800142250032X

Barbierato, E. ;, Gatti, A., Barbierato, E., & Gatti, A. (2024). The Challenges of Machine Learning: A Critical Review. Electronics 2024, Vol. 13, Page 416, 13(2), 416. DOI: 10.3390/electronics13020416

Barda, A., Horvat, C., & Hochheiser, H. (2020). A qualitative research framework for the design of user-centered displays of explanations for machine learning model predictions in healthcare. *BMC Medical Informatics and Decision Making*, 20(1), 257. DOI: 10.1186/s12911-020-01276-x PMID: 33032582

Barracliffe, L., Arandjelovic, O., & Humphris, G. (2017, March). *A Pilot Study of Breast Cancer Patients: Can Machine Learning Predict Healthcare Professionals' Responses to Patient Emotions?* Bharadiya, J. P. (2023). A tutorial on principal component analysis for dimensionality reduction in machine learning. *International Journal of Innovative Science and Research Technology*, 8(5), 2028–2032.

Barth, S. Artificial intelligence (AI) in healthcare & hospitals. Accessed from https://www.foreseemed.com/artificial-intelligence-in-healthcare. Accessed on: 27/05/2024

Barthelmann, S., Butsch, F., Lang, B. M., Stege, H., Großmann, B., Schepler, H., & Grabbe, S. (2023). Seborrheic keratosis. *JDDG: Journal der Deutschen Dermatologischen Gesellschaft*, 21(3), 265–277. DOI: 10.1111/1346-8138.16754 PMID: 36892019

Bartley, A. (n.d.). Predictiive Analytics in Healthcare. Intel Corporation. Accessed from https://www.intel.vn/content/dam/www/public/us/en/documents/white-papers/gmc-analytics-healthcare-whitepaper.pdf, Accessed on: 29/05/2024

Bassel, A., Abdulkareem, A. B., Alyasseri, Z. A. A., Sani, N. S., & Mohammed, H. J. (2022). Automatic malignant and benign skin cancer classification using a hybrid deep learning approach. *Diagnostics (Basel)*, 12(10), 2472. DOI: 10.3390/diagnostics12102472 PMID: 36292161

Bassi, P. R., & Attux, R. (2021). A deep convolutional neural network for COVID-19 detection using chest x-rays. *Research on Biomedical Engineering*, •••, 1–10. DOI: 10.1007/s42600-021-00132-9

Bates, D. W., Saria, S., Ohno-Machado, L., Shah, A., & Escobar, G. (2017). Big Data In Health Care: Using Analytics To Identify And Manage High-Risk And High-Cost Patients. Https://Doi.Org/10.1377/Hlthaff.2014.0041, 33(7), 1123–1131.

Bates, D. W., & Gawande, A. A. (2003). Improving safety with information technology. *The New England Journal of Medicine*, 348(25), 2526–2534. DOI: 10.1056/NEJMsa020847 PMID: 12815139

Batko, K., & Ślęzak, A. (2022). The use of Big Data Analytics in healthcare. *Journal of Big Data*, 9(1), 3. DOI: 10.1186/s40537-021-00553-4 PMID: 35013701

Bazgir, E., Haque, E., Maniruzzaman, M., & Hoque, R. (2024). Skin cancer classification using Inception Network. *World Journal of Advanced Research and Reviews*, 21(2), 839–849. DOI: 10.30574/wjarr.2024.21.2.0500

Behera, M. P., Sarangi, A., Mishra, D., & Sarangi, S. K. (2023). A hybrid machine learning algorithm for heart and liver disease prediction using modified particle swarm optimization with support vector machine. *Procedia Computer Science*, 218, 818–827. DOI: 10.1016/j.procs.2023.01.062

Bei, S., Xing, Z., Taocheng, L., & Qin, L. (2018). Sitting posture detection using adaptively fused 3D features. Proceedings of the 2017 IEEE 2nd Information Technology, Networking, Electronic and Automation Control Conference, ITNEC 2017, 2018-January, 1073–1077. DOI: 10.1109/ITNEC.2017.8284904

Berner, E. S., & La Lande, T. J. (2007). Overview of clinical decision support systems. In *Clinical Decision Support Systems* (pp. 3–22). Springer. DOI: 10.1007/978-0-387-38319-4_1

Berner, E. S., Webster, G. D., Shugerman, A. A., & Fenton, S. H. (1994). Performance of four computer-based diagnostic systems. *The New England Journal of Medicine*, 330(26), 1792–1796. DOI: 10.1056/NEJM199406233302506 PMID: 8190157

Bhatia, N., & Vandana. (2010). Survey of nearest neighbor techniques. [IJCSIS]. *International Journal of Computer Science and Information Security*, 8(2).

Bhattacharyya, A., Bhaik, D., Kumar, S., Thakur, P., Sharma, R., & Pachori, R. B. (2022). A deep learning-based approach for automatic detection of COVID-19 cases using chest x-ray images. *Biomedical Signal Processing and Control*, 71, 103182. DOI: 10.1016/j.bspc.2021.103182 PMID: 34580596

Bidve, V., Shafi, P. M., Sarasu, P., Pavate, A., Shaikh, A., Borde, S., Singh, V. B. P., & Raut, R. (2024). Use of explainable AI to interpret the results of NLP models for sentimental analysis. *Indonesian Journal of Electrical Engineering and Computer Science*, 35(1), 511–519. DOI: 10.11591/ijeecs.v35.i1.pp511-519

Bizimana, P. C., Zhang, Z., Asim, M., & Abd El-Latif, A. A. (2023). [Retracted] An effective machine learning-based model for early heart disease prediction. *BioMed Research International*, 2023(1), 3531420. DOI: 10.1155/2023/3531420

Boateng, E. Y., & Abaye, D. A. (2019). A review of the logistic regression model with emphasis on medical research. *Journal of Data Analysis and Information Processing*, 7(4), 190–207. DOI: 10.4236/jdaip.2019.74012

Bohr, A., & Memarzadeh, K. (2020). The rise of artificial intelligence in healthcare applications. In *Artificial Intelligence in healthcare* (pp. 25–60). Academic Press. DOI: 10.1016/B978-0-12-818438-7.00002-2

Bokori, S. A. B. A. J., & Mitani, Y. (2024, January). Skin cancer prediction using convolutional neural network. In *2024 2nd International Conference on Computer Graphics and Image Processing (CGIP)* (pp. 1–5). IEEE. https://doi.org/DOI: 10.1109/CGIP55857.2024.00009

Bouchlaghem, Y., Akhiat, Y., & Amjad, S. (2022). Feature Selection: A Review and Comparative Study. *E3S Web of Conferences, 351*, 01046. DOI: 10.1051/e3sconf/202235101046

Bozkurt, F., Coskun, H., & Aydogan, H. (2014). Effectiveness of Classroom Lighting Colors Toward Students' Attention and Meditation Extracted From Brainwaves. *Journal of Educational And Instructional Studies*, 4(2), 6–12.

Bozyel, S., Şimşek, E., Koçyiğit, D., Güler, A., Korkmaz, Y., Şeker, M., & Keser, N. (2024). Artificial intelligence-based clinical decision support systems in cardiovascular diseases. *The Anatolian Journal of Cardiology*, 28(2), 74–86. DOI: 10.14744/AnatolJCardiol.2023.3685 PMID: 38168009

Bradford, L., Aboy, M., & Liddell, K. (2020). International transfers of health data between the EU and USA: A sector-specific approach for the USA to ensure an 'adequate' level of protection. *Journal of Law and the Biosciences*, 7(1), lsaa055. Advance online publication. DOI: 10.1093/jlb/lsaa055 PMID: 34221424

Broniatowski, D. A., Paul, M. J., & Dredze, M. (2013). National and Local Influenza Surveillance through Twitter: An Analysis of the 2012-2013 Influenza Epidemic. *PLoS One*, 8(12), e83672. DOI: 10.1371/journal.pone.0083672 PMID: 24349542

BuiltIn. (n.d.). Random forest classifier in Python. Retrieved July 3, 2024, from https://builtin.com/data-science/random-forest-python-deep-dive

Bullock, M. P., Foster, N. E., & Wright, C. C. (2005). Shoulder impingement: The effect of sitting posture on shoulder pain and range of motion. *Manual Therapy*, 10(1), 28–37. DOI: 10.1016/j.math.2004.07.002 PMID: 15681266

Bustos, D. F., Narváez, D. A., Dewitte, B., Oerder, V., Vidal, M., & Tapia, F. (2024). Revisiting historical trends in the Eastern Boundary Upwelling Systems with a machine learning method. *Frontiers in Marine Science*, 11, 1446766. DOI: 10.3389/fmars.2024.1446766

Caballero, F. F., Soulis, G., Engchuan, W., Sánchez-Niubó, A., Arndt, H., Ayuso-Mateos, J. L., Haro, J. M., Chatterji, S., & Panagiotakos, D. B. (2017). Advanced analytical methodologies for measuring healthy ageing and its determinants, using factor analysis and machine learning techniques: The ATHLOS project. *Scientific Reports*, 7(1), 43955. DOI: 10.1038/srep43955 PMID: 28281663

Cai, , JLuo, , JWang, , SYang, , S. (2018). Feature selection in machine learning: A new perspective. *Neurocomputing*, 300, 70–79. DOI: 10.1016/j.neucom.2017.11.077

Canadian Centre for Occupational Health & Safety. (2017). Working in a Sitting Position -Good Body Position.

Capuano, N., Fenza, G., Loia, V., & Stanzione, C. (2022). Explainable Artificial Intelligence in CyberSecurity: A Survey. *IEEE Access : Practical Innovations, Open Solutions*, 10(September), 93575–93600. DOI: 10.1109/ACCESS.2022.3204171

Carbonell, J. G., Michalski, R. S., & Mitchell, T. M. (1983). An Overview Of Machine Learning. *Machine Learning*, 3–23. DOI: 10.1016/B978-0-08-051054-5.50005-4

Chaddad, A., Peng, J., Xu, J., & Bouridane, A. (2023). Survey of Explainable AI Techniques in Healthcare. *Sensors (Basel)*, 23(2), 1–19. DOI: 10.3390/s23020634 PMID: 36679430

Chaganti, , RRustam, , FDe La Torre Díez, , IMazón, , J. L. VRodríguez, , C. LAshraf, , I. (2022). Thyroid disease prediction using selective features and machine learning techniques. *Cancers (Basel)*, 14(16), 3914. DOI: 10.3390/cancers14163914 PMID: 36010907

Chandrasekhar, N., & Peddakrishna, S. (2023). Enhancing heart disease prediction accuracy through machine learning techniques and optimization. *Processes (Basel, Switzerland)*, 11(4), 1210. DOI: 10.3390/pr11041210

Chandre, P. R., Shendkar, B. D., Deshmukh, S., Kakade, S., & Potdukhe, S. (2023). Machine Learning-Enhanced Advancements in Quantum Cryptography: A Comprehensive Review and Future Prospects. *International Journal on Recent and Innovation Trends in Computing and Communication*, 11(11s), 642–655. DOI: 10.17762/ijritcc.v11i11s.8300

Chandre, P., Mahalle, P., & Shinde, G. (2022). Intrusion prevention system using convolutional neural network for wireless sensor network. *IAES International Journal of Artificial Intelligence*, 11(2), 504–515. DOI: 10.11591/ijai.v11.i2.pp504-515

Chaturvedi, S. S., Gupta, K., & Prasad, P. S. (2021). Skin lesion analyser: An efficient seven-way multi-class skin cancer classification using MobileNet. In *Advanced Machine Learning Technologies and Applications: Proceedings of AMLTA 2020* (pp. 165–176). Springer Singapore. https://doi.org/DOI: 10.1007/978-981-16-0186-5_15

Chaudhry, B., Wang, J., Wu, S., Maglione, M., Mojica, W., Roth, E., & Shekelle, P. G. (2006). Systematic review: Impact of health information technology on quality, efficiency, and costs of medical care. *Annals of Internal Medicine*, 144(10), 742–752. DOI: 10.7326/0003-4819-144-10-200605160-00125 PMID: 16702590

Chen, I. Y., Pierson, E., Rose, S., Joshi, S., Ferryman, K., & Ghassemi, M. (2021). Ethical Machine Learning in Healthcare. Annual Review of Biomedical Data Science, 4(Volume 4, 2021), 123–144. https://doi.org/DOI: 10.1146/ANNUREV-BIODATASCI-092820-114757/CITE/REFWORKS

Chen, Z., Liang, N., Zhang, H., Li, H., Yang, Y., Zong, X., Chen, Y., Wang, Y., & Shi, N. (2023). Harnessing the power of clinical decision support systems: Challenges and opportunities. *Open Heart*, 10(2), e002432. DOI: 10.1136/openhrt-2023-002432 PMID: 38016787

Cho, G., Yim, J., Choi, Y., Ko, J., & Lee, S.-H. (2019). Review of Machine Learning Algorithms for Diagnosing Mental Illness. *Psychiatry Investigation*, 16(4), 262–269. DOI: 10.30773/pi.2018.12.21.2 PMID: 30947496

Choi, A., Choi, S. Y., Chung, K., Chung, H. S., Song, T., Choi, B., & Kim, J. H. (2023). Development of a machine learning-based clinical decision support system to predict clinical deterioration in patients visiting the emergency department. *Scientific Reports*, 13(1), 8561. DOI: 10.1038/s41598-023-35617-3 PMID: 37237057

Chu, , CZheng, , JZhou, , Y. (2021). Ultrasonic thyroid nodule detection method based on U-Net network. *Computer Methods and Programs in Biomedicine*, 199, 105906. DOI: 10.1016/j.cmpb.2020.105906 PMID: 33360682

Chung, J., & Teo, J. (2022). Mental Health Prediction Using Machine Learning: Taxonomy, Applications, and Challenges. *Applied Computational Intelligence and Soft Computing*, 9970363, 1–19. Advance online publication. DOI: 10.1155/2022/9970363

Çınar, A. (2019). Veri madenciliğinde sınıflandırma algoritmalarının performans değerlendirmesi ve R dili ile bir uygulama. Öneri Dergisi, 14(51), 90-111. https://doi.org/DOI: 10.14783/maruoneri.vi.522168

Cirillo, D., & Valencia, A. (2019). Big data analytics for personalized medicine. *Current Opinion in Biotechnology*, 58, 161–167. DOI: 10.1016/j.copbio.2019.03.004 PMID: 30965188

Cives, M., Mannavola, F., Lospalluti, L., Sergi, M. C., Cazzato, G., Filoni, E., Cavallo, F., Giudice, G., Stucci, L. S., Porta, C., & Tucci, M. (2020). Non-melanoma skin cancers: Biological and clinical features. *International Journal of Molecular Sciences*, 21(15), 5394. DOI: 10.3390/ijms21155394 PMID: 32751327

Cleveland Clinic. (n.d.). Skin cancer. Retrieved June 29, 2024, from https://my.clevelandclinic.org/health/diseases/15818-skin-cancer

Cohen, N. M., Lifshitz, A., Jaschek, R., Rinott, E., Balicer, R., Shlush, L. I., Barbash, G. I., & Tanay, A. (2024). Longitudinal machine learning uncouples healthy aging factors from chronic disease risks. *Nature Aging*, 4(1), 129–144. DOI: 10.1038/s43587-023-00536-5 PMID: 38062254

Coleman, J., Straker, L., & Ciccarelli, M. (2009). Why do children think they get discomfort related to daily activities? *Work (Reading, Mass.)*, 32(3), 267–274. DOI: 10.3233/WOR-2009-0825 PMID: 19369719

Contreras, I., & Vehi, J. (2018). Artificial Intelligence for Diabetes Management and Decision Support: Literature Review. *Journal of Medical Internet Research*, 20(5), e10775. DOI: 10.2196/10775 PMID: 29848472

Corn, J. (2023). Balancing the Pros and Cons of AI in Healthcare. Forbes. Accessed from https://www.forbes.com/sites/forbesbusinesscouncil/2023/12/01/balancing-the-pros-and-cons-of-ai-in-healthcare/?sh=39d91e04752b Accessed on: 27/05/2024

Coskun, H., & Yigit, T. (2018). Artificial Intelligence Applications on Classification of Heart Sounds. In Nature-Inspired Intelligent Techniques for Solving Biomedical Engineering Problems (pp. 146–183). IGI Global. DOI: 10.4018/978-1-5225-4769-3.ch007

Coskun, H., Deperlioglu, O., & Yigit, T. (2017). Ekstra Sistol Kalp Seslerinin MFKK Öznitelikleriyle Yapay Sinir A lari Kullanilarak Siniflandirilmasi. 2017 25th Signal Processing and Communications Applications Conference, SIU 2017. DOI: 10.1109/SIU.2017.7960252

Coskun, H., Yiğit, T., Üncü, İ. S., Ersoy, M., & Topal, A. (2022). An Industrial Application Towards Classification and Optimization of Multi-Class Tile Surface Defects Based on Geometric and Wavelet Features. *TS. Traitement du Signal*, 39(6), 2011–2022. DOI: 10.18280/ts.390613

Cunningham, P., Cord, M., & Delany, S. J. (2008). Supervised learning. In *Machine learning techniques for multimedia* (pp. 21–49). Springer., DOI: 10.1007/978-3-540-75171-7_2

Dai, L., Zheng, T., Xu, K., Han, Y., Xu, L., Huang, E., An, Y., Cheng, Y., Li, S., Liu, M., Yang, M., Li, Y., Cheng, H., Yuan, Y., Zhang, W., Ke, C., Wong, G., Qi, J., Qin, C., & Gao, G. F. (2020). A universal design of betacoronavirus vaccines against COVID-19, MERS, and SARS. *Cell*, 182(3), 722–733. DOI: 10.1016/j.cell.2020.06.035 PMID: 32645327

Damre, S. S., Shendkar, B. D., Kulkarni, N., Chandre, P. R., & Deshmukh, S. (2024). Smart Healthcare Wearable Device for Early Disease Detection Using Machine Learning. *International Journal of Intelligent Systems and Applications in Engineering*, 12(4s), 158–166.

Das, , RSaraswat, , SChandel, , DKaran, , S. (2021). An AI-driven approach for multiclass hypothyroidism classification. In *International Conference on Advanced Network Technologies and Intelligent Computing* (pp. 319–327).

Das, A. K., Ghosh, S., Thunder, S., Dutta, R., Agarwal, S., & Chakrabarti, A. (2021). Automatic COVID-19 detection from x-ray images using ensemble learning with convolutional neural network. *Pattern Analysis & Applications*, 24(3), 1111–1124. DOI: 10.1007/s10044-021-00970-4

Das, A., Choudhury, D., & Sen, A. (2024). A collaborative empirical analysis on machine learning-based disease prediction in health care systems. *International Journal of Information Technology : an Official Journal of Bharati Vidyapeeth's Institute of Computer Applications and Management*, 16(1), 261–270. DOI: 10.1007/s41870-023-01556-5

Dash, S., Acharya, B. R., Mittal, M., Abraham, A., & Kelemen, A. (Eds.). (2020). Deep Learning Techniques for Biomedical and Health Informatics. 68. DOI: 10.1007/978-3-030-33966-1

Dash, S., Shakyawar, S. K., Sharma, M., & Kaushik, S. (2019). Big data in healthcare: Management, analysis and future prospects. *Journal of Big Data*, 6(1), 54. DOI: 10.1186/s40537-019-0217-0

Davenport, T., & Kalakota, R. (2019). The potential for artificial intelligence in healthcare. *Future Healthcare Journal*, 6(2), 94–98. DOI: 10.7861/futurehosp.6-2-94 PMID: 31363513

Delleman, N. J., & Dul, J. (2007). International standards on working postures and movements ISO 11226 and EN 1005-4. Https://Doi.Org/10.1080/00140130701674430, 50(11), 1809–1819. DOI: 10.1080/00140130701674430

Deperlıoğlu, Ö., & Köse, U. (2018). Diagnosis of diabetic retinopathy by using image processing and convolutional neural network. In 2018 2nd International Symposium on Multidisciplinary Studies and Innovative Technologies (ISMSIT) (pp. 1-5). IEEE. https://doi.org/DOI: 10.1109/ISMSIT.2018.8567055

Dhanwe, S. S., (2024). AI-driven IoT in Robotics: A Review. *Journal of Mechanisms and Robotics*, 9(1), 41–48.

Divya, K., & Kannadasan, R. (2024). A systematic review and applications of how AI evolved in healthcare. *Optical and Quantum Electronics*, 56(3), 301. Advance online publication. DOI: 10.1007/s11082-023-05798-2

Divyeshkumar, V. (2024). Predictive Analysis for Personalized Machine: Leveraging Patient Data for Enhanced Healthcare. *International Journal of Current Science Research and Review*, 07(05). Advance online publication. DOI: 10.47191/ijcsrr/V7-i5-59

Dixit, A. J. (2014). A review paper on iris recognition. *Journal GSD International society for green. Sustainable Engineering and Management*, 1(14), 71–81.

Dixit, A. J., & Kazi, M. K. (2015). Iris recognition by daugman's method. *International Journal of Latest Technology in Engineering, Management &. Applied Sciences (Basel, Switzerland)*, 4(6), 90–93.

Dixon, M. F., Halperin, I., & Bilokon, P. (2020). *Machine learning in finance* (Vol. 1170). Springer International Publishing., DOI: 10.1007/978-3-030-41068-1

Doppalapudi, S., Qiu, R. G., & Badr, Y. (2021). Lung cancer survival period prediction and understanding: Deep learning approaches. *International Journal of Medical Informatics, 148*(September 2020), 104371. DOI: 10.1016/j.ijmedinf.2020.104371

Doupe, P., Faghmous, J., & Basu, S. (2019). Machine Learning for Health Services Researchers. *Value in Health*, 22(7), 808–815. DOI: 10.1016/j.jval.2019.02.012 PMID: 31277828

Dua, S., Acharya, U. R., & Dua, P. (Eds.). (2014). Machine Learning in Healthcare Informatics. 56. DOI: 10.1007/978-3-642-40017-9

Dudani, S. A. (1976). The distance-weighted k-nearest-neighbor rule. *IEEE Transactions on Systems, Man, and Cybernetics*, SMC-6(4), 325–327. DOI: 10.1109/TSMC.1976.5408784

Durga, K. (2024). Intelligent support for cardiovascular diagnosis: The AI-CDSS approach. In *Using Traditional Design Methods to Enhance AI-Driven Decision Making* (pp. 64–76). IGI Global. DOI: 10.4018/979-8-3693-0639-0.ch002

Du, X., Zhang, W., & Zhang, X. (2023). Impact of machine learning-based clinical decision support systems on pregnancy care. *Journal of Medical Systems*, 47(8), 125.

Du, Y., McNestry, C., Wei, L., Antoniadi, A. M., McAuliffe, F. M., & Mooney, C. (2023). Machine learning-based clinical decision support systems for pregnancy care: A systematic review. *International Journal of Medical Informatics*, 173, 105040. DOI: 10.1016/j.ijmedinf.2023.105040 PMID: 36907027

El Achi, H., & Khoury, J. D. (2020). Artificial intelligence and digital microscopy applications in diagnostic hematopathology. *Cancers (Basel)*, 12(4), 797. DOI: 10.3390/cancers12040797 PMID: 32224980

El Houda, Z. A., Brik, B., & Khoukhi, L. (2022). "Why Should I Trust Your IDS?": An Explainable Deep Learning Framework for Intrusion Detection Systems in Internet of Things Networks. *IEEE Open Journal of the Communications Society*, 3(June), 1164–1176. DOI: 10.1109/OJCOMS.2022.3188750

El Naqa, I., & Murphy, M. J. (2015). *What is machine learning?* Springer.

Elam, , J. JKonsynski, , B. (1987). Using artificial intelligence techniques to enhance the capabilities of model management systems. *Decision Sciences*, 18(3), 487–502. DOI: 10.1111/j.1540-5915.1987.tb01537.x

Elliott, J. (2020). How long should I stand at my standing desk? - HealthPostures. https://healthpostures.com/how-long-should-i-stand-at-my-standing-desk/

Emre, İ. E., & Erol, Ç. S. (2017). Veri analizinde istatistik mi veri madenciliği mi? *Bilişim Teknolojileri Dergisi*, 10(2), 161–167. DOI: 10.17671/gazibtd.309297

Esteva, A., Robicquet, A., Ramsundar, B., Kuleshov, V., DePristo, M., Chou, K., Cui, C., Corrado, G., Thrun, S., & Dean, J. (2019a). A guide to deep learning in healthcare. Nature Medicine 2019 25:1, 25(1), 24–29. DOI: 10.1038/s41591-018-0316-z

Esteva, A., Kuprel, B., Novoa, R. A., Ko, J., Swetter, S. M., Blau, H. M., & Thrun, S. (2017). Dermatologist-level classification of skin cancer with deep neural networks. *Nature*, 542(7639), 115–118. DOI: 10.1038/nature21056 PMID: 28117445

Fan, D. P., Zhou, T., Ji, G. P., Zhou, Y., Chen, G., Fu, H., Shen, J., & Shao, L. (2020). Inf-Net: Automatic COVID-19 lung infection segmentation from CT images. *IEEE Transactions on Medical Imaging*, 39(8), 2626–2637. DOI: 10.1109/TMI.2020.2996645 PMID: 32730213

Fania, L., Didona, D., Morese, R., Campana, I., Coco, V., Di Pietro, F. R., Ricci, F., Pallotta, S., Candi, E., Abeni, D., & Dellambra, E. (2020). Basal cell carcinoma: From pathophysiology to novel therapeutic approaches. *Biomedicines*, 8(11), 449. DOI: 10.3390/biomedicines8110449 PMID: 33113965

Farhud, D. D., & Zokaei, S. (2021). Ethical Issues of Artificial Intelligence in Medicine and Healthcare. *Iranian Journal of Public Health*, 50(11), i–v. DOI: 10.18502/ijph.v50i11.7600 PMID: 35223619

Feero, W. G., Guttmacher, A. E., O'Donnell, C. J., & Nabel, E. G. (2011). Genomics of Cardiovascular Disease. *The New England Journal of Medicine*, 365(22), 2098–2109. DOI: 10.1056/NEJMra1105239 PMID: 22129254

Ferdous, M., Debnath, J., & Chakraborty, N. (2020). *Machine Learning Algorithms in Healthcare: A Literature Survey*. 1–6. DOI: 10.1109/ICCCNT49239.2020.9225642

Fernandes, M., Vieira, S. M., Leite, F., Palos, C., Finkelstein, S., & Sousa, J. M. C. (2020). Clinical decision support systems for triage in the emergency department using intelligent systems: A review. *Artificial Intelligence in Medicine*, 2020(102), 101762. DOI: 10.1016/j.artmed.2019.101762 PMID: 31980099

Fondazione Ergo-MTM Italia. (2021). Ergonomic Assessment Worksheet (V1.3.6). https://www.eaws.it/

Forsyth, D. A., & Ponce, J. (2003). *Computer Vision: A Modern Approach*. Prentice Hall.

Fouhy, R., Halpert, A., & Rogers, C. (2023). What is the future of AI in telemedicine? US health news. Accessed from https://www.mercer.com/en-us/insights/us-health-news/what-is-the-future-of-ai-in-telemedicine/ Accessed on: 31/05/2024

Fradkov, A. L. (2020). Early History of Machine Learning. *IFAC-PapersOnLine*, 53(2), 1385–1390. DOI: 10.1016/j.ifacol.2020.12.1888

Fraiwan, M., & Faouri, E. (2022). On the automatic detection and classification of skin cancer using deep transfer learning. *Sensors (Basel)*, 22(13), 4963. DOI: 10.3390/s22134963 PMID: 35808463

Gabriel, J., Ramírez, C., Mafiqul Islam, M., Ibnul, A., Even, H., & Islam, M. M. (2024). Machine Learning Applications in Healthcare: Current Trends and Future Prospects. Journal of Artificial Intelligence General Science, 1(1). DOI: 10.60087/jaigs.v1i1.33

Ganti, V., & Sarma, A. D. (2013). Data cleaning: A practical perspective. *Synthesis Lectures on Data Management*, 5(3), 1–85. DOI: 10.1007/978-3-031-01897-8

Gao, K., Jin, Z., & Su, J. (2021). Dual-branch combination network (DCN): Towards accurate diagnosis and lesion segmentation of COVID-19 using CT images. *Medical Image Analysis*, 67, 101836. Advance online publication. DOI: 10.1016/j.media.2020.101836 PMID: 33129141

Garcia de Lomana, , MWeber, , A. GBirk, , BLandsiedel, , RAchenbach, , JSchleifer, , K. JMathea, , MKirchmair, , J. (2020). In silico models to predict the perturbation of molecular initiating events related to thyroid hormone homeostasis. *Chemical Research in Toxicology*, 34(2), 396–411. DOI: 10.1021/acs.chemrestox.0c00304 PMID: 33185102

Garg, A. X., Adhikari, N. K., McDonald, H., Rosas-Arellano, M. P., Devereaux, P. J., Beyene, J., & Haynes, R. B. (2005). Effects of computerized clinical decision support systems on practitioner performance and patient outcomes: A systematic review. *Journal of the American Medical Association*, 293(10), 1223–1238. DOI: 10.1001/jama.293.10.1223 PMID: 15755945

Garrett, W. S., Verma, A., Thomas, D., Appel, J. M., & Mirza, O. (2023). Racial disparities in psychiatric decisional capacity consultations. *Psychiatric Services (Washington, D.C.)*, 74(1), 10–16. Advance online publication. DOI: 10.1176/appi.ps.202100685 PMID: 36004436

George, G. S., Mishra, P. R., Sinha, P., & Prusty, M. R. (2023). COVID-19 detection on chest x-ray images using homomorphic transformation and VGG inspired deep convolutional neural network. *Biocybernetics and Biomedical Engineering*, 43(1), 1–16. DOI: 10.1016/j.bbe.2022.11.003 PMID: 36447948

Gerges, C. Al, Vessies, M. B., van de Leur, R. R., & van Es, R. (2023). Deep learning-Prediction. Clinical Applications of Artificial Intelligence in Real-World Data, 189–202. DOI: 10.1007/978-3-031-36678-9_12

Ghaffar Nia, N., Kaplanoglu, E., & Nasab, A. (2023). Evaluation of artificial intelligence techniques in disease diagnosis and prediction. *Discover Artificial Intelligence*, 3(1), 5. DOI: 10.1007/s44163-023-00049-5

Gharehbaghi, A., Linden, M., & Babic, A. (2017). A decision support system for cardiac disease diagnosis based on machine learning methods. *Studies in Health Technology and Informatics*, 235, 43–47. DOI: 10.3233/978-1-61499-753-5-43 PMID: 28423752

Gitto, S., Grassi, G., DeAngelis, C., Monaco, C. G., Sdao, S., Sardanelli, F., Sconfienza, L. M., & Mauri, G. (2019). A computer-aided diagnosis system for the assessment and characterization of low-to-high suspicion thyroid nodules on ultrasound. *La Radiologia Medica*, 124(2), 118–125. DOI: 10.1007/s11547-018-0942-z PMID: 30244368

Goetz, L. H., & Schork, N. J. (2018). Personalized Medicine: Motivation, Challenges and Progress. *Fertility and Sterility*, 109(6), 952–963. DOI: 10.1016/j.fertnstert.2018.05.006 PMID: 29935653

Gonzalez, R. C., & Woods, R. E. (2008). *Digital Image Processing* (3rd ed.). Prentice Hall.

Gopatoti, A., & Vijayalakshmi, P. (2022). Optimized chest x-ray image semantic segmentation networks for COVID-19 early detection. *Journal of X-Ray Science and Technology*, 30(3), 491–512. DOI: 10.3233/XST-211113 PMID: 35213339

Gottinger, , H. WWeimann, , P. (1992). Intelligent decision support systems. *Decision Support Systems*, 8(4), 317–332. DOI: 10.1016/0167-9236(92)90053-R

Grace, M. S., Climie, R. E. D., & Dunstan, D. W. (2017). Sedentary behavior and mechanisms of cardiovascular disease-getting to the heart of the matter. *Exercise and Sport Sciences Reviews*, 45(2), 55–56. DOI: 10.1249/JES.0000000000000107 PMID: 28306676

Greenes, R. A. (2014). *Clinical decision support: The road to broad adoption*. Academic Press.

Guan, , QWang, , YDu, , JQin, , YLu, , HXiang, , JWang, , F. (2019). Deep learning based classification of ultrasound images for thyroid nodules: A large scale pilot study. *Annals of Translational Medicine*, 7(7), 137. DOI: 10.21037/atm.2019.04.34 PMID: 31157258

Guleria, V., Sharma, A., & Gupta, G. (n.d.). Biosensors in bioinformatics, biotechnology, and healthcare. Researchgate.NetA Sharma, V Guleriaresearchgate.Net. DOI: 10.52305/LDXT8191

Gulshan, V., Peng, L., Coram, M., Stumpe, M. C., Wu, D., Narayanaswamy, A., & Webster, D. R. (2016). Development and validation of a deep learning algorithm for detection of diabetic retinopathy in retinal fundus photographs. *Journal of the American Medical Association*, 316(22), 2402–2410. DOI: 10.1001/jama.2016.17216 PMID: 27898976

Gulshan, V., Rajan, R. P., & Kumar, V. (2019). Early detection of Alzheimer's disease using machine learning: An AI approach to cognitive health. *Computers in Biology and Medicine*, 110, 79–90.

Güner, Z. (2014). Veri madenciliğinde CART ve lojistik regresyon analizinin yeri: İlaç provizyon sistemi verileri üzerinde örnek bir uygulama. *Sosyal Güvence*, (6), 53–99. DOI: 10.21441/sguz.2014617906

Guo, G., Wang, H., Bell, D., Bi, Y., & Greer, K. (2003). KNN model-based approach in classification. In On The Move to Meaningful Internet Systems 2003: CoopIS, DOA, and ODBASE (pp. 986-996). Springer. https://doi.org/DOI: 10.1007/978-3-540-39964-3_62

Guo, Z., Lu, Q., Jin, Q., Li, P., Xing, G., & Zhang, G. (2024). Phylogenetically evolutionary analysis provides insights into the genetic diversity and adaptive evolution of porcine deltacoronavirus. *BMC Veterinary Research*, 20(1), 22. DOI: 10.1186/s12917-023-03863-2 PMID: 38200538

Gupta, , J. NForgionne, , G. AMora, , M. (2007). *Intelligent decision-making support systems: Foundations, applications and challenges*. Springer Science & Business Media.

Gupta, M., Sharma, S., Sakshi, & Sharma, C. (2022). Security and Privacy Issues in Blockchained IoT: Principles, Challenges and Counteracting Actions. Blockchain Technology: Exploring Opportunities, Challenges, and Applications, 27–56. https://doi.org/DOI: 10.1201/9781003138082-3/SECURITY-PRIVACY-ISSUES-BLOCKCHAINED-IOT-MANIK-GUPTA-SHAMNEESH-SHARMA-SAKSHI-CHETAN-SHARMA

Gupta, , PRustam, , FKanwal, , KAljedaani, , WAlfarhood, , SSafran, , MAshraf, , I. (2024). Detecting thyroid disease using optimized machine learning model based on differential evolution. *International Journal of Computational Intelligence Systems*, 17(3), 3. Advance online publication. DOI: 10.1007/s44196-023-00388-2

Gupta, C., Khan, V., Srikanteswara, R., Gill, N. S., Gulia, P., & Menon, S. (2024). A novel secured deep learning model for COVID detection using chest x-rays. *Journal of Cybersecurity and Information Management*, 14(01), 227–244. DOI: 10.54216/JCIM.140116

Gupta, S., & Sedamkar, R. R. (2020). Machine Learning for Healthcare: Introduction. *Learning and Analytics in Intelligent Systems*, 13, 1–25. DOI: 10.1007/978-3-030-40850-3_1

Gupta, V., Jain, N., Sachdeva, J., Gupta, M., Mohan, S., Bajuri, M. Y., & Ahmadian, A. (2022). Improved COVID-19 detection with chest x-ray images using deep learning. *Multimedia Tools and Applications*, 81(26), 37657–37680. DOI: 10.1007/s11042-022-13509-4 PMID: 35968409

Güran, A., Uysal, M., & Doğrusöz, Ö. (2014). Destek vektör makineleri parametre optimizasyonunun duygu analizi üzerindeki etkisi. *Dokuz Eylül Üniversitesi Mühendislik Fakültesi Fen ve Mühendislik Dergisi*, 16(48), 86–93.

Guzsvinecz, T., Szucs, V., & Sik-Lanyi, C. (2019). Suitability of the Kinect sensor and Leap Motion controller—A literature review. *Sensors (Basel)*, 19(5), 1072. DOI: 10.3390/s19051072 PMID: 30832385

Habehh, H., & Gohel, S. (2021). Machine Learning in Healthcare. *Current Genomics*, 22(4), 291–300. DOI: 10.2174/1389202922666210705124359 PMID: 35273459

Hafner, C., & Vogt, T. (2008). Seborrheic keratosis. *Journal der Deutschen Dermatologischen Gesellschaft*, 6(8), 664–677. DOI: 10.1111/j.1610-0387.2008.06788.x PMID: 18801147

Halli, U. M. (2022). Nanotechnology in IoT Security, *Journal of Nanoscience. Nanoengineering & Applications*, 12(3), 11–16.

Hancer, E. (2024). An improved evolutionary wrapper-filter feature selection approach with a new initialisation scheme. *Machine Learning*, 113(8), 4977–5000. DOI: 10.1007/s10994-021-05990-z

Haralick, R. M., Shanmugam, K., & Dinstein, I. H. (1973). Textural features for image classification. *. IEEE Transactions on Systems, Man, and Cybernetics*, SMC-3(6), 610–621. DOI: 10.1109/TSMC.1973.4309314

Harari, D. Y., & Macauley, R. C. (2020). Betting on CPR: A modern version of Pascal's wager. *Journal of Medical Ethics*, 46(2), 110–113. DOI: 10.1136/medethics-2019-105558 PMID: 31527140

Hasanin, T., Khoshgoftaar, T. M., Leevy, J. L., & Bauder, R. A. (2019). Severely imbalanced Big Data challenges: Investigating data sampling approaches. *Journal of Big Data*, 6(1), 107. DOI: 10.1186/s40537-019-0274-4

Hashim, M. S., & Yassin, A. A. (2023). Feature Selection Using a Hybrid Approach Depends on Filter and Wrapper Methods for Accurate Breast Cancer Diagnosis. *Journal of Basrah Researches (Sciences)*, 49(1), 45–56. DOI: 10.56714/bjrs.49.1.5

Hassan, M., Awan, F. M., Naz, A., deAndrés-Galiana, E. J., Alvarez, O., Cernea, A., Fernández-Brillet, L., Fernández-Martínez, J. L., & Kloczkowski, A. (2022). Innovations in Genomics and Big Data Analytics for Personalized Medicine and Health Care: A Review. *International Journal of Molecular Sciences*, 23(9), 9. Advance online publication. DOI: 10.3390/ijms23094645 PMID: 35563034

Hastie, T. (2009). *The elements of statistical learning: Data mining, inference, and prediction* (2nd ed.). Springer., DOI: 10.1007/978-0-387-84858-7

Hatton, C. M., Paton, L. W., McMillan, D., Cussens, J., Gilbody, S., & Tiffin, P. A. (2019). Predicting persistent depressive symptoms in older adults: A machine learning approach to personalised mental healthcare. *Journal of Affective Disorders*, 246, 857–860. DOI: 10.1016/j.jad.2018.12.095 PMID: 30795491

Healthcare Research Insight. (2024). US telemedicine industry: The AI revolution in remote healthcare. Accessed from https://www.linkedin.com/pulse/us-telemedicine-industry-ai-revolution-hpuqf/ Accessed on: 01/06/2024

Heart Disease Dataset. Available online: https://www.kaggle.com/johnsmith88/heart-disease-dataset (accessed on 1 April 2024).

Heibel, H. D., Hooey, L., & Cockerell, C. J. (2020). A review of noninvasive techniques for skin cancer detection in dermatology. *American Journal of Clinical Dermatology*, 21(4), 513–524. DOI: 10.1007/s40257-020-00517-z PMID: 32383142

He, K., Zhang, X., Ren, S., & Sun, J. (2016). Deep residual learning for image recognition. In *Proceedings of the IEEE Conference on Computer Vision and Pattern Recognition* (pp. 770–778). https://doi.org/DOI: 10.1109/CVPR.2016.90

Helaly, H. A., Badawy, M., & Haikal, A. Y. (2023). A review of deep learning approaches in clinical and healthcare systems based on medical image analysis. Multimedia Tools and Applications 2023 83:12, 83(12), 36039–36080. DOI: 10.1007/s11042-023-16605-1

Hewlett Packard Enterprise. What is AI Healthcare? Accessed from https://www.hpe.com/in/en/what-is/ai-healthcare.html, Accessed on 26/05/2024

Ho, C. W. L., & Caals, K. (2021). A Call for an Ethics and Governance Action Plan to Harness the Power of Artificial Intelligence and Digitalization in Nephrology. *Seminars in Nephrology*, 41(3), 282–293. DOI: 10.1016/j.semnephrol.2021.05.009 PMID: 34330368

Ho, E. S. L., Chan, J. C. P., Chan, D. C. K., Shum, H. P. H., Cheung, Y. M., & Yuen, P. C. (2016). Improving posture classification accuracy for depth sensor-based human activity monitoring in smart environments. *Computer Vision and Image Understanding*, 148, 97–110. DOI: 10.1016/j.cviu.2015.12.011

Holzinger, A., Goebel, R., Palade, V., & Ferri, M. (2017). Towards Integrative Machine Learning and Knowledge Extraction. Lecture Notes in Computer Science (Including Subseries Lecture Notes in Artificial Intelligence and Lecture Notes in Bioinformatics), 10344 LNAI, 1–12. DOI: 10.1007/978-3-319-69775-8_1

Holzinger, A., Malle, B., Kieseberg, P., Roth, P. M., Müller, H., Reihs, R., & Zatloukal, K. (2017), 10344 LNAI, 13–50. DOI: 10.1007/978-3-319-69775-8_2

Hosmer, D. W., Jr., Lemeshow, S., & Sturdivant, R. X. (2013). Applied logistic regression (Vol. 398). John Wiley & Sons. https://doi.org//arXiv.1007.0085 DOI: 10.48550

Hosny, A., Parmar, C., Quackenbush, J., Schwartz, L. H., & Aerts, H. J. W. L. (2018). Artificial intelligence in radiology. *Nature Reviews. Cancer*, 18(8), 500–510. DOI: 10.1038/s41568-018-0016-5 PMID: 29777175

Hossain, M. I., Maruf, M. H., Khan, M. A. R., Prity, F. S., Fatema, S., Ejaz, M. S., & Khan, M. A. S. (2023). Heart disease prediction using distinct artificial intelligence techniques: Performance analysis and comparison. *Iran Journal of Computer Science*, 6(4), 397–417. DOI: 10.1007/s42044-023-00148-7

Hosseinzadeh, , Ahmed, O. H., Ghafour, M. Y., Safara, F., hama, H., Ali, S., Vo, B., & Chiang, H.-S. (2021). A multiple multilayer perceptron neural network with an adaptive learning algorithm for thyroid disease diagnosis in the internet of medical things. *The Journal of Supercomputing*, 77(4), 3616–3637. DOI: 10.1007/s11227-020-03404-w

Huang, M.-L., & Liao, Y.-C. (2022). A lightweight CNN-based network on COVID-19 detection using x-ray and CT images. *Computers in Biology and Medicine*, 146, 105604. DOI: 10.1016/j.compbiomed.2022.105604 PMID: 35576824

Hu, B., Ge, X., Wang, L.-F., & Shi, Z. (2015). Bat origin of human coronaviruses. *Virology Journal*, 12(1), 1–10. DOI: 10.1186/s12985-015-0422-1 PMID: 26689940

Hussain, I. khan, S., & Nazir, M. Bin. (2024). Empowering Healthcare: AI, ML, and Deep Learning Innovations for Brain and Heart Health. International Journal of Advanced Engineering Technologies and Innovations, 1(4), 167–188. https://ijaeti.com/index.php/Journal/article/view/268

Hussain, E., Hasan, M., Rahman, M. A., Lee, I., Tamanna, T., & Parvez, M. Z. (2021). Corodet: A deep learning-based classification for COVID-19 detection using chest x-ray images. *Chaos, Solitons, and Fractals*, 142, 110495. DOI: 10.1016/j.chaos.2020.110495 PMID: 33250589

Hu, T., Chen, Y., Li, D., Long, C., Wen, Z., Hu, R., & Chen, G. (2023). Rice Variety Identification Based on the Leaf Hyperspectral Feature via LPP-SVM. *International Journal of Pattern Recognition and Artificial Intelligence*, 36(15), 2350001. DOI: 10.1142/S0218001423500015

HyScaler. (2024). Scope of AI in healthcare: 7 powerful advantages unlocked. Available at: https://hyscaler.com/insights/scope-of-ai-in-healthcare-7-advantages/ Accessed on: 26/05/2024

Idarraga, , A. JLuong, , GHsiao, , VSchneider, , D. F. (2021). False negative rates in benign thyroid nodule diagnosis: Machine learning for detecting malignancy. *The Journal of Surgical Research*, 268, 562–569. DOI: 10.1016/j.jss.2021.06.076 PMID: 34464894

Ikonomakis, M., Kotsiantis, S., & Tampakas, V. (2005). Text classification using machine learning techniques. *WSEAS Transactions on Computers*, 4(8), 966–974.

Internet of Things (IoT). A Review of Integration of Precedent, Existing & Inevitable Technologies. (n.d.). Retrieved October 4, 2024, from https://www.researchgate.net/publication/317231159_Internet_of_Things_IoT_A_Review_of_Integration_of_Precedent_Existing_Inevitable_Technologies

Islam, , S. SHaque, , M. SMiah, , M. S. USarwar, , T. BNugraha, , R. (2022). Application of machine learning algorithms to predict the thyroid disease risk: An experimental comparative study. *PeerJ. Computer Science*, 8, 898. DOI: 10.7717/peerj-cs.898

Islam, , Haque, M. R., Iqbal, H., Hasan, M. M., Hasan, M., & Kabir, M. N. (2020). Breast Cancer Prediction: A Comparative Study Using Machine Learning Techniques. *SN Computer Science*, 1(5), 290. https://doi.org/. DOI: 10.1007/s42979-020-00305-w

Islam, S. R., Eberle, W., Ghafoor, S. K., Siraj, A., & Rogers, M. (2020). Domain knowledge aided explainable artificial intelligence for intrusion detection and response. *CEUR Workshop Proceedings*, •••, 2600.

Islam, S., Liu, D., Wang, K., Zhou, P., Yu, L., & Wu, D. (2019). A Case Study of HealthCare Platform using Big Data Analytics and Machine Learning. *HPCCT 2019: Proceedings of the 2019 3rd High Performance Computing and Cluster Technologies Conference*, 139–146. DOI: 10.1145/3341069.3342980

Ismael, A. M., & Sengur, A. (2021). Deep learning approaches for COVID-19 detection based on chest x-ray images. *Expert Systems with Applications*, 164, 114054. DOI: 10.1016/j.eswa.2020.114054 PMID: 33013005

Ismail, M. A., Hameed, N., & Clos, J. (2021). Deep learning-based algorithm for skin cancer classification. In *Proceedings of International Conference on Trends in Computational and Cognitive Engineering: Proceedings of TCCE 2020* (pp. 709–719). Springer Singapore. DOI: 10.1007/978-981-33-4673-4_58

ISO. (2017). ISO 7250-1:2017. Basic Human Body Measurements for Technological Design — Part 1: Body Measurement Definitions and Landmarks. https://www.iso.org/standard/65246.html

Janda, M., Cust, A. E., Neale, R. E., & Smith, K. (2015). Cancer epidemiology and prevention. *Australian Family Physician*, 44(1), 16–20. https://www.racgp.org.au

Javaid, M., Haleem, A., Singh, R., Suman, R., & Rab, S. (2022). Significance of machine learning in healthcare: Features, pillars and applications. *International Journal of Intelligent Networks*, 3, 58–73. Advance online publication. DOI: 10.1016/j.ijin.2022.05.002

Jayalakshmi, T., & Santhakumaran, A. (2011). Statistical normalization and back propagation for classification. *International Journal of Computer Theory and Engineering*, 3(1), 89–93. DOI: 10.7763/IJCTE.2011.V3.288

Jayeb, A. W., Hore, A. R., Anjum, R., Sadeque, S. S., & Auqib, S. T. (2022). *Computer vision based skin disease detection using machine learning* (Doctoral dissertation, Brac University).

Jha, , RBhattacharjee, , VMustafi, , A. (2022). Increasing the prediction accuracy for thyroid disease: A step towards better health for society. *Wireless Personal Communications*, 122(2), 1921–1938. DOI: 10.1007/s11277-021-08974-3

Jiang, F., Jiang, Y., Zhi, H., Dong, Y., Li, H., Ma, S., Wang, Y., Dong, Q., Shen, H., & Wang, Y. (2017). Artificial intelligence in healthcare: Past, present, and future. *Stroke and Vascular Neurology*, 2(4), 230–243. DOI: 10.1136/svn-2017-000101 PMID: 29507784

Jiang, L., Cai, Z., Wang, D., & Jiang, S. (2007, August). Survey of improving k-nearest-neighbor for classification. In *Fourth international conference on fuzzy systems and knowledge discovery (FSKD 2007)* (Vol. 1, pp. 679-683). IEEE. https://doi.org/DOI: 10.1109/FSKD.2007.552

Jiang, P., Sinha, S., Aldape, K., Hannenhalli, S., Sahinalp, C., & Ruppin, E. (2022). Big data in basic and translational cancer research. *Nature Reviews. Cancer*, 22(11), 625–639. DOI: 10.1038/s41568-022-00502-0 PMID: 36064595

Jijo, B. T., & Abdulazeez, A. M. (2021).*Journal of Applied Science and Technology Trends*, 2(01), 20–28. DOI: 10.38094/jastt20165

Jin, X. (2024). Editorial: Intelligent Systematics: A New Transactions. *IEEE Transactions on Intelligent Systematics*, 1(1), 1–2. DOI: 10.62762/TIS.2024.100001

Johnson, A. E. W., Pollard, T. J., Shen, L., Lehman, L. W. H., Feng, M., Ghassemi, M., Moody, B., Szolovits, P., Anthony Celi, L., & Mark, R. G. (2016). MIMIC-III, a freely accessible critical care database. Scientific Data 2016 3:1, 3(1), 1–9. DOI: 10.1038/sdata.2016.35

Johnson, K. B., Wei, W., Weeraratne, D., Frisse, M. E., Misulis, K., Rhee, K., Zhao, J., & Snowdon, J. L. (2021). Precision Medicine, AI, and the Future of Personalized Health Care. *Clinical and Translational Science*, 14(1), 86–93. DOI: 10.1111/cts.12884 PMID: 32961010

Jordanabukasis (2024). The future of AI in healthcare: Trends and innovations. Cprime. CPRIME. Accessed from https://www.cprime.com/resources/blog/the-future-of-ai-in-healthcare-trends-and-innovations/ Accessed on: 05/06/2024

Jordan, M. I., & Mitchell, T. M. (2015). Machine learning: Trends, perspectives, and prospects. *Science*, 349(6245), 255–260. DOI: 10.1126/science.aaa8415 PMID: 26185243

Jothi, K. A., Subburam, S., Umadevi, V., & Hemavathy, K. (2021). WITHDRAWN: Heart disease prediction system using machine learning. *Materials Today: Proceedings*. Advance online publication. DOI: 10.1016/j.matpr.2020.12.901

Jović, A., Stančin, I., Friganović, K., & Cifrek, M. (2020, September). Clinical decision support systems in practice: Current status and challenges. In *2020 43rd International Convention on Information, Communication and Electronic Technology (MIPRO)* (pp. 355-360). IEEE.

Jutzi, T. B., Krieghoff-Henning, E. I., Holland-Letz, T., Utikal, J. S., Hauschild, A., Schadendorf, D., Sondermann, W., Fröhling, S., Hekler, A., Schmitt, M., Maron, R. C., & Brinker, T. J. (2020). Artificial intelligence in skin cancer diagnostics: The patients' perspective. *Frontiers in Medicine*, 7, 233. DOI: 10.3389/fmed.2020.00233 PMID: 32671078

K Sayyad L. (2018). Significance of Projection and Rotation of Image in Color Matching for High-Quality Panoramic Images used for Aquatic study. *International Journal of Aquatic Science*, 9(2), 130–145.

Kabir, M. F., Chen, T., & Ludwig, S. A. (2023). A performance analysis of dimensionality reduction algorithms in machine learning models for cancer prediction. *Healthcare Analytics*, 3, 100125. DOI: 10.1016/j.health.2022.100125

Kaggle projects, (2023) https://www.kaggle.com/code/sumitnayek/sudeshna-project

Kalaiselvi, K., & Deepika, M. (2020). Machine Learning for Healthcare Diagnostics. *Learning and Analytics in Intelligent Systems*, 13, 91–105. DOI: 10.1007/978-3-030-40850-3_5

Kamala, S. P. R., Gayathri, S., Pillai, N. M., Gracious, L. A., Varun, C. M., & Subramanian, R. S. (2023, July). Predictive Analytics for Heart Disease Detection: A Machine Learning Approach. In 2023 4th International Conference on Electronics and Sustainable Communication Systems (ICESC) (pp. 1583-1589). IEEE.

Kan, H., Kharrazi, H., Chang, H.-Y., Bodycombe, D., Lemke, K., & Weiner, J. (2019). Exploring the use of machine learning for risk adjustment: A comparison of standard and penalized linear regression models in predicting health care costs in older adults. *PLoS One*, 14(3), e0213258. DOI: 10.1371/journal.pone.0213258 PMID: 30840682

Kansagara, D., Englander, H., Salanitro, A., Kagen, D., Theobald, C., Freeman, M., & Kripalani, S. (2011). Risk Prediction Models for Hospital Readmission: A Systematic Review. *Journal of the American Medical Association*, 306(15), 1688–1698. DOI: 10.1001/jama.2011.1515 PMID: 22009101

Kapadiya, K., Patel, U., Gupta, R., Alshehri, M. D., Tanwar, S., Sharma, G., & Bokoro, P. N. (2022). Blockchain and AI-empowered healthcare insurance fraud detection: An analysis, architecture, and future prospects. *IEEE Access: Practical Innovations, Open Solutions*, 10, 79606–79627. DOI: 10.1109/ACCESS.2022.3194569

Kar, Y. E., Basgumus, A., & Namdar, M. (2021, October). Machine learning assisted autonomous vehicle design and control. In 2021 5th International Symposium on Multidisciplinary Studies and Innovative Technologies (ISMSIT) (pp. 462-466). IEEE. DOI: 10.1109/ISMSIT52890.2021.9604621

Karale Aishwarya, A., (2023). Smart Billing Cart Using RFID, YOLO and Deep Learning for Mall Administration. *International Journal of Instrumentation and Innovation Sciences*, 8(2).

Kasat, K., Shaikh, N., Rayabharapu, V. K., & Nayak, M. (2023). Implementation and Recognition of Waste Management System with Mobility Solution in Smart Cities using Internet of Things, *2023 Second International Conference on Augmented Intelligence and Sustainable Systems (ICAISS)*, Trichy, India, 2023, pp. 1661-1665, DOI: 10.1109/ICAISS58487.2023.10250690

Kaul, D., Raju, H., & Tripathy, B. K. (2022). Deep Learning in Healthcare. *Studies in Big Data*, 91, 97–115. DOI: 10.1007/978-3-030-75855-4_6

Kaur, G., & Oberai, E. N. (2014). A review article on Naive Bayes classifier with various smoothing techniques. *International Journal of Computer Science and Mobile Computing*, 3(10), 864–868.

Kaur, R., Jain, M., McAdams, R. M., Sun, Y., Gupta, S., Mutharaju, R., & Singh, H. (2023). An ontology and rule-based clinical decision support system for personalized nutrition recommendations in the neonatal intensive care unit. *IEEE Access : Practical Innovations, Open Solutions*, 11, 142433–142446. DOI: 10.1109/ACCESS.2023.3341403

Kavitha, C., Priyanka, S., Kumar, M. P., & Kusuma, V. (2024). Skin cancer detection and classification using deep learning techniques. *Procedia Computer Science*, 235, 2793–2802. DOI: 10.1016/j.procs.2024.04.264

Kavzoğlu, T., & Çölkesen, İ. (2010). Karar ağaçları ile uydu görüntülerinin sınıflandırılması. *Harita Teknolojileri Elektronik Dergisi*, 2(1), 36–45.

Kawamoto, K., Houlihan, C. A., Balas, E. A., & Lobach, D. F. (2005). Improving clinical practice using clinical decision support systems: A systematic review of trials to identify features critical to success. *BMJ (Clinical Research Ed.)*, 330(7494), 765. DOI: 10.1136/bmj.38398.500764.8F PMID: 15767266

Kazi, K. (2024b). Modelling and Simulation of Electric Vehicle for Performance Analysis: BEV and HEV Electrical Vehicle Implementation Using Simulink for E-Mobility Ecosystems. *In L. D., N. Nagpal, N. Kassarwani, V. Varthanan G., & P. Siano (Eds.), E-Mobility in Electrical Energy Systems for Sustainability (pp. 295-320). IGI Global.* Available at: https://www.igi-global.com/gateway/chapter/full-text-pdf/341172 DOI: 10.4018/979-8-3693-2611-4.ch014

Kazi, K. (2025d). AI-Powered-IoT (AIIoT) based Decision Making System for BP Patient's Healthcare Monitoring: KSK Approach for BP Patient Healthcare Monitoring. In *Sourour Aouadni, Ismahene Aouadni (Eds.), Recent Theories and Applications for Multi-Criteria Decision-Making, IGI Global,* Prasad, Santoshachandra Rao Karanam (2024). AI in public-private partnership for IT infrastructure development, *Journal of High Technology Management Research*, Volume 35, Issue 1, May 2024, 100496. DOI: 10.1016/j.hitech.2024.100496

Kazi, K. S. L. (2025). IoT Technologies for the Intelligent Dairy Industry: A New Challenge. In *Designing Sustainable Internet of Things Solutions for Smart Industries* (pp. 321-350). IGI Global.

Kazi, K. (2024a). Machine Learning (ML)-Based Braille Lippi Characters and Numbers Detection and Announcement System for Blind Children in Learning. In Sart, G. (Ed.), *Social Reflections of Human-Computer Interaction in Education, Management, and Economics*. IGI Global., DOI: 10.4018/979-8-3693-3033-3.ch002

Kazi, K. (2025b). Machine Learning-Driven-Internet of Things(MLIoT) Based Healthcare Monitoring System. In Wickramasinghe, N. (Ed.), *Impact of Digital Solutions for Improved Healthcare Delivery*. IGI Global.

Kazi, K. (2025c). Moonlighting in Carrier. In Tunio, M. N. (Ed.), *Applications of Career Transitions and Entrepreneurship*. IGI Global.

Kazi, K. (2025d). AI-Driven-IoT (AIIoT) based Decision-Making in Drones for Climate Change: KSK Approach. In Aouadni, S., & Aouadni, I. (Eds.), *Recent Theories and Applications for Multi-Criteria Decision-Making*. IGI Global.

Kazi, K. S. (2024a). Computer-Aided Diagnosis in Ophthalmology: A Technical Review of Deep Learning Applications. In Garcia, M., & de Almeida, R. (Eds.), *Transformative Approaches to Patient Literacy and Healthcare Innovation* (pp. 112–135). IGI Global., Available at https://www.igi-global.com/chapter/computer-aided-diagnosis-in-ophthalmology/342823, DOI: 10.4018/979-8-3693-3661-8.ch006

Kazi, K. S. (2024f). Machine Learning-Based Pomegranate Disease Detection and Treatment. In Zia Ul Haq, M., & Ali, I. (Eds.), *Revolutionizing Pest Management for Sustainable Agriculture* (pp. 469–498). IGI Global., DOI: 10.4018/979-8-3693-3061-6.ch019

Keçeli, A. S., & Can, A. B. (2014). Recognition of Basic Human Actions Using Depth Information. *International Journal of Pattern Recognition and Artificial Intelligence*, 28(2), 1450004. Advance online publication. DOI: 10.1142/S0218001414500049

Kelly, J. (2014). Proper Height For Standing Desks. https://notsitting.com/proper-height/

Kesavaraj, G., & Sukumaran, S. (2013, July). A study on classification techniques in data mining. In *2013 fourth international conference on computing, communications and networking technologies (ICCCNT)* (pp. 1-7). IEEE. DOI: 10.1109/ICCCNT.2013.6726842

Keskin, S., Aydın, F., & Yurdugül, H. (2019). Eğitsel veri madenciliği ve öğrenme analitikleri bağlamında e-öğrenme verilerinde aykırı gözlemlerin belirlenmesi. *Eğitim Teknolojisi Kuram ve Uygulama*, 9(1), 292–309. DOI: 10.17943/etku.475149

Khalifa, M., Albadawy, M., & Iqbal, U. (2024). Advancing clinical decision support: The role of artificial intelligence across six domains. *Computer Methods and Programs in Biomedicine Update*, 5, 100142. DOI: 10.1016/j.cmpbup.2024.100142

Khan, A. I., Shah, J. L., & Bhat, M. M. (2020). CoroNet: A deep neural network for detection and diagnosis of COVID-19 from chest X-ray images. *Computer Methods and Programs in Biomedicine*, 196, 105581. Advance online publication. DOI: 10.1016/j.cmpb.2020.105581 PMID: 32534344

Khan, V., & Meenai, T. A. (2021). Pretrained natural language processing model for intent recognition (BERT-IR). *Human Centric Intelligent Systems*, 1(3), 66–74. DOI: 10.2991/hcis.k.211109.001

Khan, V., Patel, D., Azfar Meenai, T., & Shukla, R. (2020). Application of deep learning techniques for automating the detection of diabetic retinopathy in retinal fundus photographs. In *Proceedings of the 2nd International Conference on Data, Engineering and Applications (IDEA)* (pp. 1–7). https://doi.org/DOI: 10.1109/IDEA49133.2020.9170712

Khan, V., Sharma, S., Ramesh, J. V. N., Pareek, P. K., Shukla, P. K., & Pandit, S. V. (2024). Enhancing tomato leaf disease detection through generative adversarial networks and genetic algorithm-based convolutional neural network. Fusion. *Practice and Applications*, 16(2), 147–177. DOI: 10.54216/FPA.160210

Khemani, B., Patil, S., Kotecha, K., & Tanwar, S. (2024). A review of graph neural networks: Concepts, architectures, techniques, challenges, datasets, applications, and future directions. *Journal of Big Data*, 11(1), 18. DOI: 10.1186/s40537-023-00876-4

Khosravi, M., Zare, Z., Mojtabaeian, S. M., & Izadi, R. (2024). Artificial Intelligence and Decision-Making in Healthcare: A Thematic Analysis of a Systematic Review of reviews. *Health Services Research and Managerial Epidemiology*, 11, 23333928241234863. Advance online publication. DOI: 10.1177/23333928241234863 PMID: 38449840

Khurana, D., Koli, A., Khatter, K., & Singh, S. (2023). Natural language processing: State of the art, current trends and challenges. *Multimedia Tools and Applications*, 82(3), 3713–3744. DOI: 10.1007/s11042-022-13428-4 PMID: 35855771

Kılınç, D., Borandağ, E., Yücala, F., Tunalı, V., Şimşek, M., & Özçift, A. (2016). KNN algoritması ve R dili ile metin madenciliği kullanılarak bilimsel makale tasnifi. *Marmara Fen Bilimleri Dergisi*, 28(3), 89–94. DOI: 10.7240/mufbed.69674

Kiran, N., Sapna, F., Kiran, F., Kumar, D., Raja, F., Shiwlani, S., Paladini, A., Sonam, F., Bendari, A., Perkash, R. S., Anjali, F., & Varrassi, G. (2023, September 3). (n.d.). Digital Pathology: Transforming Diagnosis in the Digital Age. *Cureus*, 15(9), e44620. DOI: 10.7759/cureus.44620 PMID: 37799211

Kıran, Z. B. (2010). *Lojistik regresyon ve CART analizi teknikleriyle sosyal güvenlik kurumu ilaç provizyon sistemi verileri üzerinde bir uygulama* [An application on pharmacy provision system data of social security institution by logistic regression and CART analysis techniques]. Gazi Üniversitesi Fen Bilimleri Enstitüsü.

Kishor, A., & Chakraborty, C. (2022). Artificial intelligence and internet of things based healthcare 4.0 monitoring system. *Wireless Personal Communications*, 127(2), 1615–1631. DOI: 10.1007/s11277-021-08708-5

Kobylińska, K., Orłowski, T., Adamek, M., & Biecek, P. (2022). Explainable Machine Learning for Lung Cancer Screening Models. *Applied Sciences (Basel, Switzerland)*, 12(4), 1926. Advance online publication. DOI: 10.3390/app12041926

Kolasa, K., Admassu, B., Hołownia-Voloskova, M., Kędzior, K. J., Poirrier, J. E., & Perni, S. (2024). Systematic reviews of machine learning in healthcare: A literature review. *Expert Review of Pharmacoeconomics & Outcomes Research*, 24(1), 63–115. DOI: 10.1080/14737167.2023.2279107 PMID: 37955147

Kong, Y.-K., Lee, S., Lee, K.-S., & Kim, D.-M. (2018). Comparisons of ergonomic evaluation tools (ALLA, RULA, REBA and OWAS) for farm work. *International Journal of Occupational Safety and Ergonomics*, 24(2), 218–223. DOI: 10.1080/10803548.2017.1306960 PMID: 28301984

Kononenko, I. (2001). Machine learning for medical diagnosis: History, state of the art and perspective. *Artificial Intelligence in Medicine*, 23(1), 89–109. DOI: 10.1016/S0933-3657(01)00077-X PMID: 11470218

Korneenko, E. V., Samoilov, A. E., Chudinov, I. K., Butenko, I. O., Sonets, I. V., Artyushin, I. V., Yusefovich, A. P., Kruskop, S. V., Safonova, M. V., & Sinitsyn, S. O. (2024). Alphacoronaviruses from Pipistrellus bats captured in European Russia in 2015 and 2021 are closely related to those of Northern Europe. *Frontiers in Ecology and Evolution*, 12, 1324605. DOI: 10.3389/fevo.2024.1324605

Köse, G., & Köse, U. (2022). Sağlıkta zeki karar destek sistemleri: Günümüz ve gelecek.

Kotsiantis, S. B. (2013). Decision trees: A recent overview. *Artificial Intelligence Review*, 39(4), 261–283. DOI: 10.1007/s10462-011-9272-4

Kotwal, J., Kashyap, D. R., & Pathan, D. S. (2023). Agricultural plant diseases identification: From traditional approach to deep learning. *Materials Today: Proceedings, 80*(xxxx), 344–356. DOI: 10.1016/j.matpr.2023.02.370

Koyuncugil, A., & Özgülbaş, N. (2009). Veri madenciliği: Tıp ve sağlık hizmetlerinde kullanımı ve uygulamaları. Bilişim Teknolojileri Dergisi, 2(2).

Kumar, A., Rathor, K., Vaddi, S., Patel, D., Vanjarapu, P., & Maddi, M. (2022, August). ECG Based Early Heart Attack Prediction Using Neural Networks. In 2022 3rd International Conference on Electronics and Sustainable Communication Systems (ICESC) (pp. 1080-1083). IEEE. DOI: 10.1109/ICESC54411.2022.9885448

Kumar, R., & Sharma, A. (2023). Computational strategies and tools for protein tertiary structure prediction. Basic Biotechniques for Bioprocess and Bioentrepreneurship, 225–242. DOI: 10.1016/B978-0-12-816109-8.00015-5

Kumar, A., Satheesha, T. Y., Salvador, B. B. L., Mithileysh, S., & Ahmed, S. T. (2023). Augmented intelligence enabled deep neural networking (AuDNN) framework for skin cancer classification and prediction using multi-dimensional datasets on industrial IoT standards. *Microprocessors and Microsystems*, 97, 104755. Advance online publication. DOI: 10.1016/j.micpro.2023.104755

Kumar, N., Gupta, M., Gupta, D., & Tiwari, S. (2023). Novel deep transfer learning model for COVID-19 patient detection using X-ray chest images. *Journal of Ambient Intelligence and Humanized Computing*, 14(1), 469–478. DOI: 10.1007/s12652-021-03306-6 PMID: 34025813

Kuppusamy, S., & Thangavel, R. (2023). Deep Non-linear and Unbiased Deep Decisive Pooling Learning–Based Opinion Mining of Customer Review. *Cognitive Computation*, 15(2), 1–13. DOI: 10.1007/s12559-022-10089-1

Kutubuddin (2023j). Nanotechnology in Precision Farming: The Role of Research, *International Journal of Nanomaterials and Nanostructures*, 9(2). https://doi.org/ DOI: 10.37628/ijnn.v9i2.1051

Kutubuddin (2024v). Smart Agriculture based on AI-Driven-IoT(AIIoT): A KSK Approach, *Advance Research in Communication Engineering and its Innovations*, 1(2), 23-32.

Kutubuddin, (2023h). *IoT based Healthcare Monitoring for COVID- Subvariant JN-1,* Journal of Electronic Design Technology, 4(3).

Kutubuddin, K. (2024c). Vehicle Health Monitoring System (VHMS) by Employing IoT and Sensors, *Grenze International Journal of Engineering and Technology,* Vol 10, Issue 2, pp- 5367-5374. Available at: https://thegrenze.com/index.php?display =page&view=journalabstract&absid=3371&id=8

Kutubuddin, K. (2024e). A Novel Approach on ML based Palmistry, *Grenze International Journal of Engineering and Technology,* Vol 10, Issue 2, pp- 5186-5193. Available at: https://thegrenze.com/index.php?display=page&view=journalabstract &absid=3344&id=8

Kutubuddin, K. (2022a). Predict the Severity of Diabetes cases, using K-Means and Decision Tree Approach. *Journal of Advances in Shell Programming*, 9(2), 24–31.

Kutubuddin, K. (2022b). A novel Design of IoT based 'Love Representation and Remembrance' System to Loved One's. *Gradiva Review Journal*, 8(12), 377–383.

Kutubuddin, K. (2022d). Detection of Malicious Nodes in IoT Networks based on packet loss using ML, *Journal of Mobile Computing, Communication & mobile. Networks*, 9(3), 9–16.

Kutubuddin, K. (2024e). IoT based Boiler Health Monitoring for Sugar Industries, *Grenze. IACSIT International Journal of Engineering and Technology*, 10(2), 5178–5185. https://thegrenze.com/index.php?display=page&view=journalabstract &absid=3343&id=8

Kutubuddin, S. L. (2023i). Smart Motion Detection System using IoT: A NodeMCU and Blynk Framework. *Journal of Microelectronics and Solid State Devices*, 10(3).

Laishram, A., & Padmanabhan, V. (2019). Discovery of user-item subgroups via genetic algorithm for effective prediction of ratings in collaborative filtering. *Applied Intelligence*, 49(11), 3990–4006. DOI: 10.1007/s10489-019-01495-4

Lankadasu, N. V. Y., Pesarlanka, D. B., Sharma, A., Sharma, S., & Gochhait, S. (2024). Skin Cancer Classification Using a Convolutional Neural Network: An Exploration into Deep Learning. *2024 ASU International Conference in Emerging Technologies for Sustainability and Intelligent Systems, ICETSIS 2024*, 1047–1052. DOI: 10.1109/ICETSIS61505.2024.10459368

Learning, E. M. (2012). Ensemble. *Machine Learning*. Advance online publication. DOI: 10.1007/978-1-4419-9326-7

Lee, C. H., & Yoon, H. J. (2017). Medical big data: Promise and challenges. *Kidney Research and Clinical Practice*, 36(1), 3–11. DOI: 10.23876/j.krcp.2017.36.1.3 PMID: 28392994

Lee, S.-K., Son, Y.-J., Kim, J., Kim, H.-G., Lee, J.-I., Kang, B.-Y., Cho, H.-S., & Lee, S. (2014). Prediction Model for Health-Related Quality of Life of Elderly with Chronic Diseases using Machine Learning Techniques. *Healthcare Informatics Research*, 20(2), 125–134. DOI: 10.4258/hir.2014.20.2.125 PMID: 24872911

Li, T., Zhou, M., Travieso-González, C. M., & Alonso-Hernández, J. B. (2016). ECG Classification Using Wavelet Packet Entropy and Random Forests. Entropy 2016, Vol. 18, Page 285, 18(8), 285. DOI: 10.3390/e18080285

Liang, , XYu, , JLiao, , JChen, , Z. (2020). Convolutional neural network for breast and thyroid nodules diagnosis in ultrasound imaging. *BioMed Research International*.

Liang, Z., Zhang, G., Huang, J. X., & Hu, Q. V. (2014). Deep learning for healthcare decision making with EMRs. Proceedings - 2014 IEEE International Conference on Bioinformatics and Biomedicine, IEEE BIBM 2014, 556–559. DOI: 10.1109/BIBM.2014.6999219

Liao, S. H., Chu, P. H., & Hsiao, P. Y. (2012). Data mining techniques and applications–A decade review from 2000 to 2011. *Expert Systems with Applications*, 39(12), 11303–11311. DOI: 10.1016/j.eswa.2012.02.063

Li, B., Bai, B., Han, C., Long, H., & Zhao, L. (2017). Novel hybrid method for human posture recognition based on Kinect V2. *Communications in Computer and Information Science*, 771, 331–342. DOI: 10.1007/978-981-10-7299-4_27

Linardatos, P., Papastefanopoulos, V., & Kotsiantis, S. (2021). Explainable ai: A review of machine learning interpretability methods. *Entropy (Basel, Switzerland)*, 23(1), 1–45. DOI: 10.3390/e23010018 PMID: 33375658

Lin, C. F., & Wang, S. D. (2002). Fuzzy Support Vector Machines. *IEEE Transactions on Neural Networks*, 13(2), 464–471. DOI: 10.1109/72.991432 PMID: 18244447

Liu, H., & Zhang, S. (2012). Noisy data elimination using mutual k-nearest neighbor for classification mining. *Journal of Systems and Software*, 85(5), 1067–1074. DOI: 10.1016/j.jss.2011.12.019

Liu, H., Zhong, C., Alnusair, A., & Islam, S. R. (2021). FAIXID: A Framework for Enhancing AI Explainability of Intrusion Detection Results Using Data Cleaning Techniques. *Journal of Network and Systems Management*, 29(4), 1–30. DOI: 10.1007/s10922-021-09606-8

Liu, J., & Zhang, Y. (2020). An Attribute-Weighted Bayes Classifier Based on Asymmetric Correlation Coefficient. *International Journal of Pattern Recognition and Artificial Intelligence*, 34(10), 2050025. Advance online publication. DOI: 10.1142/S0218001420500251

Li, W., Chai, Y., Khan, F., Jan, S., Verma, P., Menon, V. K., & Li, X. (2021). A Comprehensive Survey on Machine Learning-Based Big Data Analytics for IoT-Enabled Smart Healthcare System. *Mobile Networks and Applications*, 26(1), 234–252. Advance online publication. DOI: 10.1007/s11036-020-01700-6

Li, X., Tian, D., Li, W., Dong, B., Wang, H., Yuan, J., Li, B., Shi, L., Lin, X., Zhao, L., & Liu, S. (2021). Artificial intelligence-assisted reduction in patients' waiting time for outpatient process: A retrospective cohort study. *BMC Health Services Research*, 21(1), 237. DOI: 10.1186/s12913-021-06248-z PMID: 33731096

Liyakat, K. K. S. (2023b, March). Machine learning approach using artificial neural networks to detect malicious nodes in IoT networks. In *International Conference on Machine Learning, IoT and Big Data* (pp. 123-134). Singapore: Springer Nature Singapore.

Liyakat, S. (2024). Explainable AI in Healthcare. In: Explainable Artificial Intelligence in healthcare System, editors: *A. Anitha Kamaraj, Debi Prasanna Acharjya*. ISBN: 979-8-89113-598-7. doi: https://doi.org/DOI: 10.52305/GOMR8163

Liyakat, K. (2024). Explainable AI in healthcare. *Explainable Artificial Intelligence in Healthcare Systems*, 2024, 271–284.

Liyakat, K. K. S. (2023a, March). Detecting Malicious Nodes in IoT Networks Using Machine Learning and Artificial Neural Networks. In *2023 International Conference on Emerging Smart Computing and Informatics (ESCI)* (pp. 1-5). IEEE.

Liyakat, K. K. S. (2024). Machine Learning Approach Using Artificial Neural Networks to Detect Malicious Nodes in IoT Networks. In Udgata, S. K., Sethi, S., & Gao, X. Z. (Eds.), *Intelligent Systems. ICMIB 2023. Lecture Notes in Networks and Systems* (Vol. 728). Springer., available at https://link.springer.com/chapter/10.1007/978-981-99-3932-9_12, DOI: 10.1007/978-981-99-3932-9_12

Liyakat, S. (2024d). ChatGPT: An Automated Teacher's Guide to Learning. In Bansal, R., Chakir, A., Hafaz Ngah, A., Rabby, F., & Jain, A. (Eds.), *AI Algorithms and ChatGPT for Student Engagement in Online Learning* (pp. 1–20). IGI Global., DOI: 10.4018/979-8-3693-4268-8.ch001

Liyakat, S. (2025). Heart Health Monitoring Using IoT and Machine Learning Methods. In Shaik, A. (Ed.), *AI-Powered Advances in Pharmacology* (pp. 257–282). IGI Global., DOI: 10.4018/979-8-3693-3212-2.ch010

Loftus, T. J., Shickel, B., Ruppert, M. M., Balch, J. A., Ozrazgat-Baslanti, T., Tighe, P. J., Efron, P. A., Hogan, W. R., Rashidi, P., Upchurch, G. R., & Bihorac, A. (2022). Uncertainty-aware deep learning in healthcare: A scoping review. *PLOS Digital Health*, 1(8), e0000085. DOI: 10.1371/journal.pdig.0000085 PMID: 36590140

Lopes, J., Guimarães, T., & Santos, M. F. (2020). Predictive and Prescriptive Analytics in Healthcare: A Survey, Procedia Computer Science, Volume 170, Pages 1029-1034, ISSN 1877-0509, DOI: 10.1016/j.procs.2020.03.078

Luca, A. R., Ursuleanu, T. F., Gheorghe, L., Grigorovici, R., Iancu, S., Hlusneac, M., & Grigorovici, A. (2022). Impact of quality, type and volume of data used by deep learning models in the analysis of medical images. *Informatics in Medicine Unlocked*, 29, 100911. DOI: 10.1016/j.imu.2022.100911

Lu, H., & Uddin, S. (2023, April). Disease prediction using graph machine learning based on electronic health data: A review of approaches and trends. [). MDPI.]. *Health Care*, 11(7), 1031. PMID: 37046958

Luján, M. Á., Sotos, J. M., Santos, J. L., & Borja, A. L. (2022). Accurate neural network classification model for schizophrenia disease based on electroencephalogram data. *International Journal of Machine Learning and Cybernetics*, •••, 1–12. DOI: 10.1007/S13042-022-01668-7/TABLES/9

Machha Babitha, C Sushma, et al. (2022). Trends of Artificial Intelligence for online exams in education, *International journal of Early Childhood special. Education*, 14(01), 2457–2463.

Maharana, K., Mondal, S., & Nemade, B. (2022). A review: Data pre-processing and data augmentation techniques. *Global Transitions Proceedings*, 3(1), 91–99. DOI: 10.1016/j.gltp.2022.04.020

Mahbooba, B., Timilsina, M., Sahal, R., & Serrano, M. (2021). Explainable Artificial Intelligence (XAI) to Enhance Trust Management in Intrusion Detection Systems Using Decision Tree Model. *Complexity*, 2021(1), 6634811. Advance online publication. DOI: 10.1155/2021/6634811

Mahmood, S. S., Levy, D., Vasan, R. S., & Wang, T. J. (2014). The Framingham Heart Study and the Epidemiology of Cardiovascular Diseases: A Historical Perspective. *Lancet*, 383(9921), 999–1008. DOI: 10.1016/S0140-6736(13)61752-3 PMID: 24084292

Makris, A., Kontopoulos, I., & Tserpes, K. (2020). COVID-19 detection from chest x-ray images using deep learning and convolutional neural networks. In *Proceedings of the 11th Hellenic Conference on Artificial Intelligence* (pp. 60–66), https://doi.org/DOI: 10.1145/3411408.3411416

Makubhai, S. S., Pathak, G. R., & Chandre, P. R. (2024). Predicting lung cancer risk using explainable artificial intelligence. *Bulletin of Electrical Engineering and Informatics*, 13(2), 1276–1285. DOI: 10.11591/eei.v13i2.6280

Maleki Varnosfaderani, S., & Forouzanfar, M. (2024). The Role of AI in Hospitals and Clinics: Transforming Healthcare in the 21st Century. *Bioengineering (Basel, Switzerland)*, 11(4), 337. DOI: 10.3390/bioengineering11040337 PMID: 38671759

Malik, A., Sharma, S., Batra, I., Sharma, C., Kaswan, M. S., & Garza-Reyes, J. A. (2024). Industrial revolution and environmental sustainability: An analytical interpretation of research constituents in Industry 4.0. *International Journal of Lean Six Sigma*, 15(1), 22–49. DOI: 10.1108/IJLSS-02-2023-0030

Mall, S., Srivastava, A., Mazumdar, B. D., Mishra, M., Bangare, S. L., & Deepak, A. (2022). Implementation of machine learning techniques for disease diagnosis. *Materials Today: Proceedings*, 51, 2198–2201. DOI: 10.1016/j.matpr.2021.11.274

Manikis, G., Simos, N. J., Kourou, K., Kondylakis, H., Poikonen-Saksela, P., Mazzocco, K., & Fotiadis, D. (2023). Personalized risk analysis to improve the psychological resilience of women undergoing treatment for breast cancer: Development of a machine learning-driven clinical decision support tool. *Journal of Medical Internet Research*, 25, e43838. DOI: 10.2196/43838 PMID: 37307043

Manogaran, G., & Lopez, D. (2017). A survey of big data architectures and machine learning algorithms in healthcare. *International Journal of Biomedical Engineering and Technology*, 25(2–4), 182–211. DOI: 10.1504/IJBET.2017.087722

Marcos, M., Juarez, J. M., Lenz, R., Peleg, M., Stefanowski, J., Stiglic, G., & Goebel, R. (2019). Artificial Intelligence in Medicine : Knowledge Representation and Transparent and Explainable Systems. In *7th Conference on Artificial Intelligence in Medicine International Workshops (AIME 2019), KR4HC/ProHealth and TEAAM, Poznan, Poland, June 26–29, 2019*. DOI: 10.1007/978-3-030-37446-4

Mathur, P., Srivastava, S., Xu, X., & Mehta, J. L. (2020). Artificial intelligence, machine learning, and cardiovascular disease. *Clinical Medicine Insights. Cardiology*, 14, 1179546820927404. DOI: 10.1177/1179546820927404 PMID: 32952403

Mathur, S., Glaeser, H., & Hack, J. B. (2021). Predicting Alzheimer's disease using machine learning: Advancing the frontier of early diagnosis and treatment. *Journal of Alzheimer's Disease*, 81(2), 427–437. PMID: 33814449

Mayo Clinic. (n.d.). *Skin cancer*. https://www.mayoclinic.org/diseases-conditions/skin-cancer/symptoms-causes/syc-20377605

Mcgonagle, D. (2020). Since January 2020 Elsevier has created a COVID-19 resource centre with free information in English and Mandarin on the novel coronavirus COVID-19. *The COVID-19 resource centre is hosted on Elsevier Connect, the company's public news and information*.

McGraw, D. (2013). Building public trust in uses of Health Insurance Portability and Accountability Act de-identified data. *Journal of the American Medical Informatics Association : JAMIA*, 20(1), 29–34. DOI: 10.1136/amiajnl-2012-000936 PMID: 22735615

Medical News Today. (2018, April 17). *What to know about dermatofibromas*. https://www.medicalnewstoday.com/articles/318870

Meenai, A., & Khan, V. (2020). Survey of methods applying deep learning to distinguish between computer-generated and natural images. In Shukla, R. K., Agrawal, J., Sharma, S., Chaudhari, N. S., & Shukla, K. K. (Eds.), *Social Networking and Computational Intelligence* (pp. 217–225). Springer., DOI: 10.1007/978-981-15-2071-6_18

Mehrotra, P. (2016). Biosensors and their applications – A review. *Journal of Oral Biology and Craniofacial Research*, 6(2), 153–159. DOI: 10.1016/j.jobcr.2015.12.002 PMID: 27195214

Merkert, J., Mueller, M., & Hubl, M. (2015). A survey of the application of machine learning in decision support systems.

Metlek, S., & Kayaalp, K. (2020). Derin öğrenme ve destek vektör makineleri ile görüntüden cinsiyet tahmini. *Düzce Üniversitesi Bilim ve Teknoloji Dergisi*, 8(3), 2208–2228. DOI: 10.29130/dubited.707316

Mian Qaisar, S., & Subasi, A. (2022). Effective Epileptic Seizure Detection Based on the Event-Driven Processing and Machine Learning for Mobile Healthcare. *Journal of Ambient Intelligence and Humanized Computing*, 13(7), 3619–3631. Advance online publication. DOI: 10.1007/s12652-020-02024-9

Michael, R. MacIntyre, Richard G. Cockerill, Omar F. Mirza, Jacob M. (2023). Appel, Ethical considerations for the use of artificial intelligence in medical decision-making capacity assessments, Psychiatry Research, Volume 328, 115466, ISSN 0165-1781, DOI: 10.1016/j.psychres.2023.115466

Miller, R. A., & Masarie, F. E.Jr. (1990). The demise of the "Greek Oracle" model for medical diagnostic systems. *Methods of Information in Medicine*, 29(1), 1–2. DOI: 10.1055/s-0038-1634767 PMID: 2407929

Miotto, R., Wang, F., Wang, S., Jiang, X., & Dudley, J. T. (2018). Deep learning for healthcare: Review, opportunities and challenges. *Briefings in Bioinformatics*, 19(6), 1236–1246. DOI: 10.1093/bib/bbx044 PMID: 28481991

Mishra Sunil, B., (2024). Nanotechnology's Importance in Mechanical Engineering. *Journal of Fluid Mechanics and Mechanical Design*, 6(1), 1–9.

Mishra Sunil, B., (2024a). AI-Driven IoT (AI IoT) in Thermodynamic Engineering. *Journal of Modern Thermodynamics in Mechanical System*, 6(1), 1–8.

Mitra, U., & Rehman, S. U. (2024). ML-powered handwriting analysis for early detection of Alzheimer's disease. *IEEE Access : Practical Innovations, Open Solutions*, 12, 69031–69050. DOI: 10.1109/ACCESS.2024.3401104

Mittal, S., & Hasija, Y. (2020). Applications of Deep Learning in Healthcare and Biomedicine. *Studies in Big Data*, 68, 57–77. DOI: 10.1007/978-3-030-33966-1_4

Molnar, C., Casalicchio, G., & Bischl, B. (2020). Interpretable Machine Learning – A Brief History, State-of-the-Art and Challenges. *Communications in Computer and Information Science*, 1323, 417–431. DOI: 10.1007/978-3-030-65965-3_28

Morris, A. H., Horvat, C., Stagg, B., Grainger, D. W., Lanspa, M., Orme, J.Jr, & Berwick, D. M. (2023). Computer clinical decision support that automates personalized clinical care: A challenging but needed healthcare delivery strategy. *Journal of the American Medical Informatics Association : JAMIA*, 30(1), 178–194. DOI: 10.1093/jamia/ocac143 PMID: 36125018

Mousavi, Z., Shahini, N., Sheykhivand, S., Mojtahedi, S., & Arshadi, A. (2022). COVID-19 detection using chest x-ray images based on a developed deep neural network. *SLAS Technology*, 27(1), 63–75. DOI: 10.1016/j.slast.2021.10.011 PMID: 35058196

Mowbray, F., Zargoush, M., Jones, A., Wit, K., & Costa, A. (2020). Predicting Hospital Admission for Older Emergency Department Patients: Insights from Machine Learning. *International Journal of Medical Informatics*, 140, 104163. DOI: 10.1016/j.ijmedinf.2020.104163 PMID: 32474393

Mucaki, E. J., Baranova, K., Pham, H. Q., Rezaeian, I., Angelov, D., Ngom, A., Rueda, L., & Rogan, P. K. (2017). Predicting Outcomes of Hormone and Chemotherapy in the Molecular Taxonomy of Breast Cancer International Consortium (METABRIC) Study by Biochemically-inspired Machine Learning. *F1000 Research*, 5, 2124. DOI: 10.12688/f1000research.9417.3 PMID: 28620450

Muhammad, S. S., & Alrikabi, J. M. (2024). Fire detection by using DenseNet 201 algorithm and surveillance cameras images. *Journal of Al-Qadisiyah for Computer Science and Mathematics*, 16(1), 81–91. DOI: 10.29304/jqcsm.2024.16.11437

Murathan, T., & Devecioğlu, S. (2018). Veri madenciliği ve spor alanındaki uygulamaları. *Spor Bilimleri Dergisi*, 29(3), 147–156. DOI: 10.17644/sbd.371590

Murdoch, B. (2021). Privacy and artificial intelligence: Challenges for protecting health information in a new era. *BMC Medical Ethics*, 22(1), 122. DOI: 10.1186/s12910-021-00687-3 PMID: 34525993

Musen, M. A., Shahar, Y., & Shortliffe, E. H. (2014). Clinical decision-support systems. In *Biomedical Informatics* (pp. 643–674). Springer. DOI: 10.1007/978-1-4471-4474-8_22

Nagrale, M., Pol, R. S., Birajadar, G. B., & Mulani, A. O. (2024). Internet of Robotic Things in Cardiac Surgery: An Innovative Approach. *African Journal of Biological Sciences*, 6(6), 709–725. DOI: 10.33472/AFJBS.6.6.2024.709-725

Narin, A., Kaya, C., & Pamuk, Z. (2021). Automatic detection of coronavirus disease (COVID-19) using x-ray images and deep convolutional neural networks. *Pattern Analysis & Applications*, 24(4), 1207–1220. DOI: 10.1007/s10044-021-00984-y PMID: 33994847

Nayak, D. K., Mishra, P., Das, P., Jamader, A. R., & Acharya, B. (2022). Application of Deep Learning in Biomedical Informatics and Healthcare. *Intelligent Systems Reference Library*, 213, 113–132. DOI: 10.1007/978-981-16-5304-9_9

Neeraja, P., Kumar, R. G., & Kumar, M. S. Liyakat and M. S. Vani. (2024), DL-Based Somnolence Detection for Improved Driver Safety and Alertness Monitoring. *2024 IEEE International Conference on Computing, Power and Communication Technologies (IC2PCT)*, Greater Noida, India, 2024, pp. 589-594, . Available at: https://ieeexplore.ieee.org/document/10486714DOI: 10.1109/IC2PCT60090.2024.10486714

Nerkar, P. M., & Dhaware, B. U. (2023). Predictive Data Analytics Framework Based on Heart Healthcare System (HHS) Using Machine Learning, *Journal of Advanced Zoology*, 2023, Volume 44, Special Issue -2. Page, 3673, 3686.

Neupane, S., Ables, J., Anderson, W., Mittal, S., Rahimi, S., Banicescu, I., & Seale, M. (2022). Explainable Intrusion Detection Systems (X-IDS): A Survey of Current Methods, Challenges, and Opportunities. *IEEE Access : Practical Innovations, Open Solutions*, 10, 112392–112415. DOI: 10.1109/ACCESS.2022.3216617

Newman-Toker, D. E., Nassery, N., Schaffer, A. C., Yu-Moe, C. W., Clemens, G. D., Wang, Z., & Siegal, D. (2024). Burden of serious harms from diagnostic error in the USA. *BMJ Quality & Safety*, 33(2), 109–120. DOI: 10.1136/bmjqs-2021-014130 PMID: 37460118

Newman-Toker, D. E., Peterson, S. M., Badihian, S., Hassoon, A., Nassery, N., Parizadeh, D., & Robinson, K. A. (2023). Diagnostic errors in the emergency department. *Systematic Reviews*.

Ngai, E. W., & Wu, Y. (2022). Machine learning in marketing: A literature review, conceptual framework, and research agenda. *Journal of Business Research*, 145, 35–48. DOI: 10.1016/j.jbusres.2022.02.049

Niculet, E., Craescu, M., Rebegea, L., Bobeica, C., Năstase, F., Lupa teanu, G., & Tatu, A. L. (2022). Basal cell carcinoma: Comprehensive clinical and histopathological aspects, novel imaging tools, and therapeutic approaches. *Experimental and Therapeutic Medicine*, 23(1), 1–8. DOI: 10.3892/etm.2021.11234 PMID: 34917186

Nikhar, S., & Karandikar, A. M. (2016). Prediction of heart disease using machine learning algorithms. International Journal of Advanced Engineering. *Management Science*, 2(6), 239–484.

Nishat, N., Raasetti, M. M., Shoaib, A. S., & Ali, B. (2024). Machine learning and the study of language change: A review of methodologies and application. *International Journal of Management Information Systems and Data Science*, 1(2), 48–57. DOI: 10.62304/ijmisds.v1i2.144

Nithya, T., Kumar, V. N., Gayathri, S., Deepa, S., Varun, C. M., & Subramanian, R. S. (2023, August). A comprehensive survey of machine learning: Advancements, applications, and challenges. In *2023 Second International Conference on Augmented Intelligence and Sustainable Systems (ICAISS)* (pp. 354-361). IEEE. DOI: 10.1109/ICAISS58487.2023.10250547

Norgeot, B., Glicksberg, B. S., & Butte, A. J. (2019). A call for deep-learning healthcare. Nature Medicine, 25(1), 14–15. DOI: 10.1038/s41591-018-0320-3

Obermeyer, Z., & Emanuel, E. J. (2016). Predicting the future—Big data, machine learning, and clinical medicine. *The New England Journal of Medicine*, 375(13), 1216–1219. DOI: 10.1056/NEJMp1606181 PMID: 27682033

Obermeyer, Z., Powers, B., Vogeli, C., & Mullainathan, S. (2019a). Dissecting racial bias in an algorithm used to manage the health of populations. *Science*, 366(6464), 447–453. DOI: 10.1126/science.aax2342 PMID: 31649194

Ohlendorf, D., Wanke, E. M., Filmann, N., Groneberg, D. A., & Gerber, A. (2017). Fit to play: Posture and seating position analysis with professional musicians - a study protocol. *Journal of Occupational Medicine and Toxicology (London, England)*, 12(1), 1–14. DOI: 10.1186/s12995-017-0151-z PMID: 28265296

Ouartani, S., & Taleb, N. (2024). Decision support system for thyroid disease prediction using decision tree algorithm and ontology. *International Journal of Artificial Intelligence Tools and Applications*.

Ovla, H. D., & Taşdelen, B. (2012). Aykırı değer yönetimi. *Mersin Üniversitesi Saglik Bilimleri Dergisi*, 5(3).

Owida, H. A. (2022). Developments and clinical applications of noninvasive optical technologies for skin cancer diagnosis. *Journal of Skin Cancer*, 2022(1), 9218847. Advance online publication. DOI: 10.1155/2022/9218847 PMID: 36437851

Oyebode, O., Fowles, J., Steeves, D., & Orji, R. (2023). Machine learning techniques in adaptive and personalized systems for health and wellness. *International Journal of Human-Computer Interaction*, 39(9), 1938–1962. DOI: 10.1080/10447318.2022.2089085

Özcan, B., Kayapınar, K., & Adem, K. (2023). Gelişen teknoloji ile bankacılık sektöründe veri analitiği: Müşteri kaybı tahmini için makine öğrenmesi yaklaşımları. *Uluslararası Sivas Bilim ve Teknoloji Üniversitesi Dergisi*, 2(1), 74–84.

Ozer, J., Alon, G., Leykin, D., Varon, J., Aharonson-Daniel, L., & Einav, S. (2019). Culture and personal influences on cardiopulmonary resuscitation—Results of international survey. *BMC Medical Ethics*, 20(1), 102. DOI: 10.1186/s12910-019-0439-x PMID: 31878920

Paganelli, A. I., Mondéjar, A. G., da Silva, A. C., Silva-Calpa, G., Teixeira, M. F., Carvalho, F., Raposo, A., & Endler, M. (2022). Real-time data analysis in health monitoring systems: A comprehensive systematic literature review. *Journal of Biomedical Informatics*, 127, 104009. DOI: 10.1016/j.jbi.2022.104009 PMID: 35196579

Pajila, P. B., Sudha, K., Selvi, D. K., Kumar, V. N., Gayathri, S., & Subramanian, R. S. (2023, July). A Survey on Natural Language Processing and its Applications. In 2023 4th International Conference on Electronics and Sustainable Communication Systems (ICESC) (pp. 996-1001). IEEE.

Paliyawan, P., Nukoolkit, C., & Mongkolnam, P. (2014). Prolonged sitting detection for office workers syndrome prevention using Kinect. 2014 11th International Conference on Electrical Engineering/Electronics, Computer, Telecommunications and Information Technology, ECTI-CON 2014. DOI: 10.1109/ECTICon.2014.6839785

Pal, M., Saha, S., & Konar, A. (2016). Distance matching based gesture recognition for healthcare using Microsoft's Kinect sensor. *International Conference on Microelectronics, Computing and Communication, MicroCom 2016*. DOI: 10.1109/MicroCom.2016.7522586

Papadopoulos, P., Soflano, M., Chaudy, Y., Adejo, W., & Connolly, T. M. (2022). A systematic review of technologies and standards used in the development of rule-based clinical decision support systems. *Health and Technology*, 12(4), 713–727. DOI: 10.1007/s12553-022-00672-9

Pardeshi, K. P., (2022a). Development of Machine Learning based Epileptic Seizureprediction using Web of Things (WoT). *NeuroQuantology : An Interdisciplinary Journal of Neuroscience and Quantum Physics*, 20(8), 9394–9409.

Pardeshi, K. P., (2022b). Implementation of Fault Detection Framework for Healthcare Monitoring System Using IoT, Sensors in Wireless Environment. *Telematique*, 21(1), 5451–5460.

Parry, S., & Straker, L. (2013). The contribution of office work to sedentary behaviour associated risk. *BMC Public Health*, 13(1), 1–10. DOI: 10.1186/1471-2458-13-296 PMID: 23557495

Patel, R. K., Aggarwal, E., Solanki, K., Dahiya, O., & Yadav, S. A. (2023, April). A Logistic Regression and Decision Tree Based Hybrid Approach to Predict Alzheimer's Disease. In *2023 International Conference on Computational Intelligence and Sustainable Engineering Solutions (CISES)* (pp. 722-726). IEEE.

Pathak, G. R., & Patil, S. H. (2016). Mathematical Model of Security Framework for Routing Layer Protocol in Wireless Sensor Networks. *Physics Procedia, 78*(December 2015), 579–586. DOI: 10.1016/j.procs.2016.02.121

Pathak, G. R., Premi, M. S. G., & Patil, S. H. (2019). LSSCW: A lightweight security scheme for cluster based Wireless Sensor Network. *International Journal of Advanced Computer Science and Applications*, 10(10), 448–460. DOI: 10.14569/IJACSA.2019.0101062

Paul, A. K., Shill, P. C., Rabin, M. R. I., & Akhand, M. A. H. (2016). Genetic algorithm based fuzzy decision support system for the diagnosis of heart disease. In 2016 5th International Conference on Informatics, Electronics and Vision (ICIEV) (pp. 145-150). IEEE. DOI: 10.1109/ICIEV.2016.7759984

Paul, D., Sanap, G., Shenoy, S., Kalyane, D., Kalia, K., & Tekade, R. K. (2021). Artificial intelligence in drug discovery and development. *Drug Discovery Today*, 26(1), 80–93. DOI: 10.1016/j.drudis.2020.10.010 PMID: 33099022

Pavithra, , GYamuna, , & Arunkumar, , R. (2022). Deep learning method for classifying thyroid nodules using ultrasound images. In *2022 International Conference on Smart Technologies and Systems for Next Generation Computing (ICSTSN)* (pp. 1–6).

Pehlivan, G. (2006). CHAID analizi ve bir uygulama. Yayınlanmamış Yüksek Lisans Tezi. İstanbul: Yıldız Teknik Üniversitesi, FBE.

Peleg, M., Shahar, Y., Quaglini, S., Broens, T., Budasu, R., Fung, N., & Greenes, R. A. (2017). Assessment of a personalized and distributed patient guidance system. *International Journal of Medical Informatics*, 101, 108–130. DOI: 10.1016/j.ijmedinf.2017.02.010 PMID: 28347441

Piccolo, V., Russo, T., Moscarella, E., Brancaccio, G., Alfano, R., & Argenziano, G. (2018). Dermatoscopy of vascular lesions. *Dermatologic Clinics*, 36(4), 389–395. DOI: 10.1016/j.det.2018.05.006 PMID: 30201148

Pisner, D. A., & Schnyer, D. M. (2020). Support vector machine. In Mechelli, A., & Vieira, S. (Eds.), *Machine Learning* (pp. 101–121). Academic Press., DOI: 10.1016/B978-0-12-815739-8.00006-7

Pombo, , NAraújo, , PViana, , J. (2014). Knowledge discovery in clinical decision support systems for pain management: A systematic review. *Artificial Intelligence in Medicine*, 60(1), 1–11. DOI: 10.1016/j.artmed.2013.11.005 PMID: 24370382

Poongodi, T., Krishnamurthi, R., Indrakumari, R., Suresh, P., & Balusamy, B. (2020). Wearable devices and IoT. A handbook of Internet of Things in biomedical and cyber physical system, 245-273.

Potdar, K., Pardawala, T., & Pai, C. (2017). A comparative study of categorical variable encoding techniques for neural network classifiers. *International Journal of Computer Applications*, 175(4), 7–9. DOI: 10.5120/ijca2017915495

Pradeepa, M., (2022). Student Health Detection using a Machine Learning Approach and IoT, *2022 IEEE 2nd Mysore sub section International Conference (MysuruCon)*, 2022.

Pramanik, S., & Khang, A. (2024). Cardiovascular diseases: Artificial intelligence clinical decision support system. In *AI-Driven Innovations in Digital Healthcare: Emerging Trends, Challenges, and Applications* (pp. 274-287). IGI Global.

Prashant, K. Magadum (2024). Machine Learning for Predicting Wind Turbine Output Power in Wind Energy Conversion Systems, *Grenze International Journal of Engineering and Technology*, Jan Issue, Vol 10, Issue 1, pp. 2074-2080. Grenze ID: 01.GIJET.10.1.4_1 Available at: https://thegrenze.com/index.php?display=page&view=journalabstract&absid=2514&id=8

Prathibha, , SDahiya, , DRobin, , CNishkala, , C. V. (2023). A novel technique for detecting various thyroid diseases using deep learning. *Intelligent Automation & Soft Computing*, 35(1), 199–214. DOI: 10.32604/iasc.2023.025819

Proudlove, N. C., Vaderá, S., & Kobbacy, K A H. (1998). Intelligent management systems in operations: A review. *The Journal of the Operational Research Society*, 49(7), 682–699. DOI: 10.1057/palgrave.jors.2600519

Pulat, M., & Deveci Kocakoç, İ. (2021). Türkiye'de Makine Öğrenmesi ve Karar Ağaçları Alanında Yayınlanmış Tezlerin Bibliyometrik Analizi. *Yönetim Ve Ekonomi Dergisi*, 28(2), 287–308. DOI: 10.18657/yonveek.870190

Qayyum, A., Qadir, J., Bilal, M., & Al-Fuqaha, A. (2021). Secure and Robust Machine Learning for Healthcare: A Survey. *IEEE Reviews in Biomedical Engineering*, 14, 156–180. DOI: 10.1109/RBME.2020.3013489 PMID: 32746371

Qin, J., Chen, L., Liu, Y., Liu, C., Feng, C., & Chen, B. (2019). A Machine Learning Methodology for Diagnosing Chronic Kidney Disease. *IEEE Access, PP*, 1–1. DOI: 10.1109/ACCESS.2019.2963053

Qin, Y., Zhang, S., Zhu, X., Zhang, J., & Zhang, C. (2007). Semi-parametric optimization for missing data imputation. *Applied Intelligence*, 27(1), 79–88. DOI: 10.1007/s10489-006-0032-0

Qi, Z., Tian, Y., & Shi, Y. (2013). Robust twin support vector machine for pattern classification. *Pattern Recognition*, 46(1), 305–316. DOI: 10.1016/j.patcog.2012.06.019

Quinlan, R. (1987). Thyroid disease. *UCI Machine Learning Repository.* https://doi.org/DOI: 10.24432/C5D010

Ragab, M., Albukhari, A., Alyami, J., & Mansour, R. F. (2022). Ensemble deep-learning-enabled clinical decision support system for breast cancer diagnosis and classification on ultrasound images. *Biology (Basel)*, 11(3), 439. DOI: 10.3390/biology11030439 PMID: 35336813

Raghupathi, W., & Raghupathi, V. (2014). Big data analytics in healthcare: Promise and potential. *Health Information Science and Systems*, 2(1), 3. DOI: 10.1186/2047-2501-2-3 PMID: 25825667

Rahman, A., & Hossain, Md. S., Muhammad, G., Kundu, D., Debnath, T., Rahman, M., Khan, Md. S. I., Tiwari, P., & Band, S. S. (. (2022). Federated learning-based AI approaches in smart healthcare: Concepts, taxonomies, challenges and open issues. *Cluster Computing*, •••, 1–41. DOI: 10.1007/s10586-022-03658-4 PMID: 35996680

Rahmani, A. M., Yousefpoor, E., Yousefpoor, M. S., Mehmood, Z., Haider, A., Hosseinzadeh, M., & Ali Naqvi, R. (2021). Machine Learning (ML) in Medicine: Review, Applications, and Challenges. Mathematics, 9(22), 2970. DOI: 10.3390/math9222970

Rahman, T., Khandakar, A., Qiblawey, Y., Tahir, A., Kiranyaz, S., Kashem, S. B. A., Islam, M. T., Al Maadeed, S., Zughaier, S. M., & Khan, M. S.(2021). Exploring the effect of image enhancement techniques on COVID-19 detection using chest x-ray images. *Computers in Biology and Medicine*, 132, 104319. DOI: 10.1016/j.compbiomed.2021.104319 PMID: 33799220

Rajkomar, A., Dean, J., & Kohane, I. (2019). Machine learning in medicine. *The New England Journal of Medicine*, 380(14), 1347–1358. DOI: 10.1056/NEJMra1814259 PMID: 30943338

Ramos, B., Pereira, T., Moranguinho, J., Morgado, J., Costa, J. L., & Oliveira, H. P. (2021). An Interpretable Approach for Lung Cancer Prediction and Subtype Classification using Gene Expression. *Proceedings of the Annual International Conference of the IEEE Engineering in Medicine and Biology Society, EMBS*, 1707–1710. DOI: 10.1109/EMBC46164.2021.9630775

Ramudu, K., Mohan, V. M., Jyothirmai, D., Prasad, D. V. S. S. S. V., Agrawal, R., & Boopathi, S. (2023). Machine learning and artificial intelligence in disease prediction: Applications, challenges, limitations, case studies, and future directions. In *Contemporary Applications of Data Fusion for Advanced Healthcare Informatics* (pp. 297–318). IGI Global. DOI: 10.4018/978-1-6684-8913-0.ch013

Rao, D., Gudivada, V. N., & Raghavan, V. V. (2015). Data quality issues in big data. Proceedings - 2015 IEEE International Conference on Big Data, IEEE. *Big Data*, 2015, 2654–2660. DOI: 10.1109/BigData.2015.7364065

Ravi, A., (2022). *Pattern Recognition- An Approach towards Machine Learning, Lambert Publications, 2022.* ISBN.

Ray, S. J., & Teizer, J. (2012). Real-time construction worker posture analysis for ergonomics training. *Advanced Engineering Informatics*, 26(2), 439–455. DOI: 10.1016/j.aei.2012.02.011

Razia, S., Kumar, P. S., & Rao, A. S. (2020). Machine learning techniques for thyroid disease diagnosis: A systematic review. In *Modern Approaches in Machine Learning and Cognitive Science: A Walkthrough* (pp. 203–212).

Razia, , SRao, , M. N. (2016). Machine learning techniques for thyroid disease diagnosis—A review. *Indian Journal of Science and Technology*, 9(28), 1–9. DOI: 10.17485/ijst/2016/v9i28/97853

Reddy, G. T., Reddy, M. P. K., Lakshmanna, K., Kaluri, R., Rajput, D. S., Srivastava, G., & Baker, T. (2020). Analysis of dimensionality reduction techniques on big data. *IEEE Access : Practical Innovations, Open Solutions*, 8, 54776–54788. DOI: 10.1109/ACCESS.2020.2980942

Redie, D. K., Sirko, A. E., Demissie, T. M., Teferi, S. S., Shrivastava, V. K., Verma, O. P., & Sharma, T. K. (2023). Diagnosis of COVID-19 using chest x-ray images based on modified DarkCovidNet model. *Evolutionary Intelligence*, 16(3), 729–738. DOI: 10.1007/s12065-021-00679-7 PMID: 35281292

Rehman, S. U., & Manickam, S. (2024). Application of smart sensors for internet of things healthcare environment: Study and prospects. In *Next-Generation Smart Biosensing* (pp. 287–305). Academic Press. DOI: 10.1016/B978-0-323-98805-6.00006-3

Rehman, S. U., Sadek, I., Huang, B., Manickam, S., & Mahmoud, L. N. (2024). IoT-based emergency cardiac death risk rescue alert system. *MethodsX*, 13, 102834. DOI: 10.1016/j.mex.2024.102834 PMID: 39071997

Rehman, S. U., Tarek, N., Magdy, C., Kamel, M., Abdelhalim, M., Melek, A., & Sadek, I. (2024). AI-based tool for early detection of Alzheimer's disease. *Heliyon*, 10(8). Advance online publication. DOI: 10.1016/j.heliyon.2024.e29375 PMID: 38644855

Reinehr, C. P. H., & Bakos, R. M. (2020). Actinic keratoses: Review of clinical, dermoscopic, and therapeutic aspects. *Anais Brasileiros de Dermatologia*, 94(6), 637–657. DOI: 10.1016/j.abd.2019.10.004 PMID: 31789244

Renukadevi, N. T. (2021). Performance Evaluation of Hybrid Machine Learning Algorithms for Medical Image Classification. In Dash, S., Pani, S. K., Abraham, A., & Liang, Y. (Eds.), *Advanced Soft Computing Techniques in Data Science, IoT and Cloud Computing* (pp. 281–299). Springer International Publishing., DOI: 10.1007/978-3-030-75657-4_12

Riajuliislam, , MRahim, , K. ZMahmud, , A. (2021). Prediction of thyroid disease (hypothyroid) in early stage using feature selection and classification techniques. In *2021 International Conference on Information and Communication Technology for Sustainable Development (ICICT4SD)* (pp. 60–64). DOI: 10.1109/ICICT4SD50815.2021.9397052

Richter, K., Kellner, S., & Licht, C. (2023). rTMS in mental health disorders. *Frontiers in Network Physiology*, 3, 943223. Advance online publication. DOI: 10.3389/fnetp.2023.943223 PMID: 37577037

Ringer, J. M. (2023). Legal consequences of the misdiagnosed patient. In *The Misdiagnosis Casebook in Clinical Medicine: A Case-Based Guide* (pp. 515–530). Springer International Publishing. DOI: 10.1007/978-3-031-28296-6_69

Rokach, L., & Maimon, O. Z. (2008). *Data mining with decision trees: Theory and applications* (Vol. 69). World Scientific.

Roopashree, S., & Anitha, J. (2021). Deepherb: A vision-based system for medicinal plants using Xception features. *IEEE Access: Practical Innovations, Open Solutions*, 9, 135927–135941. DOI: 10.1109/ACCESS.2021.3116207

Saber, H.-A., Younes, A., Osman, M., & Elkabani, I. (2024). Quran reciter identification using NASNetLarge. *Neural Computing & Applications*, 36(12), 6559–6573. DOI: 10.1007/s00521-023-09392-1

Sabry, F., Eltaras, T., Labda, W., Alzoubi, K., & Malluhi, Q. (2022). Machine Learning for Healthcare Wearable Devices: The Big Picture. *Journal of Healthcare Engineering*, 2022(1), 4653923. DOI: 10.1155/2022/4653923 PMID: 35480146

Sadeghi, Z., Alizadehsani, R., Kausar, S., Rehman, R., Mahanta, P., Bora, P. K., Almasri, A., Alkhawaldeh, R. S., Hussain, S., Alatas, B., Shoeibi, A., Moosaei, H., Nahavandi, S., Branch, E., Science, D., Republic, C., & Republic, C. (n.d.). Panos M. *Pardalos*, 16, 1.

Sahu, B., Panigrahi, A., Sukla, S., & Biswal, B. B. (2020). MRMR-BAT-HS: A clinical decision support system for cancer diagnosis. *Leukemia*, 7129(73), 48. DOI: 10.1038/s41375-020-0724-0

Saleh, M. D., & Eswaran, C. (2012). An automated decision-support system for non-proliferative diabetic retinopathy disease based on MAs and HAs detection. *Computer Methods and Programs in Biomedicine*, 108(1), 186–196. DOI: 10.1016/j.cmpb.2012.03.004 PMID: 22551841

Salman, , KSonuç, , E. (2021). Thyroid disease classification using machine learning algorithms. *Journal of Physics: Conference Series*, 1963(1), 012140. DOI: 10.1088/1742-6596/1963/1/012140

Sankar, , SPotti, , AChandrika, , G. NRamasubbareddy, , S. (2022). Thyroid disease prediction using XGBoost algorithms. *Journal of Mobile Multimedia*, 18(3), 1–18.

Saraswathi, K., Renukadevi, N. T., Nandhini, S. S., Sushmitha, E., & Arundhathi, R. (2024). Implementation of Machine Learning Algorithms in Diabetes Prediction. In Asokan, R., Ruiz, D. P., & Piramuthu, S. (Eds.), *Smart Data Intelligence* (pp. 169–186). Springer Nature Singapore. DOI: 10.1007/978-981-97-3191-6_13

Sarker, M. (2024). Revolutionizing Healthcare: The Role of Machine Learning in the Health Sector. Journal of Artificial Intelligence General Science, 2(1), 36–61. DOI: 10.60087/jaigs.v2i1.96

Sarker, I. H. (2021). Machine Learning: Algorithms, Real-World Applications and Research Directions. *SN Computer Science*, 2(3), 160. DOI: 10.1007/s42979-021-00592-x PMID: 33778771

Sathishkumar, R., Govindarajan, M., & Dhivyasri, R. (2023). Detection and classification of neurodegenerative disease via EfficientNetB7. In *International Conference on Mobile Radio Communications & 5G Networks* (pp. 223–234), https://doi.org/ DOI: 10.1007/978-981-97-0700-3_17

Satti, S. R., Lankadasu, J. S. K., Sharma, A., Sharma, S., & Gochhait, S. (2024). Deep Learning in Medical Image Diagnosis for COVID-19. *2024 ASU International Conference in Emerging Technologies for Sustainability and Intelligent Systems, ICETSIS 2024*, 1858–1865. DOI: 10.1109/ICETSIS61505.2024.10459430

Sau, A., & Bhakta, I. (2017). Predicting anxiety and depression in elderly patients using machine learning technology. *Healthcare Technology Letters*, 4(6), 238–243. DOI: 10.1049/htl.2016.0096

Saygın, E., & Baykara, M. (2021). Karaciğer yetmezliği teşhisinde özellik seçimi kullanarak makine öğrenmesi yöntemlerinin başarılarının ölçülmesi. *Fırat Üniversitesi Mühendislik Bilimleri Dergisi*, 33(2), 367–377. DOI: 10.35234/fumbd.832264

Sayyad(2024l). Nanotechnology in Medical Applications: A Study. *Nano Trends-A Journal of Nano Technology & Its Applications*. 26(02):1-11.

Sayyad. (2024). Artificial Intelligence (AI)-Driven IoT (AIIoT)-Based Agriculture Automation. In S. Satapathy & K. Muduli (Eds.), *Advanced Computational Methods for Agri-Business Sustainability* (pp. 72-94). IGI Global. https://doi.org/DOI: 10.4018/979-8-3693-3583-3.ch005

Sayyad, K. (2017). Significance and Usage of Face Recognition System. *Scholarly Journal for Humanity Science and English Language*, 4(20), 4764–4772.

Sayyad, K. (2022a). IoT-Based Healthcare Monitoring for COVID-19 Home Quarantined Patients. *Recent Trends in Sensor Research & Technology*, 9(3), 26–32.

Sayyad, K. (2023a). Detection of Malicious Nodes in IoT Networks based on Throughput and ML. *Journal of Electrical and Power System Engineering*, 9(1), 22–29.

Sayyad, K. (2024b). IoT Driven by Machine Learning (MLIoT) for the Retail Apparel Sector. In Tarnanidis, T., Papachristou, E., Karypidis, M., & Ismyrlis, V. (Eds.), *Driving Green Marketing in Fashion and Retail* (pp. 63–81). IGI Global., DOI: 10.4018/979-8-3693-3049-4.ch004

Sayyad, L. (2023a). IoT-based weather Prototype using WeMos. *Journal of Control and Instrumentation Engineering*, 9(1), 10–22.

Sebastian, A. M., & Peter, D. (2022). Artificial Intelligence in Cancer Research: Trends, Challenges and Future Directions. *Life (Chicago, Ill.)*, 12(12), 1991. DOI: 10.3390/life12121991 PMID: 36556356

Sedlakova, J., Daniore, P., Wintsch, A. H., Wolf, M., Stanikic, M., Haag, C., Sieber, C., Schneider, G., Staub, K., Ettlin, D. A., Grübner, O., Rinaldi, F., Wyl, V., & von, . (2023). Challenges and best practices for digital unstructured data enrichment in health research: A systematic narrative review. *PLOS Digital Health*, 2(10), e0000347. Advance online publication. DOI: 10.1371/journal.pdig.0000347 PMID: 37819910

Seiffert, C., Khoshgoftaar, T. M., van Hulse, J., & Napolitano, A. (2008). RUSBoost: Improving classification performance when training data is skewed. 2008 19th International Conference on Pattern Recognition, 1–4.

Sendak, M., Gao, M., Nichols, M., Lin, A., & Balu, S. (2019a). Machine Learning in Health Care: A Critical Appraisal of Challenges and Opportunities. EGEMs (Generating Evidence & Methods to Improve Patient Outcomes), 7(1), 1. DOI: 10.5334/egems.287

Sendak, M. P., D'Arcy, J., Kashyap, S., Gao, M., Nichols, M., Corey, K., & Balu, S. (2020). A path for translation of machine learning products into healthcare delivery. *npj. Digital Medicine*, 3(1), 1–8.

Sengupta, S., & Das, S. (2024). Statistical approaches for healthcare recommendation systems enhancing personalized healthcare. In *Revolutionizing Healthcare Treatment With Sensor Technology* (pp. 238–264). IGI Global. DOI: 10.4018/979-8-3693-2762-3.ch016

Serles, U., & Fensel, D. (2024). The Five Levels of Representing Knowledge. *An Introduction to Knowledge Graphs*, 93–96, 93–96. Advance online publication. DOI: 10.1007/978-3-031-45256-7_12

Sethy, P. K., & Behera, S. K., & Others. (2020). Detection of coronavirus disease (COVID-19) based on deep features and SVM. International Journal of Mathematical. *Engineering and Management Sciences*, 5(4), 643–651. DOI: 10.47981/ijmems.5.4.181

Sevinç, E. (2022). An empowered AdaBoost algorithm implementation: A COVID-19 dataset study. *Computers & Industrial Engineering*, 165, 107912. DOI: 10.1016/j.cie.2021.107912 PMID: 35013637

Sevli, O. (2019). Göğüs kanseri teşhisinde farklı makine öğrenmesi tekniklerinin performans karşılaştırması. *Avrupa Bilim ve Teknoloji Dergisi*, (16), 176–185. DOI: 10.31590/ejosat.553549

Shailaja, K., Seetharamulu, B., & Jabbar, M. (2018). Machine learning in healthcare: A review. *2018 Second International Conference on Electronics, Communication and Aerospace Technology (ICECA)*, 910–914. DOI: 10.1109/ICECA.2018.8474918

Shams, I., Ajorlou, S., & Yang, K. (2015). A predictive analytics approach to reducing 30-day avoidable readmissions among patients with heart failure, acute myocardial infarction, pneumonia, or COPD. *Health Care Management Science*, 18(1), 19–34. DOI: 10.1007/s10729-014-9278-y PMID: 24792081

Shankar, , KLakshmanaprabu, , SGupta, , DMaseleno, , ADe Albuquerque, , V. H. C. (2020). Optimal feature-based multi-kernel SVM approach for thyroid disease classification. *The Journal of Supercomputing*, 76(2), 1128–1143. DOI: 10.1007/s11227-018-2469-4

Sharma, A. (2024). Artificial Intelligence in Healthcare. 1–25. DOI: 10.4018/979-8-3693-3731-8.ch001

Sharma, A., Kala, S., Guleria, V., & Jaiswal, V. (2021). IoT-based data management and systems for public healthcare. Assistive Technology Intervention in Healthcare, 189–224. https://doi.org/DOI: 10.1201/9781003207856-13/IOT-BASED-DATA-MANAGEMENT-SYSTEMS-PUBLIC-HEALTHCARE-AJAY-SHARMA-SHASHI-KALA-VANDANA-GULERIA-VARUN-JAISWAL

Sharma, A., Kumar, R., & Jaiswal, V. (2021). Classification of Heart Disease from MRI Images Using Convolutional Neural Network. Proceedings of IEEE International Conference on Signal Processing,Computing and Control, 2021-October, 358–363. DOI: 10.1109/ISPCC53510.2021.9609408

Sharma, A., Pal, T., & Jaiswal, V. (2021). Decision support algorithms for data analysis (pp. 31–95). Nova Science Publishers, Inc. https://cris.bgu.ac.il/en/publications/decision-support-algorithms-for-data-analysis

Sharma, , K. AArya, , RMehta, , RSharma, , RSharma, , K. A. (2013). Hypothyroidism and cardiovascular disease: Factors, mechanism, and future perspectives. *Current Medicinal Chemistry*, 20(35), 4411–4418. DOI: 10.2174/09298673113206660255 PMID: 24152286

Sharma, A., Badea, M., Tiwari, S., & Marty, J. L. (2021). Wearable Biosensors: An Alternative and Practical Approach in Healthcare and Disease Monitoring. *Molecules (Basel, Switzerland)*, 26(3), 748. DOI: 10.3390/molecules26030748 PMID: 33535493

Sharma, A., Guleria, V., & Jaiswal, V. (2022a). The Future of Blockchain Technology, Recent Advancement and Challenges. *Studies in Big Data*, 105, 329–349. DOI: 10.1007/978-3-030-95419-2_15

Sharma, A., & Kumar, R. (2022). Recent Advancement and Challenges in Deep Learning, Big Data in Bioinformatics. *Studies in Big Data*, 105, 251–284. DOI: 10.1007/978-3-030-95419-2_12

Sharma, A., Pal, T., & Jaiswal, V. (2022). Heart disease prediction using convolutional neural network. *Cardiovascular and Coronary Artery Imaging*, 1, 245–272. DOI: 10.1016/B978-0-12-822706-0.00012-3

Sharma, S., Rawal, R., & Shah, D. (2023, September 29). Addressing the challenges of AI-based telemedicine: Best practices and lessons learned. *Journal of Education and Health Promotion*, 12(1), 338. DOI: 10.4103/jehp.jehp_402_23 PMID: 38023098

Shei, R.-J., Holder, I. G., Oumsang, A. S., Paris, B. A., & Paris, H. L. (2022). Wearable activity trackers–advanced technology or advanced marketing? *European Journal of Applied Physiology*, 122(9), 1975–1990. DOI: 10.1007/s00421-022-04951-1 PMID: 35445837

Sheu, R. K., & Pardeshi, M. S. (2022). A Survey on Medical Explainable AI (XAI): Recent Progress, Explainability Approach, Human Interaction and Scoring System. *Sensors (Basel)*, 22(20), 8068. Advance online publication. DOI: 10.3390/s22208068 PMID: 36298417

Shin, H. C., Roth, H. R., Gao, M., Lu, L., Xu, Z., Nogues, I., Yao, J., Mollura, D., & Summers, R. M. (2016). Deep Convolutional Neural Networks for Computer-Aided Detection: CNN Architectures, Dataset Characteristics and Transfer Learning. *IEEE Transactions on Medical Imaging*, 35(5), 1285–1298. DOI: 10.1109/TMI.2016.2528162 PMID: 26886976

Shorewala, V. (2021). Early detection of coronary heart disease using ensemble techniques. *Informatics in Medicine Unlocked*, 26, 100655. DOI: 10.1016/j.imu.2021.100655

Shorten, C., & Khoshgoftaar, T. M. (2019). A survey on image data augmentation for deep learning. *Journal of Big Data*, 6(1), 1–48. DOI: 10.1186/s40537-019-0197-0

Shweta Nagare, , (2014). Different Segmentation Techniques for brain tumor detection: A Survey, *MM- International society for green. Sustainable Engineering and Management*, 1(14), 29–35.

Shweta Nagare, et al., (2015). An Efficient Algorithm brain tumor detection based on Segmentation and Thresholding, *Journal of Management in Manufacturing and services*, 2(17), pp.19 - 27.

Siegel, R. L., Giaquinto, A. N., & Jemal, A. (2024). Cancer statistics, 2024. *CA: a Cancer Journal for Clinicians*, 74(1), 1–23. DOI: 10.3322/caac.21820 PMID: 38230766

Simonyan, K., & Zisserman, A. (2015). Very deep convolutional networks for large-scale image recognition. In *Proceedings of the International Conference on Learning Representations (ICLR)*. https://arxiv.org/abs/1409.1556

Singh, A. K., Kumar, A., Kumar, V., & Prakash, S. (2024). COVID-19 detection using adopted convolutional neural networks and high-performance computing. *Multimedia Tools and Applications*, 83(1), 593–608. DOI: 10.1007/s11042-023-15640-2 PMID: 37362712

Singh, P., Singh, S. P., & Singh, D. S. (2019). An introduction and review on machine learning applications in medicine and healthcare. *2019 IEEE Conference on Information and Communication Technology, CICT 2019*. DOI: 10.1109/CICT48419.2019.9066250

Sirisha Devi, J., Mr. B. Sreedhar, et al. (2022). A path towards child-centric Artificial Intelligence based Education, *International Journal of Early Childhood special. Education*, 14(03), 9915–9922.

Siwicki, B. (2023). The intersection of Telehealth and AI: How can they reinforce each other? Accessed from https://www.healthcareitnews.com/news/intersection-telehealth-and-ai-how-can-they-reinforce-each-other, Accessed on: 27/09/2024

Skin Cancer Foundation. (n.d.). *Skin cancer 101*. https://www.skincancer.org/skin-cancer-information/

Soglia, S., Pérez-Anker, J., Lobos Guede, N., Giavedoni, P., Puig, S., & Malvehy, J. (2022). Diagnostics using non-invasive technologies in dermatological oncology. *Cancers (Basel)*, 14(23), 5886. Advance online publication. DOI: 10.3390/cancers14235886 PMID: 36497368

Solano, F. (2020). Photoprotection and skin pigmentation: Melanin-related molecules and some other new agents obtained from natural sources. *Molecules (Basel, Switzerland)*, 25(7), 1537. DOI: 10.3390/molecules25071537 PMID: 32230973

Song, Y., Zheng, S., Li, L., Zhang, X., Zhang, X., Huang, Z., Chen, J., Wang, R., Zhao, H., Chong, Y., Shen, J., Zha, Y., & Yang, Y. (2021). Deep learning enables accurate diagnosis of novel coronavirus (COVID-19) with CT images. *IEEE/ACM Transactions on Computational Biology and Bioinformatics*, 18(6), 2775–2780. DOI: 10.1109/TCBB.2021.3065361 PMID: 33705321

Spicuzza, L., Montineri, A., Manuele, R., Crimi, C., Pistorio, M. P., Campisi, R., Vancheri, C., & Crimi, N. (2020). Reliability and usefulness of a rapid IgM-IgG antibody test for the diagnosis of SARS-CoV-2 infection: A preliminary report. *The Journal of Infection*, 81(2), 53–59. DOI: 10.1016/j.jinf.2020.04.022 PMID: 32335175

Sreenivasulu, D., Dr. J. Sirishadevi, et al. (2022). Implementation of Latest machine learning approaches for students Grade Prediction, *International Journal of Early Childhood special. Education*, 14(03), 9887–9894.

Srinivas, K., Gagana Sri, R., Pravallika, K., Nishitha, K., & Polamuri, S. R. (2024). COVID-19 prediction based on hybrid Inception V3 with VGG16 using chest X-ray images. *Multimedia Tools and Applications*, 83(12), 36665–36682. DOI: 10.1007/s11042-023-15903-y PMID: 37362699

Srinivasu, P. N., Sandhya, N., Jhaveri, R. H., & Raut, R. (2022). From Blackbox to Explainable AI in Healthcare: Existing Tools and Case Studies. *Mobile Information Systems*, 2022, 1–20. Advance online publication. DOI: 10.1155/2022/8167821

Steinhubl, S. R., Muse, E. D., & Topol, E. J. (2015). The emerging field of mobile health. *Science Translational Medicine*, 7(283). Advance online publication. DOI: 10.1126/scitranslmed.aaa3487 PMID: 25877894

Stephenson, B., Cook, D., Dixon, P., Duckworth, W., Kaiser, M., Koehler, K., & Meeker, W. (2008). Binary response and logistic regression analysis. Available from https://www.example.com

Subramanian, R. S., Yamini, B., Sudha, K., & Sivakumar, S. (2024). Ensemble-based deep learning techniques for customer churn prediction model. *Kybernetes*. Advance online publication. DOI: 10.1108/K-08-2023-1516

Subramani, S., Varshney, N., Anand, M. V., Soudagar, M. E. M., Al-Keridis, L. A., Upadhyay, T. K., & Rohini, K. (2023). Cardiovascular diseases prediction by machine learning incorporation with deep learning. *Frontiers in Medicine*, 10, 1150933. DOI: 10.3389/fmed.2023.1150933 PMID: 37138750

Sudha, K., Ambhika, C., Maheswari, B., Girija, P., & Nalini, M. (2023). AI and IoT Applications in Medical Domain Enhancing Healthcare Through Technology Integration. In AI and IoT-Based Technologies for Precision Medicine (pp. 280-294). IGI Global.

Sudha, K., Balakrishnan, C., Anish, T. P., Nithya, T., Yamini, B., Subramanian, R. S., & Nalini, M. (2024). Data Insight Unveiled: Navigating Critical Approaches and Challenges in Diverse Domains Through Advanced Data Analysis. *Critical Approaches to Data Engineering Systems and Analysis*, 90-114.

Sudha, K., Lakshmipriya, C., Pajila, P. B., Venitha, E., & Anita, M. (2024, January). Enhancing Diabetes Prediction and Management through Machine Learning: A Comparative Study. In *2024 Fourth International Conference on Advances in Electrical, Computing, Communication and Sustainable Technologies (ICAECT)* (pp. 1-6). IEEE. DOI: 10.1109/ICAECT60202.2024.10468773

Sukums, F., Mzurikwao, D., Sabas, D., Chaula, R., Mbuke, J., Kabika, T., Kaswija, J., Ngowi, B., Noll, J., Winkler, A. S., & Andersson, S. W. (2023). The use of artificial intelligence-based innovations in the health sector in Tanzania: A scoping review. *Health Policy and Technology*, 12(1), 100728. DOI: 10.1016/j.hlpt.2023.100728

Suleimenov, I., Vitulyova, Y., Bakirov, A. S., & Gabrielyan, O. A. (2020). Artificial Intelligence: what is it? *ICCTA '20: Proceedings of the 2020 6th International Conference on Computer and Technology Applications*. Association for Computing Machinery, New York, NY, USA, pp. 22-25, DOI: 10.1145/3397125.3397141

Sultanabanu, (2023n). Nanomedicine as a Potential Therapeutic Approach to COVID-19. *International Journal of Applied Nanotechnology.* 9(2): 27–35p.

Sulymka, A. (2023). Healthcare technology trends and digital innovations in 2023. Accessed from https://mobidev.biz/blog/technology-trends-healthcare-digital-transformation Accessed on 28/05/2024

Sumathi, M., & B, D. (2016). Prediction of Mental Health Problems Among Children Using Machine Learning Techniques. *International Journal of Advanced Computer Science and Applications*, 7(1). Advance online publication. DOI: 10.14569/IJACSA.2016.070176

Sun, B., & Wei, H.-L. (2022). *Machine Learning for Medical and Healthcare Data Analysis and Modelling: Case Studies and Performance Comparisons of Different Methods.* 1–6. DOI: 10.1109/ICAC55051.2022.9911176

Sun, H., Zhu, G. A., Cui, X., & Wang, J. X. (2021). Kinect-based intelligent monitoring and warning of students' sitting posture. Proceedings - 2021 6th International Conference on Automation, Control and Robotics Engineering, CACRE 2021, 338–342. DOI: 10.1109/CACRE52464.2021.9501372

Sundar, K. S., Rajamani, K. T., & Sai, S. S. S. (2018). Exploring image classification of thyroid ultrasound images using deep learning. In *International Conference on ISMAC in Computational Vision and Bio-Engineering* (pp. 1635–1641). Springer.

Sunita Sunil Shinde, et al, (2023). Monitoring Fresh Fruit and Food Using IoT and Machine Learning to Improve Food Safety and Quality, *Tuijin Jishu/Journal of Propulsion Technology,* 44(3), pp. 2927 – 2931.

Susanto, A. P., Lyell, D., Widyantoro, B., Berkovsky, S., & Magrabi, F. (2023). Effects of machine learning-based clinical decision support systems on decision-making, care delivery, and patient outcomes: A scoping review. *Journal of the American Medical Informatics Association : JAMIA*, 30(12), 2050–2063. DOI: 10.1093/jamia/ocad180 PMID: 37647865

Sutton, R. T., Pincock, D., Baumgart, D. C., Sadowski, D. C., Fedorak, R. N., & Kroeker, K. I. (2020). An overview of clinical decision support systems: Benefits, risks, and strategies for success. *NPJ Digital Medicine*, 3(1), 1–10. DOI: 10.1038/s41746-020-0221-y PMID: 32047862

Sutton, R. T., Pincock, D., Baumgart, D. C., Sadowski, D. C., Fedorak, R. N., & Kroeker, K. I. (2020). An overview of clinical decision support systems: Benefits, risks, and strategies for success. *npj. Digital Medicine*, 3(1), 1–10. PMID: 32047862

Swain, M. J., & Ballard, D. H. (1991). Color indexing. *International Journal of Computer Vision*, 7(1), 11–32. DOI: 10.1007/BF00130487

Szolovits, P., Patil, R. S., & Schwartz, W. B. (1988). Artificial intelligence in medical diagnosis. *Annals of Internal Medicine*, 108(1), 80–87. DOI: 10.7326/0003-4819-108-1-80 PMID: 3276267

Tabachnick, B. G., Fidell, L. S., & Ullman, J. B. (2013). *Using multivariate statistics* (Vol. 6). Pearson.

Tabakan, G., & Avcı, O. (2021). Vergiye gönüllü uyumu etkileyen faktörlerin lojistik regresyon analizi ile belirlenmesi. *Sosyoekonomi*, 29(48), 541–561. DOI: 10.17233/sosyoekonomi.2021.02.25

Tahir, A. M. (2022). COVID-QU-Ex [non-COVID infections, and normal chest X-ray images dataset. Kaggle. https://www.kaggle.com/datasets/anasmohammedtahir/covidqu.]. *COVID*, 19, •••.

Takale, D. G., Mahalle, P. N., Sakhare, S. R., Gawali, P. P., Deshmukh, G., Khan, V., & Maral, V. B. (2023, August). Analysis of clinical decision support system in healthcare industry using machine learning approach. In *International Conference on ICT for Sustainable Development* (pp. 571-587). Springer, Singapore. DOI: 10.1007/978-981-99-5652-4_51

Talukder, M. A., Layek, M. A., Kazi, M., Uddin, M. A., & Aryal, S. (2024). Empowering COVID-19 detection: Optimizing performance through fine-tuned EfficientNet deep learning architecture. *Computers in Biology and Medicine*, 168, 107789. DOI: 10.1016/j.compbiomed.2023.107789 PMID: 38042105

Tantuğ, A. C. (2012). Metin sınıflandırma (Text Classification). *Türkiye Bilişim Vakfı Bilgi, Bilim ve Mühendisliği Dergisi*, 5(2).

Tariq, M. U., Poulin, M., & Abonamah, A. A. (2021). Achieving Operational Excellence Through Artificial Intelligence: Driving Forces and Barriers. *Frontiers in Psychology*, 12(July), 686624. Advance online publication. DOI: 10.3389/fpsyg.2021.686624 PMID: 34305744

Tariq, M., Majeed, H., Beg, M. O., Khan, F. A., & Derhab, A. (2019). Accurate detection of sitting posture activities in a secure IoT based assisted living environment. *Future Generation Computer Systems*, 92, 745–757. DOI: 10.1016/j.future.2018.02.013

Taşcı, M. E., & Şamlı, R. (2020). Veri madenciliği ile kalp hastalığı teşhisi. Avrupa Bilim ve Teknoloji Dergisi, 88-95. https://doi.org/DOI: 10.31590/ejosat.araconf12

Taşkın, G. G. E. V. Ç. (2005). Veri madenciliğinde karar ağaçları ve bir satış analizi uygulaması. *Eskişehir Osmangazi Üniversitesi Sosyal Bilimler Dergisi*, 6(2), 221–239.

Teo, Z. L., Jin, L., Li, S., Miao, D., Zhang, X., Ng, W. Y., Tan, T. F., Lee, D. M., Chua, K. J., Heng, J., Liu, Y., Goh, R. S. M., & Ting, D. S. W. (2024). Federated machine learning in healthcare: A systematic review on clinical applications and technical architecture. *Cell Reports Medicine*, 5(2), 101419. Advance online publication. DOI: 10.1016/j.xcrm.2024.101419 PMID: 38340728

Testa, C. B., Godoi, L. G., Monroy, N. A. J., Bortolotto, M. R. F. L., Rodrigues, A. S., & Francisco, R. P. V. (2024). Impact of Gamma COVID-19 variant on the prognosis of hospitalized pregnant and postpartum women with cardiovascular disease. *Clinics (São Paulo)*, 79, 100454. DOI: 10.1016/j.clinsp.2024.100454 PMID: 39121513

Teufel, A., & Binder, H. (2021). Clinical decision support systems. *Visceral Medicine*, 37(6), 491–498. DOI: 10.1159/000519420 PMID: 35087899

Thakur, A., Sharma, S., & Sharma, T. (2023). Design of Semantic Segmentation Algorithm to Classify Forged Pixels. Proceedings - 2023 12th IEEE International Conference on Communication Systems and Network Technologies, CSNT 2023, 409–413. DOI: 10.1109/CSNT57126.2023.10134649

Thomas, L. C. (2000). A survey of credit and behavioral scoring: Forecasting financial risk of lending to consumers. *International Journal of Forecasting*, 16(2), 149–172. DOI: 10.1016/S0169-2070(00)00034-0

Tolun, S. (2008). *Destek vektör makineleri: Banka başarısızlığının tahmini üzerine bir uygulama*. İktisadî Araştırmalar Vakfı.

Tomberlin, C. (2023). Revolutionizing healthcare: How is AI being used in the healthcare industry? Los Angeles Pacific University. Available at: https://www.lapu.edu/ai-health-care-industry/ Accessed on: 27/05/2024

Topol, E. J. (2019a). *Deep medicine: How artificial intelligence can make healthcare human again*. Basic Books.

Topol, E. J. (2019b). High-performance medicine: The convergence of human and artificial intelligence. *Nature Medicine*, 25(1), 44–56. DOI: 10.1038/s41591-018-0300-7 PMID: 30617339

Tosun, S. (2007). Sınıflandırmada yapay sinir ağları ve karar ağaçları karşılaştırması: Öğrenci başarıları üzerine bir uygulama [Doctoral dissertation, Fen Bilimleri Enstitüsü].

Tremblay, M. S., Colley, R. C., Saunders, T. J., Healy, G. N., & Owen, N. (2010). Physiological and health implications of a sedentary lifestyle. Https://Doi.Org/10.1139/H10-079, 35(6), 725–740. DOI: 10.1139/H10-079

Tunali, I., Gillies, R. J., & Schabath, M. B. (2021). Application of radiomics and artificial intelligence for lung cancer precision medicine. *Cold Spring Harbor Perspectives in Medicine*, 11(8), a039537. Advance online publication. DOI: 10.1101/cshperspect.a039537 PMID: 33431509

Tushar, A. M., Wazed, A., Shawon, E., Rahman, M., Hossen, M. I., & Jesmeen, M. Z. H. (2022). A review of commonly used machine learning classifiers in heart disease prediction. In 2022 IEEE 10th Conference on Systems, Process & Control (ICSPC), pp. 319-323. https://doi.org/DOI: 10.1109/ICSPC55597.2022.10001742

Uddin, S., Haque, I., Lu, H., Moni, M. A., & Gide, E. (2022). Comparative performance analysis of K-nearest neighbour (KNN) algorithm and its different variants for disease prediction. *Scientific Reports*, 12(1), 6256. DOI: 10.1038/s41598-022-10358-x PMID: 35428863

Uğurlu, M., Doğru, İ., & Arslan, R. S. (2023). Karanlık ağ trafiğinin makine öğrenmesi yöntemleri kullanılarak tespiti ve sınıflandırılması. *Gazi Üniversitesi Mühendislik Mimarlık Fakültesi Dergisi*, 38(3), 1737–1746. DOI: 10.17341/gazimmfd.1023147

Ullas, T. R., Begom, M., Ahmed, A., & Sultana, R. (2020). A Machine Learning Approach to detect Depression and Anxiety using Supervised Learning. *2020 IEEE Asia-Pacific Conference on Computer Science and Data Engineering (CSDE)*, 1–6.

Upadhyay, M., & Rawat, J. (2023). A review of recent machine learning techniques used for skin lesion image classification. *Advancements in Bio-Medical Image Processing and Authentication in Telemedicine*, 76–90.

Uslu, O., & Özmen-Akyol, S. (2021). Türkçe haber metinlerinin makine öğrenmesi yöntemleri kullanılarak sınıflandırılması. *Eskişehir Türk Dünyası Uygulama ve Araştırma Merkezi Bilişim Dergisi*, 2(1), 15–20.

Uyanık, F., & Kasapbaşı, M. C. (2021). Telekomünikasyon sektörü için veri madenciliği ve makine öğrenmesi teknikleri ile ayrılan müşteri analizi. *Düzce Üniversitesi Bilim ve Teknoloji Dergisi*, 9(3), 172–191. DOI: 10.29130/dubited.807922

Vahida, . (2023). Deep Learning, YOLO and RFID based smart Billing Handcart. *Journal of Communication Engineering & Systems*, 13(1), 1–8.

van der Sijs, H., Aarts, J., Vulto, A., & Berg, M. (2006). Overriding of drug safety alerts in computerized physician order entry. *Journal of the American Medical Informatics Association : JAMIA*, 13(2), 138–147. DOI: 10.1197/jamia.M1809 PMID: 16357358

Veena, C., Sridevi, M., & Liyakat, B. Saha, S. R. Reddy and N. Shirisha,(2023). HEECCNB: An Efficient IoT-Cloud Architecture for Secure Patient Data Transmission and Accurate Disease Prediction in Healthcare Systems, *2023 Seventh International Conference on Image Information Processing (ICIIP)*, Solan, India, 2023, pp. 407-410, . Available at: https://ieeexplore.ieee.org/document/10537627DOI: 10.1109/ICIIP61524.2023.10537627

Vembandasamy, K., Sasipriya, R., & Deepa, E. (2015). Heart diseases detection using Naive Bayes algorithm. International Journal of Innovative Science. *Engineering & Technology*, 2(9), 441–444.

Venu, K., & Natesan, P. (2023). Optimized Deep Learning Model Using Modified Whale's Optimization Algorithm for EEG Signal Classification. *Information Technology and Control*, 52(3), 744–760. DOI: 10.5755/j01.itc.52.3.33320

Verboven, L., Callens, S., Black, J., Maartens, G., Dooley, K. E., Potgieter, S., & Van Rie, A. (2023). A machine-learning based model for automated recommendation of individualized treatment of rifampicin-resistant tuberculosis. *Research Square*. DOI: 10.21203/rs.3.rs-2525765/v1

Vilhekar, R. S., & Rawekar, A. (2024, January 10). (n.d.). Artificial Intelligence in Genetics. *Cureus*, 16(1), e52035. DOI: 10.7759/cureus.52035 PMID: 38344556

Vincent, J. L., Moreno, R., Takala, J., Willatts, S., De Mendonça, A., Bruining, H., & Thijs, L. G. (1996). The SOFA (Sepsis-related Organ Failure Assessment) score to describe organ dysfunction/failure. *Intensive Care Medicine*, 22(7), 707–710. DOI: 10.1007/BF01709751 PMID: 8844239

Visseren, F. L. J., Mach, F., Smulders, Y. M., Carballo, D., Koskinas, K. C., Back, M., Benetos, A., Biffi, A., Boavida, J.-M., Capodanno, D., Cosyns, B., Crawford, C., Davos, C. H., Desormais, I., Di Angelantonio, E., Franco, O. H., Halvorsen, S., Hobbs, F. D. R., Hollander, M., & Williams, B. (2021). ESC guidelines on cardiovascular disease prevention in clinical practice. *European Heart Journal*, 42(34), 3227–3337. DOI: 10.1093/eurheartj/ehab484 PMID: 34458905

Vora, L. K., Gholap, A. D., Jetha, K., Thakur, R. R. S., Solanki, H. K., & Chavda, V. P. (2023). Artificial Intelligence in Pharmaceutical Technology and Drug Delivery Design. *Pharmaceutics*, 15(7), 1916. DOI: 10.3390/pharmaceutics15071916 PMID: 37514102

Wale, A. D., & Dipali, R., (2019). Smart Agriculture System using IoT. *International Journal of Innovative Research in Technology*, 5(10), 493–497.

Wali, S., Khan, I. A., & Member, S. (2021). Explainable AI and Random Forest Based Reliable Intrusion Detection system. *TecharXiv*. DOI: 10.36227/techrxiv.17169080.v1

Wang, H. (2002). *Nearest neighbours without k: A classification formalism based on probability*. Faculty of Informatics, University of Ulster.

Wang, L., Byrum, B., & Zhang, Y. (2014). Detection and genetic characterization of delta coronavirus in pigs, Ohio, USA, 2014. *Emerging Infectious Diseases*, 20(7), 1227–1230. DOI: 10.3201/eid2007.140296 PMID: 24964136

Wang, L., & Wong, A. (2020). COVID-Net: A tailored deep convolutional neural network design for detection of COVID-19 cases from chest X-ray images. *Scientific Reports*, 10(1), 19549. DOI: 10.1038/s41598-020-76550-z PMID: 33177550

Wang, S., Kang, B., & Zhang, J. (2021). A deep learning algorithm using CT images to screen for coronavirus disease (COVID-19). *European Radiology*, 31(8), 6096–6104. DOI: 10.1007/s00330-021-07715-1 PMID: 33629156

Wang, Y., Kang, H., Liu, X., & Tong, Z. (2020). Combination of RT-qPCR testing and clinical features for diagnosis of COVID-19 facilitates management of SARS-CoV-2 outbreak. *Journal of Medical Virology*, 92(6), 538–539. DOI: 10.1002/jmv.25721 PMID: 32096564

Wang, Z., Keane, P. A., Chiang, M., Cheung, C. Y., Wong, T. Y., & Ting, D. S. W. (2022). Artificial Intelligence and Deep Learning in Ophthalmology. In Lidströmer, N., & Ashrafian, H. (Eds.), *Artificial Intelligence in Medicine* (pp. 1519–1552). Springer International Publishing., DOI: 10.1007/978-3-030-64573-1_200

Wehbe, R. M., Sheng, J., & Dutta, S. (2021). DeepCOVID-XR: An AI algorithm to detect COVID-19 on chest radiographs. *Radiology*, 299(1). Advance online publication. DOI: 10.1148/radiol.2020203511 PMID: 33231531

Weingart, S. N., Simchowitz, B., Shiman, L., Brouillard, D., Cyrulik, A., Davis, R. B., & Seger, A. C. (2009). Clinicians' assessments of electronic medication safety alerts in ambulatory care. *Archives of Internal Medicine*, 169(17), 1627–1632. DOI: 10.1001/archinternmed.2009.300 PMID: 19786683

Weissman, S., Xueying, Y., Zhang, J., Chen, S., Olatosi, B., & Li, X. (2021). Using a Machine Learning Approach to Explore Predictors of Health Care Visits as Missed Opportunities for HIV Diagnosis. *AIDS (London, England)*, 35(Supplement 1), S7–S18. Advance online publication. DOI: 10.1097/QAD.0000000000002735 PMID: 33867485

Werner de Vargas, V., Schneider Aranda, J. A., dos Santos Costa, R., da Silva Pereira, P. R., & Victória Barbosa, J. L. (2023). Imbalanced data preprocessing techniques for machine learning: A systematic mapping study. *Knowledge and Information Systems*, 65(1), 31–57. DOI: 10.1007/s10115-022-01772-8 PMID: 36405957

Whisman, M. A., & South, S. C. (2017). Gene–environment interplay in the context of romantic relationships. *Current Opinion in Psychology*, 13, 136–141. DOI: 10.1016/j.copsyc.2016.08.002

WHO. 2023. Cardiovascular diseases. Retrieved from https://www.who.int/health-topics/cardiovascular-diseases#tab=tab_1 (Accessed 01/09/2024)

Wiens, J., & Shenoy, E. S. (2018). Machine Learning for Healthcare: On the Verge of a Major Shift in Healthcare Epidemiology. *Clinical Infectious Diseases*, 66(1), 149–153. DOI: 10.1093/cid/cix731 PMID: 29020316

Winge, M. C., Kellman, L. N., Guo, K., Tang, J. Y., Swetter, S. M., Aasi, S. Z., Sarin, K. Y., Chang, A. L. S., & Khavari, P. A. (2023). Advances in cutaneous squamous cell carcinoma. *Nature Reviews. Cancer*, 23(7), 430–449. DOI: 10.1038/s41568-023-00583-5 PMID: 37286893

World Health Organization. (2024). Patient safety fact sheet. *WHO*. https://www.who.int/news-room/fact-sheets/detail/patient-safety

Wright, A., & Sittig, D. F. (2008). A four-phase model of the evolution of clinical decision support architectures. *International Journal of Medical Informatics*, 77(10), 641–649. DOI: 10.1016/j.ijmedinf.2008.01.004 PMID: 18353713

Xu, Y., Liu, X., Cao, X., Huang, C., Liu, E., Qian, S., Liu, X., Wu, Y., Dong, F., Qiu, C.-W., Qiu, J., Hua, K., Su, W., Wu, J., Xu, H., Han, Y., Fu, C., Yin, Z., Liu, M., & Zhang, J. (2021). Artificial intelligence: A powerful paradigm for scientific research. *Innovation (Cambridge (Mass.))*, 2(4), 100179. DOI: 10.1016/j.xinn.2021.100179 PMID: 34877560

Yale Medicine. (n.d.). *Melanocytic nevi (moles)*. https://www.yalemedicine.org/conditions/melanocytic-nevi-moles

Yamini, B., Sudha, K., Nalini, M., Kavitha, G., Subramanian, R. S., & Sugumar, R. (2023, June). Predictive Modelling for Lung Cancer Detection using Machine Learning Techniques. In 2023 8th International Conference on Communication and Electronics Systems (ICCES) (pp. 1220-1226). IEEE. DOI: 10.1109/ICCES57224.2023.10192648

Yamini, B., Prasanna, V., Ambhika, C., M, A., Maheswari, B., R, S. S., & Nalini, M. (2023). A Comprehensive Survey of Deep Learning: Advancements, Applications, and Challenges. *International Journal on Recent and Innovation Trends in Computing and Communication*, 11(8s), 445–453. DOI: 10.17762/ijritcc.v11i8s.7225

Yan, Q., Wang, D. G., & Yang, B. (2021). COVID-19 chest CT image segmentation network by multiscale fusion and enhancement operations. *IEEE Transactions on Big Data*, 7(1), 13–24. DOI: 10.1109/TBDATA.2021.3056564 PMID: 36811064

Yan, Y., Shin, W. I., Pang, Y. X., Meng, Y., Lai, J., You, C., Zhao, H., Lester, E., Wu, T., & Pang, C. H. (2020). The first 75 days of novel coronavirus (SARS-CoV-2) outbreak: Recent advances, prevention, and treatment. *International Journal of Environmental Research and Public Health*, 17(7), 2323. DOI: 10.3390/ijerph17072323 PMID: 32235575

Yao, L., Min, W., & Cui, H. (2017). A new Kinect approach to judge unhealthy sitting posture based on neck angle and torso angle. Lecture Notes in Computer Science (Including Subseries Lecture Notes in Artificial Intelligence and Lecture Notes in Bioinformatics), 10666 LNCS, 340–350. DOI: 10.1007/978-3-319-71607-7_30

Yelne, S., Chaudhary, M., Dod, K., Sayyad, A., & Sharma, R. (2023, November 22). Harnessing the Power of AI: A Comprehensive Review of Its Impact and Challenges in Nursing Science and Healthcare. *Cureus*, 15(11), e49252. DOI: 10.7759/cureus.49252 PMID: 38143615

Yıldız, A., & Hasan, Z. A. N. (2019). Segmantasyon yapmadan patolojik kalp sesi kayıtlarının tespiti için bir örüntü sınıflandırma algoritması. *Dicle Üniversitesi Mühendislik Fakültesi Mühendislik Dergisi*, 10(1), 77–91.

Yin, R. (2022). Examining the Impact of Design Features of Electronic Health Records Patient Portals on the Usability and Information Communication for Shared Decision Making. All Dissertations. https://open.clemson.edu/all_dissertations/3050

Ylmaz, Ö., Boz, H., & Arslan, A. (2017). The validity and reliability of depression stress and anxiety scale (DASS-21) Turkish short form. *Research of Financial Economic and Social Studies*, 2(2), 78–91.

Yoon, S., & Amadiegwu, A. (2023). Emerging tech, like AI, is poised to make healthcare more accurate, accessible and sustainable. Accessed from https://www.weforum.org/agenda/2023/06/emerging-tech-like-ai-are-poised-to-make-healthcare-more-accurate-accessible-and-sustainable/, Accessed on: 27/09/2024

Zaccheus, J., Atogwe, V., Oyejide, A., & Salau, A. O. (2024). *Towards successful aging classification using machine learning algorithms.*.

Zhang, , XLee, , V. C. S. (2024). Deep learning empowered decision support systems for thyroid cancer detection and management. *Procedia Computer Science*, 237, 945–954. DOI: 10.1016/j.procs.2024.05.183

Zhang, S., Li, X., Zong, M., Zhu, X., & Cheng, D. (2017). Learning k for KNN classification. [TIST]. *ACM Transactions on Intelligent Systems and Technology*, 8(3), 1–19. DOI: 10.1145/2990508

Zhao, , ZYang, , CWang, , QZhang, , HShi, , LZhang, , Z. (2021). A deep learning-based method for detecting and classifying the ultrasound images of suspicious thyroid nodules. *Medical Physics*, 48(12), 7959–7970. DOI: 10.1002/mp.15319 PMID: 34719057

Zheng, C., Deng, X., Fu, Q., Zhou, Q., Feng, J., Ma, H., . . . Wang, X. (2020). Deep learning-based detection for COVID-19 from chest CT using weak label. MedRxiv, 2020-03, https://doi.org/DOI: 10.1101/2020.03.12.20027185

Zhou, X., Leung, C. K., Wang, K. I. K., & Fortino, G. (2024). Editorial Deep Learning-Empowered Big Data Analytics in Biomedical Applications and Digital Healthcare. *IEEE/ACM Transactions on Computational Biology and Bioinformatics*, 21(4), 516–520. DOI: 10.1109/TCBB.2024.3371808

About the Contributors

Leyla Özgür Polat serves as an Assistant Professor in the Department of Management Information Systems at Pamukkale University, Turkey. She obtained her Bachelor's, MSc, and PhD degrees from the Department of Industrial Engineering at Pamukkale University. Her research interests encompass a broad spectrum, including decision-making techniques, green supply chain management, mathematical modeling, optimization, artificial intelligence, and management information systems.

Olcay Polat received his Industrial Engineering PhD degree from the Technical University of Berlin (Germany) with the scholarship of German Academic Exchange Service (DAAD) in 2013. He has been working as Professor in the Department of Industrial Engineering at Pamukkale University (Turkey). He has a special interest in supply chain management, logistics and transportation optimization, production management and risk management. He has been published more that 100 papers in respected journals, conference proceedings and books.

***

Olayinka Racheal Adelegan joined the Nigerian Defence Academy in 2009 as a System Analyst/Programmer II and has since evolved into a dedicated and highly proficient Assistant Chief System Analyst Programmer. With more than ten years of experience at the Academy, she is passionate about Machine Learning and Deep Learning. Her strong academic foundation is complemented by an impressive record of contributions to these fields, evidenced by numerous publications. Adelegan has earned a B.Sc. and an M.Sc. in Computer Science, underscoring her deep expertise in the domain.

Olalekan Awujoola is a seasoned Chief Systems Analyst Programmer for the Nigerian Defence Academy, boasting over two decades of experience. His expertise spans a broad spectrum of skills acquired through dedicated work in the field. His passion for academia knows no bounds, as evidenced by his acquisition of the following degrees: a National Certificate in Education (NCE) in Mathematics/Physics from the Institute of Education at ABU in Zaria, a Bachelor of Technology (B.Tech) in Mathematics with Computer Science from the Federal University of Technology Minna, a Master of Science (M.Sc) in Computer Science from Ahmadu Bello University in Zaria, a Master of Science (M.Sc) in Nuclear and Radiation Physics from the Nigerian Defence Academy, and a Master of Science (M.Sc) in Information Technology from the National Open University of Nigeria. He completed his PhD in Computer Science. He also lectures Cadets of computer science in the department of computer science. Awujoola is deeply entrenched in the pragmatic application of machine learning, deep learning, artificial intelligence, the Internet of Things, and computer vision—an enthusiasm that is reflected in his specialization in Python-based machine learning. This dedication is further substantiated by his contributions to an array of research papers and book chapters. In terms of technical proficiency, he excels in developing and implementing machine learning models to tackle real-world challenges. His formidable toolkit includes expertise in Python, R, and Java, complemented by hands-on experience with frameworks such as TensorFlow, PyTorch, and scikit-learn.

Manjunatha Badiger is an Assistant Professor in the Department of VLSI Design & Technology at NMAM Institute of Technology, Nitte. He has over 12 years of experience in academics, research, and administration. Dr. Badiger holds a Ph.D. from Visvesvaraya Technological University, an M.Tech in VLSI & Embedded System Design from Reva Institute of Technology and Management, and a B.E. in Electronics & Communication Engineering from NMAM Institute of Technology, Nitte. His research interests span Machine Learning, Deep Learning, Image Processing, and VLSI. Dr. Badiger has made significant contributions to national and international journals, book chapters, and has completed various NPTEL courses. Previously, he served as an Assistant Professor in the Department of Electronics and Communication Engineering at Sahyadri College of Engineering & Management and Shree Devi Institute of Technology. Dr. Badiger is accessible via email at manjunatha.badiger@nitte.edu.in or badiger_manju@yahoo.com.

Pawan Bhaladhare working as a professor & Head of Department of Computer Science & Engineering at Sandip University, Nasik, having 25 years of teaching experience. My area of research is in information security and privacy. In the same domain, I have published 70+ papers. All Papers are published in various reputed journals with standard indexing like IEEE, Scopus, Web of Science etc.

Anyanwu Obinna Bright is an MSc Holder in Computer Science and currently works and studies at the Nigerian Defence Academy, Kaduna. He is from Abia State in the Eastern Part of Nigeria. His hobbies include sports and nature study. He is married with 4 Children.

Mehnaz Fathima C, working as an Assistant Professor in the Department of Electronics & Communication Engineering, Sahyadri College of Engineering & Management. The areas of interest are VLSI & Embedded System, Signal Processing.

Pankaj R. Chandre obtained his B.E degree in Information Technology from Sant Gadge Baba Amravati University, Amravati, India, his M.E. degree in Computer Engineering from from Mumbai University Maharashtra, India in the year 2011, and PhD in Computer Engineering from Savitribai Phule Pune University, Pune, India in the year 2021. He is currently working as an Associate Professor in the Department of Computer Science and Engineering, MIT School of Computing, MIT ADT, Pune, India. He has published 60-plus papers in international journals and conferences. He has guided more than 30 undergraduate students and 20-plus postgraduate students for projects. He is guiding 2+ PhD scholars. His research interests are Network Security & Information Security. He can be contacted at: pankaj.chandre@mituniversity.edu.in

Archana Kedar Chaudhari has competed PhD in Biomedical Instrumentation from Savitribai Phule Pune University. She is currently working as Assistant Professor in Instrumentation Engineering Department, Vishwakarma Institute of Technology, Pune India. She has more than 20 years experience in Industry and Academia. She has several Indian patents published and granted. She has published many papers in referred international journals and conferences. Her filed of Interest include Image and Signal processing, Biomedical, Health Care, Internet of Things, Wireless Sensor Networks, Artificial Intelligence, Machine Learning and Deep Learning.

Huseyin Coskun is a Asst. Prof. at Computer Engineering Department of Kutahya Health Sciences University. He is also head of Medical Informatics Department at Postgraduate education institute of Kutahya Health Sciences University. He received the B.S degree computer engineering (CE) from Süleyman Demirel University (SDU) in Isparta, Turkey. He also received the M.S. and Ph.D. degrees in CE from SDU at 2016 and 2022 respectively. His research interests include machine learning, medical informatics, audio processing, computer vision, biomedical signals, mobile programming, technical education, e-learning.

Abraham Evwiekpaefe is a Senior Lecturer in the Department of Computer Science, Nigerian Defence Academy, Kaduna. He obtained a Bachelor of Science degree in Computer Science in 1998 and a Master of Science degree in Computer Science in 2007 both from the University of Benin, Benin City. He received his Doctor of Philosophy (PhD) degree in Computer Science in 2017, also from the same prestigious University of Benin, Benin City, Edo State, Nigeria. Dr Evwiekpaefe began his professional career as a Systems Analyst/Programmer II in August 2001 and was later laterally converted to the lecturing cadre in March 2002 as a Graduate Assistant. He rose to the position of a Senior Lecturer in 2018. His area of specialization includes Software Engineering, IT adoption and Data Science. He is currently the Head of Department from January 2022 till date. He is a member of the Nigerian Computer Society. He is also a member of the International Association of Engineers (IAENG). He has served in various administrative capacities both in the Nigerian Defence Academy and beyond. He was formerly the Postgraduate Coordinator for all PG programmes in the Department of Computer Science, Nigerian Defence Academy, Kaduna. Dr Abraham has served in several ad-hoc committees in the Nigerian Defence Academy. He is the Chairman, Seminar and Public Lecture Committee, Faculty of Military Science and Interdisciplinary Studies, Jan 2019 – Date. He is the Postgraduate School External Defence Representative for the Department of Mathematics, Jan 2019 – Jan 2022. He was Postgraduate Representative, Faculty of Military Science and Interdisciplinary Studies, Jan 2019 – Jan 2022. He has supervised over 80 (eighty) BSc cadets (students), seven (7) students for the Master of Science Degree and currently a major supervisor for a doctoral degree student in the Nigerian Defence Academy. He has attended many conferences, seminars and workshops both at national and international level. He has published over fifty (50) research articles and presented scientific papers at local and International Conferences held within and outside Nigeria.

G. Mariammal is an Assistant Professor in the Department of Computer Science and Engineering at Vel Tech Rangarajan Dr. Sagunthala R&D Institute of Science and Technology, Avadi. She specializes in computer science education and research, contributing to advancements in areas like data science and software development. Mariammal is committed to fostering innovation and academic growth in her students and research community.

K. Saraswathi received the MSc Degree in Computer Science from Bharathiar University and M.Phil Degree in Computer Science from Bharathidhasan University, India in 2004 and 2006 respectively. She received Ph.D. degree in Computer Applications from Anna University, India in 2018. Since 2008, she is working as an Assistant Professor in the Department of Computer Technology, Kongu Engineering

College. Her research interests include Data Mining and Machine Learning. She has published 20 research works in referred journals and presented 10 papers in International Conferences.

Kazi Kutubuddin Sayyad Liyakat has completed his B.E., M.E., and Ph.D. in E&TC Engineering and is nowadays working as a Professor & Head of Department, E&TC Engineering Department and was Dean R&D. He is Post-Doctoral Fellow working on "IoT in Healthcare Applications". His area of Interest is IoT, AI and ML. He has published more than 110+ papers in various Journals. Also published 11 books in the field of Engineering. He has published 15 Indian Patents, 2 South African Grant Patent, 2 Indian Copyright Patents and 8 UK Grant Patent. He worked as a Reviewer for Scopus Conferences and Journal. Also work as Editorial Board Member for various Journals. He got 2 Best Researcher Award, Best Faculty Award and Appreciation Letter from MoE's Innovation Cell, Govt. of India.

Vasima Khan has a unique blend of technical expertise with student-focused teaching, a dedicated and hardworking professional who is committed to providing a well-balanced, supportive and learning environment for all students. Done Bachelors, Masters and Doctorate in Computer Science and Engineering and has more than Twelve years of experience of teaching in both UG and PG engineering colleges. Taught various important technical subjects out of which conceptual skills are Operating System, Theory of Computing, Statistics, Computer Programming, Software Engineering, Compiler Design, Databases, Computer Architecture and Data Structure & Algorithms. Also taught few recent subjects like Machine Learning, Deep Learning, Natural Language Processing etc. Doing research work in the area of Machine Learning, Deep Learning, GAN, NLP, Wireless Sensor Network and others. Participated and lead various events like Faculty Development Program, Workshops, Conferences, Cultural and Sports functions etc. Always ready to learn, teach and innovate as well as tries to incorporate new ways into teaching.

Ezhilvendan is working as Assistant Professor in Panimalar Engineering College. His research interests are network security

Shahin Shoukat Makubhai is a Reserach Scholar in the Department of Computer Science and Engineering at MIT School of Computing, MIT ADT, and Pune, India. She received her B.E. degree in Computer Science and Engineering from DKTE Society's Textile & Engineering Institute (An Autonomous Institute), Ichalkaranji, India, and her M.Tech. degree in Computer Engineering with a specialization in Cloud Computing from Vellore Institute of Technology - VIT Chennai, India in 2020. She is currently pursuing her PhD in Computer Science at MIT-ADT University, Pune, India. Shahin has earned several global certifications and has also contributed to research through patents and copyrights. Her research interests include Artificial Intelligence and Cloud Computing and Healthcare, Medical services. She can be contacted at: shahin.makubhai@mituniversity.edu.in

Uddalak Mitra received the Ph.D. degree from Visva-Bharati University, Santiniketan, India. He is currently an Assistant Professor with JIS College of Engineering, Kalyani, West Bengal. He is also a specialized professional in bioinformatics, computational biology, machine learning and deep learning, and applied artificial intelligence (ML/DL) in the field of agriculture and medical diagnosis. He has authored and coauthored more than 18 papers in journals, conference proceedings, and book chapters, and supervises Ph.D. students, in addition to master's and undergraduate students. He is also a regular reviewer in reputed international and peer-reviewed journals.

PO Odion was employed into the services of Nigerian Defence Academy on 16th April, 1999. He has a BSc in Computer Science from University of Benin in Benin City in 1996, MSc degree in Computer Science from Abubakar Tafawa Balewa University in 2006 and PhD degree in Computer Science from the Nigerian Defence Academy in 2013. Dr Odion had served in several capacities as departmental examination Officer and Registration Officer, Departmental and faculty time-table officer, departmental and faculty postgraduate coordinator, Chairman of faculty curriculum; departmental Seminar/project coordinator and so on. He was the Head of Department from November 2015 to January 2022. His research area is software engineering and project management. He is a member of the Nigeria Computer Society (NCS). He has intended both Local and International Conferences

Oluwasegun Abiodun Abioye is an experienced System Analyst and Programmer at the Nigerian Defence Academy in Kaduna, Nigeria. He embarked on his career as a System Analyst Programmer II in 2013 and has since risen to the position of Principal System/Analyst Programmer. Oluwasegun holds a Master of Science in Information Technology from the National Open University, along with a Postgraduate Diploma in Computer Science. His foundational education includes a Higher National Diploma in Computer Science from Kaduna Polytechnic and a National Diploma from Federal Polytechnic, Bida, Niger State. Oluwasegun's expertise lies in machine learning and deep learning, where he has made notable contributions. He is recognized for his research in medical imaging and various other domains. Beyond his professional endeavors, Oluwasegun enjoys reading and writing. Oluwasegun is deeply engaged in the practical application of machine learning, deep learning, artificial intelligence, the Internet of Things, and computer vision. His specialization in Python-based machine learning reflects this passion.

He has contributed to numerous research papers and book chapters, demonstrating his dedication to the field. Technically proficient, he excels in developing and implementing machine learning models to address real-world problems. His skill set includes Python, R, and Java, with hands-on experience in frameworks such as TensorFlow, PyTorch, and scikit-learn.

Ganesh R. Pathak received Bachelor of Engineering (B.E. - Computer) from Walchand Institute of Technology, Maharashtra, India, Master of Engineering (M.E. - CSEIT) from Savitribai Phule Pune University (formerly University of Pune), Maharashtra, India and PhD degree in Computer Science and Engineering at Sathyabama Institute of Science and Technology (Deemed to be University), Chennai, Tamil Nadu, India. He is presently working as a Professor in the Department of Computer Science and Engineering, School of Computing, MIT Art, Design and Technology University, Pune. His research interests include Artificial Intelligence, Machine Learning, Data Science, Computer Networks, Wireless Communication, Wireless Sensor Networks, especially security in wireless sensor networks. His teaching areas include Mobile Computing, Pervasive Computing, Healthcare, Medical services, and Security and Usability Engineering. He is a member of IEEE and CSI. He can be contacted at: ganesh.pathak@mituniversity.edu.in

Pesarlanka Devendra Babu is an accomplished final-year B.Tech student in Computer Science and Engineering, specializing in Artificial Intelligence and Machine Learning. As a proactive leader in the National Service Scheme (NSS) at Lovely Professional University (LPU), he has actively participated in numerous village development camps, demonstrating his commitment to social upliftment. His academic journey includes significant contributions to various research projects, notably a published study on skin cancer classification using convolutional neural networks. Additionally, Devendra has showcased his leadership skills as a team leader in AIESEC in India, managing and guiding teams to success. With hands-on experience in diverse data science projects, he has honed his expertise and remains passionate about exploring new frontiers in technology and research.

Siva Subramanian R is a distinguished member of R.M.K. College of Engineering and Technology in Puduvoyal, Tamil Nadu. Known for his dedication to advancing academic and technical knowledge, he plays a pivotal role at the institution

D. Ravindran is an Associate Professor at the School of Management, Kristu Jayanti College, Autonomous, Bengaluru. He has extensive experience in management education, with a focus on research and teaching in areas such as marketing and business strategy. Dr. Ravindran is dedicated to academic excellence and contributes actively to both teaching and research in the management field.

N.T. Renukadevi received the M.C.A and M.Phil Degrees in Computer Science from Bharathiar University, India in 2003 and 2008 respectively. She received Ph.D. degree in Computer Applications from Anna University, India in 2014. Since 2008, she is working as an Assistant Professor in the Department of Computer Technology, Kongu Engineering College. Her research interests include Data Mining and Image Processing. She is also a reviewer in reputed journals. She has published 20 research works in referred journals and presented 12 papers in International Conferences.

Dhivya Devi S is an Assistant Professor at SRM Institute of Science and Technology. She specializes in computer science education and research, contributing to advancements in areas like data science and software development. Dhivya Devi S is committed to fostering innovation and academic growth in her students and research community.

Ajay Sharma is currently working as a Technical Consultant in UpGrad Education Pvt Ltd and is currently posted in the School of Computing at Lovely Professional University (LPU) Jalandhar Punjab. Before joining UpGrad, he worked as a junior research fellow in the Department of Biotechnology and Bioinformatics at Jaypee University of Information Technology Solan Himachal Pradesh. He has obtained his master's degree in Computer Science (Deep Learning) in the Domain of Biomedical Image Processing and a bachelor's degree in Bioinformatics from Shoolini University Himachal Pradesh. During his bachelor's, he got a certificate of merit. Mr. Ajay has completed his Computer Science Diploma from Lovely Professional University Jalandhar Punjab. During his bachelor's and master, he has presented, Demonstrated his work at different international conferences at AIIMS Rishikesh and PGIMER Chandigarh, IHBT Palampur.

Shamneesh Sharma is currently serving as Senior Manager- Programs at upGrad Education Private Limited, Bangalore, India. and prior to this he was at iNurture Education Solution, Bangalore as Senior Faculty (Cloud Technology and Information Security) and deputed as Head in the Department of Computer Application, School of Computer Science & Engineering, Poornima University, Jaipur. He has worked as IT-Head and Associate Professor (CSE) at Alakh Prakash Goyal Shimla University, Shimla (H.P.). He has played a vital role in the implementation of New IT-Infrastructure, ERP System and Website Development along with its maintenance in the University. He is having more than 9 Years of academic and administrative experience in the field of Computer Science & Information Technology. He is B. Tech & M. Tech and presently pursuing Ph. D (Computer Science & Engineering). He has published more than 20 research manuscripts in various International & National journals & conferences. He has also presented papers in International and National conferences. He is a member of various International & National professional & academic bodies.

Sumiksha Shetty, currently working as an Assistant Professor in the department of Electronics and Communication Engineering at Sahyadri College of Engineering & Management, Mangaluru.

Ahmad Tasnim Siddiqui is an Associate Professor at the Department of Computer Science and Engineering, Sandip University, Nashik, India. He is Ph.D. in Computer Science. He also holds a Master of Computer Applications, and an M. Phil (Computer Science) from Madurai Kamaraj University, Madurai, India. He has many publications in reputed journals indexed at SCI, SCIE, and SCOPUS. He has also published book chapters in EMERALD insight, Taylors & Francis, SPRINGER, ELSEVIER, and IGI Global publications. His research interest includes e-commerce, e-learning, active learning, web mining, IoT, ICT, e-health, and cloud computing. He has a total of 18+ years of experience including 4.7 years of software industry experience. His favorite subjects are E-commerce and web Technologies using .net.

Chandra Singh is currently working as a Assistant Professor Grade II of Department of Electronics & Communication Engineering at NMAM Institute of Technology,(Nitte Deemed to be University). He pursued his Bachelors in Electronics & Communication Engineering at SSE, Mukka, M.Tech from NMAM Institute of Technology,Nitte and Pursuing PhD from VTU Belagavi. He has 4 Patents (3 Australia, 1 South Africa), 25+ peer-reviewed publications and editor of 11 research books(6 Books Published). His research interests include communication, wireless communication,IoT AI/ML,CPS,Robotics

Komal Tahiliani is an Associate Professor in the Department of Computer Science and Engineering with 19 years of academic experience. I had a substantial number of paper publications in various reputed journals and conferences. my research interests span across multiple domains of computer science, reflecting a commitment to advancing knowledge and innovation in the field. Throughout my career, I have been dedicated to fostering academic excellence and contributing to the growth and development of both undergraduate and postgraduate students.

Shafiq Ul Rehman received a Ph.D. degree from Universiti Sains Malaysia (USM), Malaysia, in 2017. He was a Postdoctoral Research Fellow with Singapore University of Technology and Design (SUTD), Singapore, from 2017 to 2020. He is currently the Chairperson of the Department of Computer Science, College of Information Technology, Kingdom University, Bahrain. He is also an Assistant Professor specializing in cyber security, artificial intelligence, the Internet of Things

(IoT), industry 4.0, and cloud/edge computing. He has authored and coauthored more than 50 papers in journals, conference proceedings, and book chapters, and supervises Ph.D., postgraduate, and undergraduate students. He is involved in various research projects related to secure machine-to-machine communication, the IoT in healthcare, industry 4.0, and emerging technologies using open-source platforms. He has experience building AI tools for healthcare, security systems for communication protocols, the IoT devices, and cloud/edge computing architecture

Celestine Ozoemenam Uwa worked in the industry for 8 years before joining the services of NDA in the year 2000. He obtained a BSc in Computer Science from University of Benin, Edo State, in 1992, an MSc in Applied Mathematics (Operations Research) from the Nigerian Defence Academy, Kaduna in 2011 and an MSc in Computer Science from Nnamdi Azikiwe Univeristy, Awka, Anambra State in 2015. He currently a PhD student in NDA. His research areas include Internet of Things, Artificial Intelligence, Operations Research, Machine Learning and Computer Vision

V.Sathya is an Assistant Professor in the Department of Computer Science and Engineering at Vel Tech Rangarajan Dr. Sagunthala R&D Institute of Science and Technology, Avadi. She specializes in computer science education and research, contributing to advancements in areas like data science and software development.

Index

A

accurate and faster interpretations 399
AIIoT 277, 283, 285, 286, 287, 301, 302, 303, 305
Artificial Intelligence 2, 3, 7, 8, 10, 11, 12, 13, 15, 16, 17, 18, 20, 23, 24, 25, 26, 28, 29, 30, 31, 37, 39, 40, 41, 45, 46, 47, 48, 49, 50, 51, 52, 53, 54, 55, 67, 69, 71, 72, 73, 74, 76, 78, 80, 83, 84, 85, 86, 88, 89, 90, 91, 92, 104, 105, 106, 107, 108, 109, 110, 114, 115, 116, 122, 138, 139, 140, 142, 161, 162, 163, 165, 167, 168, 191, 194, 195, 196, 198, 205, 210, 211, 215, 231, 237, 272, 273, 274, 277, 283, 285, 286, 287, 288, 289, 290, 292, 293, 294, 295, 296, 300, 303, 304, 305, 306, 328, 364, 365, 366, 367, 370, 378, 385, 390, 391, 392, 393, 395, 396, 397, 399, 400, 402, 403, 404, 407, 408, 409, 412, 413, 414, 415, 416, 417, 418
Augmentation 61, 81, 148, 220, 221, 226, 236, 245, 247, 248, 249, 252, 253, 254, 256, 259, 263, 266, 270, 275, 381, 397

B

Big Data 2, 5, 6, 8, 9, 27, 31, 38, 40, 48, 49, 50, 54, 55, 56, 58, 62, 69, 70, 76, 79, 81, 108, 138, 168, 169, 234, 275, 304, 315, 329, 330, 380, 390, 393, 394, 395, 396, 397, 398
Blockchain 1, 30, 78, 80, 392, 396

C

CDSS 3, 38, 39, 43, 44, 66, 83, 84, 85, 86, 87, 88, 89, 90, 91, 92, 94, 95, 96, 97, 98, 99, 100, 101, 104, 106, 141, 142, 147, 152, 154, 155, 158, 159
Classification Accuracy 246, 311, 312, 315, 324, 325, 354, 355, 357, 358, 359, 360, 363, 365
Clinical decision support system 39, 86, 105, 107, 108, 110, 142, 145, 147, 158, 159, 197
Clinician Decision Support 1
Color Histogram 236, 243, 244, 250, 251, 253, 257, 263, 264, 270
Confusion Matrix 176, 177, 178, 255, 257, 259, 260, 262, 263, 265, 266, 269, 351
COVID-19 26, 28, 140, 201, 202, 203, 204, 205, 206, 209, 210, 211, 212, 213, 219, 221, 222, 223, 224, 226, 227, 228, 229, 230, 231, 232, 233, 234, 305, 306, 367, 396, 404, 410

D

Data Protection 1, 12, 37, 44, 55, 61, 77, 380
Data Science 201, 331, 390, 395
Decision Making 7, 19, 24, 43, 57, 58, 66, 68, 70, 76, 77, 78, 106, 123, 142, 277, 282, 283, 286, 287, 288, 289, 296, 300, 301, 302, 316, 320, 328, 394, 398, 406, 407
Decision Tree 81, 93, 97, 113, 131, 132, 133, 134, 135, 139, 154, 156, 157, 162, 167, 170, 171, 172, 178, 181, 190, 292, 294, 302, 307, 320, 324, 333, 335, 347, 348, 353, 356, 358, 378
Deep Learning 2, 18, 19, 20, 21, 22, 27, 30, 32, 40, 41, 45, 48, 50, 52, 61, 65, 66, 74, 78, 81, 82, 92, 93, 94, 106, 109, 121, 122, 124, 138, 139, 144, 145, 146, 147, 159, 160, 161, 163, 164, 201, 203, 204, 205, 206, 207, 209, 210, 211, 212, 214, 216, 228, 229, 230, 231, 232, 233, 234, 237, 245, 246, 248, 249, 272, 274, 275, 291, 301, 302, 306, 317, 332, 346, 369, 370, 371, 373, 374, 375, 380, 381, 388, 389, 390, 391, 392, 393, 394, 395, 396, 397, 398, 402
Digital Medical System 201

E

emerging trends 45, 78, 108, 399, 400, 415
Enhanced Diagnostics 92
Explainable AI 1, 100, 113, 114, 115, 117, 118, 119, 122, 123, 124, 137, 138, 139, 140, 303

F

Feature Extraction 101, 121, 123, 204, 206, 217, 236, 237, 244, 246, 247, 249, 250, 251, 253, 257, 260, 271, 310, 358
Federated Learning 1, 36, 37, 38, 51, 78, 389

G

Genomics 1, 3, 22, 27, 31, 32, 34, 45, 46, 49, 54, 74, 75, 78, 329, 369, 373, 374, 391, 392
Gray level Co-occurrence Matrix 236, 237, 260, 266, 267, 270

H

Healthcare 1, 2, 3, 4, 5, 6, 7, 9, 10, 15, 17, 18, 23, 25, 26, 31, 34, 35, 36, 37, 38, 39, 42, 43, 44, 45, 46, 47, 48, 49, 50, 51, 53, 54, 55, 56, 57, 58, 59, 60, 61, 62, 63, 64, 65, 66, 67, 68, 69, 70, 71, 72, 73, 74, 75, 76, 77, 78, 79, 80, 81, 83, 84, 85, 86, 87, 88, 89, 90, 91, 92, 93, 94, 95, 96, 98, 99, 100, 101, 102, 103, 104, 107, 108, 109, 110, 113, 114, 115, 116, 117, 118, 119, 122, 123, 124, 137, 138, 140, 141, 142, 165, 166, 167, 168, 169, 180, 190, 191, 201, 202, 203, 226, 235, 236, 237, 238, 244, 246, 256, 257, 272, 277, 278, 279, 280, 281, 282, 283, 284, 285, 286, 287, 290, 291, 292, 293, 300, 301, 302, 303, 304, 305, 306, 307, 309, 311, 314, 315, 316, 328, 329, 330, 331, 332, 366, 369, 370, 371, 372, 373, 374, 375, 376, 377, 378, 379, 380, 381, 382, 383, 384, 385, 386, 387, 388, 389, 390, 391, 392, 393, 394, 395, 396, 397, 398, 399, 400, 401, 402, 403, 404, 405, 406, 407, 408, 409, 410, 411, 412, 413, 414, 415, 416, 417, 418
healthcare Industry 3, 23, 45, 53, 70, 78, 110, 114, 115, 116, 118, 237, 281, 287, 291, 300, 370, 374, 376, 378, 379, 380, 381, 383, 384, 385, 386, 388, 400, 403, 411, 412, 418
Heart disease 10, 15, 18, 65, 80, 93, 94, 98, 103, 105, 144, 165, 166, 167, 168, 169, 170, 172, 173, 178, 179, 180, 181, 183, 189, 190, 191, 192, 193, 194, 196, 197, 198, 315, 372, 397
Heart disease prediction 93, 94, 98, 105, 165, 167, 168, 170, 178, 179, 190, 192, 193, 194, 198, 315, 397
Hyperthyroidism 143, 144
Hypothyroidism 143, 144, 145, 161, 162, 164

I

Image Classification 164, 203, 213, 215, 249, 263, 266, 270, 273, 275, 331
Image Processing 27, 193, 235, 236, 237, 243, 246, 256, 272, 273, 275
Internet of Things 73, 78, 80, 81, 93, 109, 138, 277, 283, 285, 286, 287, 288, 289, 290, 291, 292, 293, 295, 301, 302, 380, 389, 393

K

Kidney Diseases 277, 278, 279, 281, 296, 298, 299, 300, 315
Kinect 333, 334, 335, 336, 338, 340, 343, 344, 352, 365, 366, 367
K-Nearest Neighbour 332
KSK Approach 277, 286, 289, 290, 296, 299, 302, 303

M

machine learning 2, 6, 7, 8, 12, 15, 16, 18, 20, 22, 27, 28, 32, 34, 36, 39, 40, 41,

42, 43, 45, 50, 53, 54, 55, 66, 67, 69, 70, 71, 72, 73, 74, 75, 76, 80, 81, 82, 83, 84, 85, 86, 88, 89, 90, 91, 92, 93, 94, 97, 101, 102, 104, 105, 106, 107, 108, 109, 110, 113, 116, 118, 119, 120, 121, 122, 123, 124, 131, 134, 138, 139, 141, 142, 145, 146, 147, 148, 152, 154, 155, 156, 157, 158, 160, 161, 162, 163, 165, 166, 167, 168, 169, 171, 175, 177, 180, 181, 182, 188, 190, 191, 192, 193, 194, 195, 196, 198, 201, 203, 211, 212, 216, 220, 224, 228, 237, 244, 249, 254, 256, 272, 274, 275, 292, 301, 302, 303, 304, 305, 306, 307, 308, 309, 311, 312, 313, 314, 316, 317, 323, 328, 329, 330, 331, 332, 339, 345, 346, 348, 366, 369, 370, 371, 372, 373, 375, 376, 377, 378, 379, 380, 381, 382, 383, 384, 385, 386, 387, 388, 390, 391, 392, 393, 394, 395, 396, 397, 398, 399, 400, 402, 405, 406, 408, 411, 413

Machine Learning 2, 6, 7, 8, 12, 15, 16, 18, 20, 22, 27, 28, 32, 34, 36, 39, 40, 41, 42, 43, 45, 50, 53, 54, 55, 66, 67, 69, 70, 71, 72, 73, 74, 75, 76, 80, 81, 82, 83, 84, 85, 86, 88, 89, 90, 91, 92, 93, 94, 97, 101, 102, 104, 105, 106, 107, 108, 109, 110, 113, 116, 118, 119, 120, 121, 122, 123, 124, 131, 134, 138, 139, 141, 142, 145, 146, 147, 148, 152, 154, 155, 156, 157, 158, 160, 161, 162, 163, 165, 166, 167, 168, 169, 171, 175, 177, 180, 181, 182, 188, 190, 191, 192, 193, 194, 195, 196, 198, 201, 203, 211, 212, 216, 220, 224, 228, 237, 244, 249, 254, 256, 272, 274, 275, 292, 301, 302, 303, 304, 305, 306, 307, 308, 309, 311, 312, 313, 314, 316, 317, 323, 328, 329, 330, 331, 332, 339, 345, 346, 348, 366, 369, 370, 371, 372, 373, 375, 376, 377, 378, 379, 380, 381, 382, 383, 384, 385, 386, 387, 388, 390, 391, 392, 393, 394, 395, 396, 397, 398, 399, 400, 402, 405, 406, 408, 411, 413

Medical Practices 113, 137

N

Natural Language Processing 20, 27, 40, 41, 43, 47, 49, 81, 123, 230, 309, 373, 388, 401, 402

P

Personalized Treatment Recommendations 94, 95

pneumonia 201, 202, 203, 204, 205, 206, 207, 212, 213, 396

Precision 1, 4, 13, 22, 23, 28, 31, 35, 40, 45, 49, 64, 74, 78, 81, 92, 95, 96, 116, 120, 121, 122, 125, 140, 155, 171, 175, 176, 183, 190, 203, 223, 224, 225, 226, 237, 248, 249, 253, 255, 257, 258, 260, 261, 262, 264, 265, 267, 268, 270, 277, 284, 292, 298, 299, 300, 303, 312, 351, 356, 372, 400, 401, 412

Precision Medicine 1, 4, 22, 23, 28, 31, 45, 49, 74, 78, 81, 122, 140, 284, 372, 401

R

Random Forest 93, 96, 113, 134, 135, 137, 140, 145, 147, 154, 156, 157, 167, 170, 236, 237, 244, 250, 251, 253, 257, 259, 260, 262, 263, 265, 266, 269, 272, 307, 313, 315, 316, 323, 333, 347, 348, 353, 354, 356

Random Forest Classifier 134, 137, 236, 244, 250, 251, 253, 259, 262, 265, 269, 272, 315, 323, 354

revolutionizing healthcare 1, 48, 109, 137, 237, 272, 395, 399, 416, 418

ROC-Curve 255

S

sitting posture 333, 335, 336, 338, 339, 342, 344, 357, 358, 359, 361, 362, 363, 364, 367

Sleep disorder 307, 308, 325
Stress 15, 16, 18, 119, 166, 180, 307, 317, 318, 325, 327, 367, 403
Support Vector Machine 80, 93, 97, 113, 124, 154, 156, 157, 167, 174, 181, 190, 197, 291, 312, 316, 331, 333, 348, 378

T

telemedicine 13, 15, 18, 46, 60, 78, 275, 375, 385, 387, 399, 408, 409, 410, 412, 414, 416, 417, 418
Thyroid detection 145, 158, 159
Thyroid prediction 145, 152, 154
transforming diagnostics 399